Essential Clinical Anesthesia Review: Keywords, Questions and Answers for the Boards

Essential Clinical Anesthesia Review: Keywords, Questions and Answers for the Boards

Edited by

Linda S. Aglio
Harvard Medical School and the Brigham and Women's Hospital, Boston, MA, USA.

Robert W. Lekowski
The Brigham and Women's Hospital and Harvard Medical School, Boston, MA, USA.

Richard D. Urman
The Brigham and Women's Hospital, Center for Perioperative Management and Medical Informatics, and Harvard Medical School, Boston, MA, USA.

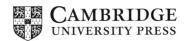
CAMBRIDGE
UNIVERSITY PRESS

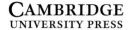

University Printing House, Cambridge CB2 8BS, United Kingdom

Cambridge University Press is part of the University of Cambridge.

It furthers the University's mission by disseminating knowledge
in the pursuit of education, learning and research at the highest international levels of excellence.

www.cambridge.org
Information on this title: www.cambridge.org/9781107681309

First published 2015

Printed in the United Kingdom by T. J. International Ltd, Padstow

A catalogue record for this publication is available from the British Library

Library of Congress Cataloguing in Publication data
Essential clinical anesthesia review : keywords, questions and answers for
the boards / edited by Linda S. Aglio, Robert W. Lekowski, Richard D.
Urman.
        p. ; cm.
Includes bibliographical references and index.
ISBN 978-1-107-68130-9 (Hardback)
I. Aglio, Linda S., editor.   II. Lekowski, Robert W., editor.
III. Urman, Richard D., editor.
[DNLM: 1. Anesthesia–Examination Questions.   2. Anesthesia–
Outlines.   3. Anesthetics–administration & dosage–Examination
Questions.   4. Anesthetics–administration & dosage–Outlines.
WO 218.2]
RD82.3
617.9′6076–dc23   2014014929

ISBN 978-1-107-68130-9 Paperback

....

Contents

Contributors

Linda S. Aglio, MD MS
Associate Professor of Anesthesia at Harvard Medical School, the current and founding Director of Neuroanesthesia, Director of Otorhinolaryngeal Anesthesia, and Associate Director of Intraoperative Neurophysiological Monitoring in the Department of Anesthesiology, Perioperative and Pain Medicine at Brigham and Women's Hospital, Boston, MA, USA

Cyrus Ahmadi Yazdi, MD DOHNS (Eng)
Clinical Fellow of Anaesthesia, Harvard Medical School
Resident, Department of Anesthesiology, Perioperative and Pain Medicine
Brigham and Women's Hospital, Boston, MA, USA

Syed Irfan Qasim Ali, MD
Clinical Fellow of Anaesthesia, Harvard Medical School
Resident, Department of Anesthesiology, Perioperative and Pain Medicine
Brigham and Women's Hospital, Boston, MA, USA

Caryn Barnet, MD
Clinical Fellow of Anaesthesia, Harvard Medical School
Resident, Department of Anesthesiology, Perioperative and Pain Medicine
Brigham and Women's Hospital, Boston, MA, USA

Jessica Bauerle, MD
Clinical Fellow of Anaesthesia, Harvard Medical School
Resident, Department of Anesthesiology, Perioperative and Pain Medicine
Brigham and Women's Hospital, Boston, MA, USA

Felicity Billings, MD
Instructor of Anaesthesia, Harvard Medical School
Anesthesiologist, Department of Anesthesiology, Perioperative and Pain Medicine
Brigham and Women's Hospital, Boston, MA, USA

Evan Blaney, MD
Instructor of Anaesthesia, Harvard Medical School
Anesthesiologist, Department of Anesthesiology, Perioperative and Pain Medicine
Brigham and Women's Hospital, Boston, MA, USA

Beverly Chang, MD
Clinical Fellow of Anaesthesia, Harvard Medical School
Resident, Department of Anesthesiology, Perioperative and Pain Medicine
Brigham and Women's Hospital, Boston, MA, USA

Christopher Chen, MD
Instructor of Anaesthesia, Harvard Medical School
Anesthesiologist, Department of Anesthesiology, Perioperative and Pain Medicine
Brigham and Women's Hospital, Boston, MA, USA

Zinaida Chepurny, MD
Clinical Fellow of Anaesthesia, Harvard Medical School
Resident, Department of Anesthesiology, Perioperative and Pain Medicine
Brigham and Women's Hospital, Boston, MA, USA

Hyung Sun Choi, MD
Assistant Professor, University of Mississippi Medical Center
Department of Anesthesiology, Jackson, MS, USA

Allison Clark, MD
Clinical Fellow of Anaesthesia, Harvard Medical School
Resident, Department of Anesthesiology, Perioperative and Pain Medicine
Brigham and Women's Hospital, Boston, MA, USA

Lauren J. Cornella, MD
Instructor of Anaesthesia, Harvard Medical School
Anesthesiologist, Department of Anesthesiology, Perioperative and Pain Medicine
Brigham and Women's Hospital, Boston, MA, USA

Lisa Crossley, MD
Assistant Professor of Anaesthesia, Harvard Medical School
Anesthesiologist, Department of Anesthesiology, Perioperative and Pain Medicine
Brigham and Women's Hospital, Boston, MA, USA

Michael D'Ambra, MD
Associate Professor of Anaesthesia, Harvard Medical School
Anesthesiologist, Department of Anesthesiology, Perioperative

and Pain Medicine
Brigham and Women's Hospital, Boston, MA, USA

Galina Davidyuk, MD PhD
Instructor of Anaesthesia, Harvard Medical School
Anesthesiologist, Department of Anesthesiology, Perioperative
and Pain Medicine
Brigham and Women's Hospital, Boston, MA, USA

Whitney de Luna, MD
Clinical Fellow of Anaesthesia, Johns Hopkins University
School of Medicine
Resident, The Johns Hopkins Hospital, Baltimore, MD, USA

Manisha S. Desai, MD
Clinical Associate Professor of Anesthesiology
University of Massachusetts School of Medicine
Worcester, MA, USA

Sukumar P. Desai, MD
Assistant Professor of Anaesthesia, Harvard Medical School
Anesthesiologist, Department of Anesthesiology, Perioperative
and Pain Medicine
Brigham and Women's Hospital, Boston, MA, USA

Kelly G. Elterman, MD
Clinical Fellow of Anaesthesia, Harvard Medical School
Resident, Department of Anesthesiology, Perioperative and
Pain Medicine
Brigham and Women's Hospital, Boston, MA, USA

Michaela K. Farber, MD MS
Instructor of Anaesthesia, Harvard Medical School
Anesthesiologist, Department of Anesthesiology, Perioperative
and Pain Medicine
Brigham and Women's Hospital, Boston, MA, USA

Iuliu Fat, MD PhD FRCP
Clinical Fellow of Anaesthesia, Harvard Medical School
Resident, Department of Anesthesiology, Perioperative and
Pain Medicine
Brigham and Women's Hospital, Boston, MA, USA

Jaida Fitzgerald, MD
Clinical Fellow of Anaesthesia, Harvard Medical School
Resident, Department of Anesthesiology, Perioperative and
Pain Medicine
Brigham and Women's Hospital, Boston, MA, USA

Devon Flaherty, MD MPH
Instructor of Anaesthesia, Harvard Medical School
Anesthesiologist, Department of Anesthesiology, Perioperative
and Pain Medicine
Brigham and Women's Hospital, Boston, MA, USA

John A. Fox, MD
Assistant Professor of Anaesthesia, Harvard Medical School
Anesthesiologist, Department of Anesthesiology, Perioperative

and Pain Medicine
Brigham and Women's Hospital, Boston, MA, USA

Gyorgy Frendl, MD PhD
Associate Professor of Anaesthesia, Harvard Medical School
Anesthesiologist, Department of Anesthesiology, Perioperative
and Pain Medicine
Brigham and Women's Hospital, Boston, MA, USA

Rejean Gareau, MD FRCP(C)
Clinical Fellow of Anaesthesia, Harvard Medical School
Resident, Department of Anesthesiology, Perioperative and
Pain Medicine
Brigham and Women's Hospital, Boston, MA, USA

Joseph M. Garfield, MD
Associate Professor of Anaesthesia, Harvard Medical School
Anesthesiologist, Department of Anesthesiology, Perioperative
and Pain Medicine
Brigham and Women's Hospital, Boston, MA, USA

Andrea Girnius, MD
Clinical Fellow of Anaesthesia, Harvard Medical School
Resident, Department of Anesthesiology, Perioperative and
Pain Medicine
Brigham and Women's Hospital, Boston, MA, USA

Laverne D. Gugino, MD PhD
Associate Professor of Anaesthesia, Harvard Medical School
Director of Intraoperative Neurophysiological Monitoring
Department of Anesthesiology, Perioperative and Pain
Medicine
Brigham and Women's Hospital, Boston, MA, USA

J. Tasker Gundy, MD
Clinical Fellow of Anaesthesia, Harvard Medical School
Resident, Department of Anesthesiology, Perioperative and
Pain Medicine
Brigham and Women's Hospital, Boston, MA, USA

Carly C. Guthrie, MD
Clinical Fellow of Anaesthesia, Harvard Medical School
Resident, Department of Anesthesiology, Perioperative and
Pain Medicine
Brigham and Women's Hospital, Boston, MA, USA

Lisa M. Hammond, MD
Clinical Fellow of Anaesthesia, Harvard Medical School
Resident, Department of Anesthesiology, Perioperative and
Pain Medicine
Brigham and Women's Hospital, Boston, MA, USA

M. Tariq Hanifi, MD
Clinical Fellow of Anaesthesia, Harvard Medical School
Resident, Department of Anesthesiology, Perioperative and
Pain Medicine
Brigham and Women's Hospital, Boston, MA, USA

James Hardy, MB BS
Instructor of Anaesthesia, Harvard Medical School
Anesthesiologist, Department of Anesthesiology, Perioperative
and Pain Medicine
Brigham and Women's Hospital, Boston, MA, USA

Philip M. Hartigan, MD
Assistant Professor of Anaesthesia, Harvard Medical School
Director of Thoracic Anesthesia
Department of Anesthesiology, Perioperative and Pain Medicine
Brigham and Women's Hospital, Boston, MA, USA

Thomas Hickey, MD MS
Clinical Fellow of Anaesthesia, Harvard Medical School
Resident, Department of Anesthesiology, Perioperative and
Pain Medicine
Brigham and Women's Hospital, Boston, MA, USA

Richard Hsu, MD
Clinical Fellow of Anaesthesia, Harvard Medical School
Resident, Department of Anesthesiology, Perioperative and
Pain Medicine
Brigham and Women's Hospital, Boston, MA, USA

Mohab Ibrahim, MD PhD
Assistant Professor of Anesthesiology and Pharmacology,
University of Arizona Medical School
Director of the Pain Clinic, University of Arizona Medical
Center, Tucson, AZ, USA

David Janfaza, MD
Instructor of Anaesthesia, Harvard Medical School
Anesthesiologist, Department of Anesthesiology, Perioperative
and Pain Medicine
Brigham and Women's Hospital, Boston, MA, USA

Yuka Kiyota, MD MPH
Clinical Fellow of Anaesthesia, Harvard Medical School
Resident, Department of Anesthesiology, Perioperative and
Pain Medicine
Brigham and Women's Hospital, Boston, MA, USA

Suzanne Klainer, MD
Instructor of Anaesthesia, Harvard Medical School
Anesthesiologist, Department of Anesthesiology, Perioperative
and Pain Medicine
Brigham and Women's Hospital, Boston, MA, USA

Benjamin Kloesel, MD MSBS
Clinical Fellow of Anaesthesia, Harvard Medical School
Resident, Department of Anesthesiology, Perioperative and
Pain Medicine
Brigham and Women's Hospital, Boston, MA, USA

Hanjo Ko, MD MSc
Clinical Fellow of Anaesthesia, Harvard Medical School
Resident, Department of Anesthesiology, Perioperative and

Pain Medicine
Brigham and Women's Hospital, Boston, MA, USA

Bhavani Kodali, MD
Associate Professor of Anaesthesia, Harvard Medical School
Vice Chair of Clinical Affairs
Department of Anesthesiology, Perioperative and Pain Medicine
Brigham and Women's Hospital, Boston, MA, USA

Vesela Kovacheva, MD PhD
Instructor of Anaesthesia, Harvard Medical School
Anesthesiologist, Department of Anesthesiology,
Perioperative and Pain Medicine
Brigham and Women's Hospital, Boston, MA, USA

J. Matthew Kynes, MD
Clinical Fellow of Anaesthesia, Harvard Medical School
Resident, Department of Anesthesiology, Perioperative and
Pain Medicine
Brigham and Women's Hospital, Boston, MA, USA

Robert W. Lekowski, MD
Residency Program Director at the Department of
Anesthesiology, Perioperative and Pain Medicine, Brigham
and Women's Hospital and Assistant Professor of Anesthesia,
Harvard Medical School, Boston, MA, USA

Joyce Lo, MD
Clinical Fellow of Anaesthesia, Harvard Medical School
Resident, Department of Anesthesiology, Perioperative and
Pain Medicine
Brigham and Women's Hospital, Boston, MA, USA

Jeffrey Lu, MD
Instructor of Anaesthesia, Harvard Medical School
Anesthesiologist, Department of Anesthesiology, Perioperative
and Pain Medicine
Brigham and Women's Hospital, Boston, MA, USA

Alvaro A. Macias, MD
Instructor of Anaesthesia, Harvard Medical School
Anesthesiologist, Department of Anesthesiology, Perioperative
and Pain Medicine
Brigham and Women's Hospital, Boston, MA, USA

Zahra M. Malik, MD
Clinical Fellow of Anaesthesia, Harvard Medical School
Resident, Department of Anesthesiology, Perioperative and
Pain Medicine
Brigham and Women's Hospital, Boston, MA, USA

Erich N. Marks, MD
Assistant Professor at the Department of Anesthesiology,
University of Wisconsin, Madison, WI, USA

Brendan McGinn, MD
Clinical Fellow of Anaesthesia, Harvard Medical School
Resident, Department of Anesthesiology, Perioperative and

Pain Medicine
Brigham and Women's Hospital, Boston, MA, USA

Jonathan R. Meserve, MD
Clinical Fellow of Anaesthesia, Harvard Medical School
Resident, Department of Anesthesiology, Perioperative and
Pain Medicine
Brigham and Women's Hospital, Boston, MA, USA

Annette Mizuguchi, MD
Assistant Professor of Anaesthesia, Harvard Medical School
Anesthesiologist, Department of Anesthesiology, Perioperative
and Pain Medicine
Brigham and Women's Hospital, Boston, MA, USA

Srdjan S. Nedeljkovic, MD
Assistant Professor of Anaesthesia, Harvard Medical School
Anesthesiologist, Department of Anesthesiology, Perioperative
and Pain Medicine
Fellowship Director, Pain Medicine
Brigham and Women's Hospital, Boston, MA, USA

Ju-Mei Ng
Instructor of Anaesthesia, Harvard Medical School
Anesthesiologist, Department of Anesthesiology, Perioperative
and Pain Medicine
Brigham and Women's Hospital, Boston, MA, USA

Michael Nguyen, MD
Instructor of Anaesthesia, Harvard Medical School
Anesthesiologist, Department of Anesthesiology, Perioperative
and Pain Medicine
Brigham and Women's Hospital, Boston, MA, USA

Olutoyin Okanlawon, MD MPH
Clinical Fellow of Anaesthesia, Harvard Medical School
Resident, Department of Anesthesiology, Perioperative and
Pain Medicine
Brigham and Women's Hospital, Boston, MA, USA

Jennifer Oliver, DO MPH
Clinical Fellow of Anaesthesia, Harvard Medical School
Resident, Department of Anesthesiology, Perioperative and
Pain Medicine
Brigham and Women's Hospital, Boston, MA, USA

Krishna Parekh, MD
Clinical Fellow of Anaesthesia, Harvard Medical School
Resident, Department of Anesthesiology, Perioperative and
Pain Medicine
Brigham and Women's Hospital, Boston, MA, USA

Jessica Patterson, MD
Clinical Fellow of Anaesthesia, Harvard Medical School
Resident, Department of Anesthesiology, Perioperative and
Pain Medicine
Brigham and Women's Hospital, Boston, MA, USA

Christian Peccora, MD
Clinical Fellow of Anaesthesia, Harvard Medical School
Resident, Department of Anesthesiology, Perioperative and
Pain Medicine
Brigham and Women's Hospital, Boston, MA, USA

Pete Pelletier, MD
Clinical Fellow of Anaesthesia, Harvard Medical School
Resident, Department of Anesthesiology, Perioperative and
Pain Medicine
Brigham and Women's Hospital, Boston, MA, USA

Sujatha Pentakota, MD
Instructor of Anaesthesia, Harvard Medical School
Anesthesiologist, Department of Anesthesiology, Perioperative
and Pain Medicine
Brigham and Women's Hospital, Boston, MA, USA

James H. Philip, ME(E) MD
Professor of Anaesthesia, Harvard Medical School
Anesthesiologist and Director of Clinical Bioengineering
Department of Anesthesiology, Perioperative and Pain
Medicine
Brigham and Women's Hospital, Boston, MA, USA

Marc Philip T. Pimentel, MD
Clinical Fellow of Anaesthesia, Harvard Medical School
Resident, Department of Anesthesiology, Perioperative and
Pain Medicine
Brigham and Women's Hospital, Boston, MA, USA

Timothy D. Quinn, MD
Clinical Fellow of Anaesthesia, Harvard Medical School
Resident, Department of Anesthesiology, Perioperative and
Pain Medicine
Brigham and Women's Hospital, Boston, MA, USA

Elizabeth M. Rickerson, MD
Instructor of Anaesthesia, Harvard Medical School
Anesthesiologist, Department of Anesthesiology, Perioperative
and Pain Medicine
Brigham and Women's Hospital, Boston, MA, USA
Palliative Care Physician, Department of Psychosocial
Oncology and Palliative Care
Dana Farber Cancer Institute, Boston, MA, USA

Susan L. Sager, MD
Instructor of Anaesthesia, Harvard Medical School
Anesthesiologist, Department of Anesthesiology, Perioperative
and Pain Medicine
Boston Children's Hospital, Boston, MA, USA

Julia Serber, MD
Clinical Fellow of Anaesthesia, Harvard Medical School
Resident, Department of Anesthesiology, Perioperative and
Pain Medicine, Brigham and Women's Hospital, Boston,
MA, USA

Shaheen Shaikh, MD
Assistant Professor of Anaesthesia
University of Massachusetts Medical School
Director of Neuroanesthesia
University of Massachusetts Medical Center, Worcester, MA, USA

Stanton Shernan, MD
Professor of Anaesthesia, Harvard Medical School
Director of Cardiac Anesthesia, Department of Anesthesiology,
Perioperative and Pain Medicine Brigham and Women's
Hospital, Boston, MA, USA

David Silver, MD
Associate Professor of Anaesthesia, Harvard Medical School
Anesthesiologist, Department of Anesthesiology, Perioperative
and Pain Medicine
Brigham and Women's Hospital, Boston, MA, USA

Alissa Sodickson, MD
Clinical Fellow of Anaesthesia, Harvard Medical School
Resident, Department of Anesthesiology, Perioperative and
Pain Medicine
Brigham and Women's Hospital, Boston, MA, USA

Pingping Song, MD
Clinical Fellow of Anaesthesia, Harvard Medical School
Resident, Department of Anesthesiology, Perioperative and
Pain Medicine
Brigham and Women's Hospital, Boston, MA, USA

George P. Topulos, MD
Associate Professor of Anaesthesia, Harvard Medical School
Anesthesiologist, Department of Anesthesiology, Perioperative
and Pain Medicine
Brigham and Women's Hospital, Boston, MA, USA

Agnieszka Trzcinka, MD
Clinical Fellow of Anaesthesia, Harvard Medical School
Resident, Department of Anesthesiology, Perioperative and
Pain Medicine
Brigham and Women's Hospital, Boston, MA, USA

Richard D. Urman, MD MBA CPE
Medical Director of Procedural Sedation at the Brigham and
Women's Hospital, Co-Director of the Center for
Perioperative Management and Medical Informatics, and
Assistant Professor of Anesthesia at Harvard Medical School,
Boston, MA, USA

Rosemary Uzomba, MD
Clinical Fellow of Anaesthesia, Harvard Medical School
Resident, Department of Anesthesiology, Perioperative and
Pain Medicine
Brigham and Women's Hospital, Boston, MA, USA

Joshua Vacanti, MD
Instructor of Anaesthesia, Harvard Medical School
Anesthesiologist, Department of Anesthesiology, Perioperative
and Pain Medicine
Brigham and Women's Hospital, Boston, MA, USA

Assia Valovska, MD
Instructor of Anaesthesia, Harvard Medical School
Anesthesiologist, Department of Anesthesiology, Perioperative
and Pain Medicine
Brigham and Women's Hospital, Boston, MA, USA

Michael Vaninetti, MD
Clinical Fellow of Anaesthesia, Harvard Medical School
Resident, Department of Anesthesiology, Perioperative and
Pain Medicine
Brigham and Women's Hospital, Boston, MA, USA

Scott W. Vaughan, DO
Clinical Fellow of Anaesthesia, Harvard Medical School
Resident, Department of Anesthesiology, Perioperative and
Pain Medicine
Brigham and Women's Hospital, Boston, MA, USA

Kamen Vlassakov, DO
Assistant Professor of Anaesthesia, Harvard Medical School
Director of Orthopedic Anesthesia
Anesthesiologist, Department of Anesthesiology, Perioperative
and Pain Medicine
Brigham and Women's Hospital, Boston, MA, USA

Christopher Voscopoulos, MD
Clinical Fellow of Anaesthesia, Harvard Medical School
Resident, Department of Anesthesiology, Perioperative and
Pain Medicine
Brigham and Women's Hospital, Boston, MA, USA

Emily L. Wang, MD
Clinical Fellow of Anaesthesia, Harvard Medical School
Resident, Department of Anesthesiology, Perioperative and
Pain Medicine
Brigham and Women's Hospital, Boston, MA, USA

Laura Westfall, MD
Clinical Fellow of Anaesthesia, Harvard Medical School
Resident, Department of Anesthesiology, Perioperative and
Pain Medicine
Brigham and Women's Hospital, Boston, MA, USA

Zhiling Xiong, MD PhD
Assistant Professor of Anaesthesia, Harvard Medical School
Director of General Surgery Anesthesia, Department of
Anesthesiology, Perioperative and Pain Medicine, Brigham
and Women's Hospital, Boston, MA, USA

Stephanie Yacoubian, MD
Clinical Fellow of Anaesthesia, Harvard Medical School
Resident, Department of Anesthesiology, Perioperative and
Pain Medicine
Brigham and Women's Hospital, Boston, MA, USA

Dongdong Yao, MD PhD
Instructor of Anaesthesia, Harvard Medical School
Anesthesiologist, Department of Anesthesiology, Perioperative and Pain Medicine
Brigham and Women's Hospital, Boston, MA, USA

Martin Zammert, MD
Instructor of Anaesthesia, Harvard Medical School
Director of Vascular Anesthesia, Department of Anesthesiology, Perioperative and Pain Medicine, Brigham and Women's Hospital, Boston, MA, USA

Maksim Zayaruzny, MD
Assistant Professor of Anaesthesia, University of Massachusetts Medical School
Anesthesiologist, University of Massachusetts Medical Center, Worcester, MA, USA

Jose Luis Zeballos, MD
Instructor of Anaesthesia, Harvard Medical School
Anesthesiologist, Department of Anesthesiology, Perioperative and Pain Medicine
Brigham and Women's Hospital, Boston, MA, USA

Natthasorn Zinboonyahgoon, MD
Clinical Fellow of Anaesthesia, Harvard Medical School
Resident, Department of Anesthesiology, Perioperative and Pain Medicine
Brigham and Women's Hospital, Boston, MA, USA

Jie Zhou, MD MS MBA
Instructor of Anaesthesia, Harvard Medical School
Anesthesiologist, Department of Anesthesiology, Perioperative and Pain Medicine
Brigham and Women's Hospital, Boston, MA, USA

Preface

Significant advances in basic science and the clinical practice of anesthesiology over the past decade have contributed exponentially to our specialty and necessitated the writing of this book. Our aim has been to provide a comprehensive and readily available reference and training source, prepared by a team of experts in their field, to clarify the basics of anesthetic management, including all new guidelines and recently developed standards of care.

Essential Clinical Anesthesia Review: Keywords, Questions and Answers for the Boards is the first review book of its kind published to serve as a companion for the written and re-certification board examinations, based on *Essential Clinical Anesthesia* and other authoritative sources.

In addition, it presents a group of important clinical entities covering critical anesthetic scenarios. It is an invaluable resource to any practicing anesthesia provider looking for an up-to-date review of problem-oriented patient management issues.

The material in this book will serve a wide range of learners and practitioners: medical students during their anesthesia rotation; residents and fellows studying for ABA (American Board of Anesthesiology) boards; student nurse anesthetists and certified registered nurse anesthetists (CRNAs); and practicing physicians. It will also serve as a source of review for the continuing education and ABA re-certification for the practicing anesthesiologist.

This book is organized into 29 sections and reflects the content of *Essential Clinical Anesthesia* and other Cambridge University Press resources. Each section has several chapters organized according to the ABA keyword list for a particular problem or clinical case scenario. The keyword list is followed by a concise discussion that includes preoperative assessment, intraoperative management, and postoperative pain management.

The book is designed to emphasize the fundamental concepts or keywords that are required to pass an exam and gives the reader the opportunity to see the application of these concepts in everyday practice. The text reflects the opinions and the clinical experiences of anesthesia experts at Harvard Medical School as well as individually known national experts in the field of anesthesiology.

History of anesthesia

Manisha S. Desai and Sukumar P. Desai

Keywords

Morton
Wells
Long
Jackson

Although anesthetic properties of nitrous oxide and ether were discovered in the 1800s, surgical operations were likely carried out under varied degrees of analgesia from times immemorial. Opiates, alcohol, cannabinoids, belladona derivatives, soporific sponges, and mesmerism were used to offer relief during surgery and are a testament to man's ingenuity.

Joseph Priestley (1733–1804, UK) discovered oxygen in 1771, and nitrous oxide in 1772. Humphry Davy (1778–1829, UK) discovered the analgesic properties of nitrous oxide in 1800 and termed it "laughing gas"; however, he did not use it in any clinical setting. In the United States, recreational use of ether and nitrous oxide was common in the 1840s (ether frolics and laughing gas parties). William E. Clarke (1819–1898, USA), while a medical student, was the first to administer ether for dental extraction in January 1842. On March 30, 1842, *Crawford W. Long* (1815–1878, USA) administered ether to James Venable during removal of a tumor from his back. Long continued using ether during surgery, but did not publish his findings until 1849. During an evening of public entertainment in 1844, Gardner Quincy Colton (1814–1898, USA) administered nitrous oxide to Samuel A. Cooley. Cooley injured himself as he was returning to his seat but did not feel any pain for a few minutes. *Horace Wells* (1815–1848, USA) attended the same demonstration and believed this was due to the analgesic effects of nitrous oxide. The next morning, fellow dentist John M. Riggs (1811–1885, USA) removed one of Wells' teeth painlessly while Colton administered nitrous oxide. Wells used nitrous oxide for pain relief in his own dental practice, but when he attempted to demonstrate this effect at Massachusetts General Hospital in 1845, the subject cried out in pain during the procedure, although later admitting that he did not remember any pain.

However, Wells' reputation never recovered from this apparent fiasco, and his life ended tragically in 1848. *William Thomas Green Morton* (1819–1868, USA), an associate of Wells, was present during the failed demonstration. He consulted with Harvard professor *Charles T. Jackson* (1805–1880, USA) and conducted experiments with ether. On October 16, 1846 Morton performed the first successful public demonstration of ether anesthesia while surgeon John Collins Warren (1778–1856, USA) removed a vascular tumor from the neck of Edward Gilbert Abbott. October 16 has thereafter been celebrated as Ether Day, and the amphitheater in which the procedure took place, Ether Dome, has been preserved as a museum at Massachusetts General Hospital, Boston.

News about the anesthetic properties of ether and nitrous oxide spread rapidly, and other agents were investigated for such properties. Obstetrician James Y. Simpson (1811–1870, UK) introduced chloroform for relief of labor pain in Edinburgh in 1847. John Snow (1813–1858, UK) is recognized as the first physician to work full time as an anesthetist. Relief of labor pain remained controversial until Snow administered chloroform to Queen Victoria (1819–1901) during the birth of Prince Leopold in 1853, and Princess Beatrice in 1857. Equipment to administer anesthetics developed over the next several decades, and the risk of anesthesia became evident as reports of anesthesia-related deaths appeared in newspapers and medical journals.

Karl Koller (1857–1944, Austria) discovered the local anesthetic properties of cocaine, when applied to the conjunctiva, in 1884. William S. Halsted (1852–1922, USA) used it for a nerve block later that year, and August Bier (1861–1949, Germany) performed the first clinical spinal anesthetic in 1898, and introduced intravenous regional anesthesia in 1908. Harvey W. Cushing (1869–1939, USA) and Ernest A. Codman (1869–1940, USA), while medical students, introduced anesthetic records in 1894. Caudal epidural anesthesia was introduced independently by Jean A. Sicard (1872–1929, France) and Fernand Cathelin (1873–1945, France) in 1901. Henry Edmund Gaskin Boyle (1875–1941, UK) introduced a

Essential Clinical Anesthesia Review: Keywords, Questions and Answers for the Boards, ed. Linda S. Aglio, Robert W. Lekowski, and Richard D. Urman. Published by Cambridge University Press. © Cambridge University Press 2015.

portable apparatus to administer nitrous oxide and oxygen in 1917. Lumbar epidural anesthesia was introduced by Fidel Pagés (1886–1923, Spain) in 1921. Torsten Gordh (1907–2010, Sweden) introduced lidocaine into clinical use in 1944. The routine use of intravenous barbiturate anesthesia (with agent pernoston) was introduced by Rudolph Bumm (1899–1942, Germany) in 1927. Harold R. Griffith (1894–1985, Canada) and Enid Johnson (1909–2001, Canada) introduced curare in 1942. The use of neuromuscular blockers greatly facilitated surgery in major body cavities, and mechanical ventilation. Laryngoscopy and tracheal intubation became routine procedures, and new drugs (local anesthetics, intravenous agents, and inhalation anesthetics) were introduced in subsequent decades. Comprehensive anesthesia machines and routine monitoring equipment were introduced in the 1960s and 1970s. Automatic blood pressure measuring devices, capnography, and pulse oximetry were introduced in the 1980s. Standards for intraoperative monitoring were developed at Harvard Medical School, and adopted by the American Society of Anesthesiologists in 1986. Technological changes have introduced ultrasound and echocardiography to our specialty, and anesthesiologists have expanded their scope of practice to include perioperative care, critical care, and the treatment of chronic pain. Ambulatory surgery and delivery of anesthesia care outside the operating rooms are recent developments.

Credit for the discovery of general anesthesia ought to be divided as follows – Clarke for the first use of ether for dental extraction, Long for introducing ether for general surgery, Wells for the introduction of nitrous oxide, Morton for the first successful public demonstration of ether, and

Jackson for the instruction he provided to Morton. Anesthesia is truly one of the most important discoveries in medicine, and it is unique in that the discovery occurred over a very brief period in the 1840s and events related to its discovery took place in America.

Question

Which one of the following statements is TRUE about individuals deserving credit for the discovery of anesthesia?

a. William Thomas Green Morton was the first to use nitrous oxide successfully during a surgical operation.
b. Horace Wells successfully demonstrated the use of ether for dental extraction.
c. Charles T. Jackson was the first to discover the anesthetic properties of nitrous oxide.
d. Crawford W. Long was the first to use ether successfully during a surgical operation.

Answer

d. Crawford W. Long was the first to use ether during a surgical operation in 1842. William E. Clarke used ether during a tooth extraction a few months earlier. Horace Wells' administration of nitrous oxide anesthesia during dental surgery was only partially successful since the patient cried out during the procedure. Charles T. Jackson advised Morton about the use of ether, and did not play a role in the discovery of the anesthetic properties of nitrous oxide. Morton was the first to publicly demonstrate the efficacy of ether as an anesthetic, four years after Long.

Preoperative anesthetic assessment

Emily L. Wang and Jeffrey Lu

Keywords

Preoperative assessment
Cardiovascular system evaluation
Functional capacity
ACC/AHA Guidelines on Perioperative
    Cardiovascular Evaluation and Care for Noncardiac
    Surgery
Active cardiac conditions
Clinical risk factors
Classification of cardiac risk for noncardiac surgery
Perioperative β-blockade
Percutaneous coronary intervention
Hypertension: perioperative management
Pulmonary system evaluation
Airway and anesthetic history
Gastrointestinal reflux
Neurologic conditions
Diabetes mellitus
Renal conditions
Hepatic conditions
Pregnancy
Allergies
Social history
Family history evaluation
Medications
Physical exam
Preoperative laboratory testing
ASA Physical Status Classification System
ASA NPO Guidelines for Fasting

Preoperative assessment: provides an evaluation of the patient's anesthetic risk for the proposed procedure, and allows recommendations to be made that help maximize patient safety. The anesthetic risk evaluation is based on the knowledge of the patient and the surgery. The goals of a preoperative assessment include a history and physical examination (including airway evaluation, medication usage, and past anesthetic and surgical experiences), control of comorbidities and perioperative

diseases, laboratory and cardiac testing as indicated, anesthetic risk assessment, anesthetic plan formulation, and patient education and informed consent. Significant abnormalities detected by the patient's history, physical exam, and associate risk factors may necessitate further testing and evaluation if it will affect the patient's treatment, management, or outcomes.

Cardiovascular system evaluation: cardiovascular status should be evaluated for all routine preoperative evaluations. Cardiovascular disease has a high prevalence in most patient populations, and cardiovascular complications may result in significant morbidity and mortality. It is important to assess functional capacity, symptoms that may indicate significant cardiac disease, and obtain information regarding prior cardiac events and test results.

Functional capacity: a patient's functional capacity is based on history, and is expressed in the form "metabolic equivalent of task" (MET). MET is defined as the ratio of metabolic rate during a specific physical activity to a reference metabolic rate at rest, set by convention to 3.5ml O_2/kg/min or equivalently, 1 kcal/kg/h. There is an increased perioperative cardiac risk for patients unable to achieve a 4 MET functional capacity, which is roughly equivalent to climbing two flights of stairs or walking two city blocks.

American College of Cardiology (ACC) and American Heart Association (AHA) Guidelines on Perioperative Cardiovascular Evaluation and Care for Noncardiac Surgery: offers a step-wise approach in the following algorithm: "Cardiac evaluation and care algorithm for noncardiac surgery based on active clinical conditions, known cardiovascular disease, or cardiac risk factors for patients 50 years of age or greater."

"*Active cardiac conditions*" definition:

1. Unstable coronary syndromes: unstable or severe angina, may include stable angina in unusually sedentary patients, recent MI (within 30 days).
2. Decompensated heart failure, or worsening or new-onset heart failure.
3. Significant arrhythmias: Mobitz II or third-degree AV block, symptomatic ventricular arrhythmias, supraventricular arrhythmias with uncontrolled ventricular rate, symptomatic bradycardia.

Essential Clinical Anesthesia Review: Keywords, Questions and Answers for the Boards, ed. Linda S. Aglio, Robert W. Lekowski, and Richard D. Urman. Published by Cambridge University Press. © Cambridge University Press 2015.

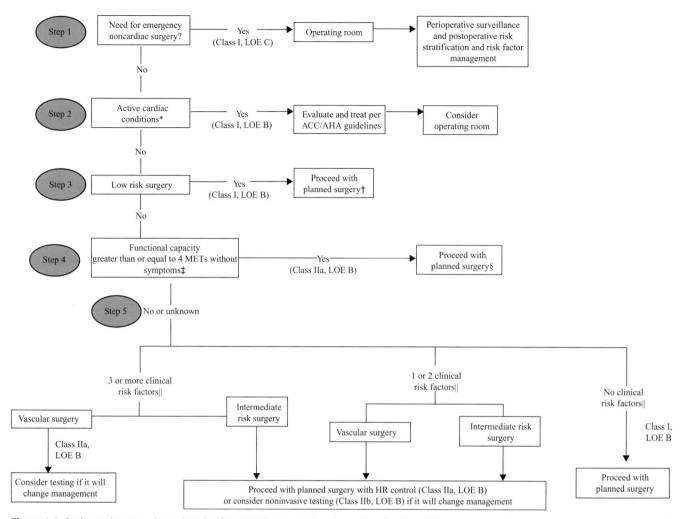

Figure 1.1 Cardiac evaluation and care algorithm for noncardiac surgery based on active clinical conditions, known cardiovascular disease, or cardiac risk factors for patients ≥50 years of age. *See Table 23 for active clinical conditions. †See class III recommendations in Table 2.6, Noninvasive Stress Testing. ‡See Table 2.1 for estimated MET level equivalent. §Noninvasive testing may be considered before surgery in specific patients with risk factors if it will change management. ‖Clinical risk factors include ischemic heart disease, compensated or prior heart failure, diabetes mellitus, renal insufficiency, and cerebrovascular disease. Consider perioperative β-blockade for populations in which this has been shown to reduce cardiac morbidity/mortality. HR, heart rate; LOE, level of evidence. (Modified from Fleisher, L. A., Beckman, J. A., Brown, K. A. et al. 2007. ACC/AHA 2007. Guidelines on Perioperative Cardiovascular Evaluation and Care for Noncardiac Surgery: Executive Summary: A Report of the American College of Cardiology/American Heart Association Task Force on Practice Guidelines. *Circulation* 116: 1971–1996.)

4. Severe valvular disease: severe aortic stenosis (valve area <1cm², pressure gradient >40 mm Hg, or symptomatic), symptomatic mitral stenosis.

"Clinical risk factors" definition:

1. diabetes mellitus
2. renal insufficiency
3. history of cerebrovascular disease
4. history of ischemic heart disease
5. history of compensated or prior heart failure

Classification of cardiac risk for noncardiac surgery:

1. High risk (>5%): emergent (especially in the elderly), aortic and other major vascular, peripheral vascular, and prolonged procedures with major blood loss or fluid shifts.

2. Intermediate risk (<5%): carotid endarterectomy, head and neck, intraperitoneal and intrathoracic, orthopedic, and prostate procedures.

3. Low risk (<1%): endoscopic, superficial, cataract, and breast procedures.

Based on ACC/AHA guidelines, further testing is directed by clinical assessment findings in relation to the complexity and invasiveness of the proposed procedure. However, emergency surgical procedures preclude preoperative evaluation, and risk factor management may require intensive care or postoperative invasive cardiac interventions.

Perioperative β-blockade: two groups mandated for β-blockade according to AHA/ACC guidelines are patients already taking β-blockers, and vascular patients with recent positive provocative cardiac testing. It is also likely recommended for intermediate risk or vascular surgical procedures with the presence of more than one clinical risk factor.

Patients with previous history of *percutaneous coronary intervention* (PCI), balloon angioplasty, bare metal stents (BMS), or drug-eluting stents (DES) require antiplatelet therapy to prevent thrombosis. Patients with BMS are required to have at least four weeks of antiplatelet therapy (clopidogrel), and patients with DES are required to have 12 months of dual antiplatelet therapy (aspirin and clopidogrel). It is recommended to delay elective, planned surgical procedures for at least 14 days after balloon angioplasty, 30 to 45 days after BMS placement, and one year after DES placement.

In patients with *hypertension*, the physician should evaluate for a history of end-organ disease such as myocardial ischemia or infarction, renal failure, and cerebrovascular disease. Although blood pressure should be optimally controlled preoperatively, there are no absolute contraindications based on blood pressure that necessitate cancellation of an elective procedure.

Pulmonary system evaluation: history taking in patients with asthma or COPD should include details about duration, therapy, baseline condition, history of intubations, hospitalizations, and recent changes in medications such as steroids or antibiotics. Notably, sleep apnea is associated with an increased incidence of postoperative apnea, respiratory failure, and poorer outcomes, especially with the administration of opioids.

Airway and anesthetic history: a key feature of the preoperative assessment, it should include details on previous intubations – especially if the patient has a history of difficult intubations – and the patient's prior anesthetic experience. History taking of prolonged intubations or possible tracheostomies should include etiology, and potential residual damage such as symptomatic tracheal stenosis. Attempts to retrieve the medical records and communicate the details to the anesthetizing team may be lifesaving. A history of previous postoperative nausea or vomiting, poor venous access, and other anxiety surrounding anesthesia such as mask "phobia" may predict future difficulties.

Allergies: allergy documentation must include the drug and reaction exhibited when administered. Appropriate history taking can help distinguish between a true drug allergy (often manifested as dyspnea or skin rashes) or a drug intolerance or side effect (typically gastrointestinal upset).

Medications: a detailed list of the patient's current medications and dosing schedule must be confirmed. It is important to document both prescribed and nonprescribed medications, as there is potential for drug interactions with anesthetic agents. In general, most medications should be continued until the night before the surgery. It is typically recommended to discontinue all alternative and complementary medications prior to the procedure. Anticoagulants should not be discontinued without a discussion with the cardiologist or physician prescribing them. Chronic pain medications often result in

tolerance and create challenges with postoperative pain management.

Gastrointestinal conditions: as pulmonary aspiration may lead to severe complications during anesthesia, the preoperative assessment includes evaluation of gastroesophageal reflux disease, dysphagia symptoms, gastrointestinal motility disorders, and metabolic disorders (e.g. diabetes mellitus) that may increase the risk of regurgitation. Gastrointestinal reflux details should include severity, frequency, impact of treatment if prescribed, current symptoms, and onset of symptoms during the night when lying flat.

Diabetes mellitus: diabetes is the most common endocrinopathy encountered preoperatively. A patient's history of the disease should include the type of diabetes, insulin status, possible end-organ damage, and previous diabetic comas. Oral hypoglycemic medications should be continued until the evening before surgery. Patients on insulin therapy will likely need to have their doses adjusted in preparation for the procedure and associated fasting. Generally, short-acting insulin is held on the morning of the surgery, and long-acting insulin is continued at the usual or reduced dose. Serum glucose levels can be checked during the fasting period, and regular insulin can be administered as needed. Insulin pumps are usually continued perioperatively at the basal rate.

Neurologic conditions: for patients with neurologic conditions, such as a history of cerebrovascular disease, multiple sclerosis, dementia, or epilepsy, it is important to document baseline functional and neurologic impairments, as well as a description of the symptoms.

Renal conditions: for renal disease patients, an assessment of their baseline renal condition should be determined. For dialysis patients, the frequency and mode of administration of the dialysis should be documented, and a plan for timing of dialysis perioperatively should be discussed.

Hepatic conditions: for hepatic disease patients, an assessment of their liver function and condition should be ascertained. Acute and chronic hepatic disease can lead to increased anesthetic and surgical risk, which can manifest as coagulopathies, ascites, encephalopathy, and alterations in drug distribution and metabolism.

Pregnancy: women of childbearing age should have their last menstrual period documented, and asked if there is any change of pregnancy. For patients who are reliable historians, routine pregnancy testing is not warranted.

Social history: this should include details about tobacco use, alcohol intake, and illegal drug use. Drug abuse and alcoholism may lead to significant changes in tolerance of anesthetic agents, and potential for withdrawal perioperatively.

Family history evaluation: all preoperative assessments should discuss the patient's familial history disposition for the life-threatening disease malignant hyperthermia. Pseudocholinesterase deficiency is another familial disease that may be suggested by a history of unexplained prolonged weakness or postoperative intubation in an otherwise healthy patient.

Physical exam: involves a general assessment of the patient, and a targeted exam focusing on the airway and cardiopulmonary system. Height, weight, blood pressure, heart rate, respiratory rate, temperature, and oxygen saturation (and if on supplemental oxygen) should be recorded. Auscultation of the heart and lungs should be noted for presence of murmurs, and abnormalities in cardiac rhythms or lung sounds. It is also recommended to do a brief baseline neurologic exam, as well as physical exam of the patient's anatomy when procedures such as a nerve block, regional anesthesia, or invasive monitoring are planned. The airway exam should include evaluation of the patient's mouth opening, ability to visualize the posterior pharyngeal structures, degree of neck mobility, thyromental distance, and dentition. Signs that a challenging tracheal intubation may be encountered include a short neck, limited range of motion of the neck, large tongue, and small mouth opening.

Preoperative laboratory testing: specific preoperative testing should be decided on an individual basis, and is appropriate depending on the nature of the procedure and the patient's medical comorbidities. Routine laboratory testing for healthy, asymptomatic patients is not recommended when the history and physical exam do not detect any abnormalities. In order for a preoperative test to be considered valuable, the results would need to alter perioperative management.

A hemoglobin or hematocrit test is indicated if the surgery is associated with significant blood loss potential, fluid shifts, or if the patient has a complex systemic disease resulting in anemia. Platelet counts are indicated if the patient has a history of low platelets, or has a disease associated with diminished platelets such as preeclampsia. Coagulation studies are indicated if the patient has significant liver disease or known coagulopathic conditions.

EKG should be obtained if the patient has cardiac risk factors and a history of cardiac disease. There is no definitive recommendation for screening EKGs to be done, but most institutions use 50 or 60 years old as the age requirement. In the absence of ongoing symptoms or changes in cardiac status, a prior EKG within three to six months is generally acceptable.

Patients with chronic renal failure should have electrolytes, blood urea nitrogen, and creatinine tested prior to any significant surgery. Renal dialysis patients should have their potassium level drawn immediately prior to the procedure.

ASA Physical Status Classification System: this classification system reflects the patient's condition and underlying disease complexity, and a patient's ASA status generally correlates with their perioperative morbidity and mortality rate. More significant comorbidities may increase perioperative morbidity. For example, a relative risk of serious perioperative complications is 2.2 and 4.4 for ASA patient status 3 and 4 respectively.

Class 1: A normal, healthy patient; no disease outside surgical process

Class 2: A patient with mild to moderate systemic disease, medically well controlled, with no functional limitation

Class 3: A patient with severe systemic disease that results in functional limitation

Table 1.1 Guidelines for fasting

	Minimum fasting period
Clear liquids (water, fruit juices without pulp, clear tea, carbonated beverages, black coffee – does not include alcohol)	2 hours
Breast milk	4 hours
Infant formula	6 hours
Nonhuman milk	6 hours
Light meal (e.g., toast and a clear liquid)	6 hours
Fried or fatty foods, meat	8 hours

(Adapted from: Vacanti et al., 2011, p. 14.)

Class 4: A patient with severe, incapacitating systemic disease that is a constant threat to life (functionally incapacitated)

Class 5: A moribund patient who is not expected to survive without the operation

Class 6: A declared brain-dead patient whose organs are being removed for donor purposes

An "E" is added to the classification to designate a patient in whom surgery is emergent.

ASA NPO guidelines for fasting: patients are required to be nil per os (NPO) prior to undergoing anesthesia to minimize the risk of aspiration. These guidelines are for elective procedures requiring general anesthesia, regional anesthesia, or sedation/analgesia (i.e., monitored anesthesia care), but are not for women in labor. In considering NPO times, both the type and amount of food ingested should be taken into account (see Table 1.1). Also, the type of liquid ingested is typically more important than the volume of liquid ingested. If the following guidelines are not met, the patient is considered to be at an increased aspiration risk. NPO guidelines for fasting do not apply for emergency surgical procedures.

Questions

1. A 55-year-old gentleman is seen in the preoperative clinic in anticipation of an upcoming hip replacement surgery. His current medical conditions are well controlled, and his vital signs are stable in the clinic. It is appropriate to continue his outpatient medications as currently prescribed until his day of surgery, except for the following medication:

   a. baby aspirin
   b. regular insulin
   c. simvastatin
   d. metoprolol
   e. omeprazole

2. An anesthetic preoperative evaluation appropriately involves the following except:

a. baseline functional capacity assessment
b. an EKG for a patient with a history of hypertension and hypercholesteremia
c. coagulation studies for a laparoscopic cholecystectomy
d. platelet count for a preeclamptic patient
e. potassium level check for a renal dialysis patient

3. A 62-year-old woman with a past medical history of compensated CHF, atrial fibrillation, and angina with activity, and peripheral vascular disease has a recent diagnosis of breast adenocarcinoma. She presents for preoperative evaluation for a modified mastectomy. Her functional capacity at baseline is 2 METs. Her vital signs include a heart rate of 90, blood pressure 135/88, respiratory rate 16, with oxygen saturation of 98% on room air. Based on the current ACC/AHA guidelines and care algorithm, which of the following would be the most appropriate course of action?
a. proceed with planned surgery
b. obtain noninvasive cardiac testing for further evaluation
c. after improvement in heart rate control, proceed with the planned surgery
d. obtain a chest radiograph
e. postpone the surgery until her cardiologist approves her for the procedure

Answers

1. b. Patients who are on insulin therapy will need to have their doses adjusted because of the fasting period that is associated with their procedure preparation. As they should be appropriately NPO the day of their surgery, short-acting insulin is generally held on the morning of the procedure. Long-acting insulin is typically continued at the usual or reduced dose. Serum glucose levels can be checked, and regular insulin can be given as needed. However, it is not appropriate to continue the currently prescribed regular insulin dose as currently when the patient will be fasting.

2. c. The need for preoperative laboratory testing is based on the patient's comorbidities and the proposed surgical procedure. It is not recommended to undergo routine laboratory testing for asymptomatic patients who have no abnormalities suspected on history or physical exam. Coagulation studies are indicated for patients who have known hepatic disease or coagulopathies. Furthermore, laparoscopic cholecystectomy procedures are not typically procedures that are associated with inducing significant coagulation abnormalities.

3. a. Based on the ACC/AHA Guidelines on Perioperative Cardiovascular Evaluation and Care for Noncardiac Surgery, this patient would proceed with the planned procedure. Applying the step-wise algorithm to the scenario, this is not an emergency noncardiac surgery. Also, it is important to note that this patient does not have any "active cardiac conditions" as defined by the ACC/AHA guidelines – she does not have decompensated heart failure, nor unstable or severe angina, and her atrial fibrillation is not associated with an uncontrolled ventricular rate. Moreover, as her breast procedure is classified as having low cardiac risk, she may proceed with the planned elective surgery.

Further reading

American Society of Anesthesiologists Task Force on Preanesthesia Evaluation. (2002). Practice advisory for preanesthesia evaluation: a report by the American Society of Anesthesiologists Task Force on Preanesthesia Evaluation. *Anesthesiology* 96, 485.

Eagle, K. A. et al. (2002). ACC/AHA Guideline Update for Perioperative Cardiovascular Evaluation for Non-cardiac Surgery – Executive Summary. A report of the American College of Cardiology/American Heart Association Task Force on Practice Guidelines (Committee to Update the 1996 Guidelines on Perioperative Cardiovascular Evaluation for Noncardiac Surgery). *Anesthesia and Analgesia* 94, 1052–1064.

Faust, R. J. (2002). *Anesthesiology Review*, 3rd edn. Philadelphia: W.B. Saunders Company, pp. 337–339 and 517–518.

Morgan, G. E., Mikhail, M. S., and Murray, M. J. (2007). *Clinical Anesthesiology*, 4th edn. McGraw-Hill Medical, pp. 1–16 and 441–463

Vacanti, C. A., Sikka, P. K., Urman, R. U., Dershwitz, M., and Segal, B. S. (2011). *Essential Clinical Anesthesia*. New York: Cambridge University Press, pp. 7–15.

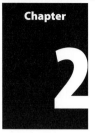

Chapter 2

Obstructive and restrictive lung disease

Emily L. Wang and Jeffrey Lu

Keywords

Obstructive lung disease
Chronic obstructive pulmonary disease (COPD)
Definition and classification of COPD
Emphysema
Chronic bronchitis
Pathophysiology of COPD
Treatment of COPD
Perioperative risk assessment of COPD
Preoperative optimization of COPD
Smoking cessation and COPD
Intraoperative management of COPD
Dynamic hyperinflation
Postoperative care of COPD
Asthma
Pathophysiology of asthma
Treatment of asthma
Preoperative optimization of asthma
Intraoperative management of asthma
Diagnosis of intraoperative bronchospasm
Restrictive lung disease
Causes of restrictive lung disease
Pathophysiology of restrictive lung disease
Treatment of restrictive lung diseases
Perioperative care of restrictive lung disease

Obstructive lung disease: the two primary obstructive lung diseases often encountered perioperatively are chronic obstructive pulmonary disease (COPD) and asthma.

COPD: the most common pulmonary disease in the perioperative setting. It is the fourth leading cause of death in the United States. Tobacco exposure causes 85% of cases.

Definition and classification of COPD: COPD is a chronic lung disease characterized by expiratory airflow limitation, which is progressive over time. The airflow limitation is not fully reversible (in contrast to asthma), and it is associated with abnormal inflammatory response in the lungs.

Table 2.1 Global Initiative for Chronic Obstructive Lung Disease staging criteria

Stage	Spirometry
0 (at risk)	$FEV_1/FVC \geq 70\%$ $FEV_1 \geq 80\%$
1 (mild)	$FEV_1/FVC < 70\%$ $FEV_1 \geq 80\%$
2 (moderate)	$FEV_1/FVC < 70\%$ FEV_1 50%–80%
3 (severe)	$FEV_1/FVC < 70\%$ FEV_1 30%–50%
4 (very severe)	$FEV_1/FVC < 70\%$ $FEV_1 < 30\%$

From: Vacanti. et al., 2011. *Essential Clinical Anesthesia*, Cambridge University Press, p. 16.

- Symptoms of COPD include chronic cough, sputum production, dyspnea, and progressive exercise intolerance with dyspnea on exertion.
- Physical examination findings may include decreased breath sounds, wheezes, rhonchi, rales, and prolonged expiratory phase. Oxygen saturation is also useful to help stratify the patient's surgical risk.
- Spirometry is used to confirm the diagnosis and classify the severity. Accepted criterion for COPD is the ratio of forced expiratory volume in the first second of expiration to forced vital capacity (FEV_1/ FVC) <70% of predicted, and postbronchodilator FEV_1 <80% of predicted. The staging system used to classify disease severity is based on the percent of FEV_1.

Historically, COPD is subdivided into emphysema and chronic bronchitis, although many patients exhibit features of both processes.

Emphysema: characterized by the destruction of lung parenchyma with normal airways. It includes destruction of collagen and elastin in the alveolar walls (so the elastic recoil

Essential Clinical Anesthesia Review: Keywords, Questions and Answers for the Boards, ed. Linda S. Aglio, Robert W. Lekowski, and Richard D. Urman. Published by Cambridge University Press.

of the lungs is decreased), which leads to airspace enlargement distal to the terminal bronchioles. This results in increased lung compliance, and hyperinflation and distortion of the chest wall.

Chronic bronchitis: characterized by inflammation of the airways, which is associated with increased mucus secretions and airway mucosa thickening. Chronic bronchitis produces airway obstruction, which can cause V/Q mismatch, hypoxia, and CO_2 retention.

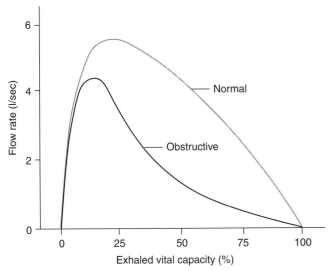

Figure 2.1 Flow–volume curve in normal and COPD patients. (From Vacanti et al. 2011. *Essential Clinical Anesthesia*, Cambridge University Press, p. 17.)

Pathophysiology of COPD: the pathogenesis of COPD derives from the combined effects of inflammation, increased oxidative stress, and imbalance in the activity of proteinases and antiproteinases. The pathologic changes are present throughout the lung, and progress over time. In the large central airways, there is enlargement of mucous glands, hyperplasia of goblet cells, loss of cilia, and decreased ciliary function, which results in such symptoms of increased mucus production and abnormal mucus clearance. In the airway walls, there is infiltration of inflammatory cells, increased smooth muscle, and deposition of connective tissue. In the small airways, there is also chronic inflammation, which causes collagen deposition and airway remodeling. The pulmonary vasculature can also be affected by vessel wall inflammation, smooth muscle deposition, and fibrosis.

Expiratory airflow limitation occurs as a result of airway inflammation, edema, mucus accumulation, airway hyperplasia and fibrosis, bronchospasm, and loss of radial traction as connective tissue is destroyed. Expiratory flow is significantly reduced throughout expiration, and expiratory time is increased.

Changes in lung volumes and capacities of COPD patients include increased total lung capacity (TLC), functional residual capacity (FRC), and residual volume (RV).

Hyperinflation occurs with COPD, which can be manifested by diaphragm flattening, rib elevation, and increase in the cross-sectional thoracic area. Ventilation–perfusion (V/Q) mismatching also occurs, and gas exchange is impaired. There is an increase in both physiologic dead space and shunt. Varying degrees of hypercarbia and hypoxemia occur in different patients.

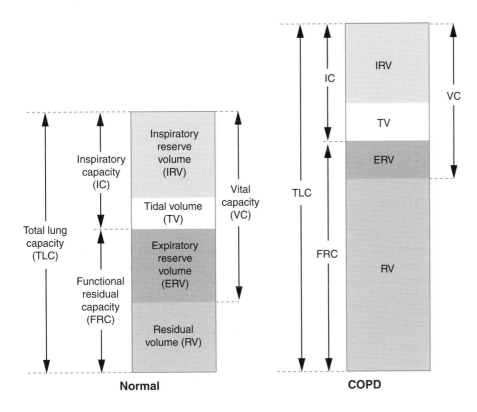

Figure 2.2 Changes in lung volumes and capacities with COPD. (From Vacanti et al. 2011. *Essential Clinical Anesthesia*, Cambridge University Press, p. 17.)

Pulmonary hypertension may result from the combined effects of chronic hypoxia and the direct pathologic changes of the pulmonary vasculature. Progressive pulmonary hypertension can cause right ventricular dysfunction and cor pulmonale.

Treatment of COPD:

- Treatment of stable COPD: smoking cessation is the only intervention that slows the progression of COPD. Yearly influenza vaccinations significantly decrease morbidity and mortality. Pharmacologic management is aimed at providing symptom relief, but does not change the disease progression. It is approached in a step-wise fashion. For early-stage COPD, short-acting inhaled bronchodilators are used for symptomatic relief. For more severe COPD, long-acting inhaled bronchodilators are used to help relieve dyspnea, and improve lung function and exercise tolerance. In severe COPD, inhaled corticosteroids help reduce the frequency of acute exacerbations. In patients with moderate to severe disease, combination therapy with long-acting β_2-agonists and inhaled corticosteroids may have additive benefits. Comprehensive, multidisciplinary pulmonary rehabilitation programs may provide improvement in exercise capacity and quality of life during all stages of COPD.

- Treatment of acute exacerbations of COPD: symptoms of acute exacerbations include worsened dyspnea, wheezing, cough, increased sputum, a change in the sputum characteristics, chest tightness, fever, and malaise. Acute exacerbations are often triggered by respiratory tract infections. Initial treatment includes escalation of bronchodilator therapy, oxygen therapy for hypoxia, antibiotics if there is evidence of bacterial infection, and possible systemic corticosteroids. The patient should be admitted to the hospital if they have progressive hypoxemia, hypercarbia, respiratory distress, or evidence of new heart failure. The highest risk of mortality is with progressive hypercarbia and respiratory acidosis. Noninvasive mechanical ventilation may be effective to decrease the need for intubation as well as the mortality. However, patients with refractory hypoxemia, severe acidosis, or respiratory arrest require intubation and mechanical ventilation.

- Treatment of end-stage COPD disease: limited treatment options for advanced COPD include domiciliary oxygen therapy, lung volume reduction surgery (LVRS), and lung transplantation. Oxygen therapy increases exercise capacity and improves survival, and is recommended for patients with PaO_2 <55 mm Hg or an arterial oxygen saturation (SaO_2) <89%; or a PaO_2 <60 mm Hg if the patient has pulmonary hypertension. Contrary to common belief, oxygen will not increase $PaCO_2$; any increases are most likely caused by changes in ventilation–perfusion distribution rather than decreased hypoxic ventilatory drive. LVRS is thought to improve chest wall mechanics in

Table 2.2 Commonly used bronchodilator drugs

Drug	Routes	Duration of action, h
β2-agonists:		
Fenoterol	MDI, Neb	4–6
Albuterol	MDI, Neb, oral	4–6
Levalbuterol	MDI, Neb	4–6
Terbutaline	MDI, Neb, oral	4–6
Formoterol	MDI	12
Salmeterol	MDI	12
Anticholinergics:		
Ipratropium bromide	MDI, Neb	6–8
Tiotropium	MDI	24+ hours
Methylxanthines:		
Aminophylline	IV, oral	variable
Theophylline	Oral	variable

IV, intravenous; MDI, metered-dose inhaler; Neb, nebulizer.
From: Vacanti. et al., 2011. *Essential Clinical Anesthesia*, Cambridge University Press, p. 18.

patients with severe hyperinflation. It is a high-risk palliative treatment, and few patients qualify.

Perioperative risk assessment of COPD: patients with COPD have a 2.7 to 4.7-fold increased risk of perioperative pulmonary complications. The degree of risk correlates with the severity of COPD. Common pulmonary complications are atelectasis, pneumonia, respiratory failure, and acute exacerbation of underlying chronic pulmonary disease.

Other risk factors for perioperative pulmonary complications include patient's age >60 years, ASA status II or higher, history of congestive heart failure, current smoking, and type of surgery. Highest risk surgeries are associated with aortic, thoracic, and upper abdominal procedures. Other increased risk surgeries include neurosurgery, head and neck surgery, emergency surgery, and prolonged surgery (>3 hours).

Current recommendations include pulmonary function tests (PFTs) for all lung resection candidates, and obtaining a chest radiograph for patients with known cardiopulmonary disease or those older than 50 years who are undergoing high-risk operations. Spirometry may be used to predict long-term functional status after a major lung resection. However, preoperative spirometry does not predict the risk of postoperative pulmonary complications. For other procedures, lab testing is an adjunct to clinical assessment and should be obtained in selected patients. Potential lab tests include chest radiographs, exercise testing, arterial blood gas analysis, and PFTs.

The potential benefit of a surgery should be weighed against the risk, especially if patients have an increased risk of perioperative pulmonary complications. However, even very high-risk patients may proceed to surgery if there is compelling indication. There is no prohibitive level of pulmonary function below which surgery is absolutely contraindicated.

Preoperative optimization of COPD: pulmonary function should be optimized in COPD patients, which includes the appropriate use of bronchodilators, treatment of active infections and acute exacerbations, and ideally the cessation of smoking. Preoperative bronchodilators help optimize airflow, and may decrease perioperative complications. However, routine preoperative administration of inhaled or oral corticosteroids is not recommended. It is beneficial to treat acute COPD exacerbations preoperatively, and it may be appropriate to delay an elective surgery until the patient is fully recovered from an acute exacerbation.

Smoking cessation and COPD: tobacco exposure is the most important cause of COPD, and smoking cessation is the only intervention that slows COPD progression. All COPD patients should be counseled on smoking cessation.

Smoking accelerates normal age-related declines in pulmonary function, and is a trigger for lung inflammation. Smoking is an independent risk factor for postoperative pulmonary complications even in the absence of chronic lung disease (including pneumonia, prolonged mechanical ventilation, and increased duration of ICU stay).

The impact of the duration of smoking abstinence on pulmonary complication rates is controversial, but there seems to be significant risk reductions when smoking has been stopped. Smoking cessation at least four to eight weeks prior to surgery lowers the patient's risk of pulmonary complications. Benefits include return of normal mucociliary function, airway secretion and reactivity, and immune function. Smoking cessation 24 to 48 hours prior to elective surgery normalizes carboxyhemoglobin levels and normalizes the oxyhemoglobin dissociation curve (i.e., corrects the left shift). Smoking cessation includes discontinuing use of non-tobacco products such as marijuana. Moreover, abstinence from smoking during the perioperative period may provide a great opportunity for long-term smoking cessation.

Intraoperative management of COPD: there exists evidence of variable quality that helps guide the choice of anesthetic technique for patients with COPD. Some studies report lower rates of postoperative pulmonary complications with the use of regional anesthesia and analgesia, as compared to general anesthesia and other postoperative pain relief strategies. It is reasonable to pursue regional techniques, especially if the patient has significant baseline pulmonary impairment. During general anesthesia, V/Q mismatching in COPD patients may be further worsened. It can cause wider alveolar–arterial oxygen gradients, as well as end-tidal and arterial carbon dioxide gradients.

- *Dynamic hyperinflation* is one of the most significant consequences of general anesthesia in COPD patients, and extreme caution should be taken to prevent it during assisted ventilation. Dynamic hyperinflation occurs when inspiration is initiated prior to the complete exhalation of the previous tidal volume; which causes the end-expiratory volume and pressures (auto-PEEP) to rise progressively with each subsequent inhalation until a new steady state is reached. The result is decreased lung compliance, further gas exchange impairment, venous return decrease, and possible barotrauma and alveolar rupture. The decrease in venous return may be significant enough to cause hypotension, decreased cardiac output, and even pulseless electrical activity. If dynamic hyperinflation is thought to be the culprit for severe hypotension, ventilation should be held to allow for unobstructed exhalation. Adequate hydration also helps ameliorate the decreased venous return. Dynamic hyperinflation can be prevented by using a slow respiratory rate, long expiratory time, and minimal tidal volume settings. Extrinsic PEEP can help keep small airways open and allow for more complete exhalation to occur.
- Bronchospasm may occur intraoperatively, and cause worsening of airflow obstruction and an abrupt increase in airway resistance. Acute bronchospasm may be treated with inhaled β_2-agonists, anticholinergics, and increased volatile anesthetics; and rarely, intravenous corticosteroid or low-dose continuous epinephrine intravenous infusion (0.25–0.5 µg/min) may be necessary to break severe refractory bronchospasm. Albuterol is not contraindicated in the management of acute bronchospasm in a patient with a history of ventricular tachycardia.
- Inspissation of pulmonary secretions may occur intraoperatively, and cause occlusion of bronchi or the endotracheal tube. Use of humidified inspiratory gases and

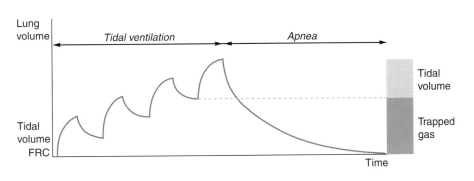

Figure 2.3 Dynamic hyperinflation during mechanical ventilation. (From Vacanti et al. 2011. *Essential Clinical Anesthesia*, Cambridge University Press, p. 19.)

maintaining adequate hydration may help prevent this. Use of a large diameter endotracheal tube (8.0 mm or larger) facilitates endotracheal tube suctioning and fiberoptic bronchoscopy if necessary. Mucolytics (N-acetylcysteine, dornase alpha) may be helpful to clear mucous plugging.

- COPD patients are sensitive to the respiratory depressant effects of commonly used medications such as benzodiazepines, narcotics, barbiturates, and propofol. Inefficient clearance of volatile agents is due to increased dead space, V/Q mismatch, and the long expiratory time-constant. Use of total intravenous anesthesia is reasonable, as it allows for timely emergence independent of underlying lung function. Analgesia should be aimed at minimizing postoperative respiratory depression.

Postoperative care of COPD: postoperative care should focus on facilitating the patient's rapid return to baseline levels of pulmonary function, i.e., awake and alert with sufficient pain control. Postoperative pulmonary complications can be prevented with the aid of lung expansion techniques (deep breathing, chest physiotherapy, and incentive spirometry). Early ambulation also facilitates secretion clearance and venous thromboembolism prevention. Patients should continue their baseline medical therapy for COPD. Acute COPD exacerbations in the perioperative period may require temporary escalation of bronchodilator therapy, antibiotics, or intravenous corticosteroids.

Asthma: obstructive pulmonary disease with prevalence of 5% in the United States. Approximately 4,000 people per year die in the United States from asthma.

Pathophysiology of asthma: chronic inflammatory disease of the airways resulting in airflow obstruction. The airflow limitation is reversible (in contrast to COPD). Asthma is characterized by airway hyperactivity and bronchospasm. It involves smooth muscle constriction, airway edema, mucus accumulation, airway inflammation, and abnormal deposition of collagen in basement membranes. Triggers may include cold air, infections, histamine, and environmental substances.

Treatment of asthma: aimed at reducing the frequency and severity of symptoms, associated functional limitations, and long-term morbidity. Patient management is based on avoidance of triggers, regular monitoring, and patient education. Pharmacologic management is approached in a step-wise fashion. Acute exacerbations often require systemic glucocorticoid administration.

Preoperative optimization of asthma: perioperative respiratory complications occur at 1–2% among asthmatics. Preoperative assessment includes the patient's asthma history (baseline activity level, frequency and severity of symptoms, degree of compliance of medication, emergency room visits, hospital admissions, previous intubations, and systemic glucocorticoid use) and lung auscultation exam. Baseline medications should be continued up to the time of surgery.

Table 2.3 Step-wise approach to baseline asthma treatment

Asthma severity	Typical features	Recommended treatment
Intermittent (step 1)	Sx 2 d/wk or less; normal FEV_1 at baseline; oral steroids once a year at most	Short-acting inhaled β_2-agonist prn (for step 1 and all other steps)
Mild persistent (step 2)	Sx >2 d/wk; β-agonists use >2 d/wk; oral steroids twice a year or more	Daily inhaled steroid or alternate controller (leukotriene inhibitor, theophylline, cromoglycates)
Moderate persistent (step 3)	Daily symptoms and β-agonist use; some activity limitation; reduced baseline FEV_1	Daily inhaled steroid (or alternate) plus daily long-acting β_2-agonist
Severe persistent (steps 4–6)	Sx throughout day; multiple uses of β-agonist each day; extreme activity limitation; FEV_1 <60%	Daily long-acting β_2-agonist plus moderate-dose (step 4) or high-dose (step 5) inhaled steroid; standing oral steroids added (step 6)

prn, as needed; Sx, symptoms.
From: Vacanti. et al., 2011. *Essential Clinical Anesthesia*, Cambridge University Press, p. 20.

Patients with poor control of their symptoms should have their treatment regimen optimized by their pulmonologist or primary care physician prior to the surgery if possible. Patients that have moderate persistent or severe persistent asthma are likely at higher risk for perioperative complications. These patients may benefit from a short course of oral steroids preoperatively. However, there have been studies that suggest patients with well-controlled asthma who have a peak flow measurement >80% of predicted have average pulmonary risk. Patients with chronic steroid treatments are at risk for adrenal suppression, and consideration should be given to administer stress-dose steroids perioperatively.

Intraoperative management of asthma: short-acting bronchodilators may be administered prophylactically immediately prior to anesthesia. Endotracheal intubation is a major stimulus for bronchospasm. If endotracheal intubation is performed, ensure that sufficient depth of anesthesia to suppress airway reflexes is achieved prior to laryngoscopy. Of note, ketamine is the only induction agent that produces smooth muscle relaxation. Intravenous lidocaine (1.5 mg/kg) also produces smooth muscle relaxation, and may be given prior to induction.

Intraoperative management goals for asthmatics are to maintain adequate anesthetic depth, avoid histamine-releasing drugs, and monitor for bronchospasm.

Diagnosis of intraoperative bronchospasm: involves the signs shown in Table 2.4.

Table 2.4 Signs of bronchospasm during general anesthesia. From: Vacanti. et al., 2011. *Essential Clinical Anesthesia*, Cambridge University Press, p. 21.

Wheezing on auscultation

Increased peak airway pressure with unchanged plateau pressure

Decreased expiratory tidal volumes

Upsloping capnography waveform

Failure of expiratory flow to reach zero (flow vs. time waveform)

Hypotension due to impaired venous return (dynamic hyperinflation)

Table 2.5 Causes of restrictive pulmonary physiology

Intrinsic to the lung parenchyma:
  Pulmonary edema
  Acute respiratory distress syndrome
  Pneumonia
  Autoimmune and collagen vascular diseases
  Pulmonary fibrosis
  Pneumonitis

Pleural space:
  Tumor (mesothelioma)
  Pneumothorax
  Pleural effusion and hemothorax
  Infection and inflammation/fibrosis (emphysema)

Chest wall:
  Obesity
  Ascites
  Anasarca
  Pregnancy
  Congenital malformations of chest wall/spine
  Circumferential burns

Neuromuscular diseases:
  High spinal cord injury
  Muscular dystrophy
  Myasthenia gravis and Eaton–Lambert syndrome
  Guillain–Barré syndrome
  Flail chest

From: Vacanti. et al., 2011. *Essential Clinical Anesthesia*, Cambridge University Press, p. 21.

If bronchospasm occurs, reassess the depth of anesthesia and administer a short-acting inhaled β_2-agonist. Severe and persistent bronchospasm may require a repeat dose of inhaled bronchodilators, intravenous corticosteroids, or use of low-dose continuous epinephrine intravenous infusion (0.25–0.5 μg/min). Extubation is also a major stimulus for bronchospasm. Consider deep extubation technique in appropriate patients. Otherwise, pretreatment with an inhaled short-acting β_2-agonist and intravenous lidocaine prior to emergence may help prevent bronchospasm.

Restrictive lung disease: restrictive lung disease impairs lung expansion, and is associated with decreased lung volumes. Restrictive lungs diseases are characterized by a decrease in TLC, RV, and FRC, and a normal FEV_1%.

Causes of restrictive lung disease: impaired lung expansion associated with restrictive lung diseases may be due to pathology located in the lung parenchyma, pleural space, or chest wall, and neuromuscular diseases may prevent respiratory muscles from effectively functioning.

Pathophysiology of restrictive lung disease: with the impaired lung expansion of restrictive lung disease, there is decreased compliance and vital capacity of the pulmonary system. The pathology is variable, and the signs and symptoms are specific to the underlying disease process. Classic symptoms typically include dyspnea and decreased exercise capacity. Pulmonary function tests (PFTs) show decreased volumes and capacities. FEV_1 is reduced, but because FVC is also reduced, the FEV_1/FVC ratio is normal. Primary parenchymal diseases often require biopsy for definitive diagnosis.

Treatment of restrictive lung diseases: treatment and chronic management is specific to the underlying disease process. The patient with restrictive disease may be presenting for operative diagnosis.

Perioperative care of restrictive lung disease: perioperative management varies with the etiology of restriction, and involves optimization of preoperative function. Treatable contributors to pulmonary restriction should be addressed preoperatively when possible (i.e., large pleural effusions, acute infection, pulmonary edema).

Assessment of the severity of the restrictive disease involves the patient's history (symptoms, degree of exercise impairment) and evaluation of PFTs. Baseline hypoxia should be identified with oxygen saturation measurement. For major pulmonary resections, a preoperative exercise test may be appropriate.

As patients have decreased FRC, ensure adequate preoxygenation prior to induction in order to avoid desaturation. Patients requiring mechanical ventilation may only tolerate relatively low tidal volumes due to decrease in pulmonary compliance, and a higher respiratory rate may be necessary to maintain adequate minute ventilation. Use of PEEP with positive pressure ventilation will help avoid atelectasis and maintain FRC. High inspired oxygen concentrations may be needed to avoid hypoxemia.

The cause of the patient's restrictive lung disease may be associated with pulmonary hypertension. Worsening pulmonary pressures can be prevented by avoiding hypoxia, hypercapnia, acidosis, hypothermia, and catecholamine surges.

Patients with respiratory muscle weakness may require prolonged postoperative ventilatory support to help overcome the normal decrease in pulmonary function associated with surgery and anesthesia. Risk of postoperative respiratory failure is more likely with significant restrictive disease. Anesthetic drug choices should be aimed at minimizing postoperative respiratory depression. Regional anesthesia and analgesia should be considered when applicable.

Questions

1. In regards to chronic obstructive and restrictive pulmonary disease, the following statements are true except:

   a. An increased total lung capacity is observed in both emphysema and chronic bronchitis.

   b. A decreased FRC is observed in restrictive lung disease.

   c. A decreased FEV_1/FVC ratio is seen in chronic obstructive pulmonary disease.

   d. An increased FEV_1/FVC ratio is observed in chronic bronchitis.

   e. A decreased FEV_1 and normal FEV_1/FVC is observed in restrictive lung disease.

2. Which of the following statements is false?

   a. While the airflow obstruction experienced by asthmatics is reversible, the expiratory airflow limitation experienced by COPD patients is not fully reversible.

   b. Dynamic hyperinflation occurs when expiration is initiated prior to the complete inhalation of the previous tidal volume, and a new steady state is reached.

   c. Smoking cessation is the only intervention that slows the progression of COPD.

   d. Ketamine is the only induction agent that produces smooth muscle relaxation.

   e. Intraoperative bronchospasm management includes inhaled β_2-agonists and anticholinergics, and intravenous corticosteroid or epinephrine.

3. Normal FEV_1/FVC ratio is approximately:

   a. 0.5

   b. 0.6

   c. 0.7

   d. 0.8

   e. 0.95

Answers

1. d. In patients with COPD (which includes emphysema and chronic bronchitis), there is an increase in total lung capacity (TLC), residual volume (RV), and functional residual capacity (FRC); and a decrease in forced expiratory volume in one second normalized to forced vital capacity ratio ($FEV_1\%$). Restrictive lung diseases are associated with impaired lung expansion, and are characterized by a decrease in TLC, RV, and FRC, and a normal $FEV_1\%$.

2. b. Dynamic hyperinflation occurs when inspiration is initiated prior to the complete exhalation of the previous tidal volume. This causes the end-expiratory volume and pressures to rise progressively with each subsequent inspiration, which leads to decreased lung compliance.

3. d. The forced expiratory volume in one second (or FEV_1) is the amount of air expired in one second and is commonly expressed as a percentage of the forced vital capacity, or FEV_1/FVC. The normal FEV_1/FVC is 75% to 80%. Accepted criterion for COPD is FEV_1/FVC <70% of predicted, and postbronchodilator FEV_1 <80% of predicted.

Further reading

Faust, R. J. (2002). *Anesthesiology Review*, 3rd edn. Philadelphia: W.B. Saunders Company, pp. 3–7, 87–90, 174–177, and 551–552.

Morgan, G. E., Mikhail, M. S., and Murray, M. J. (2007). *Clinical Anesthesiology*,

4th edn. McGraw-Hill Medical, pp. 571–580.

Smetana, W. (1999). Preoperative pulmonary evaluation. *New England Journal of Medicine* 340, 937.

Warner, D. O. (2006). Perioperative abstinence from cigarettes: physiologic

and clinical consequences. *Anesthesiology* 104, 356.

Vacanti, C. A., Sikka, P. K., Urman, R. U., Dershwitz, M., and Segal, B. S. (2011). *Essential Clinical Anesthesia*. New York: Cambridge University Press, pp. 16–22.

Chapter

3

Anesthetic goals in patients with myocardial ischemia and heart failure

Thomas Hickey and Linda S. Aglio

Keywords

Cardiac morbidity: preoperative factors
Old MI: preoperative risk assessment
Pre-hospital management: acute heart failure
Myocardial O_2 consumption
LV coronary perfusion pressure
LV filling physiology
Ventricular hypertrophy
CV physiology: LV
CHF: Frank–Starling curve
CHF Frank–Starling curve: milrinone effect
CHF Frank–Starling curve: phenylephrine
IABP: contraindications

Overview

Generally, goals aim at decreasing the significant perioperative mortality and morbidity associated with these comorbidities by careful preoperative assessment and medical optimization, an anesthetic plan that best assures hemodynamic stability, and provision for careful postoperative care including effective pain management. Practically speaking, preoperative assessment is according to ACC/AHA guidelines, and medical optimization in this population would include β-blockade and appropriate antiplatelet therapy if there is a history of PCI. Preoperative management of decompensated heart failure is complex but may include diuresis, afterload reduction, inotropic agents, rate and/or rhythm control if comorbid atrial fibrillation, intra-aortic balloon pump (IABP), and or noninvasive positive pressure ventilation (NIPPV). Operative considerations include neuraxial anesthesia, invasive blood pressure monitoring, pulmonary arterial catheters or TEE, careful fluid management, and a relatively liberal transfusion threshold. Many of these points are addressed in detail in other chapters.

Cardiac morbidity: preoperative factors. ACC/AHA guidelines suggest that the following "active cardiac conditions" be evaluated and treated before proceeding to the OR for non-emergency surgery: unstable coronary syndrome, decompensated heart failure, unstable arrhythmias, and severe valvular disease. The cardiac risk index can be calculated to predict cardiac complications by assessing the number of the following clinical risk factors: CAD, CHF, stroke, IDDM, CKD (Cr >2.0).

Table 3.1 Risk factors and complications

Risk factors	% complications
0	0.4
1	0.9
2	7
3	11

Old MI: preoperative risk assessment. "Acute" indicates MI within one week, whereas "recent" occurred 7 to 30 days prior. Acute or recent MI is considered an unstable coronary syndrome. An older MI is considered a cardiac risk index clinical risk factor.

Pre-hospital management: acute heart failure. Appropriate work-up includes EKG, cardiac enzymes, and BNP. Management strategies for ACS, if identified, are described elsewhere. NIPPV should be initiated, with consideration of the medical management per SBP shown in Table 3.2.

Table 3.2 Medical management per SBP

SBP (mm Hg)	Medical therapy
>140	Nitrates (i.e., nitroglycerin)
100–140	Nitrates plus diuretics if edema
<100	Inotropes (i.e., dopamine, dobutamine); consider careful fluid challenge

Myocardial O_2 consumption: The heart requires 8 to 10 ml of oxygen per 100 grams myocardium per minute, one of the highest requirements of any organ, with the subendothelial requirement 20% greater than epicardial. Determinants are HR, wall tension, and contractility. Increased HR not only

Essential Clinical Anesthesia Review: Keywords, Questions and Answers for the Boards, ed. Linda S. Aglio, Robert W. Lekowski, and Richard D. Urman. Published by Cambridge University Press. © Cambridge University Press 2015.

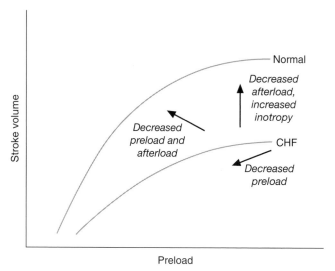

Figure 3.1 Relationship between preload and stroke volume in congestive heart failure. (Source: Steele, L. and Webster, N.R. 2001. Altered cardiac function. *Journal of the Royal College of Surgeons of Edinburgh* 46(1): 29–34.)

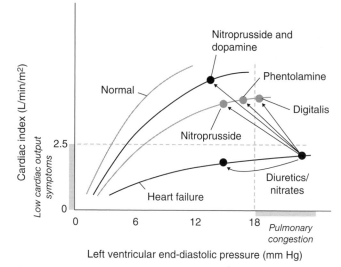

Figure 3.2 Medical management of heart failure. (From Vacanti et al. 2011. *Essential Clinical Anesthesia*, Cambridge University Press, p. 25.)

increases consumption but limits time for diastolic perfusion. Wall tension is given by Laplace's law:

Tension = (pressure × radius)/(2 × wall thickness)

LV coronary perfusion pressure: (LAD and circumflex distributions) corresponds to the gradient between diastolic aortic root pressure and LVEDP. Generally, compensatory mechanisms are able to maintain distal perfusion up to a 90% coronary occlusion.

LV filling physiology: Filling occurs during diastole. Ventricular relaxation is an active process requiring ATP. Atrial "kick" contributes roughly 15% of LVEDV, and assumes greater importance in the context of tachycardia and/or ventricular hypertrophy.

Ventricular hypertrophy: Chronic increases in pressure and volume can increase ventricular size. In chronic pressure overload (i.e., HTN, AS), sarcomeres are added in parallel resulting in concentric hypertrophy (increased wall thickness), while in chronic volume overload (i.e., valvular regurgitation), sarcomeres are added in series resulting in eccentric hypertrophy (chamber enlargement). A mixed picture typically follows myocardial infarction.

CV physiology: LV. The Frank–Starling curve describes the relationship between stroke volume (SV) and LVEDV. In a healthy heart, the SV will increase with increasing preload until there is excessive stretch on the myocardium past the optimal overlap of thin and thick myofilaments.

CHF: Frank–Starling curve. In systolic failure, the Frank–Starling curve is shifted down and to the right. That is, the failing heart will produce a lower SV at the same LVEDV. In this context, increased preload has a limited ability to augment stroke volume and may precipitate pulmonary congestion. Increases in contractility will shift the curve up and to the left. Interventions including inotropes, preload reduction (i.e., diuretic), and or afterload reduction may be useful.

Diastolic dysfunction accounts for approximately one-third of heart failure and describes the impaired filling with preserved EF that occurs when there is impaired ventricular relaxation. In this context, elevated LVEDP can quickly result in pulmonary edema. Reduced LV compliance can result from ischemia (remember that myocardial relaxation requires energy) and or hypertrophy from chronic elevated afterload (i.e., HTN or AS).

CHF Frank–Starling curve: milrinone effect. Milrinone is an "inodilator" that works via PDE III inhibition with consequent increases in myocardial cAMP. Along with the inotropic effect come improved lusitropy, and systemic and pulmonary vasodilation. As above, this agent would be expected to shift the Frank–Starling curve up and to the left.

CHF Frank–Starling curve: phenylephrine. As above, inotropes along with afterload and preload reduction are proven strategies in heart failure. Phenylephrine is an α-1 agonist causing venous greater than arterial constriction. It is not a standard therapy in CHF and would have a variable effect on the Frank–Starling curve. While the initial increase in preload resulting from splanchnic constriction may (or may not) augment stroke volume depending on where the patient is on the Frank–Starling curve, continued use of phenylephrine will act to decrease venous return and preload. Meanwhile, increases in myocardial oxygen demand in the context of increased afterload could precipitate ischemia in patients with coronary disease.

IABP: contraindications. IABP is considered if the response to medical management is inadequate. Insertion is through the femoral artery. Placement is distal to the origin of the left subclavian artery and superior to the renal arteries. Inflation (during diastole) and deflation (during systole) are synchronized with the EKG or arterial pressure waveform. Contraindications include: aortic insufficiency (would be worsened by the pump), sepsis, and severe PVD.

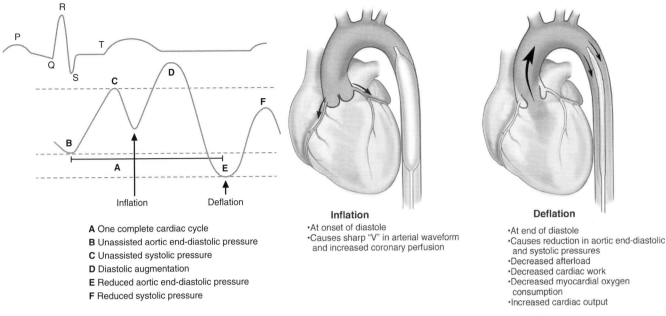

A One complete cardiac cycle
B Unassisted aortic end-diastolic pressure
C Unassisted systolic pressure
D Diastolic augmentation
E Reduced aortic end-diastolic pressure
F Reduced systolic pressure

Inflation
• At onset of diastole
• Causes sharp "V" in arterial waveform and increased coronary perfusion

Deflation
• At end of diastole
• Causes reduction in aortic end-diastolic and systolic pressures
• Decreased afterload
• Decreased cardiac work
• Decreased myocardial oxygen consumption
• Increased cardiac output

Figure 3.3 IABP timing: inflation/deflation. (From Vacanti et al. 2011. *Essential Clinical Anesthesia*, Cambridge University Press, p. 26.)

Questions

1. A 68-year-old man presents for preoperative evaluation for planned femoral to popliteal bypass surgery. Despite his vascular disease he is able to walk a flight of stairs without symptoms. Records indicate ejection fraction of 30% and prior myocardial infarct. Baseline creatinine is 2.4. Which best approximates his risk of major perioperative cardiac complications?

   a. 0.1%
   b. 1%
   c. 10%
   d. 20%

2. The same patient checks into the hospital on the day of surgery. In the preoperative area, he is clearly dyspneic at rest. Over the past few nights he has been increasingly short of breath, unable to lie flat at night. EKG shows new atrial fibrillation. CXR shows cardiomegaly with diffuse lung field opacities compatible with pulmonary venous congestion. Cardiac enzymes and a BNP are pending. What is the best course of action?

   a. Proceed with case only after preoperative IV Lasix and initiation of dobutamine drip.

   b. Proceed with case only after initiation of milrinone drip.
   c. Proceed with case only after he is ruled out for ACS.
   d. Postpone case and arrange for cardiology consult.

Answers

1. c. As described above, this patient would have a total of three clinical risk factors, correlating with an 11% risk of major perioperative cardiac complications.
2. d. This patient has acutely decompensated systolic heart failure, which doubles his already high perioperative risk of major cardiac complications. It would be irresponsible to proceed with this noncardiac case. ACS should be ruled out and the patient should be seen by cardiology before discharge.

Further reading

Vacanti, C. A., Sikka, P. K., Urman, R. U., Dershwitz, R., and Segal, B.S. (eds) (2011). *Essential Clinical Anesthesia*, 1st edn. New York, NY: Cambridge University Press, Chapter 4.

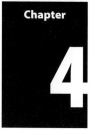

Anesthetic goals in patients with valvular heart disease

Zahra M. Malik and Martin Zammert

Keywords

Endocarditis prophylaxis
Mitral stenosis: pathophysiology
Mitral stenosis: anesthetic management
Acute intraoperative atrial fibrillation in mitral
    stenosis: treatment
Mitral regurgitation
Mitral regurgitation: hemodynamic management
Acute mitral regurgitation: management
Mitral valve prolapse: anesthetic implications
Aortic stenosis
Aortic stenosis: anesthetic considerations
Aortic stenosis and spinal anesthesia
Aortic regurgitation
Acute aortic regurgitation: management
Cardiac pressure–volume relationship

The 2007 AHA guidelines recommend *endocarditis prophylaxis* for moderate to high-risk patients:

- prosthetic valve or history of infective endocarditis
- complex cyanotic heart disease
- surgically reconstructed systemic pulmonary shunts/conduits
- congenital cardiac valve malformations
- history of surgical valve repair
- hypertrophic cardiomyopathy with obstruction
- MVP and auscultatory evidence of regurgitation and/ or echocardiography evidence of thickened leaflets

Undergoing these procedures:

- respiratory tract (tonsillectomy/adenoidectomy, respiratory tract procedures, rigid bronchoscopy)
- GI tract (esophageal varices sclerotherapy, esophageal stricture dilatations, ERCP with biliary obstruction, biliary tract surgery, operations involving intestinal mucosa) if proven GI tract infection or if non-elective procedure
- genitourinary tract (prostate surgery, cystoscopy, urethral dilatation) if proven GU tract infection or if non-elective procedure

Additionally, antibiotic prophylaxis for dental procedures that involved manipulation of gingival tissue, the periapical region of teeth, or perforation of the oral mucosa was deemed reasonable in the following cardiac conditions:

- prosthetic cardiac valve or prosthetic material used for valve repair
- previous history of infective endocarditis
- congenital heart disease (CHD)
  - unrepaired cyanotic CHD, including palliative shunts and conduits
  - completely repaired congenital heart defect with prosthetic material or device, whether placed by surgery or by catheter intervention, during the first six months after the procedure
  - repaired CHD with residual defects at the site or adjacent to the site of a prosthetic patch or prosthetic device (which inhibit endothelialization)
- cardiac transplant recipients who develop cardiac valvulopathy

Aortic stenosis is characterized by a narrowed valve causing a pressure gradient from the left ventricle to the aorta (normally

Table 4.1 Hemodynamic goals for the intraoperative management of valvular heart disease

Lesion	Preload	Systemic vascular resistance	Heart rate	Contractility
Aortic stenosis	↑	↑	↓	→
Hypertrophic cardiomyopathy	↑	↑	↓	↓
Mitral stenosis	↑	→ or ↑	↓	→
Mitral regurgitation	↑	↓	↑	→
Aortic regurgitation	↓	↓	↑	→

(From: Vacanti et al., 2011, p. 32.)

Essential Clinical Anesthesia Review: Keywords, Questions and Answers for the Boards, ed. Linda S. Aglio, Robert W. Lekowski, and Richard D. Urman. Published by Cambridge University Press. © Cambridge University Press 2015.

there is minimal gradient between both chambers). As the stenosis progresses, an increasing pressure gradient develops across the aortic valve with resulting LV hypertrophy to normalize wall stress and maintain CO. Over time, the LV hypertrophy results in reduced LV diastolic compliance. Thus LVEDP increases to maintain the same LVEDV. The pulmonary capillary bed is protected from progressive increase in diastolic pressure by atrial contraction which contributes up to 40% of ventricular filling in patients with aortic stenosis (normally 15–20%). Loss of atrial kick causes decreased CO and rise in LAP. At late stages LV dilatation can occur leading to progressive LV failure.

Advanced aortic stenosis is characterized by the triad of dyspnea on exertion, angina, and orthostatic or exertional syncope. Without surgical treatment, most patients with symptomatic AS die within two to five years.

Aortic stenosis pressure–volume relationship: the high pressure gradient across the aortic valve results in a high intraventricular pressure in order to maintain a normal stroke volume. The end-diastolic pressure is higher than normal due to reduced LV compliance.

Aortic stenosis: anesthetic considerations. Maintaining NSR is essential. Tachycardia should be avoided (AS is characterized by a fixed SV and CO becomes HR dependent). Normal to high preload is needed as a stiff LV requires a higher filling pressure to maintain normal end-diastolic volume. Sudden decreases in SVR should be avoided as the stenosis limits a compensatory rise in CO. Myocardial depression should be avoided through prevention of hypercarbia, hypoxia, and acidosis. Maintaining aortic diastolic pressure is crucial in preventing ischemia in patients with preexisting CAD. Patients with mild to moderate AS may tolerate spinal or epidural anesthesia if dosed gradually. For general anesthesia, opioid-based induction techniques avoid excessive cardiac depression.

Aortic regurgitation: in chronic aortic regurgitation the LV undergoes eccentric hypertrophy and LV dilatation, which accommodates blood flowing back to the ventricle during diastole. Systemic arterial blood pressure and SVR are typically reduced. The LVEDV and stroke volume increase as the ventricle accommodates both regurgitant and left atrial blood volume. Most patients remain asymptomatic for one to two decades. Valve replacement is considered in patients who are symptomatic or asymptomatic with reduced ventricular function. In *acute aortic regurgitation*, the sudden increase in LVEDP is transmitted to the left atrium and pulmonary circulation, which can precipitate dyspnea. Forward flow of blood can be severely compromised. It is an emergency requiring immediate surgery.

The anesthetic *management of aortic regurgitation* includes preoperative medical optimization with diuretics and afterload-reducing agents, particularly ACE inhibitors. The decrease in arterial blood pressure reduces the diastolic gradient for regurgitation. Preload should be maintained, with heart rate ideally in the upper limit of normal and avoiding sudden afterload increases to minimize regurgitant volumes associated with prolonged diastole. Diastolic blood pressure should be

maintained to ensure adequate cardiac perfusion. Contractility should be maintained. Spinal and epidurals are generally well tolerated. The use of volatile anesthetics may be beneficial because of associated vasodilatation.

The *pressure–volume relationship* in acute aortic regurgitation includes increased end-diastolic volume and slightly increased end-diastolic pressure. The end-systolic volume is greater than normal due to the regurgitation volume. In contrast, in chronic aortic regurgitation the heart may undergo significant dilatation, but the end-diastolic pressure is normal as a result of cardiac remodeling.

Mitral stenosis: pathophysiology. Mitral sentosis results in obstruction of blood flow from the left atrium to the left ventricle and thus markedly affecting LV filling. The left ventricle is underfilled and the pressure within the left atrium is significantly increased. Pressures in the pulmonary vasculature and right side of the heart can also be elevated. A fixed CO state develops as there is a significant reduction in LV preload.

Risk factors for developing pulmonary edema in mitral stenosis: mitral valve area <1.5 cm²; NHYA functional class >II; prior adverse cardiac event; LVEF <0.4.

Mitral stenosis pressure–volume relationship: mitral stenosis leads to a reduction in end-diastolic, and end-systolic, volume as well as a reduction in LV pressures. LV function is normal in most people but stroke volume is decreased secondary to chronic underfilling.

Anesthetic considerations in mitral stenosis: goals are to maintain slightly reduced to normal heart rate (allowing more time in diastole to improve LV filling), maintain normal sinus rhythm (atrial kick facilitates LV filling), maintain adequate preload and afterload to generate CO and maintain coronary perfusion pressure, respectively, avoiding precipitants of pulmonary hypertension (and thus right heart failure) including hypoxemia, hypercarbia, and acidosis. *Acute intraoperative atrial fibrillation in patients with mitral stenosis* should be treated by cardioversion into normal sinus rhythm.

Mitral regurgitation involves a portion of the LV stroke volume being ejected backwards into the left atrium during systole. The direct consequences include an elevation of left atrial pressure, reduced CO, and volume-related stress on the left ventricle as it accommodates both the regurgitant volume in diastole, as well as the normal pulmonary venous return. The volume of regurgitant flow is affected by the mitral valve orifice size, time available for regurgitant flow during systole, transvalvular pressure gradient, SVR opposing forward flow, and left atrial compliance.

Mitral regurgitation *pressure–volume relationship*: in chronic mitral regurgitation the left atrium becomes dilated to accommodate the larger volume, without a substantial increase in pressure. Both left atrium and ventricle are volume overloaded resulting in an increased LV end-diastolic volume and normal end-diastolic pressure. LV end-diastolic volume is normal because of an increased stroke volume. The effective cardiac output, however, is impaired because parts of the ejected volume regurges back into the LA.

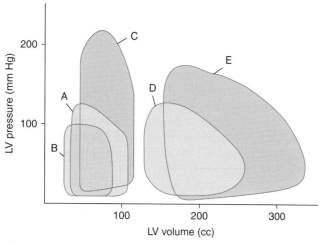

Figure 4.1 Pressure–volume loops in patients with valvular heart disease. A, normal; B, mitral stenosis; C, aortic stenosis; D, mitral regurgitation (chronic); E, aortic regurgitation (chronic). LV, left ventricular. (Reproduced, with permission, from Jackson, J. M., Thomas, S. J., and Lowenstein, E. 1982. Anesthetic management of patients with valvular heart disease. *Semin Anesth* 1: 239.)

The hemodynamic *management* of *mitral regurgitation* includes promoting forward flow and minimizing regurgitant volume. Cardiac function should be medically optimized prior to elective surgery with digoxin, diuretics, and vasodilators. Preload should be normalized to supply a dilated LV. Forward flow is promoted by maintaining a normal to high heart rate and by reducing afterload. Contractility should be maintained.

In *acute mitral regurgitation*, the left atrial compliance undergoes little immediate change. Thus left atrial pressure increases dramatically when exposed to the regurgitant volume. The pressure is transmitted backwards into the pulmonary system and the right heart, precipitating pulmonary edema, pulmonary hypertension, and right heart failure.

Mitral valve prolapse involves prolapse of the valve into the left atrium during systole. It is the most common cause of chronic MR and about 10% of patients with MVP develop progressive MR and require intervention. The natural history is generally benign and most patients have a normal life span. Complications of this lesion include infective endocarditis, CVA, arrhythmias, need for surgery, and sudden death. Only patients with MVP and auscultatory evidence of regurgitation and/or echocardiography evidence of thickened leaflets require *endocarditis prophylaxis*.

Questions

1. Which of the following clinical conditions is endocarditis prophylaxis clinically indicated according to the 2007 AHA guidelines?
   a. A 62-year-old man with a history of aortic stenosis who underwent mechanical aortic valve replacement two years ago, about to undergo tooth extraction.
   b. A 32-year-old female scheduled for an elective cystoscopy, who exercises daily, found to have an isolated I/VI holosystolic murmur in preoperative clinic.
   c. A 21-year-old male with a history of surgically uncorrected bicuspid aortic valve undergoing surveillance TEE.
   d. A 39-year-old female with echocardiographic evidence of MR with structurally normal valves undergoing ERCP.

2. Left atrial contraction contributes to approximately what percent of ventricular filling in a normal person versus a person with aortic stenosis?
   a. 40% vs. 20%
   b. 10% vs. 50%
   c. 20% vs. 40%
   d. 35% vs. 60%

3. Which of the following correctly lists the heart rate and blood pressure anesthetic goals in managing mitral regurgitation?
   a. Normal to high end heart rate, normal to reduced afterload.
   b. Normal to low end heart rate, normal to high end afterload.
   c. Normal to high end heart rate, normal to high end afterload.
   d. Normal to low end heart rate, normal to high end afterload.

Answers

1. a. Endocarditis prophylaxis is recommended in moderate to high-risk patients undergoing respiratory, GI tract, or genitourinary procedures. This includes patients with a prosthetic valve, history of infective endocarditis, surgical valve repair or surgically reconstructed pulmonary shunts/conduits, complex cyanotic heart disease, mitral regurgitation, and hypertrophic cardiomyopathy with obstruction.

2. c. Atrial contraction normally contributes 15% to 20% of ventricular filling. With left ventricular hypertrophy, there is a decrease in ventricular diastolic compliance, which can precipitate pulmonary capillary congestion. Atrial contraction in this setting contributes to up to 40% of ventricular filling.

3. a. The hemodynamic management of mitral regurgitation under general anesthesia aims to optimize forward flow and minimize regurgitant volume. Preload should be normalized to supply a dilated LV. A normal to high heart rate and reduced afterload promote forward flow. Additionally, contractility should be maintained.

Further reading

Sundar, S., Erlich, J. M., and Sundar, E. (2011). Anesthetic goals in patients with valvular heart disease. In Vacanti, C. A., Sikka, P. K., Urman, R. U., Dershwitz, M., and Segal, B. S. (eds) *Essential Clinical Anesthesia*. New York, NY: Cambridge University Press, pp. 28–36.

Townsley, M. and Martin, D. E. (2013). Anesthetic management for the surgical treatment of valvular heart disease. In Hensley, F. A., Martin, D. E., and Gravlee, G.P. (eds) *A Practical Approach to Cardiac Anesthesia*, 5th edn. Philadelphia, PA: Lippincott Williams & Wilkins, pp. 319–358.

Wilson, W., Taubert, K. A., Gewitz, M. et al. (2007). Prevention of infective endocarditis: a guideline from the American Heart Association Rheumatic Fever, Endocarditis, and Kawasaki Disease Committee, Council on Cardiovascular Disease in the Young, and the Council on Clinical Cardiology, Council on Cardiovascular Surgery and Anesthesia, and the Quality of Care and Outcomes Research Interdisciplinary Working Group. *Circulation*, 116: 1736–1754, e376–e377.

Vacanti, C. A., Sikka, P. K., Urman, R. U., Dershwitz, R., and Segal, B.S. (eds) (2011). *Essential Clinical Anesthesia*, 1st edn. New York, NY: Cambridge University Press, p. 32.

Morgan, G. E., Mikhail, M. S., and Murray, M. J. (eds) (2006). *Clinical Anesthesiology*, 4th edn. McGraw-Hill, p. 467.

Obesity

5

Kelly G. Elterman and Suzanne Klainer

Keywords

Causes of rapid desaturation: obesity
Hypoxemia in morbid obesity: cause
Morbid obesity: airway evaluation
Morbid obesity: pulmonary function
Morbid obesity: hypoxemia physiology
Morbid obesity: PFTs
Morbid obesity: pharmacokinetic considerations
Morbid obesity: rapid desaturation
Obesity: risk of aspiration

Current obesity classifications are as follows: overweight (BMI 25.00–29.99 kg/m^2); class I obesity (BMI 30.00–34.99 kg/m^2); class II obesity (BMI 35.00–39.99 kg/m^2); class III obesity (BMI $\geq$40.00 kg/m^2). Perioperative risk, as well as mortality, increases with increasing BMI. The obese patient presents unique challenges throughout the perioperative period due to changes in several organ systems.

Obesity and the cardiovascular system

Obesity results from an imbalance between energy supply and demand. Energy needs and *oxygen consumption* are increased by as much as 25%. This demand is met by an increase in minute ventilation and cardiac output.

The obese patient is more likely to have altered cardiopulmonary mechanics, which can lead to *V/Q mismatch*, and *hypoxemia*. Obese patients are more likely to have underlying heart disease, which may be undiagnosed as usual signs and symptoms (edema, increased jugular venous distention, dyspnea on exertion, orthopnea, etc.) may be difficult to identify secondary to body habitus or physical inactivity. For this reason, these patients frequently require preoperative cardiovascular evaluation, including EKG, CXR, and echocardiography.

Obesity and the pulmonary system

The obese patient may present with an increased neck circumference or excess pharyngeal tissue, which may indicate a predisposition to *upper airway obstruction and difficult mask ventilation*.

Obese patients also have *decreased functional residual capacity (FRC), decreased total lung capacity (TLC)*, and *PFTs consistent with restrictive pathology* as a result of decreased diaphragmatic mobility due to adipose tissue in the thorax and abdomen. Induction of anesthesia and the supine position further decrease FRC. This combination of *decreased FRC and increased oxygen requirements* causes obese patients to desaturate quickly when apneic. The decreased FRC also predisposes these patients to atelectasis, as closing capacity (CC) may exceed FRC.

The incidence of *obstructive sleep apnea (OSA)* is nearly 90% in the morbidly obese. Frequently, it may be undiagnosed. OSA occurs as a result of excess pharyngeal tissue, which collapses and obstructs the upper airway when the patient is asleep, sedated, or anesthetized. The presence of OSA should alert the anesthesiologist to the possibility of a *difficult airway*, specifically *difficult mask ventilation*.

Patients with OSA benefit from perioperative CPAP use. Long-term OSA, particularly if not treated with continuous positive airway pressure (CPAP), may lead to *"obesity-hypoventilation," or "Pickwickian" syndrome*, which is a condition of obesity, hypoxemia, hypercarbia, daytime somnolence, polycythemia, pulmonary hypertension, and ultimately right heart failure.

Obesity and the renal system

Obese patients have increased renal blood flow (RBF), glomerular filtration rate (GFR), and tubular reabsorption. This increase may be related to the overall *increased blood volume and cardiac output* seen in the obese state. Increases in RBF and GFR lead to *increased excretion of renally cleared drugs*. This baseline increase in GFR also makes these patients more susceptible to hypovolemia and prerenal azotemia, particularly as a result of diuretic, angiotensin-converting enzyme inhibitor (ACEI), or nonsteroidal anti-inflammatory drug (NSAID) use. Volume loading and maintenance of euvolemia is very important in these patients. Intraoperative fluid requirement may be higher than calculated for normal-weight patients.

Essential Clinical Anesthesia Review: Keywords, Questions and Answers for the Boards, ed. Linda S. Aglio, Robert W. Lekowski, and Richard D. Urman. Published by Cambridge University Press. © Cambridge University Press 2015.

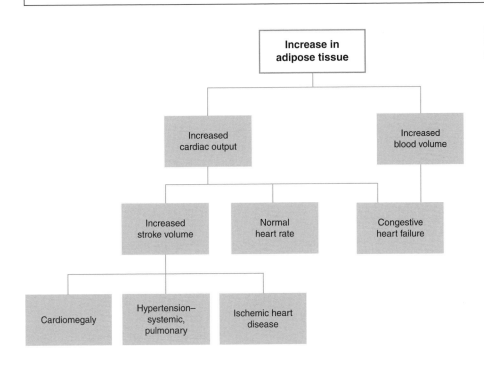

Figure 5.1 Cardiovascular changes in obesity. (From Vacanti et al. 2011. *Essential Clinical Anesthesia*, Cambridge University Press, p. 38.)

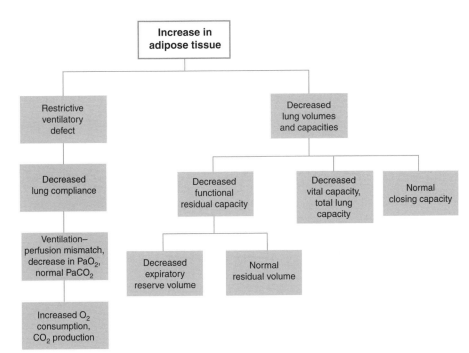

Figure 5.2 Pulmonary changes in obesity. (From Vacanti et al. 2011. *Essential Clinical Anesthesia*, Cambridge University Press, p. 39.)

Obesity and the gastrointestinal system

Obesity alone does not increase aspiration risk. Obesity does present challenges in airway management, however, which may significantly contribute to the risk of aspiration in these patients.

Obese patients frequently have hepatobiliary disease, such as fatty liver infiltration and cholelithiasis. Abnormalities in cholesterol metabolism predisposes these patients to hepatic dysfunction and postoperative gallstones.

Induction of anesthesia in the obese patient

Obese patients have many characteristics that predispose them to *difficult airway management* and *rapid oxygen desaturation*. Adequate time and preparation is crucial for safety during anesthetic induction and airway management. A ramp should be placed under the patient to optimize intubating conditions, and preoxygenation should be accomplished in a 30° reverse Trendelenburg or sitting position.

Airway equipment, including intubating laryngeal mask airway (LMA), bougie, video laryngoscope, or fiberoptic bronchoscope should be readily available. An LMA can be an effective alternative to ventilation should mask ventilation prove difficult. *BMI >26 has been shown to be a risk factor for difficult mask ventilation.* Similarly, *neck circumference >40 cm and Mallampati score of 3 or greater has been linked to difficult intubation* in the obese population.

Preinduction administration of metoclopramide or H$_2$ blockers to minimize the effects of aspiration may be considered, but has not been shown to reduce the risk of aspiration. If aspiration is of concern, rapid sequence induction with cricoid pressure should be pursued.

Obesity and pharmacokinetics

The increased cardiac output and overall hypervolemic state of obese patients may *increase drug requirements.* Lipophilic drugs, such as propofol, benzodiazepines, and opioids, often have a larger volume of distribution in these patients. Therefore *induction or loading doses of lipophilic medications should be calculated based on total body weight (TBW),* not ideal body weight (IBW). Hydrophilic drugs, such as

nondepolarizing neuromuscular blockers, do not have a larger volume of distribution and should be dosed by IBW. Succinylcholine, however, should be dosed by TBW due to *increased plasma cholinesterase activity in obese patients.* Repeat dosing, of both lipophilic and hydrophilic drugs, and calculation of infusion rates, particularly for opioids, should be based on IBW. The increased RBF and GFR, and the resultant increased renal clearance found in obese patients, should be kept in mind when dosing medications.

Sevoflurane and desflurane have been identified as optimal inhalational agents for obese patients, due to their rapid and consistent recovery profiles, hemodynamic control, decreased incidence of postoperative nausea/vomiting, and overall cost-effectiveness. More lipophylic agents such as isoflorane may have prolonged duration of action.

Obesity and regional anesthesia

Regional anesthesia, including epidural and spinal anesthesia, although more technically challenging, may safely be performed in the obese patient. Importantly, *in-dwelling catheters may be more likely to migrate, sympathetic blockade may spread*

Table 5.1 Organ system, comorbidity, and anesthetic implications

Organ system	Comorbidity	Anesthetic implications
Cardiovascular	Hypervolemic state	Increased volume of distribution, hypertension
	High cardiac output state	Cardiomegaly, CHF
	CHF (systolic and diastolic dysfuncion)	Increased risk of perioperative CHF
	Ischemic heart disease	Myocardial infarction, heart failure
	DVT	Perioperative thromboembolism, pulmonary embolism, need for DVT prophylaxis
	Hypotension	Myocardial ischemia, LV failure
	Valvular heart disease	Heart failure
	Peripheral vascular disease	Reduced blood flow, limb ischemia, poor wound healing
Pulmonary	OSA	Hypercarbia, respiratory acidosis, polycythemia, difficult ventilation
	Pulmonary hypertension	Right heart failure
	Restrictive lung volumes	Shorter time to hypoxia, difficult oxygenation
	Difficult airway management	Difficult ventilation and intubation, pulmonary aspiration
Endocrine	Diabetes and insulin resistance	Cardiovascular disease, central obesity, perioperative glucose control
	Hypercholesterolemia	Systemic cardiovascular disease
Gastrointestinal	Gastroparesis	Pulmonary aspiration, delayed gastric emptying. PONV?
	GERD	Rapid sequence intubation, risk of pulmonary aspiration
	Fatty liver	Altered liver function
	Hepatobiliary disease	Cholelithiasis, biliary obstruction, hepatic insufficiency
Renal	Increased GFR, RBF	Predisposition to renal insufficiency, greater fluid requirements, altered clearance of drugs; consider discontinuation of ACE inhibitors and/or diuretics
CNS	Hypersensitivity to CNS depressants	Hypersomnolence, central apnea, reduced drug requirement
	Cerebrovascular disease	Decreased cerebral blood flow
Hematologic	Polycythemia	Increased viscosity, platelet aggregation
	Thrombosis	DVT and pulmonary embolus
	Poor wound healing	Wound infections

(From Vacanti et al. 2011. *Essential Clinical Anesthesia*, Cambridge University Press, p. 38.)

more cephalad, and neuraxial opioids may have an increased respiratory depressant effect in these patients.

Intraoperative considerations

Maintaining oxygenation may be an intraoperative challenge in obese patients, due to *decreased FRC and respiratory compliance*. Recruitment maneuvers and use of positive end-expiratory pressure (PEEP), up to 15 cm H_2O, have been shown to improve oxygenation.

Avoidance of nitrous oxide, or limiting it to <50%, may also be beneficial in these patients.

Obese patients undergoing laparoscopy may have further reduced FRC and pulmonary mechanics due to Trendelenburg positioning and pneumoperitoneum. V/Q mismatching may worsen, leading to hypoxemia and hypercarbia, which may lead to acidosis, increased pulmonary vascular resistance, and right heart strain. Absorption of CO_2 from laparoscopic insufflation further worsens these effects.

Positioning may be another important intraoperative consideration for obese patients. Standard protective positioning equipment designed for nonobese patients may not work well for these patients, and they may suffer untoward consequences as a result. For this reason, increased vigilance and monitoring of pressure points may be necessary.

Postoperative considerations

Obese patients have increased morbidity and mortality in the postoperative period due to OSA, increased sensitivity to respiratory depressants, reduced cardiopulmonary reserve, and increased risk for thromboembolic events. Early use of BiPAP or CPAP has been shown to decrease incidence of postoperative hypoxia in these patients.

Perioperative DVT prophylaxis with either subcutaneous heparin or LMWH has been shown to decrease DVT risk.

Non-opioid-based pain management strategies, including the use of regional anesthesia, NSAIDs, and ketamine, are recommended to avoid respiratory depression and subsequent cardiopulmonary morbidity and mortality.

Questions

1. Increased energy needs and oxygen consumption found in obese patients results in which of the following?
   a. decreased cardiac output and increased minute ventilation
   b. increased cardiac output and decreased minute ventilation
   c. increased cardiac output and increased minute ventilation
   d. decreased cardiac output and decreased minute ventilation

2. A patient with long-standing untreated OSA is at risk for which of the following:
   a. hypocarbia
   b. pulmonary hypertension
   c. difficult intubation
   d. anemia

3. Which of the following statements is MOST true regarding medication dosing in obese patients?
   a. All medications should be dosed according to TBW.
   b. Lipophilic medications should be dosed according to IBW.
   c. Loading doses of hydrophilic medications should be dosed according to IBW.
   d. Repeat doses of all medications should be based on IBW.

Answers

1. c. Obese patients have increased cardiac output and minute ventilation, both of which occur as a result of increased oxygen consumption, due to increased metabolic demand.
2. b. Pulmonary hypertension occurs as a result of hypoxia and hypercarbia, which occurs in obstructive sleep apnea.
3. d. Induction or loading doses should be dosed by TBW. Repeat doses should be based on IBW.

Further reading

Nguyen, L. C. and Jones, S. B. (2011). Obesity. In Vacanti, C. A., Sikka, P. J., Urman, R. D., Dershwitz, M., and Segal, B. S. (eds) *Essential Clinical Anesthesia*. Cambridge: Cambridge University Press, p. 38.

Casati, A. and Putzu, M. (2005). Anesthesia in the obese patient: pharmacokinetic considerations. *Journal of Clinical Anesthesia* 17(2), 134–145.

Passannante, A. N. and Rock, P. (2005). Anesthetic management of patients with obesity and sleep apnea. *Anesthesiology Clinics of North America* 23(3), 479–491.

Ebert, T., Shankar, H., and Haake, R. (2006). Perioperative considerations for patients with morbid obesity. *Anesthesiology Clinics* 24, 621–636.

Passannante, A. and Tielborg, M. (2009). Anesthetic management of patients with obesity with and without sleep apnea. *Clinics in Chest Medicine* 30, 569–579.

Chapter

6

Chronic renal failure

Michael Vaninetti and Assia Valovska

Keywords

Chronic renal failure
Lab assessment of renal function
Azotemia
Uremia
Dialysis effects
Renal failure: electrolyte effects
Contrast-induced nephropathy prevention
Hyperkalemia treatment
Hypermagnesemia treatment
Renal failure: comorbidities
Renal failure: platelet function
Renal failure: pharmacokinetics

Chronic renal failure (CRF) is defined by an estimated glomerular filtration rate (GFR) <60 ml/min/1.73m^2 for at least three months. It results in impaired handling of fluids and acid loads, regulation of electrolytes, and excretion of medications.

Lab assessment of renal function: the most accurate study is the creatinine clearance rate (CCR) = (urine creatinine × urine flow rate)/(serum creatinine) based on 24-hour urine collection. However, two-hour tests are relatively accurate as well. BUN and Cr are good screening tools but not as accurate.

CRF severity is classified based on estimated GFR.

Azotemia refers to retention of nitrogenous waste products due to renal insufficiency.

Uremia is the clinical manifestation of multiorgan system derangement due to advanced renal insufficiency. Blood urea nitrogen (BUN) serves as a marker, although this can be elevated due to non-renal causes.

Renal failure comorbidities

Cardiovascular:

- congestive heart failure (CHF) from chronic fluid overload, anemia, accelerated atherosclerosis, uremia-induced pericarditis

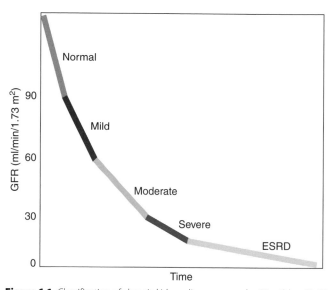

Figure 6.1 Classification of chronic kidney disease: normal >90, mild = 60–89, moderate = 30–59, severe = 15–29, ESRD/dialysis <15. Values are GFR (glomerular filtration rate) in ml/min/1.73 m^2. (From Vacanti et al. 2011. *Essential Clinical Anesthesia*, Cambridge University Press, p. 43.)

Pulmonary:

- pulmonary edema secondary to fluid overload, hypoalbuminemia and CHF
- atelectasis due to decreased muscle mass and decreased surfactant

Neurologic:

- CNS dysfunction secondary to uremic encephalitis
- peripheral and autonomic neuropathy leading to orthostatic hypotension, impaired circulatory response to anesthesia, silent ischemia, and impaired gastric emptying

Hematology/immunology:

- anemia requiring EPO and/or transfusions
- uremic coagulopathy caused by altered *platelet function* and worsened by anemia (RBCs release ADP, inactivating

Essential Clinical Anesthesia Review: Keywords, Questions and Answers for the Boards, ed. Linda S. Aglio, Robert W. Lekowski, and Richard D. Urman. Published by Cambridge University Press. © Cambridge University Press 2015.

Table 6.1 Electrolyte derangements in renal failure patients

Hyperkalemia	Hypokalemia	Hypermagnesemia	Hyperphosphatemia/Hypocalcemia
Suppresses cardiac electrical conduction	Lowers arrhythmia threshold (uncommon except if patient on dialysis or malnourished)	Causes skeletal weakness and potentiates nondepolarizing muscle relaxants	Associated with renal osteodystrophy and calciphylaxis especially in blood vessels and skin

prostacyclin and enhancing platelet–vessel wall interactions); PT, PTT, and platelet count may be normal despite uremic coagulopathy
- leukocyte and immune dysfunction due to uremia, malnutrition and dialysis-induced inflammatory response; increased exposure to infections from dialysis grafts, catheters and blood products

GI/nutrition:
- malnutrition leading to greater risk of poor wound healing, infection, prolonged recovery from illness
- uremia-induced enteropathy, peptic ulcer disease, and nausea/vomiting

Renal failure: electrolyte effects

Hyperkalemia treatment: administer calcium chloride, beta-agonists, intravenous insulin and dextrose, diuretics (e.g., furosamide), kayexalate or dialysis.

Hypermagnesemia treatment: administer intravenous calcium, loop diuretic along with 5% dextrose and ½ normal saline infusion.

Dialysis effects

Dialysis can cause a coagulopathy from anticoagulation agents required for hemodialysis. Also, blood samples taken immediately after hemodialysis can produce inaccurate results as redistribution of fluid and electrolytes takes about six hours. Lastly, dialysis "disequilibrium syndrome" (less common with peritoneal dialysis) may occur if fluid and electrolyte shifts are too rapid, leading to weakness, nausea, vomiting, convulsions, and coma.

Complications associated with chronic renal failure

Patients with CRF are at high risk of perioperative renal disease progression due to increased sensitivity to hypovolemia, nephrotoxins, and hemodynamic perturbations. They are also at risk of developing profound acidemia, particularly in the postoperative period when residual anesthetics and opioids lead to CO_2 retention, given baseline diminished buffer base reserve secondary to impaired acid excretion. Uremia-induced nausea and vomiting are also common in CRF patients, which increases the risk of aspiration during induction and emergence from anesthesia. Other risks to consider include surgical bleeding, GI bleeding, intracerebral hemorrhage, and hemorrhagic pericardial effusion.

Contrast-induced nephropathy

Prevent contrast-induced nephropathy by pretreating with oral N-acetylcysteine, sodium bicarbonate infusion, periprocedural hemofiltration, and by postponing elective surgery for at least two days after contrast administration.

Renal failure: pharmacokinetics

Chronic renal failure leads to altered pharmacokinetics due to altered volume, electrolytes, pH, decreased serum protein, impaired biotransformation and excretion. While lipid-soluble drugs are metabolized by the liver to water-soluble forms before elimination by the kidneys, ionized drugs are eliminated unchanged by the kidneys and so their duration of action may be prolonged in CRF. Opioids and sedatives, for example, more commonly cause respiratory depression in patients with CRF.

Loading doses of most drugs administered by bolus or short-term infusion do not need to be altered significantly in CRF since their duration of action is determined by redistribution not elimination. *Maintenance doses,* however, do need reduction in CRF as they depend on elimination.
Preoperative considerations:
- Avoid hemodialysis on the day of surgery due to risk of rebound anticoagulation, fluid shifts, hypokalemia, and hypoxemia.
- Consider RBC transfusion if Hb ≤8 g/dl, or if Hb <10 g/dl for major surgery.
- Minimize risk of coagulopathy by administering cryoprecipitate, dDAVP or conjugated estrogens, performing heparin-free dialysis, or treating anemia with RBC transfusion or erythropoietin.

Intraoperative considerations:
Set up
- Minimize premedication given susceptibility to excess sedation and respiratory depression.
- Utilize strict aseptic technique for all invasive procedures.
- Avoid urinary catheters if patient is anuric given increased risk of infections.
- Carefully position patients as they are at high risk for fractures from renal osteodystrophy and inability to report discomfort from sensory neuropathy.

Induction
- Manage increased risk of aspiration by reducing gastric acidity and promoting gastric emptying with H_2 blockers, metoclopramide, and citric acid/sodium citrate.

Table 6.2 Pharmacologic considerations for commonly used perioperative drugs in patients with CRF

Drug class	Pharmacokinetics	Considerations
Inhalational anesthetics	Eliminated primarily by the lungs	Sevoflurane has potentially nephrotoxic metabolite (compound A)
Lipid soluble		
Benzodiazepines	Increased free fraction in CRF	Potentiated clinical effect in CRF Certain metabolites are pharmacologically active and accumulate with repeated dosing
Barbiturates	Free fraction of induction dose is almost doubled in patients with CRF	Exaggerated clinical effect in CRF. Need to reduce induction dose
Propofol	Rapid, extensive hepatic metabolism. Pharmacokinetics unchanged in CRF	Effects are not prolonged in CRF
Etomidate	Increased free fraction in CRF	CRF does not alter clinical effects
Ketamine	Redistribution and hepatic metabolism largely responsible for termination of anesthetic effects. Minimal change in free fraction in CRF	CFR does not alter clinical effects
Opioids	Primarily metabolized in liver	May have increased and prolonged effect in CRF Active metabolites may prolong action with chronic administration: Morphine-6-glucuronide (morphine) has potent analgesic and sedative effects; Normeperidine (meperidine) has neurotoxic effects; Hydromorphone-3-glucuronide (hydromorphone) can cause cognitive dysfunction and myoclonus; Fentanyl has no active metabolites
Ionized drugs		
Muscle relaxants	Standard dose of succinylcholine raises serum K^+ 0.5–0.8 mEq/L, which is unchanged in CRF	Succinylcholine is not contraindicated in CRF if the serum K^+ is not elevated
	Many nonpolarizing NMBs result in prolonged effects due to reliance on renal excretion	Cisatracurium, mivacurium, and rocuronium are preferable in CRF
Cholinesterase inhibitors	Decreased elimination in CRF and half-life is prolonged	Half-life prolongation is similar or greater than the duration of blockade from long-acting NMBs so recurarization is rarely seen
Digoxin	Excreted in urine	Increased risk of toxicity in CRF
Vasoactive drugs		
Catecholamines		Catecholamines with α-adrenergic effects constrict renal vasculature and may reduce renal blood flow
Sodium nitroprusside	Metabolized by the kidney and excreted as thiocyanate	Toxicity from thiocyanate accumulation is more likely in CRF
Antibiotics	Penicillins, cephalosporins, aminoglycosides, and vancomycin are predominantly dependent on renal elimination	Loading dose is unchanged but maintenance doses are substantially reduced

(From Vacanti et al. 2011. *Essential Clinical Anesthesia*, Cambridge University Press, p. 46.)

- Reduce dose of induction drugs and slow rate of infusion given increased risk of hypotension.
- Anticipate hypotension and manage with fluids and vasopressors.
- Check serum K^+ concentration prior to succinylcholine administration.

Maintenance

- Reduce sedative and anesthetic doses.
- Avoid renally excreted neuromuscular blockers (NMBs).
- Administer fluids and blood to permit adequate organ perfusion even if dialysis is required postoperatively or even intraoperatively.

- Controlled ventilation is often preferable since spontaneous ventilation may result in hypercarbia, exacerbated acidemia, and hyperkalemia.

Emergence

- Anticipate potential delayed emergence, aspiration, hypertension, respiratory depression, and pulmonary edema.
- Ensure adequate reversal of neuromuscular blockade.

Postoperative considerations:

It is important to monitor for CV complications (EKG, Troponin I), pulmonary edema (CXR), and hyperkalemia in patients with chronic renal failure. In considering these results, one should also evaluate the need for postoperative dialysis.

Questions

1. Renal function is best assessed by:
   a. BUN:Cr ratio
   b. creatinine clearance rate
   c. creatinine plasma concentration
   d. urine flow rate and specific gravity

2. The following are treatments for hyperkalemia EXCEPT:
   a. dialysis
   b. beta-blocker
   c. dextrose and insulin infusion
   d. intravenous calcium chloride

3. Renal failure associated coagulopathy in a patient with anemia can be treated with:
   a. vitamin K administration
   b. fresh frozen plasma
   c. red blood cell transfusion
   d. platelet transfusion

Answers

1. b. The most accurate assessment of renal function is the creatinine clearance rate (CCR) = (urine creatinine × urine flow rate)/(serum creatinine) based on 24-hour urine collection.

2. b. Beta-agonists, not beta-blockers, are used to treat hyperkalemia by shifting potassium intracellularly.

3. c. Uremic coagulopathy is worsened by anemia, as RBCs release ADP, which normally inactivates prostacyclin and enhances platelet–vessel wall interaction. For this reason, PT, PTT, and platelet count may be normal despite uremic coagulopathy.

Further reading

Bittner, E. A. (2011). Chronic renal failure. In Vacanti, C. A., Sikka, P. J., Urman, R. D., Dershwitz, M., and Segal, B. S. (eds) *Essential Clinical Anesthesia.* Cambridge: Cambridge University Press, pp. 43–48.

ABA Key Words (2013). *Open Anesthesia.* Media Wiki. www.openanesthesia.org/ openanesthesia.org:KeywordBrowser.

McCarthy, D. and Shorten, G. (2011). Chronic kidney disease. In B.J. Pollard *Handbook of Clinical Anesthesia*, 3rd edn. CRC Press, pp. 203–206.

Chapter

7

Liver disease

Julia Serber and Evan Blaney

Keywords

Hepatic blood flow
Cirrhosis
Portal hypertension
Child–Turcotte–Pugh (CTP) classification
Model for end-stage liver disease (MELD)
Ascites
Esophageal variceal bleeding
Cirrhotic cardiomyophaty
Portopulmonary hypertension
Hepatopulmonary syndrome
Hepatic encephalopathy
Autonomic neuropathy
Fulminant hepatic failure

Anatomy and physiology

The liver is the largest of the solid organs in the body and weighs approximately 1,500 g. The anatomy of the liver can be described by using the morphology or functional aspects. The liver is made up of two lobes – right and left – which are separated by the falciform ligament. The right lobe is larger and has two additional lobes, the caudate and the quadrate lobes. The liver anatomy can also be described by functional anatomy. Claude Couinaud divided the liver into eight functionally independent segments, which each have their own vascular inflow and outflow as well as biliary drainage.

The blood supply to the liver is from the portal vein (about 75%) and the hepatic artery. Normal portal vein pressure is approximately 10 mm Hg, and normal hepatic artery pressure is arterial. Normal *hepatic blood flow* is about 1,500 ml/min, which correlates to 25% of cardiac output. The liver is supplied by sympathetic nerve fibers (T6–11). Many important functions are performed by the liver, including metabolic functions (carbohydrate, fat, protein, and drug metabolism), bile secretion, bilirubin excretion, albumin production, ammonia excretion, and synthesis of all the coagulation factors except for factor VIII and von Willebrand factor.

Hepatic blood flow is decreased by any cause that results in a lower systemic blood pressure and cardiac output. Causes include general and regional anesthesia (spinal/epidural), positive pressure ventilation, hypoxemia, and beta-blockers.

Liver cirrhosis

When providing anesthesia for a patient with liver disease, it is important to know that liver disease is a multiorgan disorder that leads to a variety of pathophysiologic derangements. Liver disease often may progress to cirrhosis. *Cirrhosis* is characterized by hepatic cell death, fibrosis, as well as regenerative nodules.

Portal hypertension is a common sequela seen in patients with chronic liver disease. Associated findings include ascites, portosystemic shunts, hepatic encephalopathy, and splenomegaly.

Risk stratification of the cirrhotic patient

The *Child–Turcotte–Pugh (CTP) classification*, the *model for end-stage liver disease (MELD)*, and the pediatric version (PELD) are liver failure classification systems that are utilized to assess prognosis. The CTP classification is based on five variables (bilirubin, albumin, INR or PT, ascites, and encephalopathy) and groups patients by score to determine their prognosis. The MELD is a statistical model based on serum bilirubin, serum creatinine, and INR to determine the severity of the liver disease as well as the need for a liver transplant.

Effects of liver disease
Gastrointestinal

Portal hypertension is defined as pressure in the portal vein >10 mm Hg. High portal pressure causes portovenous collaterals to develop. These collaterals are commonly found at four sites – esophageal, periumbilical, retroperitoneal, and hemorrhoidal.

The finding of *ascites* is one of the hallmarks of decompensated liver cirrhosis. Ascites is caused by changes in

Essential Clinical Anesthesia Review: Keywords, Questions and Answers for the Boards, ed. Linda S. Aglio, Robert W. Lekowski, and Richard D. Urman. Published by Cambridge University Press. © Cambridge University Press 2015.

the dynamics of portal blood flow, activation of the renin–angiotensin–aldosterone system, and reduction in the plasma oncotic pressure. Treatments for ascites include sodium and water restriction, diuretics, and abdominal paracentesis.

Esophageal variceal bleeding can be a lethal complication of cirrhosis. Treatment options include beta-blockers, vasopressin, somatostatin, variceal banding, sclerotherapy, and transjugular portosystemic shunting.

Metabolic derangements seen in patients with liver disease can include hypoglycemia, hypokalemia, hyponatremia, hypomagnesemia, and hypoalbuminemia.

Hemodynamic

Hemodynamic changes can also accompany liver disease. These patients commonly have a hyperdynamic circulation coupled with low peripheral vascular resistance and an increased cardiac index. Often patients with cirrhosis develop signs of high output heart failure *cirrhotic cardiomyopathy*.

Hematologic

Hematologic effects include anemia, thrombocytopenia, and coagulopathy. Causes of anemia in these patients include bone marrow suppression, red cell destruction, blood loss, and iron deficiency. Thrombocytopenia is due to splenic sequestration.

All clotting factors except for factor VIII are produced in the liver. Therefore worsening liver disease with decreased liver function causes a deficiency of clotting factors. These patients are at risk for bleeding. Fresh frozen plasma can be used to replace these clotting factors prior to surgery.

Renal

Renal dysfunction is commonly seen in patients with liver disease. Three major causes are: prerenal azotemia, acute tubular necrosis, and hepatorenal syndrome. Hepatorenal syndrome is characterized by worsening renal function in the setting of worsening liver disease. The renal function does not improve unless the liver function improves.

Pulmonary
Portopulmonary hypertension

Portopulmonary hypertension is seen in about 2% to 4% of patients with end-stage liver disease and about 5% to 10% of patients who are evaluated for orthotopic liver transplantation. Portopulmonary hypertension may complicate hepatic resection if it leads to increased central venous pressure. Portopulmonary hypertension affects eligibility for liver transplantation. Portopulmonary hypertension is characterized by a mean pulmonary artery pressure >25 mm Hg in the setting of a normal pulmonary capillary wedge pressure and an elevated pulmonary vascular resistance in the setting of portal hypertension. Symptoms include: dyspnea on exertion (most commonly seen symptom), fatigue, palpitations, chest pain,

and syncope. Transthoracic Doppler echocardiography is used to diagnose this disease. Effective management is crucial as it may facilitate hepatic resection. Vasodilators (e.g., epoprostenol, sildenafil, and nitric oxide) may be used to reduce pulmonary vascular resistance.

Hepatopulmonary syndrome

Hepatopulmonary syndrome is defined by the presence of hepatic dysfunction or portal hypertension, an increased alveolar–arterial oxygen gradient, and the finding of intrapulmonary vasodilation. Patients may present with digital clubbing, spider angiomata, arterial hypoxemia, and orthodeoxia (decrease in arterial blood oxygen level upon moving to an upright position), and platypnea (difficult breathing when moving to an upright position). See diagnostic algorithm for the diagnostic approach to hepatopulmonary syndrome. There are currently no effective medical therapies for hepatopulmonary syndrome. Liver transplantation has been shown to be the only therapy that improves survival when compared with medical therapy alone.

Neurologic
Hepatic encephalopathy

There are multiple factors that are thought to play a role in causing *hepatic encephalopathy* including elevated ammonia levels and activation of GABA receptors in the brain. Hepatic encephalopathy resembles multiple other conditions and thus it is important to differentiate amongst them. These other conditions include metabolic problems (hypoglycemia, hyponatremia, and hypernatremia), intracranial processes (subdural hematoma, intracranial hemorrhage, intracranial mass lesion), and infectious diseases (i.e., meningitis).

Autonomic neuropathy

Autonomic neuropathies have been found in up to 50% of patients with chronic liver disease. These neuropathies typically manifest as impaired cardiovascular function and impaired gastric motility. The incidence of hypotension during general anesthesia is higher in patients with autonomic neuropathies. Cirrhotic patients with autonomic neuropathy have an increased mortality. Autonomic neuropathies usually resolve after liver transplantation with the return of normal liver function.

Fulminant hepatic failure

Fulminant hepatic failure is severe hepatic dysfunction and occurs most commonly as a result of drug toxicity (most frequently from acetaminophen) that has multiple causes. Other toxins include ethanol, *Amanita phalloides* (a fungus), halothane, and phosphorus. Viral hepatitis is the second leading cause. Other causes include Budd–Chiari syndrome, acute fatty liver of pregnancy, and Wilson's disease.

Acute encephalopathy is often seen in patients with fulminant hepatic failure and is associated with progressive brain swelling and increased intracranial pressure that can lead to brain herniation and death. Bacterial infections can develop in these patients, with rates reported to be as high as 80%.

Supportive care is the treatment for fulminant hepatic failure. For patients that do not recover with supportive care, liver transplantation is the only available treatment.

Pharmacologic management in cirrhosis

Cirrhosis and liver failure may affect the distribution, duration of action, and elimination of a number of drugs. In addition to these changes in metabolism, decreases in serum albumin and altered total body water affects the volume of distribution of many drugs. It is therefore important to think about the metabolism of medications before they are given to this patient population.

Perioperative access and monitoring and postoperative care

Perioperative access and monitoring will depend on multiple factors including the severity of the patient's liver disease and the surgery being performed. In addition to the standard ASA monitors, additional preparation might include warming devices, an arterial line, large-bore IV access, central or peripheral venous pressure monitoring, pulmonary artery catheter placement (especially in patients with portopulmonary hypertension), and intraoperative transesophageal echocardiography. Caution should be used with TEE given the likely presence of varices.

Ventilation is often a critical issue for these patients. In large abdominal cases, pressure control ventilation with permissive hypercapnia may be needed to avoid high peak alveolar pressures and high PEEP, thus preventing pulmonary injury.

Patients with portopulmonary hypertension may require nitric oxide or other pulmonary arterial vasodilators.

Pain management may be challenging in this patient population. In cirrhotic patients with encephalopathy, opioids may cause pronounced sedation. Coagulopathy may prevent the use of regional anesthesia.

Questions

1. The MELD score is calculated using the following lab values:
   a. bilirubin, INR, Cr
   b. bilirubin, AST, Cr
   c. PT, INR, Cr

2. True or false: the MELD score is used to allocate donor livers for transplant?

3. Pain management in patients with cirrhosis may be affected by:
   a. coagulopathy
   b. decreased ability to metabolize drugs
   c. decreased ability to clear drugs
   d. all of the above

Answers

1. a. The model for end-stage liver disease (MELD) is based on serum bilirubin, serum creatinine, and the international normalized ratio.
2. True. The MELD score and the PELD score (the pediatric version of the MELD score) are used to determine the severity of the liver disease and the need for liver transplantation.
3. d. Liver failure or decrease in liver function may lead to coagulopathy making it unsafe to use neuraxial anesthesia. Cirrhosis and liver failure may affect the distribution, duration of action, and elimination of medications. In liver failure, morphine and meperidine have prolonged half-lives while the half-life of fentanyl appears unchanged. Ketamine has a prolonged half-life due to an increased volume of distribution.

Further reading

Modak, R. (2008). *Anesthesiology Keywords Review. Liver Transhepatic Phase: Transfusion*. Philadelphia: Lippincott Williams & Wilkins, pp. 254–255.

Morgan et al. (1996). Chapter 35. Anesthesia for patients with liver disease. In *Lange Clinical Anesthesiology*, 4th edn. New York: McGraw-Hill.

Vacanti, C. A., Sikka, P. K., Urman, R. U., Dershwitz, M., and Segal, B. S. (2011).

Brookman, J. C. and Sandberg, W. S. Liver disease. Chapter 8 in: Vacanti et al., 2011. *Essential Clinical Anesthesia*. New York: Cambridge University Press.

Chapter

8

Principles of diabetes mellitus and perioperative glucose control

Olutoyin Okanlawon and Richard D. Urman

Keywords

Types of diabetes mellitus
Stress-related diabetes
Effects of hyperglycemia
Hyperglycemia and outcomes in critically ill patients
Ketoacidosis
Intraoperative blood glucose management

Diabetes mellitus (DM) is a disease characterized by altered metabolism of carbohydrates (manifested by hyperglycemia), lipids, and proteins. In the United States, 90% of diabetic patients have type II diabetes and relative deficiency in circulating insulin. The American Diabetes Association (ADA) describes in-hospital hyperglycemia as follows:

- medical history of diabetes – DM previously diagnosed and acknowledged by the patient's treating physician.
- unrecognized diabetes – hyperglycemia (fasting blood glucose $\geq$126 mg/dL or random blood glucose $\geq$200 mg/dL) occurring during hospitalization and confirmed as diabetes after hospitalization by the treating physician.
- hospital-related hyperglycemia – hyperglycemia (fasting blood glucose $\geq$126 mg/dL or random blood glucose $\geq$200 mg/dL) occurring during hospitalization and reverting to normal after hospital discharge.

Types of diabetes mellitus

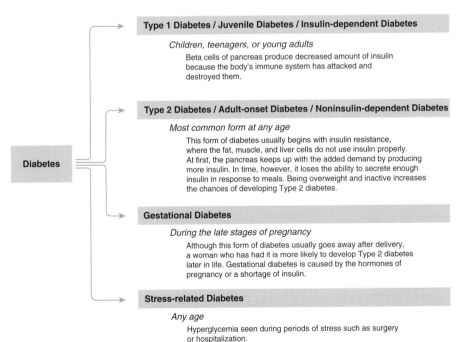

Figure 8.1 Classification of diabetes mellitus. (From Vacanti et al. 2011. *Essential Clinical Anesthesia*, Cambridge University Press, p. 57.)

Stress-related diabetes

Surgery and hospitalization are examples of the many stressful events that can occur in patients. In particular, stress affects on the HPA axis, lead to an increase in concentration of blood glucose, decrease in insulin production, and increased insulin resistance. In addition to corticosteroid production, there are a number of stress-induced hormones such as glucagon, growth hormone, epinephrine, and corticosteroids. These substances cause an increase in gluconeogenesis and glycogenolysis by the liver, ultimately leading to increase in glucose production.

Epinephrine and norepinephrine inhibit insulin release by their action on α-adrenergic receptors, while insulin secretion from β cells is prompted by an increase in blood glucose concentration.

Effects of hyperglycemia

Classified into acute vs. long-term effects, diabetes has a wide range of complications ranging from diabetic ketoacidosis to renal insufficiency, coronary artery disease, eventually affecting all organ systems. Particularly in the perioperative setting, hyperglycemia is associated with overall hospital mortality. There is an increased incidence of pneumonia, wound infection, and myocardial infarction. Hyperglycemia is associated with poor patient outcome, prolonged mechanical ventilation, sepsis, and renal failure.

Wound infection

Hyperglycemia has been associated with increased incidence of postoperative wound infection, which may be explained by microvascular changes in the tissues that limit blood supply to the tissue. Another factor is the decrease in phagocytosis and chemotaxis of the polymorphonuclear cells.

Wound healing

Adequate glycemic control in the perioperative period improves wound healing by increasing granulation tissue formation, fibroblast proliferation, and collagen synthesis. Hyperglycemia may cause nonenzymatic glycosylation with the production of abnormal proteins that decrease elastance and tensile strength. There are also decreases in capillary proliferation. All of these are proven to worsen the healing processes.

Hyperglycemia and outcomes in critically ill patients

Research has shown a reduction in mortality from 8% to 4.6% in ICU patients who maintained their blood glucose concentrations between 80 and 110 mg/dL. The largest reduction was seen in sepsis-induced multiple organ failure. There was a decrease in in-hospital mortality, bloodstream infection rate, and acute renal failure requiring dialysis.

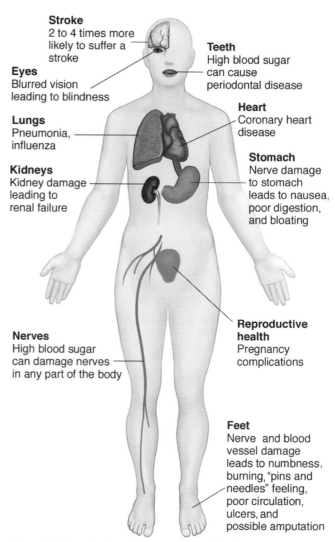

Figure 8.2 Complications of diabetes mellitus. (From Vacanti et al. 2011. *Essential Clinical Anesthesia*, Cambridge University Press, p. 59.)

Neurologic injury

Supernormal blood sugar levels at the time of cerebral injury are associated with worsened neurologic outcome. As a substrate for anaerobic metabolism, glucose increases lactate levels, thereby worsening intracellular acidosis, and leading to more deregulation of cellular homeostasis. The poor functional recovery in stroke patients with hyperglycemia is mainly attributed to the viability of the penumbra (the area surrounding the area of primary insult).

Myocardial infarction

Diabetic patients tend to suffer painless MI, which can make detection and treatment difficult. The increased production of stress hormones with preexisting insulin resistance leads to a decrease in utilization of glucose by the heart. However, since a more oxygen-expensive alternative in fatty acid metabolism/oxidation is used to fulfill energy requirements, there is ultimately more ischemia (due to the widening demand–supply gap).

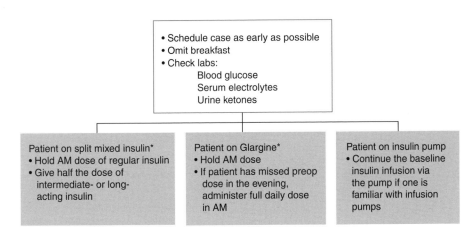

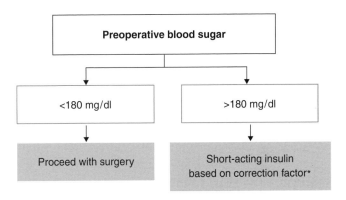

Figure 8.3 Intraoperative blood glucose management. For correction factor, see Figure 8.4. (From Vacanti et al. 2011. *Essential Clinical Anesthesia*, Cambridge University Press, p. 60.)

Ketoacidosis

Primarily occurs in type I diabetics. Diabetic *ketoacidosis* (DKA) is a life-threatening condition, which results from a lack of insulin and highly elevated blood glucose concentrations (up to 500 mg/dl). With the accumulation of ketone bodies (e.g., acetoacetate), the resulting high anion gap metabolic acidosis leads to dyspnea, nausea, and vomiting, abdominal pain, and constant urination. If blood glucose level is not corrected a coma will likely occur. Treatment: aggressive hydration, placement on an insulin drip (10 U/h or 0.1 units/kg/h to decrease glucose levels at a rate of no more than 100 mg/dl/h), and replacement of electrolytes (especially potassium). Once glucose level reaches 250 mg/dl, an infusion of 5% dextrose in water is started to prevent hypoglycemia.

Intraoperative blood glucose management

Preoperative evaluation

Preoperative evaluation should include assessment of glycemic control, early detection of electrolyte abnormalities, and determination of the extent of end-organ disease (e.g., the determination of cardiovascular disease via EKG/echo, tilt test for orthostatic hypotension).

Airway examination

The "prayer sign," which is difficulty in approximating the metacarpophalangeal joints of the two hands, is often seen in patients with chronic diabetics. They tend to also have restricted neck movement due to atlanto-occipital joint fusion, thereby posing some difficulty in intubation. Furthermore, DM II patients also tend to be obese and therefore may be difficult for mask ventilation as well.

Laboratory tests include routine laboratory tests, blood glucose, EKG, BUN, creatinine, and plasma electrolytes. To determine the extent of renal insufficiency and the active state of diabetic nephropathy, sometimes 24-hour creatinine clearance, ketones, and albumin are checked. HgA$_{1c}$ can

*Correction factor (CF) = 1500/ [Total daily dose (TDD) of insulin]
   Example: If TDD is 50 U, CF = 1500/50 = 30 U
   1 U of regular insulin will decrease the blood sugar by 30 mg/dl. Blood sugar is maintained between 100 and 150 mg/dl.

Figure 8.4 Blood glucose guidelines. (From Vacanti et al. 2011. *Essential Clinical Anesthesia*, Cambridge University Press, p. 26.)

help determine the adequacy of glucose control during the last month.

Medications

Intraoperative management: intraoperative hyperglycemia leads to poorer patient outcomes; however, there is ongoing debate about what should be the ideal target blood glucose level. The recent NICE–SUGAR (normoglycemia in intensive care evaluation – survival using glucose algorithm regulation) study suggests a moderate target of 100 to 150 mg/dl seems to have more benefits than risks. Blood glucose should be measured preoperatively and every hour intraoperatively, and in the immediate postoperative period. During a prolonged insulin infusion a background glucose infusion is used to prevent hypoglycemia, ketosis, and protein breakdown. While many electrolytes are affected by glucose deregulation, potassium should be measured periodically. Insulin and epinephrine stimulate potassium uptake while hyperosmolality and acidosis translocate potassium out of the cells.

Table 8.1 Insulin time chart

Type of insulin	Start of action	Peak of action, hours	Duration of action, hours
Humalog (rapid)	15 min	1.5–2	4
Regular (short)	30 min	2–3	5
NPH (intermediate)	1–2 h	4–8	14–20
Lente (intermediate)	2–3 h	8–12	16–24
Ultralente (long)	2–4 h	8–14	18–24
Lantus (long)	1–2 h	6	18–26

From: Vacanti et al., 2011. *Essential Clinical Anesthesia*, Cambridge University Press, p. 60.

For Type I DM requiring intraoperative insulin administration, bolus dose is calculated by dividing the daily insulin requirement by 24 (approximately 0.1 U/kg). In insulin naïve patients the dose is 0.02 U/kg IV.

Postoperative management: immediate and continuous measurement of blood glucose levels in the postoperative period is necessary. Medication management is through IV insulin or a subcutaneous insulin regimen is continued until the patient can resume caloric intake. Adequate pain control (to minimize release of catabolic hormones that increase glucose levels), treatment of nausea/vomiting, and close monitoring of hemodynamic instability, respiratory depression, and hypoglycemia are important.

Questions

1. Which of the following types of insulin preparations has the fastest onset of action if administered subcutaneously (SQ)?
   a. glargine (Lantus)
   b. lispro (Humalog)
   c. regular (Humulin-R)
   d. NPH (Humulin-N)
   e. ultralente

2. Recent studies from the NICE–SUGAR trial recommend which intraoperative blood glucose range for optimal management?
   a. 90–120 mg/dl
   b. 100–200 mg/dl
   c. 150–200 mg/dl
   d. 100–150 mg/dl

Answers

1. b. Lispro and Regular are the two main short-acting insulin types with similar peaks of action and duration of about four hours. Lispro's onset of action is 15 minutes, twice as fast as Regular.

2. d. The normoglycemia in intensive care evaluation – surviving using glucose algorithm regulation (NICE-SUGAR) trial demonstrated that among medical ICU patients, intensive glycemic control (targeting a blood glucose of 81 to 108 mg/dL) is associated with increased mortality compared to conventional glycemic control (≤180 mg/dL). Follow-up studies include a glycemic target of of ≤180 mg/dL, with 2009 recommendation by the American Association of Clinical Endocrinologist, and ADA guidelines to initiate insulin infusion in the critically ill patient with blood glucose >180mg/dL, with a goal range of 140 to 180 mg/dL.

Further reading

Dellinger, R. P., Levy, M. M., Rhodes, A., et al. (2013). Surviving sepsis campaign: international guidelines for management of severe sepsis and septic shock: 2012. *Critical Care Medicine* 41(2), 580–637.

Moghissi, E. S., Korytkowski, M. T., DiNardo, M., et al. (2009). American Association of Clinical Endocrinologists and American Diabetes Association consensus statement on inpatient glycemic control. *Endocrine Practice* 15(4), 353–369.

Chapter

9

Common blood disorders

Rosemary Uzomba, Michael D'Ambra, and Robert W. Lekowski

Keywords

Anemia (primary and secondary)
Anemia: compensatory responses
Polycythemia (primary and secondary),
  polycythemia vera
Coagulation, hemostasis (primary and secondary)
Platelet disorders (disorders of primary hemostasis),
  thrombocytopenia
von Willebrand disease (vWD)
Clotting factor disorders (disorders of secondary
  hemostasis), hemophilia A and B, vitamin
  K deficiency, prothrombin complex
  concentrate (PCC)
Fresh frozen plasma (FFP), unfractionated heparin
  (UH), warfarin, low molecular weight
  heparin (LMWH)
Disorders of thrombosis, factor V Leiden deficiency,
  protein C and S deficiencies
Heparin-induced thrombocytopenia/
  thrombosis (HITT)
Anti-cardiolipin, lupus anticoagulant
Disorder of fibrinolysis
Disseminated intravascular coagulation (DIC)

Anemia is defined as a reduced concentration of functional red blood cells (RBCs).

The causes include blood loss, decreased RBC production, or increased RBC destruction.

Dehydration may falsely elevate hemoglobin (Hb) and hematocrit (Hct) in an anemic patient. Conversely, hemodilution may falsely lower Hb and Hct in a patient with an unchanged RBC mass (thus giving the false appearance of anemia).

In acute blood loss the Hb/Hct may appear falsely normal prior to re-equilibration and resuscitation.

Compensatory responses to anemia require alterations in *regional blood flow*, *microcirculation*, and *central blood flow*.

These alterations enable the redistribution of blood flow from nonvital to vital organs, enhance tissue oxygen (O_2) extraction, and increase Hb unloading of O_2 to tissues.

During acute normovolemic anemia, cardiac output (CO) increases due to an increase in venous return, decreased afterload, decreased blood viscosity, and increased sympathetic stimulation (which results in increased inotropy).

Primary anemia is due to a structural abnormality of the Hb molecule or RBC membrane. This is a less common etiology for anemia.

- Examples include: sickle cell disease (SCD), thalassemia, hereditary spherocytosis, glucose-6-phosphate dehydrogenase (G6PD), and immune hemolytic anemia.

In *secondary anemia* the etiology is multifactorial. This is a more common reason for anemia.

- Examples include: megaloblastic anemia, iron deficiency anemia, anemia of chronic disease.

Polycythemia is defined as an elevated Hb and Hct.

Primary polycythemia is a disorder *not* caused by increased erythropoietin (EPO). (EPO stimulates RBC production.)

- Most common primary polycythemia is *polycythemia vera*, a neoplastic stem cell disorder.
- If left untreated it can cause thrombotic manifestations (MI, ischemic stroke, pulmonary embolism, deep venous thrombosis).
- Additionally, there is an increased risk of hemorrhage.
- Treatment includes correction of underlying condition, phlebotomy (to lower the Hct and prevent hyperviscosity), and myelosuppressive drugs such as hydroxyurea.

Secondary polycythemia is caused by increased EPO production in *response to chronic tissue hypoxia*.

- Examples include high altitude and cardiopulmonary disease.
- Additionally, tumors that secrete EPO (e.g., kidney tumors) can cause a secondary polycythemia.

Essential Clinical Anesthesia Review: Keywords, Questions and Answers for the Boards, ed. Linda S. Aglio, Robert W. Lekowski, and Richard D. Urman. Published by Cambridge University Press. © Cambridge University Press 2015.

- Treatment includes correction of the underlying condition and phlebotomy.

Coagulation is a complex process that requires a normal endothelium to respond to injury by forming clots (thrombus). The endothelial injury eventually initiates the coagulation cascade and hemostasis (i.e., cessation of blood loss from damaged vessel).

Hemostasis is a two-part process:

- *Primary hemostasis* involves the formation of a platelet plug.
- In *primary hemostasis,* exposed collagen binds platelets. This is facilitated by *von Willebrand Factor* (vWF). Activated platelets modify their membrane proteins leading to an increased affinity to bind fibrinogen (factor I).

Disorders of primary hemostasis

Platelet disorders are either *quantitative*, a problem of platelet number (i.e., thrombocytopenia) defined as a platelet count <150 K/μl, or *qualitative*, a problem of platelet function (which may be inherited or acquired).

- The four main etiologies for *thrombocytopenia* are: *dilutional thrombocytopenia* (e.g., as a result of massive resuscitation/transfusion), *decreased production* (e.g., drug side effects, infections, chemotherapy, radiation therapy, alcohol toxicity), increased *destruction/consumption* (e.g., disseminated intravascular coagulation (DIC), ITP, TTP, HELLP syndrome, institution of CPB, and *splenic sequestration* – as seen in hypothermic platelets or those with portal hypertension.
- The most common cause of intraoperative thrombocytopenia is *dilutional*. Interestingly, 80% of blood volume needs to be replaced before clinically significant thrombocytopenia is seen.
- The risk for increased surgical bleeding occurs at a platelet level of <50 K/μL; whereas, spontaneous bleeding occurs at a platelet level of <5–10 K/μL.
- *Qualitative inherited disorders of platelet function* are rare and usually diagnosed in childhood. They include abnormalities of the platelet membrane (e.g., Bernard–Soulier syndrome) or platelet granules.
- *Qualitative acquired disorders of platelet function* are due to drugs (e.g., aspirin, clopidigrel, glycoprotein IIb/IIIa inhibitors), systemic conditions (e.g., uremia, liver disease, myelodysplastic disorders), or cardiopulmonary bypass (CPB).

Von Willebrand Disease (vWD) is a relatively common bleeding disorder affecting 1% to 2% of the population. It is a disorder that effects platelet adhesion to injured vessels.

- Inherited vWD occurs as a result of von Willebrand factor (vWF) deficiency (Table 9.1). This can be *qualitative* (Type 2A, 2B, 2M, 2N) or *quantitative* (Type 1 or 3).

Table 9.1 Classification and treatment of vWD

Type	Mechanism of disease	Treatment of choice
1	Paritial quantitative deficiency of vWF (and factor VIII)	Desmopressin
2	Qualitative defects of vWF	
2A	Defective platelet-dependent vWF functions, associated with lack of larger multimers	Factor VIII–vWF concentrates
2B	Heightened platelet-dependent vWF functions, associated with lack of larger multimers	Factor VIII–vWF concentrates
2M	Defective platelet-dependent vWF functions	Factor VIII–vWF concentrates
2N	Defective vWF binding to factor VIII	Factor VIII–vWF concentrates
3	Severe or complete vWF deficiency and moderately severe factor VIII deficiency, without alloantibodies	Factor VIII–vWF concentrates
	Severe or complete vWF deficiency and moderately severe factor VIII deficiency, with alloantibodies	Recombinant factor VIII

(Adapted from Soliman, D. E. and Broadman, L. M. 2006. Coagulation defects. *Anesthesiology Clinics*, 24: 549–578; From Vacanti et al. 2011. *Essential Clinical Anesthesia*, Cambridge University Press, p. 66.)

- vWF is a multimeric protein produced by endothelium and platelets, which acts as a carrier for factor VIII (anti-hemophiliac factor) *and* provides an adhesive link between platelets and injured vessels.
- Acquired vWD occurs a result of lymphoproliferative disease, cardiac and valvular defects, and medications (e.g., valproic acid [Depakote®]).
- Symptoms of vWD include mucocutaneous bleeding (most common) that leads to bruising, epistaxis, gingival bleeding, and menorrhagia.

Secondary hemostasis involves the formation of fibrin strands (to strengthen the platelet plug) via the coagulation cascade.

- The coagulation cascade (Figure 9.1) involves a series of reactions to form clotting factors thrombin (factor IIa) and fibrin (factor Ia).
- Two pathways: the extrinsic pathway (tissue factor [TF]-monitored by prothrombin time [PT]) and the intrinsic pathway (contact activation – monitored by partial thromboplastin time [PTT]). These pathways converge to a common pathway (monitored by thrombin time [TT]). (Table 9.2)
- Clotting factors are serine proteases (Table 9.3) synthesized in the liver, except factors III (3-TF), IV (4-Ca^{2+}), and VIII (8-anti-hemophiliac).

Table 9.2 Common laboratory tests for hemostasis

Class	Test	Normal value
Platelet function	Platelet count Bleeding time Platelet function and aggregation analysis	100,000–400,000 cells/μl <10 min
Coagulation studies	PT–tissue pathway	Normal, 11–14 s; prolonged with low levels of factor I, II, V, VII, or X, or liver disease. INR standardizes results across laboratories
	PTT–contact activation pathway	Normal, 24–35 s; prolonged with low levels of factor I, II, V, VIII, IX, X, XI, or XII. Heparin prolongs PTT
	Thrombin time	Normal, 22–32 s; prolonged with low levels of factor I or II
	ACT	Normal, 80–180 s. Monitor heparin therapy with large doses in the operating room
	Thromboelastography	Measure of time to initial clot formation, time to clot formation, clot strength, clot lysis
Fibrinolysis tests	D-dimer levels	When plasmin cleaves cross-linked fibrin (fibrinolytic states)
	Fibrin degradation products	Excessive activity of plasmin, which degrades fibrin (DIC)

INR, international normalized ratio.
(From Vacanti et al. 2011. *Essential Clinical Anesthesia*, Cambridge University Press, p. 66.)

Table 9.3 Coagulation factors

Factor	Name	Plasma concentration, μg/ml	% of normal required for hemostasis
I	Fibrinogen	3000	30
II	Prothrombin	100	40
III	Tissue factor	–	–
IV	Calcium	–	–
V	Proaccelerin	10	10–15
VII	Proconvertin	0.5	5–10
VIII	Antihemophilic	0.1	10–40
IX	Thromboplastin	5	10–40
X	Stuart	10	10–15
XI	Prethromboplastin	5	20–30
XII	Hageman	30	0
XIII	Fibrin stabilizing	30	1–5

(From Vacanti et al. 2011. *Essential Clinical Anesthesia*, Cambridge University Press, p. 66.)

- Cascade regulators include: protein C, antithrombin III (AT III), TF pathway inhibitor (TFPI), plasmin, and prostacyclin.

Disorders of secondary hemostasis

Clotting factor disorders are either **inherited** factor deficiencies (e.g., hemophilia A and B) or **acquired** clotting factor inhibitors (e.g., autoimmune disorder, drug reactions).

- The two most common **inherited** partial or complete clotting factor deficiencies are hemophilia A and B.
- *Hemophilia A* is an X-linked recessive deficiency of factor VIII. Factor VIII (8) is a cofactor for IXa (9a), which converts factor X to its activated form (Xa). Affected

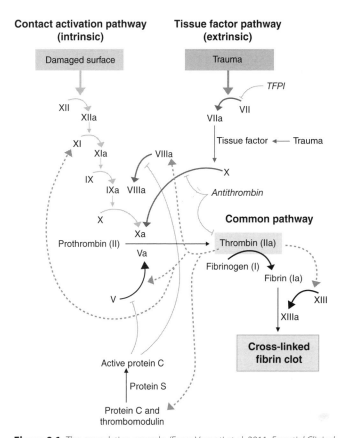

Figure 9.1 The coagulation cascade. (From Vacanti et al. 2011. *Essential Clinical Anesthesia*, Cambridge University Press, p. 26.)

platelets are diagnosed with reduced factor VIII activity, prolonged PTT with a normal PT and platelet count. About 1:5,000 male births are affected.

- *Hemophilia B* is a deficiency in factor IX. It affects 1:34,000 male births. It is diagnosed by a demonstration of reduced factor IX activity, prolonged PTT with a normal PT and platelet count.
- Hemophiliacs have symptoms of unexplained bruising, bleeding into joints (80%), muscles, and the GI tract. The severity of bleeding is dependent upon the degree of factor deficiency. Severe, spontaneous bleeding occurs when there is <1% clotting factor. Mild bleeding means that >5% of factor is present. Mild and moderate deficiency yields excessive bleeding after significant trauma or surgery.
- Treatment of hemophilia A or B involves transfusion with FFP (which carries a low risk of viral transmission) or recombinant factor concentrates (0% risk of viral transmission).
- Of note, 30% of patients with hemophilia A have alloantibodies to factor VIII (8) and therefore cannot be treated with factor concentrates. These patients must be managed with "bypass" agents (e.g., recombinant factor VIIa [7a]).

Acquired clotting disorders occur as a result of systemic disorders or drug therapies used to treat thromboembolic phenomena.

- Vitamin K is needed for synthesis of factors II, VII, IX, X, protein C and S. Vitamin K consists of two subunits: vitamin K_1 (found in leafy green vegetables) and vitamin K_2 (synthesized by intestinal bacteria).
- *Vitamin K deficiency* (which leads to deficiencies in the K-dependent clotting factors) is acquired as a result of poor diet, intestinal problems (such as, biliary obstruction, malabsorption, cystic fibrosis, small intestine resection, or use of antibiotics that destroy intestinal bacteria). Laboratory investigation reveals PT prolongation (because factor VII is depleted relatively early). Treatment is by way of oral (PO) or intravenous (IV) administration of vitamin K. If given IV, slow administration prevents hypotension. Correction of coagulopathy takes six to eight hours (IV) or 12 hours (PO).
- *Warfarin (Coumadin®)* is a systemic anticoagulant that prevents vitamin K synthesis by inhibiting vitamin K epoxide reductase.
- Treatment of excess warfarin (or reversal of warfarin effect) involves administration of *FFP* (which provides all clotting factors) and vitamin K. Urgent reversal requires the administration of *prothrombin complex concentrate (PCC)* (which provides factors 2, 7, 9, and 10).
- *Unfractionated heparin (UH)* causes its anticoagulation effect by reversibly binding to antithrombin III (AT III). AT III inhibits factors Xa and IIa (thrombin) and heparin accelerates the effect of AT III. Reversal of heparin's effect is via neutralization by protamine or by cessation of heparin. The half-life of heparin is <1 hour.

- *Low molecular weight heparin (LMWH)* binds to AT III as well, but has a greater ability to inhibit Xa (rather than IIa). LMWHs have a longer half-life than UH and are therefore given as a once-a-day dose. Examples of LMWH include enoxaparin (Lovenox®) and fondaparinux (Arixtra®).

Disorder of thrombosis

Clotting factor disorders can also manifest as hypercoaguable states that can be **inherited, acquired, or autoimmune.**

- *Factor V Leiden* (the most common **hereditary** hypercoaguable disorder, affecting 4% to 8% of the population). A mutation of the procoagulant factor V.
- *Protein C, S, or AT III deficiencies* – an inherited quantitative or qualitative decrease in activity of the regulators of the clotting cascade (proteins C and S deactivate factors V and VIII).
- Treatment of hypercoaguable disorders is six months of warfarin (after the first thrombotic event) and life-long warfarin (after a second event).
- **Acquired hypercoagulable** states in the perioperative setting, occur with orthopedic, major vascular, or oncological procedures.
- **Autoimmune**-related hypercoagulable states include: *anti-cardiolipin antibody and lupus anticoagulant.* These autoantibodies are associated with other autoimmune diseases, but may occur independently.
- These antibodies are associated with venous or arterial thrombosis, thrombocytopenia, and recurrent fetal loss. Patients are at risk for MI, valvular heart disease, cerebral infarctions, headaches, and visual disturbances.
- Treatment includes chronic anticoagulation, elastic stockings, and maintenance of normovolemia/normothermia.

A hypercoagulability work-up requires the measurement of:
- CBC/PT/PTT
- fibrinogen (I)
- factor V Leiden assay
- protein C assay
- protein S antigen
- antithrombin functional assay
- anti-cardiolipin antibody
- lupus anticoagulant panel
- homocysteine assay

These levels need to be checked two to three weeks after a thrombotic event (because proteins are consumed acutely after an event).

Heparin-induced thrombocytopenia/thrombosis (HITT)

- A paradoxical etiology of an acquired hypercoaguable state that can occur with the administration of heparin.

- Occurs when negatively charged heparin binds the positively charged platelet factor (PF4).
- HITT occurs when IgG binds to the heparin-PF4 complex → platelet activation → release of microparticles → to thrombosis, platelet consumption, and thrombocytopenia.
- The diagnosis of HITT is made by the demonstration of the HITT antibody formation (antiheparin-PF4), thrombocytopenia (usually >50% platelet decrease), and clinical evidence of thrombosis.
- Interestingly, not all patients that have antiheparin-PF4 Ab will develop HITT.
- Treatment of HITT includes immediate cessation of heparin therapy and the initiation of nonheparin anticoagulant to prevent thrombotic complication (e.g., a direct thrombin (IIa) inhibitor such as bivalrudin). Additionally, care must be taken to avoid: LMWHs (as they cross-react with HITT antibodies), heparin flushes, and heparin-coated lines.

Disorder of fibrinolysis

Disseminated intravascular coagulopathy (DIC) is the typical disorder of fibrinolysis. It is a consumptive coagulopathy characterized by inappropriate widespread systemic activation of coagulation and excessive fibrinolysis.

- Precipitating factors of DIC (Figure 9.2).
- DIC results in small vessel thrombosis and generalized bleeding.
- Laboratory investigation reveals:
  - thrombocytopenia
  - elevated fibrin split products (FSP)
  - elevated D-dimers
  - decreased fibrinogen (factor I).
- Treatment of DIC is supportive with correction of underlying cause and treatment of diffuse bleeding with FFP (to replace coagulation factors), cyroprecipitate (to replace fibrinogen), and platelets (to treat the thrombocytopenia).

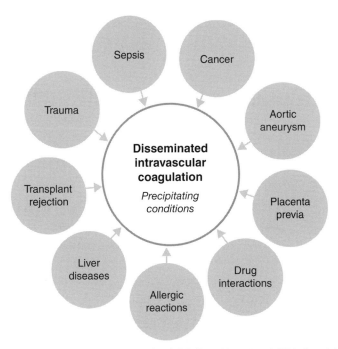

Figure 9.2 Conditions associated with DC. (From Vacanti et al. 2011. *Essential Clinical Anesthesia*, Cambridge University Press, p. 65.)

Questions

1. Thrombocytopenia can occur as a result of:
   a. massive RBC transfusion
   b. alcohol toxicity
   c. cardiopulmonary bypass
   d. hypothermia
   e. all of the above

2. Vitamin K deficiency
   a. leads to increased thrombotic phenomena
   b. laboratory investigation reveals a decreased PT because factor VII is not depleted
   c. is quickly corrected by oral administration of vitamin K
   d. causes decreased synthesis of factors V and VIII
   e. can be caused by poor nutrition

3. Heparin
   a. causes its anticoagulation effect by inhibition of factor V and protein S
   b. inhibits antithrombin III (AT III)
   c. is neutralized by a negatively charged molecule
   d. accelerates the action of AT III
   e. has a half-life that is longer than low molecular weight heparin (LMWH)

Answers

1. e. The four main etiologies for *thrombocytopenia* include: **dilutional thrombocytopenia** (e.g., as a result of massive resuscitation/transfusion), **decreased production** (e.g., drug side effects, infections, chemotherapy, radiation therapy, alcohol toxicity, vitamin B_{12}/folate deficiency), increased **destruction/consumption** (e.g., disseminated intravascular coagulation (DIC), drug exposure, ITP, TTP, hemolytic uremic syndrome (HUS), antiphospholipid antibody syndrome (AAS), HELLP syndrome, institution of CPB), and **splenic sequestration** – as seen in hypothermic patients or those with portal hypertension.

2. e. *Vitamin K deficiency* (which leads to deficiencies in the K-dependent clotting factors II, VII, IX, X, and proteins C and S) is acquired as a result of poor diet, intestinal problems (such as biliary obstruction, malabsorption, cystic fibrosis, small intestine resection, or use of antibiotics that destroy intestinal bacteria). Laboratory investigation reveals PT prolongation (because factor VII is depleted relatively

early). Treatment is via administration of vitamin K orally (takes 12 hours for correction) or intravenously (takes six to eight hours).

3.   d. *Unfractionated heparin (UH)* is a negatively charged drug that causes its anticoagulation effect by reversibly binding to antithrombin III (AT III). AT III inhibits factors Xa and IIa (thrombin) and heparin accelerates the effect of AT III. Reversal of heparin's effect is via neutralization by **positively** charged protamine or by cessation of heparin.

The half-life of heparin is <1 hour (much shorter than LMWH).

Further reading

Bethune, W. and Fitzsimons, A. E. (2011). Persistent postoperative bleeding in cardiac surgical patients. In Vacanti, C. A., Sikka, P. J., Urman, R. D., Dershwitz, M., and Segal, B. S. (eds) *Essential Clinical Anesthesia*. Cambridge: Cambridge University Press, pp. 497–502.

The elderly patient

Allison Clark and Lisa Crossley

Keywords

Age-related P50
Aging: cardiovascular physiology
Aging: pulmonary physiology
Geriatrics: autonomic function
Geriatrics: NSAID use
Geriatrics: pulmonary changes

Cardiovascular complications account for the majority of perioperative events in the elderly. Cardiovascular changes with aging are displayed in Figure 10.1.

Systolic hypertension and left ventricular hypertrophy become more prevalent with aging due to decreased vascular elasticity and compliance, and increased tissue fibrosis.

Although resting cardiac output is largely unchanged, the geriatric patient is *unable to increase stroke volume during exercise.*

Parasympathetic tone is decreased and *sympathetic tone* is increased; however, *response to beta-adrenergic stimulation* is decreased in the elderly patient. Maximal heart rate is decreased.

Pulmonary changes are noted in the Table 10.1. There is an increase in closing capacity, work of breathing, dead space, and V/Q mismatch resulting in a lower resting PaO_2. Central response to hypoxia and hypercarbia is diminished.

Renal function declines with aging as a result of decreased renal blood flow and tissue degeneration. Creatinine levels are

Table 10.1 Pulmonary changes in the elderly patient.

System	Complications
Neurologic	Pain crisis, stroke, retinopathy, neuropathy, chronic pain syndrome
Pulmonary	Acute chest syndrome, airway hyperreactivity, restrictive lung disease
Genitourinary	Hyposthenuria, chronic renal insufficiency, urinary tract infection, priapism, increased obstetric complications
Gastrointestinal	Cholelithiasis, liver disease, dyspepsia
Hematologic	Hemolytic anemia, acute aplastic anemia, splenic enlargement/fibrosis
Orthopedic	Osteonecrosis, osteomyelitis, dactylitis
Vascular	Leg ulcers
Immunologic	Immune dysfunction, erythrocyte auto/alloimmunization

(From Vacanti et al. 2011. *Essential Clinical Anesthesia*, Cambridge University Press, Table 11.1.)

typically normal due to decreased muscle mass and thus creatinine production. In general, *NSAID use* can be considered safe in the geriatric patient; however, these should be avoided in the presence of renal failure or insufficiency as they should in any patient.

Essential Clinical Anesthesia Review: Keywords, Questions and Answers for the Boards, ed. Linda S. Aglio, Robert W. Lekowski, and Richard D. Urman. Published by Cambridge University Press. © Cambridge University Press 2015.

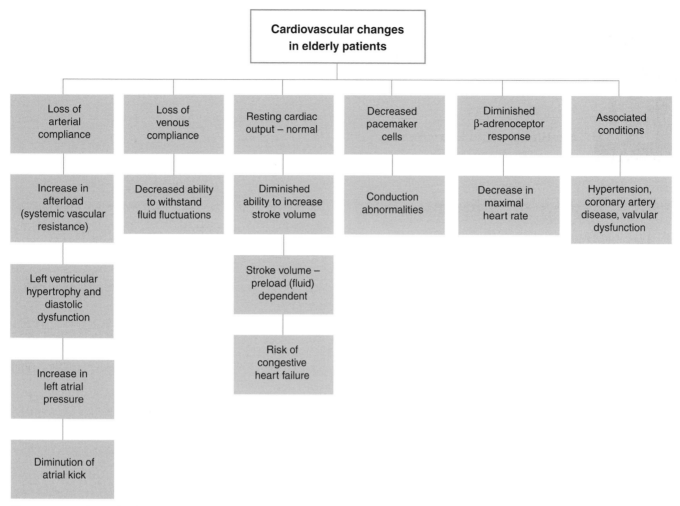

Figure 10.1 Cardiovascular changes in elderly patients. From: Vacanti et al., 2011, p. 71.

Questions

1. Which of the following is true of the elderly?

   a. cardiac output is decreased
   b. maximal heart rate is increased
   c. systolic blood pressure is increased
   d. parasympathetic tone is increased

2. Which of the following is increased in the elderly patient?

   a. FRC
   b. closing capacity

   c. PaO_2
   d. hypoxic pulmonary vasoconstriction

Answers

1. c. Systolic blood pressure is increased in the elderly patient due to atherosclerosis and decreased arterial compliance. Cardiac output is maintained, while maximal heart rate and parasympathetic tone are both decreased.
2. b. Closing capacity is increased in the elderly, while FRC, PaO_2, and hypoxic pulmonary vasoconstriction are decreased.

Further reading

Bose, R. and Barnett, S. (2011). The elderly patient. In Vacanti, C. A., Sikka, P. J., Urman, R. D., Dershwitz, M., and Segal, B. S. (eds) *Essential Clinical Anesthesia*. Cambridge: Cambridge University Press, pp. 70–76.

Hevesi, Z. (2008). Geriatric disorders. In Hines, R. and Marschall, K. (eds) *Stoelting's Anesthesia and Co-Existing Disease*, 5th edn. Philadelphia, PA: Churchill-Livingstone, pp. 639–650.

Neurologic diseases and anesthesia

Nantthasorn Zinboonyahgoon and Joseph M. Garfield

Keywords

Cerebrovascular disease: pathophysiology, preoperative evaluation and preparation, elective surgery after stroke, anesthetic management

Seizure disorders: pathophysiology, anesthetic management, management of seizure activiley

Alzheimer's disease: pathophysiology, cholinesterase inhibitors, anesthetic management

Parkinson's disease: anti-Parkinson medications and interaction with anesthesia

Huntington's disease: response to succinylcholine, anesthetic management

Multiple sclerosis: choice of anesthesia, body temperature, and exacerbation

Spinal cord injury

Acute – NEXUS criteria, immobilization of C-spine, spinal shock, anesthetic management

Chronic – pathophysiology, autonomic hyperreflexia: prevention and treatment

Syringomyelia, amylotrophic lateral sclerosis, Guillain–Barré syndrome: pathophysiology, anesthetic management

Cerebrovascular disease

Pathophysiology: cerebrovascular disease (stroke) is a consequence of the interruption of the blood supply to the brain, resulting from thrombosis, hemorrhage, or embolism. Transient ischemic attack (TIA) produces stroke symptoms lasting less than 24 hours.

Preoperative evaluation and preparation: stroke is not only considered a vascular disease but also an independent risk factor for patients to develop postoperative cardiac complications. Cardiac evaluation should be done preoperatively in this patient population. The risk of bleeding and the benefit of preventing further stroke should be assessed before deciding to continue warfarin, aspirin, or dipyridamole. *Elective surgery*

after stroke should be delayed for two to three months to allow the recovery of regional blood flow and CO_2 responsiveness.

Anesthetic management: the aim of anesthesia is to ensure rapid recovery and assessment of neurologic function in the immediate postoperative period (consider short-acting medication). Avoid succinylcholine due to possible hyperkalemic response.

Since glucose metabolizes to lactic acid, excessive lactate levels can cause tissue acidosis and increased tissue injury; hyperglycemia is associated with poor neurological outcome in acute stoke. Hypoglycemia and severe hyperglycemia should be avoided in stroke patients.

Perioperative blood pressure should be maintained at about 20% to 40% of baseline, as hypotension may result in cerebral hypoperfusion and infarction. Sustained hypertension should also be avoided, as it may cause intracranial hemorrhage.

Seizure disorders

Pathophysiology: seizures are the result of transient, paroxysmal, and synchronous discharge of groups of neurons in the brain and can result from metabolic or systemic derangements such as hypoglycemia, hyponatremia, hypoxia, or drug toxicity. Epilepsy, a relatively common seizure disorder, is characterized by recurrent episodes over relatively long intervals, i.e., months to years, with multiple causes. Seizures are classified into: (1) generalized (grand mal or tonic-clonic); (2) petit mal (staring or repeated blinking of the eyes); or (3) partial (simple or complex). A continuous seizure over many minutes to hours without recovery of consciousness is termed *status epilepticus* and considered a medical emergency requiring acute intervention, usually in the form of pharmacological agents, to terminate seizure activity.

Anesthetic management: antiepileptic drugs should be continued until surgery, and may even have to be supplemented intraoperatively. However, carbamazepine, phenytoin, barbiturates, and cytochrome P450 3A4 inducers can prolong the effects of aminosteroid neuromuscular blocking agents (rocuronium, vecuronium, pancuronium). Phenytoin administration

Essential Clinical Anesthesia Review: Keywords, Questions and Answers for the Boards, ed. Linda S. Aglio, Robert W. Lekowski, and Richard D. Urman. Published by Cambridge University Press. © Cambridge University Press 2015.

for more than seven days is sufficient to demonstrate a significantly increased requirement for vecuronium as the result of enzyme induction.

Potentially epileptogenic agents such as enflurane, methohexital, and ketamine should be avoided. Atracurium, which is metabolized to laudanosine, and meperidine to normeperidine, also have epileptogenic potential.

Management of seizure activity: if a seizure occurs, maintain the airway, ventilation, and circulation; control the seizure with intravenous drugs such as midazolam (2 to 5 mg), diazepam (5 to 10 mg), or propofol (50 to 75 mg); then administer phenytoin 500 to 1000 mg slowly, levetiracetam or valproic acid, to prevent recurrent seizure; also turn the patient to the side to prevent aspiration; an oral airway may be inserted, if tolerated, to help prevent biting of the lips or tongue.

Alzheimer's disease

Pathophysiology: Alzheimer's disease is a chronic neurodegenerative disorder characterized by irreversible impairment of cognitive function and memory. Patients also may experience gait and motor disturbances, seizures, apraxia, and aphasia. Treatment is to control symptoms and to slow their progression.

Cholinesterase inhibitors (tacrine, donepezil, and rivastigmine) are used to alleviate mental and cognitive decline. These agents will prolong the effect of succinylcholine and the relative resistance to nondepolarizing NMBAs (there can be a prolonged effect on patients on donezepil receiving atracurium).

Anesthetic management: patients may be disoriented and unable to give informed consent, in which case a valid health care proxy should be in place to provide consent for procedures. Cholinesterase inhibitors should be continued in the perioperative period.

As general anesthetics can induce long-lasting neurotoxicity (at the molecular level) and cognitive dysfunction in animal models (desflurane), regional anesthesia may be appropriate provided that the patient can remain cooperative. Light levels of short-term sedation coupled with a regional technique may be useful, provided that they are very carefully titrated to minimize disinhibition and exacerbation of preexisting disorientation.

General anesthesia: premedication should be minimized; use short-acting agents for rapid return of baseline mental status. Anticholinergics (except glycopyrrolate, which does not cross the blood–brain barrier) may make the patient more confused and impair cognition.

Parkinson's disease

Pathophysiology: Parkinson's disease (PD) is a degenerative disorder caused by the loss of dopaminergic neurons in the basal ganglia resulting in a disrupted extrapyramidal system. The classic triad of PD is tremor, cogwheel rigidity, and bradykinesia. Patients can also have abnormalities of posture and gait, but intellectual function is intact in the early course of the disease.

Anti-Parkinson drugs and anesthesia: the pharmacologic treatment of PD aims to increase central levels of dopamine. Abrupt cessation of medication is dangerous and can result in severe muscle rigidity that interferes with ventilation. In rare instances, Parkinsonian hyperpyrexic syndrome may develop, characterized by rigidity, hyperthermia, reduced level of consciousness, autonomic instability, and elevations of serum creatine kinase (CK), which may be fatal if not recognized and treated immediately and aggressively. Anti-Parkinsonian medications should therefore be continued until the day of surgery and restarted as soon as possible postoperatively, with the following caveats:

- Levodopa with decarboxylase inhibitor, e.g., Carbidopa® (inhibits the peripheral breakdown of dopamine); the half-life of levodopa is short; interruption for 6 to 12 hours can result in the loss of therapeutic effects. The dose may be repeated intraoperatively IV, through an OG or NG tube. However, levodopa can cause orthostatic hypotension, cardiac irritability, nausea, and vomiting.
- Dopamine agonists (bromocriptine, pergolide, ropinirole, pramipexole, and cabergoline) can cause precipitous hypotension during anesthesia.
- Type B monoamine oxidase inhibitors, e.g., selegiline (inhibits dopamine catabolism), can interact with meperidine, serotonergic drugs, and catecholamines.

Anesthetic management: as Parkinson's disease is associated with autonomic insufficiency (by levodopa or PD itself), hemodynamic instability and altered response to vasopressors is possible during anesthesia.

There is a case reported of hyperkalemia following succinylcholine administration, but no altered response to nondepolarizing NBMAs. Ketamine has been reported to potentiate sympathomimetic properties of levodopa. Morphine, alfentanil, and fentanyl have been reported to exacerbate muscle rigidity.

Postoperatively, patients are susceptible to symptom exacerbation, aspiration, respiratory failure, and mental confusion.

Dopamine antagonists such as metoclopramide, phenothiazines, and droperidol should be avoided as they may worsen extrapyramidal symptoms.

Finally, a rare complication of deep brain stimulation to treat Parkinson's disease is the development of Parkinsonian hyperpyrexia syndrome, where patients become acutely symptomatic. This complication is usually seen following discontinuation of anti-parkinson medications, but can occur following deep brain stimulation. It is very similar, clinically, to the neuroleptic malignant syndrome and is treated as such. Management consists of dopaminergic drug replacement, supportive measures and treatment of complications.

Huntington's disease

Pathophysiology: Huntington's disease is an inherited degenerative disorder in the caudate nucleus, characterized by a triad of choreiform movements, progressive dementia, and personality changes, with an onset age of 35 to 40 years. Unfortunately, there is no cure at this time. Treatment is symptomatic; haloperidol is used to decrease choreoathetoid movements, and fluphenazine also may relieve chorea, hallucinations, and delusions.

Anesthetic management: patients may develop dysphagia and are at risk for pulmonary aspiration. Rapid sequence induction should be employed. *Decreased plasma cholinesterase levels may lead to a prolonged response after succinylcholine administration.* Patients may also have increased sensitivity to nondepolarizing NMBAs.

Multiple sclerosis

Pathophysiology: multiple sclerosis (MS) is an autoimmune disorder causing demyelination of the brain and spinal cord, characterized by its multifocal involvement ranging from visual problems (optic neuritis), paresthesias, weakness and urinary incontinence (spinal cord), and gait disturbances (cerebellum). The course ranges from subacute with variable symptom-free intervals, punctuated by relapses, to chronic progressive.

Treatment for MS is to control damage and slow disease progression. Several immunosuppressants, including corticosteroids, interferon, glatiramer acetate, intravenous immunoglobulin, methotrexate, and cyclophosphamide, are used for acute relapses. However, neurological damage still remains after remission.

Anesthetic management: choice of anesthesia. Regardless of anesthetic technique or drug selection, there is always a risk of postoperative exacerbation due to surgical stress. Spinal anesthesia has been reported to cause exacerbations, whereas peripheral nerve blocks and epidurals have not been so described. General anesthesia can be done safely. However, if paresis or paralysis is present, succinylcholine should be avoided. Patients may also have a prolonged response to nondepolarizing NMBAs.

Body temperature should be monitored and aggressively treated because increased body temperature, even of as little as 1°C, can exacerbate the symptoms due to the interruption of nerve conductions in the region of demyelinations. Corticosteroid should be supplemented in chronic steroid users.

Spinal cord injury
Acute spinal cord injury

Cervical spine injury, especially the upper cervical spine, can lead to disasterous outcomes such as high levels of spinal cord injury and quadriplegia. About 4% to 5% of head injuries and 1% to 3% of major traumas have concurrent spine injury.

Table 11.1 The NEXUS clinical criteria

1. Tenderness at the posterior midline of the cervical spine
2. Focal neurologic deficit
3. Decreased level of alertness
4. Evidence of intoxication
5. Clinically apparent pain that might distract the patient from the pain of a cervical spine injury

(*Source*: Pasternak, J. J. and lanier, W. L. 2012. Spinal cord disorders. In Hines, R. L. and Maschall, K.E. (eds) *Stoelting's Anesthesia and Co-Existing Disease*, 6th edn. Philadelphia: Elsevier Saunders, pp. 255–256.)

Preoperative management: detection of C-spine injury. *The National Emergency X-Radiography Utilization Study criteria* (NEXUS criteria) is a clinical tool to screen cervical spine injury (see Table 11.1). If patients have any of the clinical signs listed in the table, radiographic investigation should be obtained (plain film cervical spine C1–T1, AP, lateral cross table, open mouth or CT scan, MRI). However, radiologic findings must be interpreted with clinical signs. If there is any doubt, it is prudent to treat patients as having an unstable C-spine.

Intraoperative management

Immobilization of C-spine, especially during airway manipulation and positioning before fixation. Neck collars and halo thoracic devices are used for immobilization but can cause difficult laryngoscopy. Manual in-line stabilization should be applied during all airway manipulations (even awake fiberoptic, as patients can cough and have C-spine motions).

Spinal shock: an acute spinal cord injury initially produces flaccid paralysis and loss of sensation below the level of injury. Hypotension is common due to the loss of sympathetic nervous system activity causing vasodilatation and a loss of innervation from T1 to T4 (cardiac acceleration center) causing bradycardia. This hemodynamic disturbance is called spinal shock, typically lasting one to three weeks. The treatment is fluids and vasopressor/inotrope. Hypothermia is to be carefully maintained, as patients tend to become poikilothermic below the cord lesion.

Postoperative management: an upper cervical cord injury causes phrenic nerve paralysis (C3–C5), and disturbed diaphragmatic innervation causes alveolar hypoventilation and inability to clear secretions. Patients may require endotracheal intubation and ventilatory support.

Chronic spinal cord injury

Pathophysiology: chronic spinal cord injury is associated with multiple comorbidities. Patients who have injuries above C3–C5 may have an impaired ability to clear secretions, leading to atelectasis, pneumonia. Renal failure from calculi is common, and also a common cause of death in chronic SCI patients. Patients have a high risk of deep venous thrombosis due to immobilization; heparin and pneumatic boots should be applied during the perioperative period.

Patients turn from acute flaccid paralysis to spasticity of muscles below the cord lesion, which is managed by a muscle relaxant such as bacolfen (GABA-B agonist), which should be continued perioperatively due to withdrawal symptoms that can lead to spasticity, seizure, and death.

Anesthetic management: the goal of anesthetic management in chronic spinal cord injury is prevention and early treatment of autonomic hyperreflexia, which will be mentioned. Avoid succinylcholine administration after 24 hours of SCI due to possible exaggerated hyperkalemia. Patients have the potential for labile hemodynamic, especially in high spinal cord lesions due to loss of vascular tone. Maintaining normothermia is essential as patients tend to have hypothermia from lack of compensation vasoconstriction.

Autonomic hyperreflexia (AHR)

Pathophysiology: autonomic hyperreflexia is a reaction caused by hyperstimulation of the autonomic nervous system in patients with spinal cord injuries above T6 (T6 through T10 also may be susceptible but have mild clinical presentation). Autonomic hyperreflexia can occur after the resolution of spinal shock (one to three weeks after injury) and remains afterwards.

- Sensory stimuli are usually transmitted through the spinal cord and from the reflex arch by connecting to sympathetic splanchnic outflow track to blood vessel and viscera. This reflex is normally inhibited from the higher central nervous system centers. However, spinal cord transection causes loss of this inhibitory reflex, leading to massive sympathetic response below the level of transection.
- Sympathetic response causes vasoconstriction in the splanchnic sympathetic outflow (T5–L2) leading to hypertension (15 to 20 mm Hg above baseline). Hypertension can cause pulmonary edema, headache, seizure, and cerebral hemorrhage. If not treated promptly, it may lead to seizures, stroke, myocardial infarction, and death.
- Carotid sinus and aortic arch baroreceptors sense increased blood pressure resulting in reflex bradycardia through the vagus nerve. Sympathetic stimulation also effects the vasomotor center in the medulla to release parasympathetic output resulting in vasodilation, cutaneous flushing, and nasal stuffiness above the level of the cord injury.

Any stimulation below the level of the cord lesion, including skin stimulation, decubitus ulcers, surgery, or labor contractions, can trigger autonomic hyperreflexia. (The most common triggers are distention of the rectum or bladder.)

Prevention and treatment

Prevention: even in patients who do not have sensation below the transaction level, anesthesia is still necessary to suppress painful stimuli to prevent AHR during surgery, or labor and delivery.

Local anesthesia: application of topical anesthesia to the bladder or rectal mucosa for bladder or rectal instrumentation might be helpful but is unreliable in preventing AHR, as the underlying muscular layer proprioceptors are not anesthetized.

Regional anesthesia: spinal anesthesia and epidural anesthesia are reliable methods both in surgical patients and in labor and delivery. However, spinal anesthesia has a greater advantage in preventing AHR due to denser block and a lesser degree of sacral sparing.

General anesthesia: adequate depth of general anesthesia can suppress AHR.

Treatment: removal of the stimulus (if the suspected cause is bladder distension, the catheter should be checked for any kinks or blockage).

Pharmacologic treatment of hypertension includes vasodilators (sodium nitroprusside, nitroglycerin, nifedipine, hydralazine). Bradycardia is treated with anticholinergics. Due to unopposed alpha-adrenergic activity, pure beta-adrenergic blockers are relatively contraindicated for treatment of HT from AHR.

Syringomyelia

Pathophysiology: syringomyelia is thought to occur as the result of an obstruction of the cerebrospinal fluid outflow from the fourth ventricle leading to increased pressure, and dilation and cavitation of the spinal cord. Most commonly, the cervical spine is affected, causing sensory and motor deficits in the upper extremities.

Anesthetic management: syringomyelia may be associated with Arnold–Chiari malformation. Thoracic scoliosis is common; respiratory function should be assessed. Patients who have muscle wasting will have increased sensitivity to NMBA.

Amyotrophic lateral sclerosis (ALS)

Pathophysiology: ALS is a degenerative disease of the motor ganglia in the anterior horn of the spinal cord and spinal pyramidal tracts, resulting in skeletal muscle weakness. Patients with bulbar involvement may have dysphagia and are at risk for pulmonary aspiration. Respiratory muscle involvement can result in respiratory failure and death.

Anesthetic management: respiratory function should be assessed by spirometry.

Neuraxial anesthesia can exacerbate symptoms; however, epidural anesthesia has been reported as successful without exacerbation or impairment of respiratory function.

General anesthesia can worsen respiratory function. Succinylcholine is associated with exaggerated hyperkalemia, and patients can have a prolonged response to nondepolarizing NMBAs.

Autonomic dysfunction may be present (orthostatic hypotension, resting tachycardia), and intraoperative hemodynamic instability is expected.

Table 11.2 Neurologic disease and neuromuscular blocking agents

Disease	Depolarizing agent: succinylcholine	Nondepolarizing NMBA
Alzheimer's disease (patient takes cholinesterase inhibitors)	Prolonged response	Relatively resistant
Parkinson's disease	Case report of hyperkalemia	No change
Huntington's disease	Prolonged response	Prolonged response
ALS	Hyperkalemia	Prolonged response
MS	Avoid if paresis or paralysis is present	Prolonged response
GBS	Hyperkalemia	Prolonged response

(From Vacanti et al. 2011. *Essential Clinical Anesthesia*, Cambridge University Press, p. 79.)

Peripheral nervous system disorders
Guillain–Barré syndrome

Pathophysiology: Guillain–Barré Syndrome (GBS), an acute demyelinating polyneuropathy, usually occuring after a viral illness, resulting in ascending motor paralysis. If patients have bulbar involvement they are at an increased risk for aspiration, respiratory failure, and requirement of ventilatory support. Complete spontaneous recovery occurs in a few weeks to several months in most cases.

Anesthetic management: the risk of aspiration and respiratory function should be assessed.

Regional anesthesia may exacerbate neurologic symptoms but the risk should be weighed against the benefit of preventing aspiration and respiratory failure. With general anesthesia, succinlycholine is contraindicated and patients will have a prolonged response to nondepolarizing NMBAs. Autonomic dysfunction is prominently found in GBS and can cause sudden death. Labile blood pressure during anesthesia is to be expected. Despite adequate preoperative spontaneous breathing, mechanical ventilation may be necessary postoperatively in these patients.

Questions

1. Which medication does not worsen Parkinson symptoms?
   a. droperidol
   b. haloperidol
   c. tramadol
   d. metoclopramide

2. Which statement is correct about autonomic hyperreflexia?
   a. It is preventable by applying local anesthesia during bladder or urethral instrumentation.
   b. It can happen in 24 hours to 6 weeks after spinal cord injury.
   c. Spinal or epidural analgesia can prevent AHR during labor and delivery.
   d. The treatment of choice for hypertension is beta-adrenergic blockers.

3. Which statement is true about spinal cord injury?
   a. Succinylcholine is contraindicated in all cases.
   b. A CT scan of the neck in intoxicated patients is a reliable tool to rule out cervical spine injury.
   c. Spinal shock is a result of the interruption of sympathetic innervations, which causes vasodilatation, hypotension, and bradycardia.
   d. Only the acute phase of spinal cord injury is associated with hypothermia.

4. Succinlycholine can cause exaggerated hyperkalemia in the following conditions, except:
   a. Guillain–Barré syndrome
   b. multiple sclerosis
   c. amyotrophic lateral sclerosis (ALS)
   d. Huntington's disease

5. Which conditions warrant cervical spine radiologic investigation for suspected C-spine instability?
   a. patients who have midline neck pain and quadriplegia
   b. intoxicated patients
   c. patients who have a fractured femur from a car accident
   d. all of the above

Answers

1. c. Tramadol. Medications in droperidol, haloperidol, and metoclopramide inhibit dopamine activity and worsen Parkinsonian symptoms.
2. c. RA or deep GA, but not LA, can reliably prevent autonomic hyperreflexia during procedure or labor. Autonomic hyperreflexia can occur after the resolution of spinal shock (one to three weeks) and remains thereafter. Due to unopposed alpha-adrenergic activity, pure beta-adrenergic blockers are relatively contraindicated for treatment of HT from autonomic hyperreflexia.
3. c. Succinylcholine can cause exaggerated hyperkalemia for the spinal cord injury patient, 24 to 48 hours after injury. CT scan is useful to detect spinal cord injury, but radiologic findings must be interpreted with clinical signs. Both acute and chronic spinal cord injuries are a risk for hypothermia during anesthesia.
4. d. Huntington's disease. Patients with Guillain–Barré syndrome, multiple sclerosis, and amyotrophic lateral sclerosis (ALS) can develop exaggerated hyperkalemia after

receiving succinylcholine. However, patients with Huntington's disease can develop prolonged paralysis.

5. d. According to the NEXUS criteria, all of the patients are indicated for cervical spine radiologic investigation.

Further reading

Pasternak, J. J. and Lanier, W. L. (2012). Spinal cord disorders. In Hines, R. L. and Marschall, K.E. (eds) *Stoelting's Anesthesia and Co-Existing Disease*, 6th edn. Philadelphia: Elsevier Saunders.

Pasternak, J. J. and Lanier, W. L. (2012). Diseases affecting the brain. In Hines, R. L. and Marschall, K.E. (eds) *Stoelting's Anesthesia and Co-Existing Disease*, 6th edn. Philadelphia: Elsevier Saunders.

Pasternak, J. J. and Lanier, W. L. (2012). Diseases of the autonomic and peripheral nervous systems. In Hines, R. L. and Marschall, K.E. (eds) *Stoelting's Anesthesia and Co-Existing Disease*, 6th edn. Philadelphia: Elsevier Saunders.

Spanakis, S. G., Lin, J., and Sikka, P. K. (2011). Neurologic diseases and anesthesia. In Vacanti, C. A., Sikka, P. J., Urman, R. D., Dershwitz, M., and Segal, B. S. (eds) *Essential Clinical Anesthesia*. Cambridge: Cambridge University Press.

Newman, E. J., Grosset, D. G., and Kennedy, P. G. (2009). *Neurocritical Care* 10(1), 136–140.

Chapter

12

Anesthetic considerations in psychiatric disease

Nantthasorn Zinboonyahgoon and Joseph M. Garfield

Keywords

Depression: antidepressants (tricyclic antidepressants, SSRIs, SNRIs, MAOIs), anesthetic implications, serotonin syndrome
Bipolar disorder: lithium, lithium toxicity, anesthetic considerations
Schizophrenia: antipsychotics (typical, atypical), anesthetic considerations, neuroleptic malignant syndrome

Depression

Lifetime prevalence of significant depressive symptoms is 13% to 20% and 3.7% to 6.7% for major depressive disorder. Depressive patients experience a wide range of clinical symptoms ranging from lack of pleasure and sleeping problems to psychomotor retardation or even committing suicide in extreme cases.

Antidepressants: although the exact etiology of depression remains unknown, there is experimental evidence that depletion of brain catecholamines (serotonin, norepinephrine (NE), and dopamine) plays an important role. Accordingly, pharmacologic treatment of depression involves the administration of drugs that increase levels of these brain catecholamines. In addition to the treatment of depression, antidepressants are also used to alleviate chronic pain and for other psychiatric conditions such as sleep disorders, anxiety, attention-deficit hyperactivity disorder (ADHD), obsessive–compulsive disorder (OCD), and substance abuse. Antidepressants are categorized by their mechanism.

Tricyclic antidepressants (TCAs)

Members: amitriptyline (most potent anticholinergic effect), doxepine (least cardiac effect), nortriptyline, imipramine, and desipramine

Mechanism: TCAs inhibit catecholamine reuptake (increase serotonin, NE, and dopamine in nerve synapses and the brain).

However, TCAs also interact with histamine, muscarinic, alpha-adrenergic receptors, and ion channels (sodium and calcium channels) in the heart.

Side effects: as TCAs interact with many neurotransmitters and ion channels, they have many side effects, as follows:

- Anticholinergic side effects (dry mouth, blurred vision, urinary retention, tachycardia, confusion, and delirium). Anticholinergic compounds, including benadryl, a centrally acting anticholinergic, can also cause acute urinary retention, especially in elderly males with prostatic enlargement. Quaternary anticholinergic compounds, such as glycopyrrolate, do not cross the blood–brain barrier and are far less likely to cause behavioral side effects.
- Arrhythmias, postural hypotension.
- Other, nonspecific side effects such as weight gain, sexual dysfunction, and sedation; with TCA overdoses patients can have seizures, coma, heart block, hypotension, VT, VF, and systole.

Anesthetic implications

Abrupt cessation of any antidepressant drugs are associated with a risk for patients to develop discontinuation syndrome, which includes nausea, abdominal pain and diarrhea, sleep disturbance, headaches, and affective problems. Antidepressants should therefore be continued during the perioperative period.

Increased levels of serotonin and NE resulting in increased anesthetic requirement and exaggerated responses to sympathetic stimulation and indirect-acting vasopressors such as ephedrine; direct-acting agents such as phenylephrine are a better choice, especially during acute treatment (first 14 to 21 days), but not after long-term administration, as long-term treatment is associated with downregulation of receptors.

Tricyclic antidepressants increase central cholinergic activity; co-administration with anticholinergics that can cross the blood–brain barrier, such as atropine, can lead to postoperative confusion, especially in elderly patients.

Essential Clinical Anesthesia Review: Keywords, Questions and Answers for the Boards, ed. Linda S. Aglio, Robert W. Lekowski, and Richard D. Urman. Published by Cambridge University Press. © Cambridge University Press 2015.

Table 12.1 The serotonin syndrome: associated drugs

Antidepressants	Analgesics	Antiemetic agents	Drugs of Abuse	Others	Others
SSRIs	meperidine	ondansetron	MDMA (ecstasy)	dextromethorphan	ritonavir tryptophan
SNRIs	fentanyl	metoclopramide	LSD	valproate	St. John's wort
TCAs	tramadol			sibutramine	ginseng
MAOIs	pentazocine			sumatriptan	lithium
				linezolide	

Selective serotonin reuptake inhibitors (SSRIs) and serotonin–norepinephrine reuptake inhibitors (SNRIs)

Members: SSRIs: fluoxetine, paroxitine, fluvoxamine, sertraline, and citalopram; SNRIs: venlafaxine, buproprion, and duloxetine. (Because it is believed that NE level has an important role in neuropathic pain and lower side effect profiles, SNRIs are gaining more popularity in chronic neuropathic pain over TCAs and SSRIs.)

Mechanism: SSRIs inhibit serotonin reuptake resulting in increased serotonin levels; SSRIs inhibit both serotonin and NE uptake. SNRIs increase both neurotransmitters with minimal effect on anticholinergics, antihistamines, and ion channels.

Side effects: SSRIs and SNRIs have mild side effects such as agitation, insomnia, nausea, and decreased appetite.

Anesthetic implications: SSRIs can inhibit cytochrome P450 enzymes, resulting in increased blood levels of warfarin, theophylline, phenytoin, and benzodiazepines. Fluoxetine and paroxitine have the strongest effect, whereas sertraline and citalopram have the least effect.

Miscellaneous effects: many antidepressants have more complex mechanisms, involving interactions with multiple neurotransmitters, e.g., mirtazapine, mianserin, roboxetine, and trazadone.

Monoamine oxidase inhibitors (MAOIs)

Members: isocarboxazid (Zelapar®); phenelzine (Nardil®); selegiline (Emsam®, Eldepryl®, and Zelapar®); tranylcypromine (Parnate®).

Mechanism: inhibit MAO type A, a mitochondrial enzyme that is expressed in most neurons, resulting in increased NE, dopamine, and serotonin levels (MAO type B degrades dopamine more readily than serotonin and norepinephrine; MAO type B inhibitors such as selegiline (Zelepar®), and rasagaline (Azilect®) have been used for Parkinson's disease).

Side effects: hypertensive and hyperpyrexic crisis if taken with tyramine-containing foods (cheese, wine, smoked fish, or meat), exaggerated hypertension with sympathomimetic drugs.

Anesthetic implications: current recommendation suggests no need to stop MAOIs before elective surgery due to risk of discontinuation syndrome and suicide. However, meperidine (Demerol®) should be avoided when a patient is concurrently

taking a type A MAO inhibitor. Meperidine, a synthetic opioid and member of the phenypiperidine opioid series, appears to be a weak serotonin reuptake inhibitor. However, the combination can result in an acute hypertensive–hyperpyrexic crisis, thought to be a manifestation of the serotonin syndrome, which may be fatal (see below). This, in fact, happened in the well known Libby Zion case. An overworked house officer at New York Hospital failed to heed the notice of a possible adverse drug interaction and administered meperidine to a young woman who was taking an MAOI, resulting in her death and ultimately leading to the 80-hour working week for interns and residents. Fentanyl, morphine, codeine, oxycodone, and buprenorphine, on the other hand, appear to be safe in patients taking MAOIs.

MAOIs increase serotonin and NE levels, leading to increased anesthetic requirement, and exaggerate hypertensive responses to sympathetic stimulation. Moreover, the combination of MAOIs and meperidine has been reported to cause serotonin syndrome. Serum pseudocholinesterase activity may decrease with phenelzine, and succinylcholine doses may need to be reduced. Finally, MAOIs inhibit liver enzymes responsible for opioid metabolism, which can enhance their clinical potency and duration of effect.

Serotonin syndrome is an adverse drug reaction resulting from excessive serotonin activity by serotonin-enhancing drugs (Table 12.1), not limited to only SSRIs. It can occur with overdose of a single such drug or a combination. Meperidine and tramadol should be avoided in patients taking antidepressants and medications in Table 12.1.

Clinical manifestations: serotonin syndrome has an acute onset, usually within six hours after taking medications, starting with agitation and hyperkinesias, hyperreflexia, tachycardia, hypertension, and mental status changes. As signs and symptoms of serotonin syndrome progress, patients can develop hypotension, hyperthermia, rigidity, and rhabdomyolysis, which is difficult to distinguish from neuroleptic malignant syndrome and malignant hyperthermia. Comparison between the three conditions and their management are shown in Table 12.2.

Bipolar disorder

DSM IV classified bipolar disorder into three main categories: bipolar I disorder (consisting of episodes of mania cycling with depressive episodes), bipolar II disorder (consisting of episodes of hypomania cycling with depressive episodes), and

Table 12.2 Comparison of serotonin syndrome, neuroleptic malignant syndrome, and malignant hyperthermia

Condition	Cause and triggers	Sign and symptoms	Treatment
Serotonin syndrome	**Excess serotonin** activity, triggered by serotoninergic drugs **Acute onset**, usually within six hours	1. Agitation, mental status changes 2. Tachycardia, hypertension 3. Hyperkinesias, tremor, hyperreflexia, **clonus** (helps distinguish it from NMS and MH) Severe case: hypotension, hyperthermia, rigidity, and rhabdomyolysis	Stop suspected drugs Administer benzodiazepines In severe cases use a serotonin antagonist (**Cyproheptadine**), Control hyperthermia Neuromuscular paralysis **Dantrolene is not effective**
Neuroleptic malignant syndrome	**Abrupt decrease of dopamine** activity by: rapid increase of antipsychotics, metoclopramide, or cessation of a dopamine agonist **Slow onset**, within 24 to 72 hours	1. Mental status changes 2. Autonomic instability: tachycardia, hyperthermia 3. Neuromuscular abnormalities: **bradykinesia**, rigidity Severe case: hyperthermia, rigidity, rhabdomyolysis	Stop anti-dopamine medications (or continue dopaminergic medications) Hemodynamic support Benzodiazepines **Bromocriptine** Dantrolene in severe cases
Malignant hyperthermia	Inherited disorder causes excessive release of calcium from sarcoplasmic recticulum in skeletal muscle, triggered by: anesthetic drugs (succinylcholine, inhalation agents)	Masseter muscle rigidity, muscle rigidity, **elevated ETCO$_2$,** tachycardia, tachypnea Severe case: hyperthermia, rigidity, rhabdomyolysis, metabolic acidosis Diagnosis in suspected susceptible patient: caffeine halothane contraction test	Stop triggering agents Control hyperthermia Hemodynamic support **Dantrolene**

cyclothymic disorder (consisting of hypomania and less severe episodes of depression). Lifetime prevalence of bipolar disorder ranges from 0.6% to 1.1%.

During manic episodes, bipolar patients, can display inflated self-esteem, flight of ideas, engage in risky behaviors, experience psychomotor agitation and even hallucinations. Treatment of mania includes lithium, carbamazepine, or atypical antipsychotic agents.

Lithium: lithium is used in bipolar disorder as a specific treatment in manic episodes and as prevention for relapses; the exact mechanism is not well understood.

Side effects of lithium at therapeutic levels include tremor, first-degree AV block, widening QRS complexes, hypothyroidism, leukocytosis, aplastic anemia, nephrogenic diabetes insipidus, and teratogenic effects. However, the most feared side effect is lithium toxicity.

Lithium toxicity: lithium has a very narrow therapeutic window (0.6–0.8 mEq/l; up to 1.2 mEq/l for acute episodes). A level >2 mEq/l is considered toxic. As lithium is entirely excreted by the kidney at the proximal tubule in exchange for sodium, decreased renal function, thiazide diuretics, and hypovolemia can increase lithium levels, whereas loop diuretics, i.e., furosemide, do not. Lithium levels can also be increased by co-administration with ACE inhibitors, celecoxib, and NSAIDs.

Signs and symptoms of lithium toxicity are dose dependent, beginning with increased thirst or urination, fine tremor, and edema, progressing to nausea, vomiting, diarrhea, drowsiness, slurred speech, confusion, coarse tremor and twitching, muscle weakness, seizures, coma, and death in severe unrecognized or untreated cases.

Treatment: maintain airway and provide hemodynamic support; hydration with sodium-containing solution, hemodialysis; however, forced diuresis is controversial.

Anesthetic considerations in patients taking lithium

- Recent lithium level and electrolytes should be reviewed.
- Monitor lithium level during major procedures associated with large fluid shifts.
- As dehydration and volume loss can precipitate lithium toxicity, sodium-containing fluids should be administered along with frequent evaluation of volume status.
- Co-administration of celecoxib and NSAIDs can increase lithium level and should probably be avoided.
- Sedating effects of lithium can decrease anesthetic requirement.
- Muscle weaknesses from lithium toxicity can prolong neuromuscular blockade; neuromuscular monitoring should be employed.

Schizophrenia

Schizophrenia has an estimated lifetime prevalence of 0.5% to 1.0%. Patients may experience either positive symptoms (paranoia, delusions, hallucinations, and grossly disorganized thought processes) or negative symptoms (affective flattening and social withdrawal, seen more in schizo-affective disorders). In many instances, especially with overt, uncontrolled episodes, patients may exhibit agitation and acting out violent behaviors.

In the belief that overactivity of CNS dopamine underlies schizophrenic behaviors, pharmacologic treatment of schizophrenia embodies the use of agents that antagonize the dopamine 2 (D2) receptor. Antipsychotic agents have been categorized as follows: typical antipsychotics (strong D2 antagonists) and atypical antipsychotics (weak D2 antagonists). Applications of antipsychotic agents also include bipolar disorder, delirium, and controlling of aggressive behavior (i.e., use of haloperidol, a butyrophenone, to quieten aggressive patients who disrupt an emergency room).

Typical antipsychotics

Members: haloperidol, chlorperapine, perphenazine, thioridazine, chlorprothizine.

Mechanism: dopaminergic antagonists, which will not only inhibit the mesocortico-limbic pathway (thought) but also interfere with the nigrostriatal pathway (movement), and the tubuloinfundibular pathway (pituitary).

Side effects

Central nervous: sedation, cognitive dysfunction, extrapyramidal symptoms, tardive dyskinesia, akathisia, acute dystonia, and parkinsonism.
ANS: orthostatic hypotension, anticholinergic effects (tachycardia, dry mouth, and urinary retention).
Cardiovascular: prolonged QT interval, torsades de pointes.
Others: leukopenia, pancytopenia, jaundice, galactorhea.

Atypical antipsychotics

Members: clozapine, olanzapine, risperidone.

Mechanism: weak dopamine 2 antagonist, and antagonist to some subtypes of serotonin. They not only have milder and better tolerated side effects but also are used to control both positive and negative symptoms and patients who fail to respond to typical antipsychotics.

Side effects: overall this group have minimal extrapyramidal side effects. Clozapine can cause seizure, neutropenia; also, weight gain is a common side effect with these agents.

Anesthetic considerations

CNS: continue antipsychiatric agent(s) during operative period to control psychiatric symptoms; sedating effects of antipsychotic can lead to decrease in anesthetic requirement. Patients can have abnormal temperature regulation due to dopamine blockage in the hypothalamus; temperature should be monitored frequently throughout the acute perioperative period.

Cardiovascular system: patients may exhibit orthostatic hypotension due to alpha blockade; antipsychotics can prolong QT and lead to torsades de pointes; QT interval should be

monitored. Droperidol, a butyrophenone and dopamine antagonist formerly used as an antinausea agent, now carries an FDA "black box" warning due to the possibility of its effects on QT intervals and is essentially no longer used as an antiemetic agent.

Neuroleptic malignant syndrome

Neuroleptic malignant syndrome (NMS) appears to be caused by abrupt decreases of dopaminergic activity. This can result from rapidly increasing dosages of antipsychotics, or metoclopramide, or abrupt cessation of a dopamine agonist (bromocriptine, levodopa, or amantadine).

Unlike serotonin syndrome, the clinical course of NMS has a slow onset, usually within 24 to 72 hours, beginning with bradykinesia, rather than hyperkinesia. However, in severe cases it is difficult to distinguish the signs and symptoms of NMS from those of neuroleptic malignant syndrome and malignant hyperthermia, see comparison in Table 12.2.

Questions

1. Which statement is true?
   a. Serotonin syndrome occurs only in patients taking SSRIs or SNRIs.
   b. Clonus helps distinguish serotonin syndrome from malignant hyperthermia.
   c. Dantrolene is indicated in serotonin syndrome and neuroleptic malignant syndrome.
   d. Signs and symptoms of neuroleptic malignant syndrome include acute onset (less than six hours), hyperkinesia, hypotension, tachycardia, and muscle rigidity.

2. Which statement is true?
   a. All antidepressants should be stopped one to three days before an operation to decrease the risk of cardiac arrhythmia.
   b. TCAs and MAOIs are associated with an increased anesthetic requirement.
   c. Ephedrine is the drug of choice for treating hypotension in patients who take an antidepressant.
   d. QRS interval should be monitored in patients who take an antipsychotic.

3. Which statement is true about lithium?
   a. Lithium increases anesthetic requirement.
   b. Lithium induces resistance to nondepolarizing NMBAs.
   c. Thiazide, NSAIDs, and celecoxib can decrease blood lithium levels.
   d. Adequate hydration with a sodium-containing solution can prevent lithium toxicity.

Answers

1. b. Serotonin syndrome can happen with any medications with serotoninergic activities. Clonus and hyperreflexia help distinguish serotonin syndrome from malignant

hyperthermia and NMS. Dantrolene is not indicated in serotonin syndrome. Neuroleptic malignant syndrome presents with slow onset (24 to 72 hours) of bradykinesia, tachycardia, and muscle rigidity.

2. b. Current recommendation suggests no need to stop any antidepressant before elective surgery due to risk of discontinuation syndrome and suicide. TCAs and MAOIs are associated with an increased anesthetic requirement. Ephedrine is associated with exaggerated hypertension in patients who acutely take antidepressants. QT, not QRS, interval should be monitored in patients who take an antipsychotic.

3. d. Lithium can decrease anesthetic requirement and can induce sensitivity to nondepolarizing NMBAs. Hypovolemia and certain medications (thiazide, NSAIDs, and celecoxib) can increase blood lithium levels; adequate hydration with sodium-containing solution can prevent lithium toxicity.

Further reading

Williams, M. and Turner, T. J. (2008). Adrenergic pharmacology. In Golan, D., Tashjian, A., Armstrong, E., and Armstrong, A. (eds) *Principles of Pharmacology*, 2nd edn. Philadelphia: Lippincott, p. 132.

Nadel-Vicins, M., Chyung, J. H., and Turner, T. J. (2008). Pharmacology of serotoninergic and central adrenergic transmission. In Golan, D., Tashjian, A., Armstrong, E., and Armstrong, A. (eds) *Principles of Pharmacology*, 2nd edn. Philadelphia: Lippincott.

Taniguchi, C. and Guengerich, F. P. (2008). Drug metabolism. In Golan, D., Tashjian, A., Armstrong, E., and Armstrong, A. (eds) *Principles of Pharmacology*, 2nd edn. Philadelphia: Lippincott.

Gillman, P. K. (2005). Monoamine oxidase inhibitors, opioid analgesics and serotonin toxicity. *British Journal of Anesthesia* 95, 434–441.

Lerner, B. A. (2009). A life-changing case for doctors in training. New York Times, March 3, 2009.

Boyer, E. W. and Shannon, M. (2005). The serotonin syndrome. *New England Journal of Medicine* 352, 1112–20.

Hines, R. L. and Marschall, K. E. (2012). Psychiatric disease, substance abuse and drug overdose. In Hines, R. L. and Marschall, K. E. (eds) *Stoelting's Anesthesia and Co-Existing Disease*, 6th edn. Philadelphia: Elsevier Saunders.

Amirfarzan, H. and Sikka, P. K. (2011). Anesthetic considerations in psychiatric disease. In Vacanti, C. A., Sikka, P. J., Urman, R. D., Dershwitz, M., and Segal, B. S. (eds) *Essential Clinical Anesthesia*. Cambridge: Cambridge University Press.

Loosen, P. T. and Shelton, R. C. (2008). Mood disorder. In Ebert, M. H., Loosen, P. T., Nurcombe, B., and Leckman, J.F. (eds) *Current Diagnosis and Treatment: Psychiatry*, 2nd edn. McGraw-Hill.

Timmer, R. T. and Sands, J. M. (1999). Lithium intoxication. *Journal of the American Society of Nephrology* 10, 666–674.

Strawn, J. R., Keck, P. E., and Caroff, S. N. (2007). Neuroleptic malignant syndrome. *American Journal of Psychiatry* 164(6), 870–876.

Chapter

13

Substance abuse and anesthesia

Nantthasorn Zinboonyahgoon and Joseph M. Garfield

Keywords

General considerations
Tobacco: mechanism of action, postoperative
  complications, smoking cessation
Alcohol: mechanism of action, acute intoxication,
  chronic alcohol abuse
Opioids: mechanism of action, acute effects, chronic
  effects, opioid and elective surgery, buprenorphrine
  and elective surgery, postoperative pain control
Cocaine: mechanism of action, acute effects, chronic
  effects, cocaine and elective surgery
Amphetamine: mechanism of action, acute effects,
  chronic effects, amphetamine and elective surgery
Marijuana: mechanism of action, effects, medical
  marijuana
Hallucinogens: mechanism of action, effects

General considerations

Substance abuse has a high prevalence but is usually underreported. As a history and physical examination might not gain enough information from patients, obtaining a urine test is very useful. In certain cases, e.g., emergency or trauma cases, a toxicity screen, "tox screen," as it is known colloquially, drawn preoperatively can be of great value. Even though the report may take several hours, the results can be of great help in the immediate postoperative period when a patient exhibits unusual physiological states that are otherwise difficult to diagnose.

Effects of behaviorally active substances not only alter patient physiologic status but also interact with a number of medications and anesthetic agents, which can complicate anesthesia even in young healthy people. Intoxicated patients cannot provide reliable information and often are not able to cooperate, which will limit some choices of anesthesia (regional anesthesia, awake intubation). Moreover, chronic drug abusers usually have psychological and physical comorbidities that make anesthesia more complicated. Specific concerns and anesthetic implications for individual substances will be discussed below.

Tobacco

Mechanism of action: tobacco contains more than 3,000 active substances, including nicotine and carbon monoxide. Nicotine stimulates nicotinic cholinergic receptors, causing sympathetic stimulation, increased HR, BP, and myocardial contractility. Carbon monoxide avidly binds to Hb (it has 210 times the binding capacity of oxygen) forming carboxyhemoglobin, which results in lower available stores of oxyhemoglobin, resulting in decreased tissue oxygenation. Hemoglobin, a tetramer, contains four oxygen-binding sites. The binding of carbon monoxide at one of these sites increases the oxygen affinity of the remaining three sites, which causes the hemoglobin molecule to retain oxygen that would otherwise be delivered to the tissue. This effect causes a shift to the left of the oxyhemoglobin dissociation curve. Heavy cigarette smokers, i.e., one to two packs per day, can have their oxyhemoglobin reduced by up to 8% to 9%. It is also thought that cigarette smoking may impair the viability of tissue flaps, perhaps from the effects of chronic elevated carbon monoxide levels on tissue oxygenation. Tobacco increases airway irritability and decreases mucociliary clearance. Long-term smoking also is associated with COPD, CAD, PVD, and stroke.

Smoking increases the risk of *postoperative complications*. Pulmonary complications (laryngospasm, pneumonia, respiratory failure, and ICU admission), potentially increase cardiovascular complications, impair tissue oxygenation, and lead to impaired wound healing.

Smoking cessation should be encouraged before elective surgery. Even only 12 to 24 hours of cessation will decrease carboxyhemoglobin levels and increase tissue oxygenation; 48 to 72 hours of cessation may lead to increased airway secretion and airway reactivity. One to two weeks may be enough to reduce sputum volume, but at least four to eight weeks of cessation is required to reduce pulmonary complications.

Essential Clinical Anesthesia Review: Keywords, Questions and Answers for the Boards, ed. Linda S. Aglio, Robert W. Lekowski, and Richard D. Urman. Published by Cambridge University Press. © Cambridge University Press 2015.

Alcohol

Mechanism of action: alcohol appears to act at GABA-A receptors at a specific ethanol-binding site and causes CNS depression starting from sedation and euphoria, but higher doses lead to disinhibition, impaired motor control, coma, impaired airway reflex, and aspiration. Benzodiazepines, such as oxazepam (Serax®), are useful in preventing delirium tremens (the DTs). It is thought that benzodiazepines, by binding to the benzodiazepine site at the GABA-A receptor, mimic the action of ethanol and induce a state of neuronal quiescence, thereby preventing the excitatory clinical manifestations of DTs.

Acute intoxication can delay gastric emptying time, leading to increased risks of aspiration; ethanol-induced hypoglycemia can worsen mental status; CNS depression induced by ethanol decreases anesthetic requirements during acute intoxication.

Chronic alcohol abuse is associated with gastritis, alcoholic cirrhosis, chronic pancreatitis, peripheral neuropathy, cardiac beriberi, Wernicke's encephalopathy (vitamin B_1 should be administrated to prevent worsening cardiac beriberi or Wernicke's encephalopathy). Withdrawal symptoms and delirium tremens can occur 6 to 48 hours following last alcohol consumption. Moreover, as alcohol is a liver enzyme inducer, chronic alcohol abuse tends to require higher concentrations/doses of anesthetic agents.

Opioids

Mechanism of action: opioids bind μ receptors, both $μ_1$ (analgesia) and $μ_2$ (respiratory depression), and cause euphoria, analgesia, and respiratory depression.

Acute effects: the most severe deleterious effect of strong μ agonists is opioid-induced respiratory depression, which consists of sedation, reduced respiratory rate, hypoxia, and pupillary constriction, progressing to coma and apnea in severe cases. Severe respiratory depression often results in unsuspecting clients who buy unusually potent lots of narcotic, such as heroin. Management consists of maintaining airway patency, supporting ventilation/oxygenation and, if necessary, an antidote (naloxone) can be carefully administered. It should be noted that a number of emergency facilities stock intranasal naloxone for use in suspected narcotic overdose. Opioids may delay gastric emptying time and place patients at increased risk of aspiration. Rapid sequence induction should be considered for intubation.

Chronic effects: chronic opioid users may develop tolerance and withdrawal symptoms (agitation, hypertension, tachycardia, lacrimation, and diarrhea). Naloxone and mixed agonist-antagonist agents are relatively contraindicated as they can precipitate withdrawal symptoms.

Intravenous drug users may exhibit difficult IV access, infective endocarditis, HIV, and hepatitis infection. However, chronic opioid users also include chronic pain patients and patients receiving opioid maintenance therapy for opioid dependence. It is very important in patients receiving high doses of opioids on a long-term basis for legitimate conditions (chronic pain, cancer, chronic pancreatitis) not to be judgmental and accuse them of drug-seeking behaviors when they present for emergent procedures. Although physicians are under great pressure to curb narcotic prescriptions in the case of abusers, the medical profession must be aware of legitimate narcotic use and take care not to embarrass or emotionally traumatize these patients.

Opioid and elective surgery: baseline opioids (morphine, methadone) should be maintained to control baseline pain levels and prevent withdrawal symptoms.

Buprenorphine and elective surgery: if patients who take mixed agonist–antagonist (buprenorphine or Subutex®, buprenorphine plus naloxone or suboxone) agents undergo major surgery (expecting considerable postoperative pain, as in joint replacement, laparotomy, thoracotomy), they should stop them one to three days before surgery (depending on the dose patients have been taking) to prevent their antagonist effect against postoperative opioids. Supplements of low-dose opioids may be needed at this time to prevent withdrawal symptoms. These mixed agents may be resumed postoperatively when acute pain is no longer an issue and large doses of potent narcotics are no longer needed.

For minor procedures (where severe pain is not expected, as in endoscopic procedures) patients should continue these medications until the morning of surgery to prevent withdrawal symptoms.

Postoperative pain control: as chronic opioid users usually develop opioid tolerance, postoperative pain control strategies also include the expectation of higher opioid requirements compared to opioid naïve patients, patient-controlled analgesia, and multimodal therapy (e.g., nonsteroid anti-inflammatory drugs, NMDA antagonist [ketamine, dextromethophan], antiepileptic [Gabapentin], regional anesthesia [nerve block, neuraxial block].

Cocaine

Mechanism of action: cocaine blocks dopamine, serotonin, and norepinephrine reuptake, which results in CNS stimulation, manifested as euphoria and intoxication. Cocaine also stimulates the sympathetic nervous system (SNS), causing vasoconstriction, hypertension, tachycardia, arrhythmia, and can lead to myocardial infarction, cardiomyopathy, and aortic dissection.

Acute effects: with acute cocaine use, CNS stimulation results in increased anesthetic requirements. SNS stimulation results in hypertension, but beta-blockers are relatively contraindicated for treating the hypertensive effect from cocaine, as unopposed alpha activity could worsen hypertension (labetalol, which has some alpha blockage activity, may be less problematic). On the other hand, patients might have exaggerated hypertension with ephedrine and ketamine.

Chronic effects: as chronic cocaine use leads to depletion of the aforementioned neurotransmitters, patients will experience the opposite physiologic change of acute users. Patients require less anesthetic agents and have a lack of response to ephedrine. Cocaine-induced thrombocytopenia in chronic users might complicate regional anesthesia. Moreover, cocaine smokers are prone to respiratory complications, such as perforated nasal septum, pulmonary infiltrates, and pulmonary edema.

Cocaine and elective surgery: cocaine can last in the urine for two to three days. There is clinical evidence showing that if patients test positive for urine cocaine, but are clinically non-toxic and do not have an extensive cardiac history, they are at

no greater risk, compared to drug-free patients, for proceeding to a surgical procedure.

Amphetamine

Mechanism of action: amphetamines release catecholamine, dopamine, and serotonin from presynaptic nerves, leading to euphoria, CNS stimulation, and SNS stimulation.

Acute effects: like cocaine, increased anesthetic requirements, hypertension, and tachycardia.

Chronic effects: chronic abuse causes neurotransmitter depletion (see above), resulting in decreased anesthetic requirements and downregulation of adrenergic receptors,

Table 13.1 Common substances and clinical implications

Substances	Mechanism of actions	Systemic effects	Clinical implications
Tobacco (smoked)	Nicotine, stimulates nicotinic cholinergic receptor Carbon monoxide Other substance	Nicotine stimulates SNS (increases HR, BP) CO shift of oxygen dissociation to the left Overall effects: increased airway irritability, increased mucous production, decreased mucociliary clearance Associated with COPD, CAD, PVD, stroke, and many cancers	Increased pulmonary complication (laryngospasm, bronchospasm, atelectasis, respiratory failure, mechanical ventilator) and impaired wound healing Cessation of 24 hours will reduce CO–Hb level but needs more than four to eight weeks to decrease pulmonary complications Concern for specific comorbid disease
Ethanol (ingested)	GABA-A agonist	Acute: impaired cognition, delayed gastric emptying time, hypoglycemia, hypovolemia Chronic: associated with cirrhosis, pancreatitis, cardiomyopathy, peripheral neuropathy, encephalopathy, withdrawal symptoms	Acute: uncooperative patient, at risk for aspiration, **decreased** MAC requirement Chronic: **increased** MAC and anesthetic requirement Concern for specific comorbid disease
Opioids (smoked, ingested, IV)	Mu receptor agonist	Acute: impair cognition, respiratory depression, delay gastric emptying time Chronic: tolerance to opioids for pain control, withdrawal, IVDU associated with infective endocarditis	Acute: at risk for aspiration, respiratory depression from sedating medication Chronic: avoid mu agonist or agonist/antagonist, which can precipitate withdrawal symptoms Pain control: maintain baseline opioids, multimodal therapy, anticipate increased opioid requirement
Cocaine (smoked, nasally, IV, rectally, vaginally)	Dopamine, NE, serotonin reuptake inhibitor	Acute: CNS stimulation – agitation, impaired cognition, coma, seizure Sympathetic stimulation – hypertension, tachycardia, cardiac arrhythmia, vasospasm, MI, aortic dissection Pulmonary (cocaine smoker) – crack lung: diffuse alveolar infiltration, fever Chronic: diffuse alveolar damage, noncardiogenic pulmonary edema, pulmonary infarction Cocaine-induced thrombocytopenia	Acute: uncooperative patient at risk for aspiration, **increase** MAC requirement Beta-blocker is contraindicated for cocaine-induced HT Synergetic sympathomimetic effect with ephedrine, causes exaggerated HT Chronic: **decreased** MAC requirement Resistance to ephedrine due to depletion of NE storage
Amphetamines (ingested)	Indirect sympathomimetic, CNS stimulation	Acute: CNS stimulation – agitation, seizure Sympathetic stimulation – hypertension, tachycardia, cardiac arrhythmia Chronic: psychosis, withdrawal could induce depression	Acute: uncooperative patient, **increased** MAC requirement Chronic: **decreased** MAC requirement Resistance to ephedrine due to depletion of NE storage

(From Vacanti et al. 2011. *Essential Clinical Anesthesia*, Cambridge University Press, Table 14.1.)

resulting in attenuated responses to indirect sympathomi-metics such as ephedrine. (A direct sympathomimetic such as phenylephrine is probably a better choice for hypotension.)

Amphetamine and elective surgery: some amphetamine derivatives (methyphenidrate, dextroamphetamine) are also indicated in certain medical conditions such as ADHD and narcolepsy. Even though there are case reports of safe continuations of these medications before elective surgery, this remains controversial.

Marijuana

Mechanism of action: active substances in marijuana are tetra-hydrocannabinol and cannabinoids, which stimulate cannabi-noid receptors (CB1, CB2), produce euphoria, analgesic, anxiolysis, and sedation. Low doses can stimulate the SNS, causing hypertension and tachycardia, whereas high doses inhibit SNS, leading to bradycardia and hypotension.

Effects: life-threatening cardiac arrhythmias in preexisting cardiac condition patients are potentially possible but rare. A fatal overdose is even more extremely rare, and withdrawal symptoms have been reported but mild. Marijuana smokers can have pulmonary effects similar to tobacco (airway irrita-tion, increased CO–Hb level).

Medical marijuana: marijuana is also beneficial and allowed in certain medical conditions such as chemotherapy-induced emesis, AIDS-related anorexia, glaucoma, certain psychiatric conditions, and chronic pain. There are relatively few reports discussing the risks and benefits of stopping med-ical marijuana before surgery; however, recreational use should be prohibited before elective procedure.

Hallucinogens

Hallucinogens include, but are not limited to, lysergic acid diethylamide or LSD, phencyclidine or PCP, psilocybin, and mescaline. *Mechanisms of action* include acting as partial agonist, agonist, or antagonist to serotonin, dopamine, adrenergic recep-tor, resulting in CNS stimulation and mild SNS stimulation.

Effects: as with cocaine and amphetamines, patients might exhibit hypertension, tachycardia, cardiac arrhythmia, and inadequate pressor response to ephedrine. Phenylephrine, a direct-acting adrenergic agent, may be a better choice for treating hypotension.

Questions

1. Which statement is true?
   a. Methadone and suboxone should be continued until the morning of the day of a major operation.
   b. In order to achieve the best postoperative outcome, smoking should be stopped at least two weeks before elective surgery.
   c. Buprenorphine is a drug of choice for pain control in opioid-dependent patients.
   d. Chronic amphetamine users may be resistant to the pressor effect of ephedrine.

2. Which statement is true?
   a. Labetalol is a better choice than metoprolol in cocaine-induced hypertension.
   b. Cocaine-abuse patients will always have an exaggerated response to ephedrine.
   c. Anesthetic requirements increase in acute cocaine, amphetamine, and alcohol abuse.
   d. All pulmonary effects from smoking will be reversed 24 to 48 hours after smoking cessation.

3. Which statement is true?
   a. Chronic alcohol abusers should receive vitamin B$_1$ to prevent heart failure and encephalopathy.
   b. History and physical examination are reliable tools to detect substance abuse in patients.
   c. The primary action of cocaine is to enhance GABA and dopamine receptors.
   d. Marijuana is legal in some states in the United States; medical indications include chemotherapy-induced emesis, ADHD, and narcolepsy.

Answers

1. d. Methadone, but not suboxone, should be continued until the morning of an operation. Cigarette smokers need four to eight weeks of cessation to decrease pulmonary complications. Buprenorphrine has a ceiling effect, and is not a good choice for pain control. Chronic amphetamine users may be resistant to the pressor effects of ephedrine.

2. a. Labetalol has alpha-antagonist activity, and is a better choice than metoprolol in cocaine-induced hypertension. Acute cocaine abuse, but not chronic, may have an exaggerated response to ephedrine. Anesthetic requirements increase in acute cocaine or amphetamine abuse, but decrease in acute alcoholic intoxication. After 24 to 48 hours of smoking cessation, only carboxy–Hb will be decreased, but for decreasing pulmonary complication, it needs four to eight weeks.

3. a. Chronic alcohol abuse is associated with vitamin B$_1$ deficiency and patients should receive vitamin B$_1$ to prevent cardiac beriberi and Wernicke's encephalopathy. History and physical examination are not reliable in substance abuse patients; urine toxicology screen is very useful in this population. Mechanism of action of cocaine is interaction with dopamine, NE, and serotonin. Medical marijuana is legal in some states; indication includes chemotherapy-induced emesis, chronic disease-related anorexia, and glaucoma.

Further reading

Gorman, D., Drewry, A., Huang, Y. L., and Sames, C. (2003). The clinical toxicology of carbon monoxide. *Toxicology* 187(1), 25–38.

Carbon Monoxide Poisoning, in En.wikipedia.org/wiki/carbon_monoxide_poisening

Merlin, M. A., Saybolt, M, Kapitanyan, R. et al. (2010). Intranasal naloxone delivery is an alternative to intravenous naloxone for opioid overdoses. *American Journal of Emergency Medicine* 28, 295–303.

Graetz, T. J. and Leffert, L. R. (2011). Substance abuse and anesthesia. In Vacanti, C. A., Sikka, P. J., Urman, R. D., Dershwitz, M., and Segal, B. S. (eds) *Essential Clinical Anesthesia*. Cambridge: Cambridge University Press.

Findlay, J. Y. (2009). Is there an optimum timing for smoking cessation? In Fleisher, L. A. (ed) *Evidence-based Practice of Anesthesiology*, 2nd edn. Philadelphia: Elsevier Saunders.

Elkassabany, N. (2009). Should we delay surgery in the patient with recent cocaine use? In Fleisher, L. A. (ed) *Evidence-based Practice of Anesthesiology*, 2nd edn. Philadelphia: Elsevier Saunders.

Fischer, S. P., Schmiesing, C. A., Guta, C. G., and Brock-Utne, J. G. (2006). General anesthesia and chronic amphetamine use: should the drug be stopped preoperatively? *Anesthesia and Analgesia* 103, 203–206.

Alford, D. P., Compton, P., and Samet, J. H. (2006). Acute pain management for patients receiving maintenance methadone or buprenorphine therapy. *Annals of Internal Medicine* 144, 127–134.

Anatomy of the human airway

Richard Hsu and Christopher Chen

Keywords

Nasal cavity
Oral cavity
Pharynx
Larynx
Epiglottis
Cricoid
Vallecula
Innervation of the larynx
Sensory innervation of the pharynx
Superior laryngeal nerve
Recurrent laryngeal nerve
Trachea

Nasal cavity

The general function is for the passage, filtration, humidification, and warming of inhaled air. It is bordered by the cribriform plate superiorly, hard palate inferiorly, turbinates laterally, and is divided by the septum in the midsagittal plane. The mucous membranes are supplied by the trigeminal nerve (CN V); more specifically, V1 anteriorly and V2 to the floor of the nasal cavity and posterior structures. Blood supply arises from the ophthalmic, maxillary, and facial arteries.

Oral cavity

This space includes dentition, anterior two-thirds of the tongue, floor of the mouth, as well as the undersurface of the hard and soft palates. The tongue is a special structure in this space. Its anterolateral attachment is to the mandible, and its posterior attachments are to the stylohyoid process and hyoid bone. The *vallecula* is the fossa formed by the folds where the tongue attaches to the epiglottis: the medial glossoepiglottic fold and the lateral pharyngoglottic folds. The mandible articulates with the temporal bones of the cranium, allowing for (1) rotation and (2) translation.

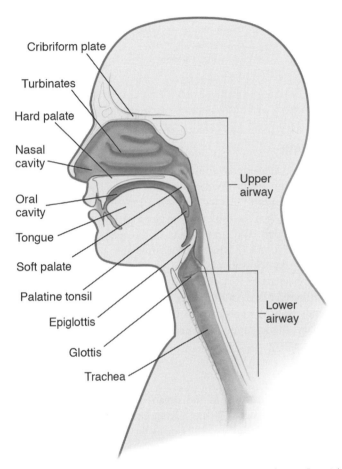

Figure 14.1 Anatomy of the upper airway. (From Vacanti et al. 2011. *Essential Clinical Anesthesia*, Cambridge University Press, p. 94.)

Sensation to the oral cavity is provided by the lingual branch of the trigeminal nerve (anterior two-thirds), glossopharyngeal nerve (posterior one-third), as well as a small component derived from the vagus nerve. Blood supply arises from a branch of the external carotid artery.

Essential Clinical Anesthesia Review: Keywords, Questions and Answers for the Boards, ed. Linda S. Aglio, Robert W. Lekowski, and Richard D. Urman. Published by Cambridge University Press. © Cambridge University Press 2015.

Table 14.1 Clinical manifestations of motor nerve injury

Nerve	Subtypes of injury	Clinical manifestation	Cord position/appearance
Superior laryngeal nerve (external branch)	Unilateral injury – Acute – Chronic	Hoarseness Generally has minimal effect (the other vocal cord compensates), but there may be residual dysphonia	Aryepiglottic fold shortened on the affected side and lengthened on the normal side; affected cord appears wavy
	Bilateral injury	Hoarseness, tiring of voice	Cords appear wavy
Recurrent laryngeal nerve	Unilateral injury	Hoarseness	Affected cord – adducted to the paramedian position
	Bilateral injury – Acute – Chronic	Stridor, respiratory distress Aphonia	Cords nearly closed Cords are paramedian
Vagus nerve (prior to branching of the nerve)	Unilateral injury Bilateral injury	Hoarseness Aphonia	Affected cord – midline Midway between abduction and adduction (cadaveric position)

(From Vacanti et al. 2011. *Essential Clinical Anesthesia*, Cambridge University Press, p. 97, Table 15.3.)

Pharynx

This is a U-shaped fibromuscular tube, which can be anatomically and functionally divided into three areas. The nasopharynx is an air conduit, and receives sensation from the trigeminal nerve (CN V) to the roof, and the glossopharyngeal (CN IX) to the remainder. The oropharynx is the main passage of the aerodigestive tract, which starts after the anterior tonsillar pillars (palatoglossal folds) and receives sensation from the glossopharyngeal (CN IX) and vagus (CN X) nerves. The hypopharynx is a continuation of the aerodigestive tract, and extends from the epiglottis to the lower border of the cricoid cartilage. Blood supply in general is derived from the external carotid artery.

Larynx

The larynx functions as the organ of phonation, and as a passageway for air into the trachea and lungs. It lies at the level of C3–C6 in adults, anterior to the hypopharynx.

It consists of three unpaired cartilages. The *epiglottis* protects the lower airways from contamination from the alimentary tract and is the functional division between the oropharynx and larynx. The prominent thyroid cartilage houses the glottic opening (the narrowest part of the adult airway), and is attached to the hyoid bone superiorly by the thyrohyoid membrane, and to the cricoid cartilage inferiorly by the cricothyroid membrane. The *cricoid* cartilage is signet ring-shaped, and is the only complete cartilaginous ring in the airway. It is the narrowest part of the pediatric airway until age five. The cricothyroid ligament continues posteriorly behind the thyroid cartilage to form the anterior commissure and subsequently to create the true vocal cords, which attach between the arytenoids.

There are also three paired cartilages. The arytenoids are attached to the epiglottis laterally by the aryepiglottic ligaments, and have articular facets inferiorly with the cricoid

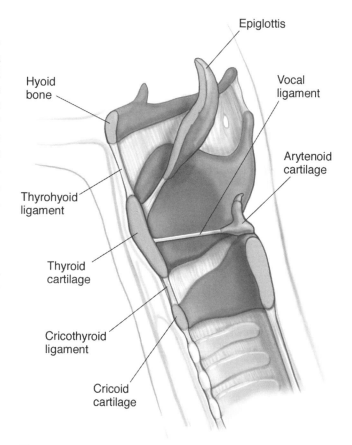

Figure 14.2 Cartilage of the larynx. (From Vacanti et al. 2011. *Essential Clinical Anesthesia*, Cambridge University Press, p. 96.)

cartilage. The remaining two paired cartilages are the cuneiform and the corniculate.

Innervation of the larynx involves different sets of branches of the vagus nerve (CN X). Starting with the superior aspect of the larynx, sensation from the base of the tongue to the vocal cords is supplied by the internal laryngeal nerve, a branch of the *superior laryngeal nerve*. Sensation from the vocal cords down to the trachea and distal airways is supplied by the *recurrent laryngeal nerves*. In terms of motor function, the external laryngeal nerve (also a branch of the superior laryngeal nerve) supplies the cricothyroid muscle, the sole adductor of the vocal cords. The recurrent laryngeal nerves supply all the other muscles of the larynx.

Blood supply of the larynx is derived from the external carotid and subclavian arteries.

Trachea

This is a tubular structure that begins at the inferior border of the cricoid cartilage at the C6 level, consisting of 16 to 20 C-shaped hyaline cartilaginous rings connected posteriorly by the membranous trachea. It is approximately 12 mm in diameter, and 9 to 15 cm in length. The carina is at the level of the sternal angle, between T4 and T5 vertebrae, at which point it divides into the shorter right mainstem bronchus (and subsequently the upper, middle, lower lobes) and the longer left mainstem bronchus (and subsequently the upper and lower lobes).

Questions

1. Which of the following motor nerve injuries would result in stridor and respiratory distress, with the cords appearing nearly closed on examination?
   a. unilateral acute superior laryngeal nerve injury
   b. unilateral chronic superior laryngeal nerve injury
   c. bilateral acute recurrent laryngeal nerve injury
   d. bilateral vagus nerve injury (prior to branching of the nerve)

2. The pharyngeal, or gag, reflex is mediated by which combination of sensory and motor nerves, respectively?
   a. CN V (sensory), CN X (motor)
   b. CN IX (sensory), CN X (motor)
   c. CN V (sensory), CN IX (motor)
   d. CN X (sensory), CN X (motor)

3. Which of the following statements is true?
   a. The cricoid cartilage is the narrowest part of the airway in a ten-year-old child.
   b. The "Adam's apple" is represented by the bony hyoid.
   c. The internal laryngeal nerve provides sensation below the vocal cords and distal airways.
   d. A cricothyroidotomy is an emergency airway maneuver that introduces a breathing tube below the level of the true vocal cords.

Answers

1. c. Acutely, the cords would appear nearly closed on examination, which would result in stridor and acute respiratory distress.
2. b. Remember that in the pharynx, CN IX supplies sensation and CN X is responsible for motor functions.
3. d. A cricothyroidotomy involves an incision through the cricothyroid membrane, which is below the level of the vocal cords.

Further reading

Vacanti, C., Sikka, P., Urman, R., Dershwitz, M., and Segal, B. (eds) (2011). *Essential Clinical Anesthesia*. Cambridge: Cambridge University Press, Chapter 15.

Chapter

15

Airway assessment

Richard Hsu and Christopher Chen

Keywords

Interincisor distance
Thyromental distance
Predictors of difficult mask ventilation
Atlanto-occipital joint extension
Sniffing position
Mallampati classification

Obtaining a pertinent patient history is of crucial importance for the assessment of any airway. A sample of associations between congenital, acquired, and traumatic disease states and problems with airway management is provided in Table 15.1. However, a known history of difficult intubation and ventilation may be the best predictor of difficulty with future attempts.

On physical examination, make note of the patient's general appearance: level of consciousness, evidence of respiratory distress, body habitus, cervical collar, external trauma, pregnancy, and body jewelry. Masking difficulties may arise with, for example, a beard, facial abnormalities, obstructed nares, or trauma. Measure the *interincisor distance* ($\geq$4 cm is desirable), as well as the ability to prognath mandibular teeth anterior to maxillary teeth. A high arched palate or a long narrow mouth may present difficulty, as may a tongue or other oral cavity piercing. Measure the *thyromental distance* ($\geq$7 cm is desirable). Be aware of any dentures, loose teeth, or prominent upper incisors or canines. Lastly, examine the neck: size, length, mobility, and ability to "sniff."

Difficult mask ventilation is defined as inadequate movement of gas in and out of the lungs due to an inadequate mask seal, excessive gas leak, or excessive resistance due to obstruction of the airway. *Predictors of difficult mask ventilation* include BMI >26 kg/m^2, age >55 years, obstructive sleep apnea or history of snoring, and the presence of a beard.

Atlanto-occipital joint extension is important for acquiring an appropriate *sniffing position* for intubation. Elevation of the head to about 10 cm with pads below the occiput and the shoulders remaining on the table helps align the laryngeal and pharyngeal axes. Subsequent head extension at the atlanto-occipital joint creates the shortest distance from the incisors to the glottic opening – it aligns the oral axis with the laryngeal axis. Note that a neck extension of less than 35° is associated with intubation difficulty.

Mallampati classification is performed as the patient sits with the head in a neutral position, mouth open, tongue protruding to its limit, without phonation. It has a 50% sensitivity for predicting difficult intubation, and has a high false-positive rate.

Essential Clinical Anesthesia Review: Keywords, Questions and Answers for the Boards, ed. Linda S. Aglio, Robert W. Lekowski, and Richard D. Urman. Published by Cambridge University Press. © Cambridge University Press 2015.

Table 15.1 Conditions associated with difficult endotracheal intubation.

Syndrome/pathology	Description/difficulty
Congenital syndromes	
Down's	Large tongue and small mouth make laryngoscopy difficult; small subglottic diameter is possible; laryngospasm is common
Klippel–Feil	Neck rigidity because of cervical vertebral fusion
Pierre Robin	Small mouth, large tongue, mandibular anomaly; awake intubation essential in neonate
Treacher Collins	Direct laryngoscopy is difficult
Turner's	High likelihood of difficult direct laryngoscopy
Acquired disease states	
Angioedema	Obstructive swelling renders ventilation and intubation difficult
Ankylosing spondylitis	Fusion of cervical spine may render direct laryngoscopy impossible
Diabetes mellitus	May have reduced mobility of atlanto-occipital joint
Hypothyroidism	Large tongue and abnormal soft tissue (myxedema) make ventilation and intubation difficult
Laryngeal edema (postintubation)	Irritable airway, narrowed laryngeal inlet
Obesity	Upper airway obstruction with loss of consciousness; tissue mass makes mask ventilation difficult
Papillomatosis	Airway obstruction
Radiation therapy	Fibrosis may distort airway or make manipulations difficult
Rheumatoid arthritis	Mandibular hypoplasia, temporomandibular joint arthritis, immobile cervical spine, laryngeal rotation, and cricoarytenoid arthritis make intubation difficult
Sarcoidosis	Airway obstruction (lymphoid tissue)
Scleroderma	Tight skin and temporomandibular joint involvement make mouth opening difficult
Soft tissue, neck injury (edema, bleeding, emphysema)	Anatomic distortion of airway, obstruction
Temporomandibular joint syndrome	Severe impairment of mouth opening
Tetanus	Trismus renders oral intubation impossible
Infection	
Abscess (submandibular, retropharyngeal, Ludwig's angina)	Distortion of airway may render mask ventilation or intubation extremely difficult
Croup, bronchitis, pneumonia (current or recent)	Airway irritability with tendency for cough, laryngospasm, bronchospasm
Epiglottitis	Laryngoscopy may worsen obstruction
Trauma	
Basilar skull fracture	Nasal intubation attempts may result in intracranial trauma
Cervical spine injury	Neck manipulation may traumatize spinal cord
Maxillary or mandibular injury	Airway obstruction, difficult mask ventilation and intubation; cricothyroidotomy may be necessary with combined injuries

(From Vacanti et al. 2011. *Essential Clinical Anesthesia*, Cambridge University Press, p. 99, Table 16.1.)

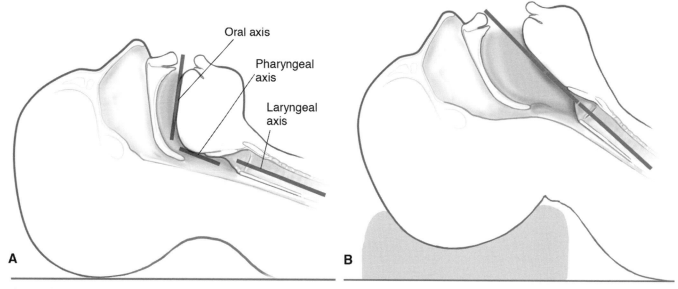

Oral axis

Pharyngeal axis

Laryngeal axis

A   B

Figure 15.1 Ideal position of the head for intubation. (From Vacanti et al. 2011. *Essential Clinical Anesthesia*, Cambridge University Press, p. 100.)

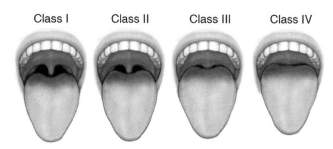

Class I   Class II   Class III   Class IV

Figure 15.2 Optimal position of the head for ventilation or intubation. (From Vacanti et al. 2011. *Essential Clinical Anesthesia*, Cambridge University Press, p. 100.)

Questions

1. Which of the following is not generally considered a predictor of difficult mask ventilation?
   a. weight
   b. age
   c. snoring
   d. beard

2. An airway examination where the soft palate is not visible would receive which Mallampati classification?
   a. Class I
   b. Class II
   c. Class III
   d. Class IV

3. Which of the following syndromes/pathologies is not commonly associated with cervical spine issues relevant to direct laryngoscopy?
   a. Klippel–Feil
   b. scleroderma
   c. ankylosing spondylitis
   d. rheumatoid arthritis

Answers

1. a. Distribution of a person's weight may be more important than the absolute weight itself, and is another reason why a thorough physical examination should be performed in every airway assessment. Again, the predictors of a difficult mask ventilation include BMI >26 kg/m^2, age >55 years, OSA or history of snoring, and the presence of a beard.
2. d. Please refer to the Mallampati classification (see Figure 15.2) for explanation.
3. b. In scleroderma, the primary concern is that tight skin and the involvement of the temporomandibular joint may make mouth opening difficult.

Further reading

Vacanti, C., Sikka, P., Urman, R., Dershwitz, M., and Segal, B. (eds) (2011). *Essential Clinical Anesthesia*. Cambridge: Cambridge University Press, Chapter 16.

16

Perioperative airway management

Richard Hsu and Maksim Zayaruzny

Keywords

Jaw thrust
Laryngeal mask airway (LMA™)
Combitube™
Preoxygenation/denitrogenation
Cormack–Lehane grades of laryngeal views
Mainstem bronchial intubation
Rapid sequence induction (RSI)
Complications of nasotracheal intubation

Invasive airway maintenance techniques

Bag-mask ventilation assists or controls ventilation in the peri-induction/emergence period of a general anesthetic, for the delivery of an anesthetic, and during resuscitation. A good mask seal is the most important aspect. Use of positive pressures in access of 20 mm Hg may result in gastric insufflation, compromise of oxygenation, regurgitation, and/or aspiration.

Jaw thrust involves (1) down-placing the mask onto the face using the thumb and index fingers around the circuit connector of the mask with (2) concurrent upward displacement of the mandible with the remainder of the fingers. Two-handed techniques may be warranted in patients who are elderly, obese, edentulous, or bearded, or have a history of OSA. Excessive force may result in dislocation of the temporo mandibular joint.

The *laryngeal mask airway (LMA™)* consists of a laryngeal mask (a bowl surrounded by an air-/fluid-tight circumferential inflatable cuff), an airway tube, and a 15 mm connector. Placed in the hypopharynx, with the opening overlying the laryngeal entrance, it allows for spontaneous or positive pressure ventilation with up to 20 cm H_2O pressure. LMA™ protects the larynx from oropharyngeal secretions, but not from regurgitated contents. Contraindications include patients with full stomach, laboring women, patients with a risk of pulmonary aspiration (hiatal hernia, significant positional GERD), patients with poor pulmonary/chest wall compliance, limited

mouth opening, as well as obstruction in the oropharyngeal, glottic, or subglottic portions of the airway. Complications include sore throat, vascular compression, mucosal injury, and neurapraxias. The lingual, hypoglossal, and recurrent laryngeal nerves are the three most commonly involved in LMA-related nerve injury.

The *Combitube™* is a double-cuffed, double-lumen tube that allows ventilation and oxygenation with either tracheal or esophageal intubation. It can be inserted without visualization of the larynx and commonly enters the esophagus, allowing ventilation through the proximal opening. The proximal oropharyngeal balloon is made of latex; the distal balloon is similar to the conventional ETT cuff. There are two sizes: original manufacturer recommendation is to use the 41F tube for patients over 5 feet tall and 37F for patients of smaller stature. There are no pediatric sizes.

Contraindications include the presence of esophageal obstruction or other pathology, upper airway foreign body, intact gag reflex, lower airway obstruction, patients with latex allergy, and patients <4 feet tall. Complications include laceration of esophageal wall and pyriform sinus, and other complications similar to those of the LMA.

Endotracheal intubation with a cuffed endotracheal tube provides airway patency and aspiration protection, allows positive pressure mechanical ventilation, and removal of tracheobronchial secretions in the anesthetized patient. It is indicated whenever an airway needs to be protected and maintained, controlled positive pressure mechanical ventilation or neuromuscular blockade is required by the nature of surgery or patient positioning, as well as in cases when postoperative mechanical ventilation is expected.

It is most commonly accomplished via the orotracheal approach, while nasotracheal route is reserved for cases where unobstructed access to the oral cavity is required, in cases of maxillo-mandibular fixation, and in emergent cases where there is limited access to the oral cavity.

Nasotracheal intubation is relatively contraindicated in cases of basal skull fractures, coagulopathy, planned systemic anticoagulation or thrombolysis, and elevated intracranial

Essential Clinical Anesthesia Review: Keywords, Questions and Answers for the Boards, ed. Linda S. Aglio, Robert W. Lekowski, and Richard D. Urman. Published by Cambridge University Press. © Cambridge University Press 2015.

pressure. *Complications of nasotracheal intubation* include epistaxis, retropharyngeal laceration/abscess, turbinectomy, submucosal passage, and sinusitis. High-pressure, low-volume cuffs may cause tracheal mucosal ischemia. Low-pressure, high-volume cuffs may cause sore throat and provide an improper seal to guard against aspiration.

The most common blades for direct laryngoscopy are described below.

- Macintosh (curved): this blade displaces the tongue and soft tissues and is advanced into the vallecula to expose the larynx. Advantages include less dental trauma, more space in the oro- and hypopharynx for ETT passage, and reduced damage to the epiglottis.
- Miller (straight): this blade directly lifts the epiglottis to expose the vocal cords, but it flattens tissue with less displacement, providing less space for ETT passage.

Preparation for general anesthesia and tracheal intubation

Ensure that appropriate airway equipment is checked for proper function, and that there is an oxygen source, suction, flowing IV line, induction agents, neuromuscular blockers, and emergency medications. Proper patient positioning improves laryngeal visualization and *preoxygenation/denitrogenation* provides more time for laryngoscopy in the apneic patient before desaturation occurs. *Preoxygenation/denitrogenation* may be accomplished by deep breathing 100% oxygen via a tight-fitting mask with high fresh gas flows for 1.5 minutes or tidal breathing for 3 minutes. End-tidal oxygen concentration of >90% should be sought.

Troubleshooting an inadequate laryngeal view

Consider adding cricoid pressure – the external laryngeal manipulation of the cricoid cartilage, usually posteriorly and to the right. Also consider using a bougie, which is placed by hooking the tip beneath the epiglottis and advancing into the trachea, after which the ETT can be passed over the bougie.

Verification of ETT placement

Direct visualization of the ETT passing between cords is the gold standard. Other methods for placement verification include bronchoscopy, sustained detection of end-tidal CO_2, auscultation of lung fields, chest expansion, condensation in the ETT during exhalation, palpation of the cuff in the suprasternal notch, and chest radiography. Each of these additional methods in isolation does not absolutely guarantee correct placement, but in combination they increase the likelihood that the placement is endotracheal. *Mainstem bronchial intubation* should be suspected if breath sounds are heard unilaterally or higher than expected increase in airway pressures during positive pressure ventilation is observed. The right mainstem bronchus is the one most commonly intubated if the endotracheal tube is advanced too far blindly.

Airway injuries

The most frequent sites of injury are the larynx (33%), pharynx (19%), and esophagus (18%). The incidence of dental injuries during airway manipulation is approximately one per 2,073 patients, with the maxillary incisors being the most frequently injured teeth.

Rapid sequence induction (RSI)

This technique involves adequate preoxygenation followed by the IV administration of an induction agent and a fast-acting neuromuscular blocking agent in rapid succession with the application of constant cricoid pressure (Sellick's maneuver). Cricoid pressure displaces the cricoid cartilage downward against the compressible esophagus or hypopharyngeal lumen, though its effectiveness is debatable. Mask ventilation should be avoided to decrease the risk of gastric distension and aspiration. This technique minimizes the time between loss of consciousness and intubation in order to theoretically increase protection against pulmonary aspiration. As such, the indication for an RSI is a patient with a high risk of gastric content aspiration.

Extubation

Risks surrounding extubation include aspiration, laryngospasm, bronchospasm, airway obstruction, vocal cord paralysis, hypertension, and hypoventilation. General criteria for extubation include return of consciousness and spontaneous respiration, the ability to follow simple commands, an intact gag reflex, a sustained head lift for five seconds, adequate pain control, and stable vital signs. Objective criteria for extubation include a respiratory rate <30/min, tidal volumes >5 ml/kg, vital capacity >10 ml/kg, peak negative inspiratory force of –20 cm H_2O, dead space to tidal volume ratio of <0.6, PaO_2 >70 mm Hg, and $PaCO_2$ <55 mm Hg on an FiO_2 of 40%.

Figure 16.1 Cormack and Lehane grades of laryngeal views. (From Vacanti et al. 2011. *Essential Clinical Anesthesia*, Cambridge University Press, p. 109.)

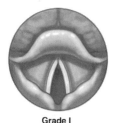

Grade I

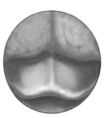

Grade II

Grade III

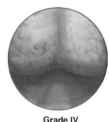

Grade IV

Questions

1. Which of the following airway devices is not appropriate for a patient with a latex allergy?

    a. LMA
    b. Combitube
    c. King laryngeal airway
    d. endotracheal tube

2. In what clinical scenario after an endotracheal tube intubation attempt should you consider mainstem bronchial intubation?

    a. absence of end-tidal CO_2 during controlled ventilation
    b. presence of breathing circuit leak during controlled ventilation
    c. absence of breath sounds over the right upper lung field during controlled ventilation
    d. visualization of the ETT tip at the level of the clavicles on chest radiograph

3. What is an appropriate way to preoxygenate (or denitrogenate) a patient?

    a. Ask the patient to take eight vital capacity breaths at 100% FiO_2 via a tightly fitting face mask.
    b. Leave a face mask attached to 6 l/min of O_2 on a patient breathing tidal volumes for five minutes.
    c. Deliver air at 15 l/min for five minutes via a tightly fitting face mask to a spontaneously breathing patient.
    d. Blow by O_2 for ten minutes.

Answers

1. b. The balloons on the Combitube are made of latex.
2. c. If the endotracheal tube were in a mainstem such that airflow to the right upper lung field is inadequate, then breath sounds would not be auscultated over that lung field. Determining correct endotracheal position requires gathering and interpreting a collection of information and clues that must be done quickly for the safe oxygenation and ventilation of an anesthetized patient.
3. a. Avoid entrainment of room air with a tight face mask seal, and use 100% O_2 during preoxygenation. Eight vital capacity breaths under these conditions will generally preoxygenate a patient well enough for most anesthesiologists to safely perform an endotracheal intubation.

Further reading

Vacanti, C., Sikka, P., Urman, R., Dershwitz, M., and Segal, B. (eds) (2011). *Essential Clinical Anesthesia*. Cambridge: Cambridge University Press, Chapter 17.

Walz, J. M., Zayaruzny, M., and Heard, S. O. (2007). Airway management in critical illness. *Chest* 131(2), 608–620.

17

Management of the difficult airway

Richard Hsu and Maksim Zayaruzny

ASA Difficult Airway Algorithm

The algorithm is provided in Figure 17.1 for ease of reference, and as a visually organized guide for these challenging clinical situations. The development of primary and alternative strategies prior to any airway management scenario is ideal. Note the early strategy of LMA insertion (denoted as a "supraglottic airway" or SGA) after failed "laryngoscopy/face mask ventilation." If a standard LMA is successfully inserted, then the scenario proceeds down the "non-emergency pathway," allowing for adequate ventilation and time to prepare alternative approaches to intubation. The LMA ProSeal has a built-in conduit allowing an orogastric tube to empty gastric contents, while the LMA Fastrach (intubating LMA or iLMA) is designed for use as a tool for blind endotracheal intubation of ETTs up to 8.5 mm in diameter.

Alternative approaches to intubation

Endotracheal tube guides are devices that serve as "Seldinger-like" conduits over which an ETT may be passed into the trachea and/or one ETT to be exchanged for another. Examples include a gum elastic bougie with a coudé tip, or an Aintree AEC ET Guide in conjunction with a flexible fiberoptic bronchoscope.

Lighted stylets transilluminate the soft tissue structures of the anterior neck to direct the ETT into the trachea.

Examples include the Trachlight, Seeing Optical Stylet, Bonfils Retromolar Intubation Fiberscope, Weiss video-optical intubation stylet, and Nanoscope. These may be inappropriate for patients with known airway abnormalities (tumors, infections, abscesses, foreign bodies, trauma), and are relatively contraindicated in obese patients and those with limited neck extension.

Indirect fiberoptic laryngoscopes are another category of useful tools. The Bullard laryngoscope incorporates an anatomically curved blade that does not require a wide mouth opening or neck extension. It has a fiberoptic bundle that allows for distal illumination as well as video output during laryngoscopy. The video Macintosh intubating laryngoscope system and the GlideScope also have video output capabilities that allow for less airway manipulation compared to traditional direct laryngoscopy.

Flexible fiberoptic intubation

Uses include the intubation of the awake or anesthetized patient (orally or nasally) with the suspected difficult airway; intubation of patients with upper or lower airway abnormalities and unstable or immobile cervical spines; means to confirm proper ETT placement, aid for placement/positioning of double-lumen tracheal tubes; and as a tool for performing pulmonary lavage or toilet. Prepare by checking for a shaft without excessive bends or curvatures, a properly functioning control lever, a working "non-clogged" channel for suction or lavage, and adequate focusing of the lens.

Technique tips:

- handle in nondominant hand
- oxygen or suction attached for clearing secretions and lens defogging
- always keep insertion cord (i.e., the shaft) straight
- Ovassapian intubating oral airway, Williams (pink) airway, jaw thrust, or gentle tongue traction from a second operator may improve visualization of the larynx with the bronchoscope

---

Essential Clinical Anesthesia Review: Keywords, Questions and Answers for the Boards, ed. Linda S. Aglio, Robert W. Lekowski, and Richard D. Urman. Published by Cambridge University Press. © Cambridge University Press 2015.

DIFFICULT AIRWAY ALGORITHM

1. **Assess the likelihood and clinical impact of basic management problems:**
   - **Difficulty with patient cooperation or consent**
   - **Difficult mask ventilation**
   - **Difficult supraglottic airway placement**
   - **Difficult laryngoscopy**
   - **Difficult intubation**
   - **Difficult surgical airway access**

2. **Actively pursue opportunities to deliver supplemental oxygen throughout the process of difficult airway management.**

3. **Consider the relative merits and feasibility of basic management choices:**
   - **Awake intubation** *vs.* **intubation after induction of general anesthesia**
   - **Non-invasive technique** *vs.* **invasive techniques for the initial approach to intubation**
   - **Video-assisted laryngoscopy as an initial approach to intubation**
   - **Preservation** *vs.* **ablation of spontaneous ventilation**

4. **Develop primary and alternative strategies:**

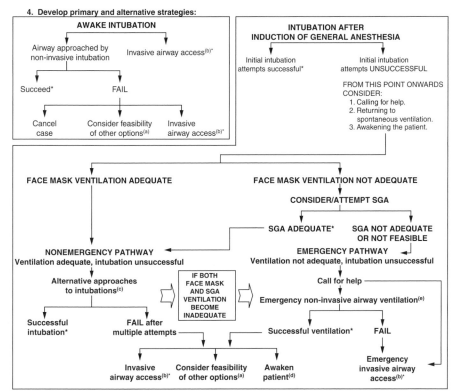

Figure 17.1 Practice guidelines for management of the difficult airway. (ASA February 2013. With permission.)

*Confirm ventilation, tracheal intubation, or SGA placement with exhaled CO_2.

a. Other options include (but are not limited to): surgery utilized face mask or supraglottic airway (SGA) anesthesia (e.g., LMA, ILMA, laryngeal tube), local anesthesia infiltration or regional nerve blockade. Pursuit of these options usually implies that mask ventilation will not be problematic. Therefore, these options may be of limited value if this step in the algorithm has been reached via the Emergency Pathway.

b. Invasive airway access includes surgical or percutaneous airway, jet ventilation, and retrograde intubation.

c. Alternative difficult intubation approaches include (but are not limited to): video-assisted laryngoscopy, alternative laryngoscope blades, SGA (e.g., LMA or ILMA) as an intubation conduit (with or without fiberoptic guidance), fiberoptic intubation, intubating stylet or tube changer, light wand, and blind oral or nasal intubation.

d. Consider re-preparation of the patient for awake intubation or canceling surgery.

e. Emergency non-invasive airway ventilation consists of a SGA.

- use the smallest clinically adequate ETT and turn its bevel 90° counterclockwise to facilitate its entrance into the larynx
- visualize the tracheal carina and ETT tip simultaneously to confirm successful intubation

Transtracheal jet ventilation (TTJV)

A percutaneous emergency airway option that is included in the difficult airway algorithm.

Basic steps include placing a large-bore nonkinking needle/catheter in the midline of the cricothyroid membrane, directed caudad, with the patient supine and neck extended. A Leur-Lok™ syringe (may contain some saline to visualize air bubbles) is attached and continuous aspiration performed once skin is punctured. The needle and catheter are advanced slightly, and then the catheter alone is advanced into the airway. Jet ventilation is then started. Complications include subcutaneous placement, subcutaneous emphysema, pneumomediastinum, pneumothorax, and esophageal puncture.

Cricothyrotomy and emergency tracheostomy

These are invasive procedures usually reserved for the "cannot intubate, cannot ventilate" scenario in which awakening the patient is not an option. Percutaneous cricothyrotomy kits are commercially available and utilize the Seldinger technique for catheter placement (usually >4 mm internal diameter to allow conventional ventilation). A cannula over needle technique with small-bore catheters may also be performed. Small internal diameter requires jet ventilation with passive exhalation. In both cases the needle is first advanced through the midline of the cricothyroid membrane in the caudad direction with aspiration until air is seen in the syringe. Alternatively, a scalpel can be used for a horizontal skin incision over the cricothyroid membrane; the membrane is then incised horizontally and the handle of the scalpel may be inserted and turned 90° to stent the incision. A tracheal hook may also be used to stabilize the trachea as the tracheal tube is inserted. Complications include bleeding, subcutaneous emphysema, pneumothorax, and injury to surrounding structures. Note that damage to the cricoid cartilage may lead to life-threatening airway collapse in children <5 years of age.

Awake intubation

Advantages include the maintenance of spontaneous ventilation, an increase in the size and patency of the pharynx and retropalatal spaces, maintenance of the tone of upper and lower esophageal sphincters, preservation of important airway reflexes, and ability to assess neurologic status in patients with vertebral and spinal cord injuries after the airway is secured and before induction.

If possible, a detailed explanation is essential to ensure patient cooperation. Mild sedation may be achieved with small doses of midazolam, fentanyl, or a dexmedetomidine infusion. Verbal communication is essential throughout the procedure. Oversedation can produce airway obstruction (e.g., an oversedated patient). Antisialagogues (e.g., glycopyrrolate 0.2–0.4 mg IV or IM) increase the effectiveness of topical anesthetics and minimize secretions. Vasoconstrictors – such as oxymetazoline, phenylephrine, and cocaine – for nasal intubation decrease the likelihood and/or extent of bleeding. Local anesthetics for topical application include lidocaine, cocaine (contraindicated in ischemic heart disease, hypertension, tachydysrhythmias, preeclampsia, concurrent MAO-inhibitor use), tetracaine (narrow therapeutic window), and benzocaine (may produce methemoglobinemia).

Topicalization techniques are employed to decrease a patient's reactivity to the procedure itself. Nebulized lidocaine is a popular choice, but its administration takes time and the resultant numbing effect is not always long lived. Local anesthetic-soaked cotton swabs may be placed in the nasal passage or at the base of the palatoglossal arches where the glossopharyngeal nerve travels. Dripping local anesthetic solution on the tongue base with the tongue tip held to promote a slow and more controlled aspiration of the local anesthetic. The superior laryngeal nerve block inhibits sensation of the larynx above the vocal cords, while the *translaryngeal nerve block* via the transtracheal technique anesthetizes the tracheal mucosa innervated by the recurrent laryngeal nerve. A small-bore needle 23/25 gauge is inserted in the midline of the cricothyroid membrane and 2 to 3 cc of 2% lidocaine is injected after intratracheal placement confirmed by aspiration of air. May produce coughing.

Intubation techniques include fiberoptic bronchoscopy (most common), direct laryngoscopy, video laryngoscopy, and blind nasotracheal intubation. Contraindications include patient refusal, inability to cooperate, and a true allergy to local anesthetics. Relative contraindications include ischemic heart disease, poorly controlled bronchospasm, and patients who cannot tolerate raised intracranial or intraocular pressures.

Questions

1. Which of the following basic management problems is not part of the initial assessment as described by the ASA Difficult Airway Algorithm?
   a. difficult ventilation
   b. difficulty with patient cooperation
   c. difficult IV access
   d. difficult tracheostomy

2. In the ASA Difficult Airway Algorithm, when is the most appropriate time to consider alternative approaches to intubation?
   a. ventilation is adequate, intubation is unsuccessful
   b. initial intubation attempts are found to be unsuccessful
   c. cannot intubate, cannot ventilate
   d. initial intubation attempts are successful

3. Which of the following is not a listed option on the ASA Difficult Airway Algorithm for emergency invasive airway access?
   a. LMA
   b. surgical or percutaneous airway
   c. retrograde intubation
   d. jet ventilation

Answers

1. c. Difficult peripheral IV access, while it can make an already challenging airway management situation more complicated, is not considered to be a part of the initial assessment per ASA guidelines.

2. a. Being able to ventilate in a situation where initial intubation is unsuccessful gives the anesthetic provider limited but precious time to consider a safe alternative approach to intubation. While answer choice (b) is a similar situation, no information on the ability to ventilate is included, so the decision to proceed with an urgent surgical airway rather than considering another approach to intubation by the anesthesiologist is a competing option.

3. a. Refer to item "b" in the fine print of the 2013 ASA Difficult Airway Algorithm (see Figure 17.1). This is a slight change in wording from that given by previous versions of the algorithm.

Further reading

Apfelbaum, J. L., Hagberg, C. A., Caplan, R. A. et al. (2013) Practice guidelines for management of the difficult airway: an updated report by the American Society of Anesthesiologists Task Force on Management of the Difficult Airway. *Anesthesiology* 118(2), 51–70.

Vacanti, C., Sikka, P., Urman, R., Dershwitz, M., and Segal, B. (eds) (2011). *Essential Clinical Anesthesia*. Cambridge: Cambridge University Press, Chapter 18.

Gibbs, M. and Walls, R. (2007). Surgical airway. In Hagberg, C.A. (ed) *Benumof's Airway Management*. Philadelphia, PA: Mosby Elsevier, pp. 678–696.

Chapter

18

Medical gas supply, vacuum, and scavenging

Marc Philip T. Pimentel and James H. Philip

Essential Clinical Anesthesia Review: Keywords, Questions and Answers for the Boards, ed. Linda S. Aglio, Robert W. Lekowski, and Richard D. Urman. Published by Cambridge University Press. © Cambridge University Press 2015.

Keywords
Common gas laws
Critical temperature
Avogadro's hypothesis
Oxygen
Nitrous oxide
Medical air
Carbon dioxide
Nitric oxide
Heliox
Manifold and pipeline network
Diameter index safety system (DISS)
Pin index safety system
Vacuum
Scavenging systems

The *common gas laws* describe ideal gases at varying volumes, pressures, and temperatures.

Boyle's law states that $P1 \times V1 = P2 \times V2$

Charles' law states that $V1 / T1 = V2 / T2$

Gay-Lussac's law states that $P1 / T1 = P2 / T2$

The ideal gas law states that $P \times V = n \times R \times T$

Above a gas' *critical temperature*, the gas cannot be liquefied by applying pressure. This is why oxygen (critical temperature –118°C) stored in a container at room temperature is entirely gaseous, but nitrous oxide in a pressurized container (critical temperature 36.5°C) exists as both liquid and gas at room temperature.

According to *Avogadro's hypothesis*, one mole of any gas occupies 22.4 liters at standard temperature and pressure (0°C, 1 Atm), or 24 liters at room temperature and pressure (20°C, 1 Atm). These definitions and constants are useful in calculating the amount of remaining gas in a container by weight.

Medical gases

Oxygen is supplied as a compressed gas through wall pipelines and also in green E-tank cylinders, which hold 660 liters of oxygen at 2,200 psi. The amount of oxygen remaining in an E-cylinder is directly proportional to the E-tank's pressure. *Nitrous oxide* is an anesthetic gas available through both wall pipelines and blue E-cylinders, which hold 1,600 liters at 745 psi. In a full tank, nitrous oxide exists as both a liquid and a gas. The amount of nitrous oxide remaining in an E-tank is estimated by its weight. One mole of nitrous oxide (44 grams per mole) occupies 24 liters at room temperature. The pressure in a nitrous oxide tank begins to fall when all the liquid is evaporated, usually at 25% of capacity. *Medical air* is supplied through wall pipelines and yellow E-cylinders, which hold 600 liters of air at 1,800 psi, comprised of 78% nitrogen, 21% oxygen, and 1% other gases. *Carbon dioxide* is used for insufflation in the operating room. It exists as both liquid and gas in gray E-cylinders containing 1,590 liters at 838 psi. To assess contents the cylinder must be weighed and the tare (empty) weight printed on the tank subtracted. The same is true for nitrous oxide.

Other less commonly used gases include *nitric oxide* (NO) and *Heliox*. *Nitric oxide* is a pulmonary vasodilator that is FDA approved for improving oxygenation in neonates with pulmonary hypertension. It is supplied as a gaseous blend of nitric oxide (800 ppm) and nitrogen (2000 psi) at 21°C. *Heliox* is a mixture of helium and oxygen (usually 70/30, respectively), which is 8% less dense than room air. Laminar airflow is improved because of its low density (decreased Reynolds number), making Heliox useful in cases of upper airway obstruction, status asthmaticus, and stridor.

Gas delivery system

The *manifold and pipeline network* delivers medical gases at 50 to 55 psi. The *diameter index safety system* (DISS) is a set of noninterchangeable connections between the anesthesia machine and the wall pipeline. Small concentric bores and shoulders inside the hose connectors are unique to each gas (e.g., the DISS prevents connection of the nitrous oxide gas outlet to the oxygen supply hose). The *pin index safety system* is a set of noninterchangeable connections between the gas cylinders (e.g., oxygen E-cylinder) and the anesthesia

Table 18.1 Medical gas cylinders

Gas	Formula	Color (US)	Color (international)	psi at 21°C	State in cylinder	E-cylinder capacity, L
Oxygen	O_2	Green	White	1900–2200	Gas	660
Carbon dioxide	CO_2	Gray	Gray	838	Gas and liquid <31°C	1590
Nitrous oxide	N_2O	Blue	Blue	745	Gas and liquid <37°C	1600
Helium	He	Brown	Brown	1600–2000	Gas	500
Nitrogen	N_2	Black	Black	1800–2200	Gas	660
Air		Yellow	White and black	1800	Gas	600

(From Vacanti et al. 2011. *Essential Clinical Anesthesia*, Cambridge University Press, Table 19.4.)

machine. Specific pin configurations are keyed to their respective gases (e.g., the pins prevent connecting the nitrous oxide tank to the oxygen yoke). *Vacuum* is typically provided through a wall pipeline or from a pump on the anesthesia machine at −40 kPa (−300 mm Hg). *Scavenging systems* collect waste anesthetic gases from the breathing system. Active gas disposal systems are most common and employ central vacuum; an interface failure may cause negative pressures in the breathing system. Passive gas disposal systems operate via the pressure of the waste gas itself; occlusion may cause excess positive pressure in the breathing system.

Questions

1. In an oxygen pipeline failure, the back-up oxygen E-cylinder is used in an anesthesia machine with an electrically driven ventilator. The tank reads 1,100 psi. You decide to utilize closed circuit ventilation. How long will the tank last with oxygen fresh gas flow of 0.25 LPM?

   a. 330 minutes
   b. 660 minutes
   b. 1,100 minutes
   d. 1,320 minutes

2. The 22 mm hose used for the passive gas disposal system becomes kinked during a long anesthetic on mechanical ventilation with a circle system breathing circuit. What is an expected consequence of this occlusion?

   a. negative pressure in the breathing system
   b. positive pressure in the breathing system
   c. increased rebreathing of carbon dioxide
   d. exposure of anesthesia provider to waste gas

3. During an anesthesia machine check, it was noted that connecting an E-cylinder to the oxygen yoke was difficult. It was later noted that the oxygen tank was mistaken for a nitrous oxide tank. What prevented this potentially devastating connection?

   a. diameter index safety system
   b. oxygen failsafe device
   c. pin index safety system
   d. scavenging system

Answers

1. d. An E-cylinder holds 660 liters of oxygen at 2,200 psi. At 1,100 psi, only 330 liters of oxygen remain, which would last 1,320 minutes at a flow rate of 0.25 LPM.
2. b. The 22 mm hose carries waste gas, and in a passive gas disposal system, the gas is driven by the patient's exhaled gases. If this hose is kinked, the waste gas will be trapped, and positive pressure will be transmitted to the breathing system.
3. c. The pin index safety system features noninterchangeable connections that are keyed to specific gases. In most cases the pin index safety system prevents misconnection of gases. Misconnection may still occur if the pins are damaged or missing.

Further reading

Eisenkraft, J. B. (2008). Anesthesia delivery systems. In Longnecker, D., Brown, D., Newman, M., and Zapol, W. (eds) *Anesthesiology*. New York: McGraw-Hill, pp. 767–820.

US Department of Labor, Occupational Safety & Health Administration (OSHA). (2014). Waste anesthetic gases. www.osha.gov/SLTC/wasteanestheticgases/ [Accessed May 9, 2014].

Chapter

19

Anesthesia machine

Marc Philip T. Pimentel and James H. Philip

The anesthesia machine can be divided into parts, according to pressure: the *high-pressure system* is exposed to the pressure of the cylinders (up to 2,200 psi), containing the yoke, pressure gauges, and pressure regulators. The *intermediate-pressure system* is exposed to the wall pipelines (55 psi), containing the pipeline connections, pressure gauges, flow meters, etc. The *low-pressure system* lies from the needle valves of the flow meters to the common gas outlet. These do not include the patient breathing circuit, which is also sometimes called the low-pressure system.

The *diameter index safety system* (DISS) and *pin index safety system* are described in Chapter 18. They ensure that air, nitrous oxide, and oxygen reach the anesthesia machine properly.

Medical gas inlets provide air, nitrous oxide, and oxygen from the wall pipeline to the operating room, usually at

50 to 55 psi. *Pressure regulators* in the anesthesia machine are used to lower the pressure of cylinder gases from >1,000 psi down to 45 to 50 psi. Because the cylinder gases are regulated to a lower pressure than the wall pipeline, the wall pipeline is used preferentially to the cylinder while both are connected. *Check valves* prevent backwards flow of gases from the cylinders into the pipeline or other cylinders.

The *oxygen failsafe device* stops the flow of nitrous oxide in case of low oxygen pressure in the anesthesia machine. *Proportioning systems* link the nitrous oxide and oxygen controls at the flow meter, with a target minimum oxygen concentration in the fresh gas flow. Although the *oxygen failsafe device* and *proportioning systems* help maintain a minimum FiO_2, an inspired oxygen monitor is required to prevent hypoxic gas mixtures from reaching the patient, especially with low fresh gas flow. The *oxygen low-pressure alarm* is triggered when the oxygen supply is critically low. In older anesthesia machines, this alarm is sounded by a whistle and may be silent when the oxygen supply decreases very slowly.

Flow meters provide the fresh gases (air, nitrous oxide, oxygen) through the vaporizers to the common gas outlet. The oxygen flow meter is always positioned last (closest to the patient) to ensure continued oxygen flow in case of a leak in the nitrous oxide or airflow meters or conduits. Inside the flow meter, the fresh gas levitates a cylindrical or a spherical bobbin (each measured at its *widest* point) that indicates the flow. At low flows, laminar flow predominates and the bobbin's height is determined by gas viscosity. At higher flows, turbulence occurs and the bobbin's height is determined by gas density.

A *variable bypass vaporizer* is commonly used to administer halothane, isoflurane, and sevoflurane. Fresh gas from the *flow meters* passes through the vaporizer. Some of the stream is diverted to the vaporizing chamber, which saturates the gas passing through it with volatile anesthetic. This active stream recombines with the bypass stream before leaving the vaporizer. The *control dial* changes the proportion of these two streams, which is called the *splitting ratio*, and determines the partial pressure of volatile agent delivered by the vaporizer.

Essential Clinical Anesthesia Review: Keywords, Questions and Answers for the Boards, ed. Linda S. Aglio, Robert W. Lekowski, and Richard D. Urman. Published by Cambridge University Press. © Cambridge University Press 2015.

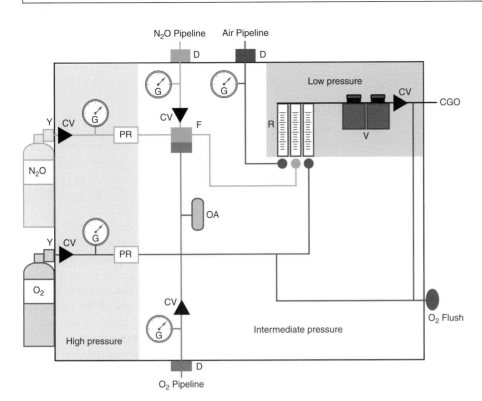

Figure 19.1 Structure of an anesthesia machine. Y, yoke; D, diameter index safety system (DISS); G, pressure gauge; PR, pressure regulator; F, oxygen failsafe device; OA, oxygen alarm; R, rotameters; V, vaporizer assembly; CV, check valve. (From Vacanti et al. 2011. *Essential Clinical Anesthesia*, Cambridge University Press, Figure 20.2.)

Each vaporizer is calibrated for specific volatile agents, each of which has a different saturated vapor pressure (SVP). For example, placing sevoflurane (SVP 157 mm Hg) in an isoflurane vaporizer (calibrated to SVP 238 mm Hg) results in lower than expected sevoflurane output. The splitting actually occurs at the outflow of the vaporization chamber according to manufacturers' user manuals and newer textbooks.

As volatile agents evaporate, the latent heat of vaporization cools the liquid and thereby decreases the saturated vapor pressure and resulting vapor output. The *variable bypass vaporizer* achieves *temperature compensation* via a bimetallic strip at the vaporization chamber inlet to adjust the effective splitting ratio to offset this temperature effect.

At high altitudes and decreased atmospheric pressure, the saturated vapor pressure of a liquid agent remains unchanged (at constant temperature). The splitting ratio remains almost unchanged, and so the partial pressure of delivered agent remains constant, as does its anesthetizing capability. However, because the atmospheric pressure has decreased and partial pressure of delivered agent remains constant, the output concentration of delivered agent is increased. In other words, the vaporizer puts out a higher fraction of a lower atmospheric pressure, resulting in the same partial pressure. Anesthetization at altitude remains unchanged.

Desflurane has a high vapor pressure (SVP 660 mm Hg), close to atmospheric pressure (760 mm Hg), which makes it prone to boiling at room temperature. To avoid the unpredictable vaporizer output from boiling desflurane (and possible volatile agent overdose), a different design is used to provide more consistent vaporization. A specially designed *desflurane vaporizer* heats and pressurizes the desflurane, providing consistent vapor flow that is added to the fresh gas flow. Constant concentration is thereby produced. At high altitudes, this results in decreased agent partial pressure and decreased anesthetization unless the vaporizer setting is increased to offset this effect.

The *Aladin vaporizing system* uses a different refillable cassette for each agent. The vaporization is controlled by a computer.

The *common gas outlet* (CGO) is the final point for gas output from the anesthesia machine to the breathing circuit. It receives low-pressure gas from the vaporizers and from the *oxygen flush* at the final exit point at a flow between 35 and 75 L/min. A check valve protects the vaporizer and flow meters from the oxygen flush. The patient breathing circuit is connected to the CGO. Older machines had an accessible CGO. Most newer machines do not; they have a direct connection to the breathing circuit.

$Vapor(ml)$

$$= Fresh\ gas\ flow\ through\ vaporizing\ chamber(ml)x\frac{SVP}{ATP-SVP}$$

Table 19.1 Approximate output concentration of an agent when administered through a different vaporizer set to deliver 1%

Agent	SVP, mm Hg at 20°C	Vaporizer	Output concentration %
Sevoflurane	157	Isoflurane	057
Isoflurane	238	Sevoflurane	1.75
Halothane	243	Isoflurane	1.03
Isoflurane	238	Halothane	0.97

(From Vacanti et al. 2011. *Essential Clinical Anesthesia*, Cambridge University Press, Table 20.1.)

Questions

1. During a medical mission, the team runs out of isoflurane. Which of the following volatile agents would be most suitable to fill an isoflurane vaporizer?

   a. sevoflurane
   b. halothane
   c. enflurane
   d. desflurane

2. While increasing the fresh gas flow during a short general anesthetic with sevoflurane at fresh gas flow of 1 LPM, it is noted that the rotameter bobbin is stuck against the side wall of the Thorpe tube. What would be the effect on the inspired concentration of sevoflurane?

   a. The observed concentration of inspired sevoflurane would be higher than expected.
   b. The observed concentration of inspired sevoflurane would be lower than expected.
   c. The observed concentration of inspired sevoflurane would be unchanged.
   d. The observed concentration of inspired sevoflurane would fall to zero.

3. A leak in the vaporizer system occurs, and fresh gas no longer flows to the common gas outlet. The patient is receiving positive pressure ventilation on an anesthesia machine with fresh gas decoupling. How can oxygen best be provided to the patient using the anesthesia machine?

   a. Use the oxygen flush valve during inspiration.
   b. Use the oxygen flush valve during expiration.
   c. Use the oxygen flush valve during both inspiration and expiration.

   d. Disconnect the anesthesia machine from the pipeline oxygen and activate the back-up oxygen cylinder.

Answers

1. b. The amount of gas delivered by a variable bypass vaporizer at a given fresh gas flow is determined by the splitting ratio. When a different gas is placed in the vaporizer, the output is affected by the saturated vapor pressure of the new gas. Halothane (SVP 243 mm Hg) would be most suitable in an isoflurane vaporizer (SVP 283 mm Hg) because it has a similar vapor pressure. Filling the vaporizer with a volatile agent with higher vapor pressure would result in increased vaporizer output.

2. a. Fresh gas flow is directly proportional to vaporizer output. Because more gas is flowing through the vaporizing chamber, more volatile agent can be carried to the breathing circuit. The rotameter bobbin is stuck in a position that is lower than the real flow. Therefore there is a higher than expected fresh gas flow. At this low fresh gas flow, the inspired concentration of volatile agent is lower than the delivered concentration because of dilution of the volatile agent in the circuit by exhaled gas. In this example, the increased fresh gas flow will raise the inspired concentration toward the vaporizer setting concentration.

3. b. The oxygen flush valve delivers high-flow oxygen at 35 to 70 LPM from the intermediate-pressure system, bypassing the vaporizers and flow meters. Activating the oxygen flush during inspiration has the potential to expose the patient to these high flows and high pressures and thereby produce barotrauma. Modern anesthesia machines feature fresh gas decoupling or pressure limiting features that protect against this injury.

Further reading

Eisenkraft, J. B. (2013). Anesthesia delivery systems. In Ehrenwerth, J., Eisenkraft, J. B., and Berry, J. M. (eds) *Anesthesia Equipment: Principles and Applications*. Elsevier.

Brockwell, R. C. and Andrews, J. J. (2009). Inhaled anesthetic delivery systems. In Miller, R. D., Eriksson, L. I., Fleisher, L. A. et al. (eds) *Miller's Anesthesia*, 7th edn. Philadelphia: Churchill-Livingstone, pp. 667–718.

Chapter

20

Anesthesia ventilators

Marc Philip T. Pimentel and James H. Philip

Keywords

Volume controlled ventilation (VCV)
Tidal volume
Pressure controlled ventilation (PCV)
Inspiratory pressure
Synchronized intermittent mandatory
    ventilation (SIMV)
Pressure support ventilation (PSV)
Positive end-expiratory pressure (PEEP)
Gas-driven ventilators
Ascending bellows
Descending bellows
Piston-driven ventilators
Fresh gas decoupling
Fresh gas compensation
Fresh gas coupling

Modes of ventilation

Volume controlled ventilation (VCV) is the most commonly used mode of ventilation in the operating room. The *tidal volume* is set by the anesthetist (usually 7–10 ml/kg ideal body mass). The ventilator delivers a constant flow until the set tidal volume is reached, with a corresponding rise in airway pressure. A pressure limit of 40 cm H_2O helps avoid barotrauma. Volume controlled ventilation is useful because it provides consistent minute ventilation, especially with changes in airway compliance (laparoscopic insufflation, position change, etc.).

Pressure controlled ventilation (PCV) is another mode of ventilation commonly used in the operating room. The *inspiratory pressure* is set by the anesthetist (usually 10–30 cm H_2O). During each breath, the ventilator tries to deliver and maintain the set inspiratory pressure. To do this it delivers high flow, then falling flow until the inspiratory pressure is reached. This produces a *tidal volume*. Pressure controlled ventilation generates larger *tidal volumes* with airway pressures

lower than peak pressures with VCV. High abdominal pressure during laparoscopic insufflation will result in diminished tidal volumes and hypoventilation. A sudden fall in insufflation pressure will result in a large tidal volume and possibly volutrauma.

Synchronized intermittent mandatory ventilation (SIMV) allows the patient to breathe between ventilator-driven breaths. The tidal volume and respiratory rate are set by the anesthetist. During a patient-initiated breath, the ventilator delays the next driven breath to avoid breath stacking. Synchronized intermittent mandatory ventilation is useful for weaning patients to spontaneous ventilation, especially during emergence from anesthesia. The driven breaths can be volume controlled or pressure controlled.

Pressure support ventilation (PSV) is a mode used during spontaneous ventilation (i.e., the patient is able to initiate breaths). The inspiratory pressure is set by the anesthetist. The ventilator delivers this pressure each time the patient initiates a breath, which decreases the work of breathing and allows the patient to set the respiratory rate. A back-up mode is included in case of apnea. PSV is useful for maintaining minute ventilation in spontaneously ventilating patients. Because low pressures can be set, this mode is commonly used with the laryngeal mask airway.

Positive end-expiratory pressure (PEEP) is the pressure the ventilator maintains during and at the end of exhalation. Positive end-expiratory pressure reduces atelectasis and maintains the patency of small airways, improving PaO_2 at a given FiO_2. Increased PEEP reduces venous return and may lead to hypotension. Excessive PEEP with high inspiratory pressures can lead to barotrauma.

Ventilator drives

Gas-driven ventilators are powered by compressed gases, such as air or oxygen. Bellows are used to drive gases into the patient's breathing circuit. *Ascending bellows* rise during exhalation and can create positive pressure in the breathing circuit. They will cease to rise in the event of a circuit disconnect.

Essential Clinical Anesthesia Review: Keywords, Questions and Answers for the Boards, ed. Linda S. Aglio, Robert W. Lekowski, and Richard D. Urman. Published by Cambridge University Press. © Cambridge University Press 2015.

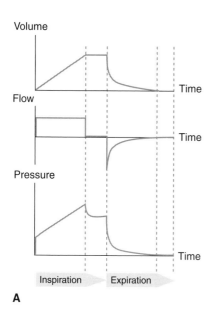

A

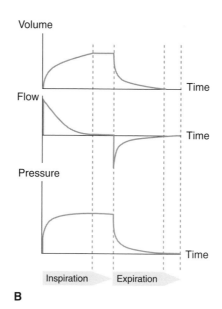

B

Figure 20.1 Relationship between tidal volume, flow, and pressure. (A) Volume controlled ventilation; (B) pressure controlled ventilation. (From Vacanti et al. 2011. *Essential Clinical Anesthesia*, Cambridge University Press, Figure 21.1.)

Descending bellows fall on exhalation. They are considered unsafe because they will continue to operate even in the presence of a circuit disconnect, with the operator unaware of the disconnect. In this situation air is entrained by the descending bellows' inward leak. Modern gas-driven ascending-bellows ventilators use feedback control of bellows movement to provide constant tidal volume despite changes in fresh gas flow. This is called *fresh gas compensation*. It originated with GE-Datex-Ohmeda and is now present on most anesthesia machines that use bellows-driven ventilation. A drawback of gas-driven ventilation is that during oxygen pipeline failure, the ventilator is driven by the back-up oxygen cylinder and depletes it.

Piston-driven ventilators use an electrically driven piston to push gases into the lungs with volume control or create pressure control through electronic feedback. *Fresh gas decoupling* is achieved by diverting the fresh gas into the reservoir bag during inspiration. These ventilators operate independently of driving gas, but they require battery back-up during power failure. These ventilators are produced by Dräger Corporation.

Fresh gas coupling occurs in older ventilators and is a popular topic for board review. Fresh gas flow occurring during inspiration is added to the tidal volume. For example, a fresh gas flow of 6 LPM results in 100 ml/s flow during each delivered inspiration. Over a two-second inspiratory time, the tidal volume is increased by 200 ml.

Questions

1. A patient with morbid obesity is undergoing laparoscopic surgery. He is being mechanically ventilated with VCV (tidal volume 500 ml, respiratory rate 12 breaths per minute, peak inspiratory pressure 30 cm H_2O). The patient is placed into the Trendelenburg position, and the abdomen is insufflated. The peak pressures reach the limit of 40 cm H_2O, and the delivered tidal volume decreases to 400 ml. Breath sounds are equal bilaterally. What might be a good alternative mode of ventilation at this time?

   a. VCV
   b. PSV
   c. PCV
   d. SIMV

2. Four hours have passed since the start of laparoscopic surgery in a morbidly obese patient. You notice the SpO_2 decreasing slowly during the case. The patient is being ventilated with PCV with inspiratory pressure 25 cm H_2O, PEEP 0 cm H_2O, and respiratory rate 12 breaths per minute with resulting tidal volumes of 500 ml. FiO_2 is already 100%. What else can be done to increase the patient's SpO_2?

   a. increase minute ventilation
   b. decrease FiO_2
   c. give recruitment breaths and increase PEEP
   d. increase the inspiratory pressure

3. Anesthesia is being delivered with an older ventilator that exhibits fresh gas coupling. The fresh gas flow is 3 LPM. The set tidal volume is 400 ml per breath. The respiratory rate is ten breaths per minute. The I:E ratio (inspiratory time:expiratory time) is 1:2. What is the resulting tidal volume?

   a. 300 ml
   b. 400 ml
   c. 500 ml
   d. 700 ml

Answers

1. c. Because of its flow characteristics, PCV tends to produce greater volumes with lower inspiratory pressures versus the

peak pressures observed with VCV. Obese patients in the Trendelenburg position are at risk for decreased tidal volumes because of the weight of soft tissues on the chest wall and diaphragm. Appropriately managed PCV may be able to maximize tidal volumes while maintaining acceptable peak pressures.

2. c. Obese patients are at increased risk for pulmonary atelectasis, especially with extended case duration. A recruitment breath of up to 40 cm H_2O for 30 to 60 seconds, followed by addition of PEEP can be helpful.

3. c. Fresh gas coupling occurs when fresh gas that flows during inspiration adds to the intended tidal volume. The respiratory rate is ten breaths per minute with an I:E ratio of 1:2 (6 seconds per breath = 2 seconds inspiration + 4 seconds expiration). A fresh gas flow of three liters per minute (50 ml per second) results in an additional 100 ml per breath over 2 seconds. 400 ml + 100 ml = 500 ml tidal volume.

Further reading

Eisenkraft, J. B. (2013). Anesthesia delivery systems. In Ehrenwerth, J., Eisenkraft, J. B., and Berry, J. M. (eds) *Anesthesia Equipment: Principles and Applications*. Elsevier.

Brockwell, R. C. and Andrews, J. J. (2009). Inhaled anesthetic delivery systems. In Miller, R. D., Eriksson, L. I., Fleisher, L. A. et al. (eds) *Miller's Anesthesia*, 7th edn. Philadelphia: Churchill-Livingstone, pp. 667–718.

Chapter 21

Anesthesia breathing apparatuses

Marc Philip T. Pimentel and James H. Philip

Keywords

CO_2 absorber
Reservoir
Adjustable pressure limiting valve (APL valve)
Rebreathing
Dead space
Mapleson circuits
Circle system
Soda lime
Baralyme
Compound A
Carbon monoxide

Anesthesia breathing apparatuses allow patients to breathe a desired gas mixture. The main parts of an anesthesia breathing apparatus are the reservoir, conduit, and a mechanism for CO_2 elimination (or *CO_2 absorber*). The *reservoir* provides sufficient gas for inhalation. A low resistance conduit carries gas to the patient. An *adjustable pressure limiting valve* (APL valve) allows gas to exit the circuit when a pressure limit is reached.

On inhalation the patient *rebreathes* a column of gas from the previous breath. This volume is known as the *dead space*. It extends from the patient to the site of CO_2 elimination (either the exhalation valve or the fresh gas source). The patient's tidal volume must be greater than the dead space in order to receive fresh gases and eliminate CO_2.

Mapleson circuits in their original forms are no longer used in clinical practice, but are still tested on examinations. They differ from each other by the positions of the fresh gas flow, APL valve, conduit, and reservoir (see Figure 21.1). During spontaneous ventilation, rebreathing is minimized by *Mapleson circuits* A > (D, F, E) > (C, B). However, during positive pressure ventilation, *rebreathing* is minimized by (D, F, E) > (B, C) > A.

The *circle system* is used in most modern anesthesia delivery systems (see Figure 21.2). The circuit contains an inspiratory limb, expiratory limb, unidirectional valves, CO_2 absorber, APL valve, and a reservoir bag. Because of the valves, gas flows only in one direction, and dead space is minimized, terminating at the wye piece (Y-piece).

Instead of venting CO_2 from the circuit, *CO_2 absorbents* are used to chemically remove CO_2 from the circuit. Two typical CO_2 absorbents are *soda lime* (e.g., Sodasorb®, W.R. Grace) and *Baralyme®* (Allied Chemical Products). *Soda lime* is a mixture of calcium hydroxide, water, sodium hydroxide, and potassium hydroxide. *Baralyme* is a similar material in which barium hydroxide is substituted for sodium hydroxide. CO_2 from the circuit combines with water to form carbonic acid, which is neutralized by the strong bases in the absorber. The final products are calcium carbonate (or barium carbonate), heat, and water. Baralyme was noted to produce the greatest amount of heat, and absorber fires were reported after using Baralyme with sevoflurane. This product was removed from the US market in 2004.

Compound A is produced when sevoflurane is used with CO_2 absorbents. Compound A is nephrotoxic in rats, but no cases of nephrotoxicity have been reported in humans. Factors that increase compound A formation are low fresh gas flow (<1 LPM), high sevoflurane concentration, high absorbent temperatures, desiccation of CO_2 absorbent, and using Baralyme rather than soda lime.

Carbon monoxide is produced when desflurane or isoflurane are used with CO_2 absorbents. Factors that increase carbon monoxide production are similar to those that produce compound A. Carbon monoxide production is greatest with desflurane > isoflurane > halothane = sevoflurane.

Several newer products absorb CO_2 at lower temperature and do not produce compound A or carbon monoxide. Examples are Amsorb®, Draegersorb Free, and Medisorb.

It is important to know when the *CO_2 absorber* is exhausted. Residual CO_2 will appear in the inspired gas mixture. pH indicators in the absorber will change color when the absorbent is exhausted; most change from white to purple.

Essential Clinical Anesthesia Review: Keywords, Questions and Answers for the Boards, ed. Linda S. Aglio, Robert W. Lekowski, and Richard D. Urman. Published by Cambridge University Press. © Cambridge University Press 2015.

Table 21.1 Classification of breathing systems

Type	Inhalation	Exhalation to	Reservoir	Rebreathing	Example
Open	Air + agent	Atmosphere	Nil	Nil	Open drop T-piece
Semi-open	Air + agent from machine	Atmosphere	Small	Minimal	T-piece with small reservoir
Semi-closed	From machine	Atmosphere + machine	Large	Possible	Magill attachment; Mapleson systems
Closed	From machine	Machine	Large	Yes + CO_2 absorbent	Circle system

(From Vacanti et al. 2011. *Essential Clinical Anesthesia*, Cambridge University Press, Table 22.1.)

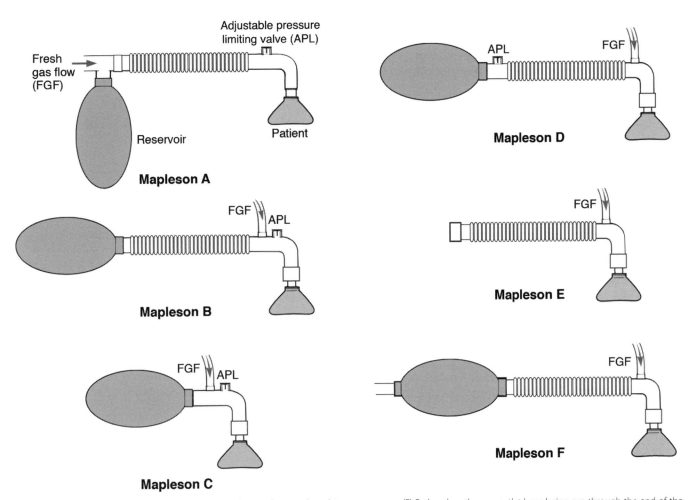

Figure 21.1 (A-D) The historical classification by Mapleson of various breathing apparatuses. (E) Rather than the gas outlet hose being run through the end of the breathing tube, it can run for a short distance outside the tube and then enter it closer to the mask. This will allow for the addition of a bag on the end of the tube to assist ventilation. (F) The gas supply hose can run external to the breathing tube and enter the tube adjacent to the mask. This is what is done in an Ayre T-piece. Again, a bag may be added to assist ventilation, making it a Mapleson F circuit or a Jackson–Rees modification to an Ayre T-piece. (From Vacanti et al. 2011. *Essential Clinical Anesthesia*, Cambridge University Press, Figure 22.4.)

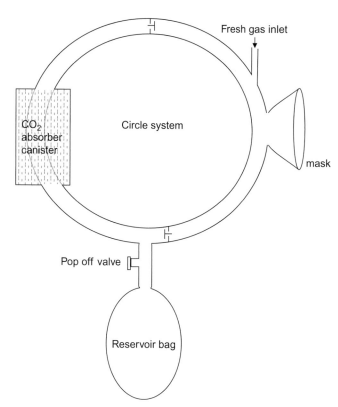

Figure 21.2. A circle system. (From Vacanti et al. 2011. *Essential Clinical Anesthesia*, Cambridge University Press, Figure 22.6.)

Absorbent temperature will also increase because the CO_2 absorbing reaction is exothermic.

Figure 21.2 shows the breathing circuit for the GE ADU anesthesia machine. In all other anesthesia machines the fresh gas inlet is between the CO_2 absorber canister and the inspiratory valve, which is shown at the top of the figure.

Questions

1. A 50-year-old man collapses in an anesthesia museum. A breathing device from the Mapleson circuit exhibit is used for controlled ventilation. What is the best choice for preventing rebreathing in this patient?
   a. Mapleson A
   b. Mapleson B
   c. Mapleson C
   d. Mapleson D

2. Ten hours into a Monday morning Whipple procedure under closed circuit desflurane with Baralyme, an ABG shows SpO_2 70%. The pulse oximeter reads SpO_2 96%. What is the best course of action?
   a. repeat the ABG
   b. flush the circuit with 100% oxygen, change the CO_2 absorber, and switch to sevoflurane with fresh gas flow >2 LPM
   c. administer methylene blue with 100% oxygen
   d. increase PEEP

3. A patient is breathing spontaneously through a circle system connected to an anesthesia machine. Fresh gas flow is 10 liters per minute. Minute ventilation is 5 liters per minute. The expiratory limb of the circle system is disconnected. What is the effect on end-tidal carbon dioxide?
   a. end-tidal carbon dioxide will increase
   b. end-tidal carbon dioxide will decrease
   c. end-tidal carbon dioxide will remain constant
   d. the patient will rebreathe carbon dioxide

Answers

1. d. Rebreathing is best minimized with Mapleson circuits D, E, and F, which position the fresh gas closest to the patient and the APL valve is positioned more distally or is missing.
2. b. The patient has been poisoned with carbon monoxide, which is evident from the difference in pulse oximetry and ABG readings. Carbon monoxide production occurs most when desflurane is used with Baralyme at low fresh gas flows.
3. c. Because of the expiratory limb disconnection, the patient's exhaled gases are not retained in the breathing circuit and do not reach the carbon dioxide absorbent. However, the fresh gas flow far exceeds the patient's minute ventilation, and rebreathing of carbon dioxide will not occur, despite the disconnect. Hence, the patient's end-tidal carbon dioxide will remain constant.

Further reading

Brockwell, R. C. and Andrews, J. J. (2009). Inhaled anesthetic delivery systems. In Miller, R. D., Eriksson, L. I., Fleisher, L. A. (eds) *Miller's Anesthesia*, 7th edn. Philadelphia: Churchill-Livingstone, pp. 667–718.

Kodali, B. S. Anesthesia breathing systems. www.capnography.com/Circuits/breathingcircuits.htm [Accessed May 9, 2014].

22

Electrical safety

Marc Philip T. Pimentel and James H. Philip

Keywords

Ohm's law
Voltage
Current
Resistance
Isolated power supply
Isolation transformer
Line isolation monitor (LIM)
Microshock
Macroshock
Unipolar electrocautery
Bipolar electrocautery

Ohm's law states that *voltage* is equal to *current* multiplied by *resistance* ($V = I \times R$). *Voltage* is the energy carried per charge that passes through a circuit, measured in volts. *Current* is the electrical charge that passes through a circuit per second, measured in amperes. *Resistance* describes how difficult it is for current to flow through the circuit, measured in ohms. Transposing Ohm's law, $I = V/R$. Thus current flows in proportion to 1/Resistance. Qualitatively and colloquially stated, current tends to flow through the path of least resistance. An electrical shock occurs when a complete circuit is made from a power source, through a patient, through a ground or other conductor, and back to the power source. A shock will not occur if the circuit is incomplete.

In the OR, an *isolated power supply* reduces the risk of accidental electrical shock in case of one electrical fault (i.e., instrument or person touching an exposed electrical wire). The *isolated power supply* does so by *not* having an electrical connection to the ground. This is achieved by the use of an *isolation transformer*. The system is said to be "ungrounded." In the case of a single fault, the current is unable to return to the power supply via the ground, so a complete circuit cannot be made. In order for a shock to occur, two faults are required (e.g., touching two short-circuited devices). A *line isolation monitor* (LIM) sounds an alarm when it detects the first electrical fault. This fault will allow significant electrical

current to flow if there were to be a second fault. There is no additional alarm for the second fault. Rather, shock, sparks, or circuit breaker opening occurs and the existence of a problem is obvious. The LIM is able to reduce the possibility of *macroshock* (milliamps and greater), but *microshock* (usually microamps) can still occur without an alarm from the LIM.

Microshock is caused by smaller currents and is important when wires or electrodes are close to the endocardium, which is especially susceptible to these smaller currents. Pacemakers and saline-filled central venous catheters are conductors that can cause arrhythmias from the passage of microamps passing through the heart.

Electrocautery is typically used in the OR. *Unipolar* electrocautery is the most common: current passes from the tip of the electrocautery device, burns through the target tissue, and then returns to the unit via a large current-dispersing return pad and return wire. *Bipolar electrocautery* causes current to pass between two closely spaced prongs with the target tissue in between. Because the current passes between the two prongs, there is no need for a return pad. In patients with pacemakers, placement of the return pad away from the pacemaker is recommended to avoid inadvertent microshock; use of bipolar electrocautery also reduces this risk. Open delivery of oxygen (e.g., loose face mask or nasal prongs) poses a fire danger whenever high heat (e.g., sparks or laser) and fuel (e.g., flammable material or patient tissue) are near each other.

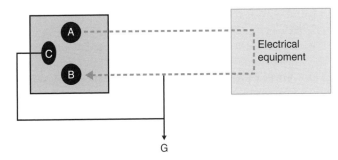

Figure 22.1 Concept of grounding. (From Vacanti et al. 2011. *Essential Clinical Anesthesia*, Cambridge University Press, Figure 23.4.)

Essential Clinical Anesthesia Review: Keywords, Questions and Answers for the Boards, ed. Linda S. Aglio, Robert W. Lekowski, and Richard D. Urman. Published by Cambridge University Press. © Cambridge University Press 2015.

Table 22.1 Effects of 60 Hz AC on an average human for a one-second duration of contact

Current	Effect
Macroshock	
1 mA (0.001 A)	Threshold of perception
5 mA (0.005 A)	Threshold of pain and accepted as maximum harmless current intensity
10–20 mA	"Let-go" current before sustained muscle contraction
50 mA	Pain, possible fainting, mechanical injury; heart and respiratory functions continue
100–300 mA	Ventricular fibrillation will start, but respiratory center remains intact
6000 mA	Sustained myocardial contractions, followed by normal heart rhythm: temporary respiratory paralysis; burns if current density is high
Microshock	
100 μA (0.1 mA)	Ventricular fibrillation
10 μA (0.01 mA)	Recommended maximum allowable 60 Hz leakage current

(Reproduced with permission from Ehrenwerth J. 1993. Electrical safety. In Ehrenwerth, J. and Eisenkraft, J. B. (eds) *Anesthesia Equipment Principles and Applications*. St. Louis: Mosby-Year Book Inc, p. 151.)

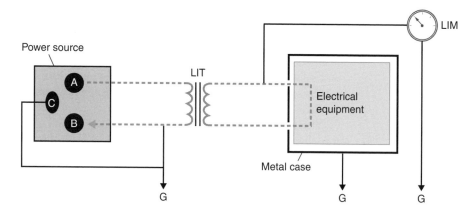

Figure 22.2 Line isolation. (From Vacanti et al. 2011. *Essential Clinical Anesthesia*, Cambridge University Press, Figure 23.5.)

Questions

1. The line isolation monitor in an OR effectively *prevents* which of the following:

    a. macroshock
    b. microshock
    c. grounding
    d. none of the above, only an alarm is sounded

2. A plastic surgeon wishes to use electrocautery near the patient's face. Which of the following is the safest course of action?

    a. Proceed with unipolar electrocautery with endotracheal intubation.
    b. Proceed with bipolar electrocautery with open face mask.
    c. Proceed with argon beam electrocautery with open face mask.
    d. Proceed with unipolar electrocautery with nasal cannula.

3. A patient with third-degree heart block and a permanent pacemaker presents for abdominal surgery. What is the most appropriate site for unipolar electrocautery return pad placement?

    a. right arm
    b. left arm
    c. left chest wall
    d. right thigh

Answers

1. d. By itself, the line isolation monitor cannot *prevent* inadvertent electrical shock from occurring in the operating room. The line isolation monitor sounds an alarm when it detects a single fault in an isolated power supply, usually at 2 milliamps. It is then advised that the operating room personnel take actions to avoid a second electrical fault with consequent macroshock, such as unplugging the last activated electrical device.

2. a. Electrocautery can cause operating room fires when used in an oxygen-enriched environment in the presence of a fuel source. Containing the flow of oxygen, separate from the site of electrocautery, helps to prevent operating room fires from occurring. Bipolar cautery does not reduce sparking at the surgical site.

3. d. When using electrocautery in patients with implanted electrical devices, such as pacemakers, it is best to direct the

current's path away from the implanted leads. Pacemakers are usually placed in the left chest, with the leads near the heart's conducting system. Directing the current away from the pacemaker (toward the leg) will help prevent interference with the pacemaker, as well as the risk of microshock.

Further reading

Litt, L. (2009). Electrical safety in the operating room. In Miller, R. D., Eriksson, L. I., Fleisher, L. A. (eds) *Miller's Anesthesia*, 7th edn. Philadelphia: Churchill-Livingstone, pp. 3041–3051.

National Fire Protection Association. (2012). Standard for health care facilities. (NFPA 99). www.nfpa.org/codes-and-standards/document-information-pages?mode=code&code=99 [Accessed May 9, 2014].

Chapter

23

Hemodynamic patient monitoring

Thomas Hickey and Linda S. Aglio

Keywords

ASA standard monitors
Noninvasive blood pressure monitoring
Invasive blood pressure monitoring
Invasive blood pressure indications
Arterial waveform: peripheral vs. central
Central venous pressure
Central venous catheters (CVC) indications
Respiratory variation-based indicators
Pulse pressure variation physiology
Pulse pressure variation pathophysiology
Stroke volume and SV index
Constrictive pericarditis: venous waveform
Pulmonary artery pressure monitoring

ASA standard monitors: a *qualified anesthesia provider* should be present throughout any GA, regional, or MAC case. At a minimum, *temperature, EKG, pulse oximeter, capnography,* and *BP* and *HR* at least every five minutes should be monitored. Circulatory function should be evaluated by continual palpation of pulses, auscultation of heart sounds, monitoring of intra-arterial pressure, ultrasound of peripheral pulse, oximetry, and/or capnograph. Invasive monitors should be considered on a case-by-case basis.

Noninvasive blood pressure monitoring: automated NIBP monitors measure blood pressure cuff oscillations via a transducer. SBP and DBP are extrapolated from the lowest cuff pressure with the greatest average oscillation amplitude, which is the MAP. An undersized cuff will overestimate SBP; an oversized cuff will underestimate SBP.

Invasive blood pressure monitoring: pressure can be measured within the cardiovascular system by connecting a hollow cannula within the vessel via high-pressure tubing to a transducer, which converts intraluminal pressure changes to an electrical signal. *Zeroing* removes the effect of atmospheric pressure on the transducer system: the transducer is exposed to atmospheric pressure and that pressure is set to zero. *Leveling* refers to placement of an already zeroed transducer at the level of the pressures we seek to measure (i.e., right atrium for blood pressure at the level of the heart; tragus for pressure in the circle of Willis). A 1 cm change in transducer height correlates with a 0.75 mm Hg pressure difference. *Underdamping* occurs when the frequency of the pressure waveform approaches that of the system, prolonging diaphragmatic oscillations within the transducer; *under*damping *over*estimates systolic pressure. *Over*damping can be thought of as too rigid a diaphragm, and will *under*estimate systolic pressure. Troubleshoot damping issues by minimizing length of tubing, removing unnecessary stopcocks, eliminating air bubbles, and continually flushing the system.

Invasive blood pressure indications: consider the following indications for arterial lines: (1) need for real-time monitoring (i.e., significant cardiovascular disease, trauma, ongoing significant resuscitation); (2) need for repeated ABG (i.e., blood loss, electrolyte, and/or acid–base disturbance); (3) unreliable NIBP (i.e., CPB, shock, LVAD, morbid obesity, burns).

Arterial waveform: peripheral vs. central. As measurements are made more peripherally, the arterial upstroke becomes steeper with exaggerated systolic and pulse pressures. MAP will be slightly greater in the aorta compared to peripheral sites.

Central venous pressure equals right atrial pressure. CVP tracing includes the positive waves: *a* (atrial systole), *c* (isovolumic RV contraction causing excursion of closed tricuspid valve), and *v* (blood filling the atrium comes up against a closed tricuspid valve during late systole to early diastole). The *x descent* represents atrial relaxation and geometrical changes in the atria caused by ventricular systole, while the *y descent* represents the atrium emptying into the RV after opening of the tricuspid valve.

Central venous catheters (CVC) indications: include: (1) measurement of CVP; (2) administration of some pressors/inotropes, chemotherapeutics, antibiotics, immunosuppressants, hypertonic solutions, TPN; (3) hemodialysis access; and (4) diagnosis of arrhythmias. Interpretation of volume status from CVP is fraught with error for a number of reasons including high right heart compliance and variations with

Essential Clinical Anesthesia Review: Keywords, Questions and Answers for the Boards, ed. Linda S. Aglio, Robert W. Lekowski, and Richard D. Urman. Published by Cambridge University Press. © Cambridge University Press 2015.

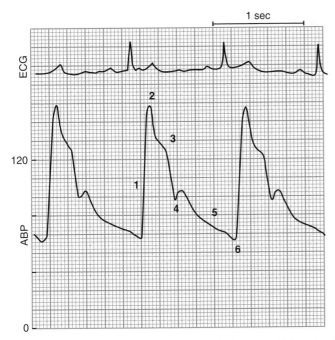

Figure 23.1 The systolic components following the R wave on EKG consist of: (1) steep pressure upstroke peak; (2) systolic peak pressure; and (3) decline, which correspond to the period of left ventricular systole. The down slope is interrupted by the (4) dicrotic notch, which reflects aortic valve closure at end systole. The remaining decay of waveform, (5) diastolic runoff, occurs during diastole following the EKG T wave and reaches its nadir at end diastole; (6) end-diastolic pressure. (Modified from Mark, J. B. 1998. *Atlas of Cardiovascular Monitoring*, Churchill Livingstone.)

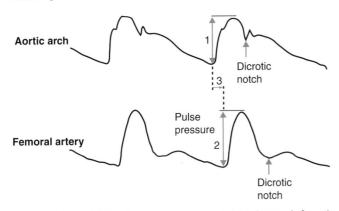

Figure 23.3 Arterial blood pressure waves recorded simultaneously from the aortic arch and femoral artery have different morphologies. In this example, the femoral artery waveform has a wider pulse pressure (1 and 2); a delayed upstroke (3); a delayed, slurred dicrotic notch (arrows); and a more prominent diastolic wave following the dicrotic notch. (Modified from Mark, J. B. 1998. *Atlas of Cardiovascular Monitoring*, Churchill Livingstone.)

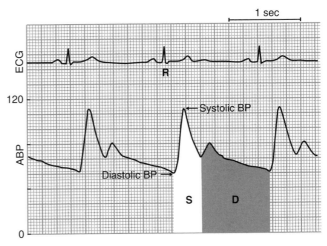

Figure 23.2 Systolic (S) and diastolic (D) pressures are shown with arrows. Mean arterial pressure (MAP) is represented by the area beneath the arterial pressure curve divided by the beat period, and it incorporates the S and D portions of the cardiac cycle. (Modified from Mark, J. B. 1998. *Atlas of Cardiovascular Monitoring*, Churchill Livingstone.)

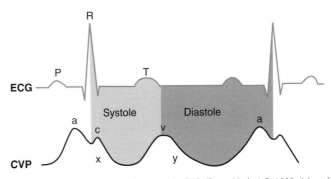

Figure 23.4 CVP waves synchronized to EKG. (From Mark, J. B. 1998. *Atlas of Cardiovascular Monitoring*, Churchill Livingstone.)

respiration and PEEP. However, CVP *trends* can be useful if measurements are made with consistent techniques and absent LV dysfunction, severe mitral regurgitation, and pulmonary hypertension. As with most clinical data, they should be considered alongside all other clinical and laboratory indicators of perfusion.

Respiratory variation-based indicators: during spontaneous breathing, blood pressure normally decreases (<5 mm Hg) during the negative intrathoracic pressure period of inspiration. Exaggerated decreases as seen in constrictive pericarditis and severe asthma exacerbation are termed "pulsus paradoxus." The reverse is seen during mechanical ventilation, where cyclic changes in intrathoracic pressure and volume cause cyclic changes in LV preload and, therefore, in stroke volume (SV) and blood pressure. In preload-dependent patients (i.e., patients on the steep portion of the Frank–Starling curve), these changes are more pronounced. Thus variations in systolic pressure, pulse pressure (PP), SV, and pulse oximetry plethysmography amplitude during mechanical ventilation can be predictive of volume responsiveness.

Pulse pressure variation physiology: physiologic changes during mechanical ventilation are complex; however, major changes during positive pressure (i.e., inspiration) include: (1) decreased venous return, which within several beats of end inspiration results in decreased LV preload and CO; (2) increased RV afterload secondary to increased alveolar pressure transmitted to the pulmonary capillaries; (3) initial increased LV preload secondary to the squeezing out of the

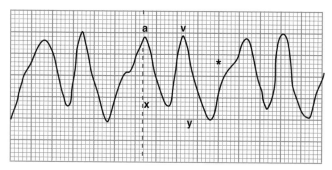

Figure 23.5 Pericardial constriction showing deep *x* and *y* descents as well as a flatter curve after they descend marked by an asterisk (*). (Modified from Mark, J. B. 1998. *Atlas of Cardiovascular Monitoring*, Churchill Livingstone.)

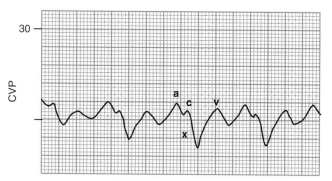

Figure 23.7 Percardial tamponade showing a dampened *y* descent. (Modified from Mark, J. B. 1998. *Atlas of Cardiovascular Monitoring*, Churchill Livingstone.)

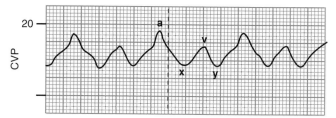

Figure 23.6 The CVP pattern for right ventricular ischemia can mimic that seen in pericardial restriction or restrictive cardiomyopathy with pronounced *x* and *y* descents. (Modified from Mark, J. B. 1998. *Atlas of Cardiovascular Monitoring*, Churchill Livingstone.)

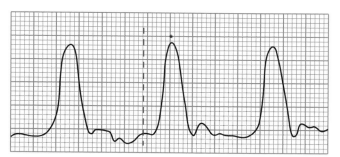

Figure 23.8 Tall cannon a waves are the results of atrial contraction against a closed tricuspid valve. * denotes an example of a cannon wave. (Modified from Mark, J. B. 1998. *Atlas of Cardiovascular Monitoring*, Churchill Livingstone.)

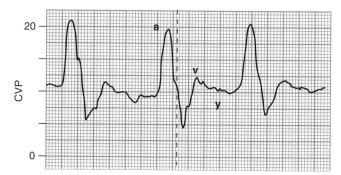

Figure 23.9 Tricuspid stenosis, with a tall a wave and a blunted descent. (Modified from Mark, J. B. 1998. *Atlas of Cardiovascular Monitoring*, Churchill Livingstone.)

pulmonary venous blood; and (4) decreased LV afterload secondary to the augmentation of transmural pressure across the heart during systole. Hence there is an inspiratory augmentation of LV SV followed several beats later by a decreased expiratory LV SV.

Pulse pressure variation pathophysiology: PP is directly proportional to LV SV. In a hypovolemic patient, PP variation is more pronounced for several reasons: (1) central veins and the right atrium are underfilled, making them more compliant (hence more collapsible), impeding RV preload; (2) the hypovolemic patient is on the steep portion of the Frank–Starling curve, meaning that preload changes for the reasons described will have exaggerated effects on SV; (3) less volume in the pulmonary circuit means a greater gradient between alveolar pressure and pulmonary arterial and venous pressures in the upper lung zones. In summary: systolic and PP are maximal during inspiration and are minimal several beats later during expiration; when hypovolemia exists during positive pressure ventilation, PP variation (owing mainly to the decreased SV during expiration) will be more pronounced.

Stroke volume and SV index: SV is EDV minus ESV. Normal volumes in a 70 kg man are EDV 120 cc, ESV 50 cc, and thus an SV of 70 cc. *Stroke index*, similar to cardiac index, relates the SV to the patient's body surface area (BSA). An average BSA for an adult male is 1.9 m^2, giving an average stroke index of approximately 37 cc/m^2.

Constrictive pericarditis: venous waveform. Restricted diastolic filling of the ventricles reduces SV and CO. A prominent *y* descent with an abrupt termination represents rapid initial ventricular filling abruptly encountering pericardial restraint. Similar patterns are seen with restrictive cardiomyopathy, RV ischemia, and tamponade. Various other pathologies are discernible from the CVP tracing as shown in Figures 23.5 to 23.9.

Pulmonary artery pressure monitoring: pulmonary arterial catheters (PACs) are a controversial but potentially useful tool in managing critically ill patients. Relative contraindications include: LBBB, mechanical valve, bacteremia, and hypercoagulable state. Measured parameters include: intracardiac pressures, thermodilution, CO, mixed venous oxygen saturation, shunt fractions and gradients, and PCWP. Derived parameters are shown in Table 23.1.

Table 23.1 Derived parameters

Derived parameter	Formula	Normal value
Cardiac index	CO/BSA	2.6–4.2 l/min/m^2
Systemic vascular resistance	(MAP – CVP)/CO × 80	900–1300 dyn*s/cm^5
Pulmonary vascular resistance	(MPAP – PAWP)/CO – 80	40–180 dyn*s/cm^5
Left ventricular stroke work	SV × (MAP – PAWP) × 0.0136	58–10 gm-m/beat
Right ventricular stroke work	SV – (MPAP – PAWP) × 0.0136	8–16 gm-m/beat
Stroke volume (SV)	CO/HR × 1000	60–100 ml/beat
Coronary artery perfusion pressure	Diastolic BP – PAWP	60–80 mm Hg
Arterial oxygen content (CaO_2)	(0.0138 × Hb × SaO_2) + (0.0031 × PaO_2)	17–20 ml/dl
Venous oxygen content (CvO_2)	(0.0138 × Hb × SvO_2) + (0.0031 × PaO2)	12–15 ml/dl
A-V oxygen content difference [C(a – v)O_2]	CaO_2 – CvO_2	4–6 ml/dl
Oxygen delivery	CaO_2 × CO × 10	950–1150 ml/min
Oxygen consumption	[C(a – v)O_2] × CO × 10	200–250 ml/min

A-V, arteriovenous; BP, blood pressure; BSA, body surface area; gm-m, gram-meter; Hb, hemoglobin; HR, heart rate; MAP, mean arterial pressure; MPAP, mean pulmonary artery pressure; SaO_2, arterial oxygen saturation; SvO_2, venous oxygen saturation.
(From Vacanti et al. 2011. *Essential Clinical Anesthesia*, Cambridge University Press, p. 166.)

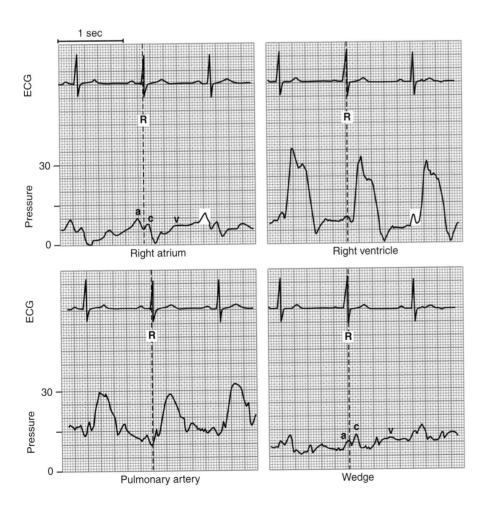

Figure 23.10 Pressure waveforms recorded from a PAC as it passes through the heart. (Modified from Mark, J. B. 1998. *Atlas of Cardiovascular Monitoring*, Churchill Livingstone.)

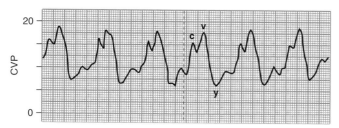

Figure 23.11

Questions

1. A previously healthy 31-year-old woman experiences significant postpartum hemorrhage. She becomes hemodynamically unstable and is intubated, paralyzed, and mechanically ventilated. Respiratory variation in arterial pressure is used to guide fluid resuscitation. She undergoes hysterectomy with resolution of hemorrhage. After several hours of aggressive fluid resuscitation with crystalloid, colloid, and blood products it is noted that the magnitude of the respiratory variation is low and that the variation now exists primarily in the inspiratory increase, whereas previously it had been mainly in the expiratory decrease. Which is the likeliest explanation for this change?

   a. persistent hypovolemia
   b. hypervolemia
   c. papillary muscle rupture
   d. acute respiratory distress syndrome

2. A 62-year-old obese man with severe COPD and untreated OSA is admitted to the MICU with sepsis from presumed pneumonia. A central venous catheter is placed and the pressure tracing shown in Figure 23.11 is noted. Which of the following is the most likely pathology?

   a. pericardial tamponade
   b. constrictive pericarditis
   c. right ventricular ischemia
   d. tricuspid regurgitation
   e. complete heart block

Answers

1. b. In conditions of supranormal intravascular volume, the pathophysiologic conditions described above for the hypovolemic patient undergoing PP variation monitoring no longer exist. RV and LV preload become adequate throughout the respiratory cycle, and the positive intrathoracic pressure seen during inspiration results in a significant increase in LV preload during each inspiration. Hence in hypervolemia, less respiratory PP variation is seen overall with the majority of variation on inspiration rather than on expiration.

2. d. The first three choices share similar hemodynamic alterations as described in the discussion above. In tricuspid regurgitation a tall "*c-v wave*" is seen with obliteration of the *x* descent, representing the rise in atrial pressure during ventricular systole. In complete heart block, atrial contraction against a closed tricuspid valve results in a large "cannon" a wave.

Further reading

Vacanti, C., Sikka, P., Urman, R., Dershwitz, M., and Segal, B. (eds) (2011). *Essential Clinical Anesthesia*. Cambridge: Cambridge University Press Chapter 24.

Chapter

24

The electrocardiogram and approach to diagnosis of common abnormalities

Thomas Hickey and Linda S. Aglio

Keywords

Localization of an MI
Cardiac cycle: EKG correlation
Pacer lead placement: EKG morphology
EKG leads: P-wave detection
EKG loose lead effect
Myocardial ischemia intraop Dx/Rx
Complete heart block (CHB): Rx
Hypocalcemia: EKG effects
Subarachnoid bleed: EKG effects

Overview

The cardiac cycle consists of a P, Q, R, S, and T wave:

EKG interpretation involves: (1) rate, (2) rhythm, (3) axis, (4) intervals, (5) chambers, and (6) ischemia:

1. Normal ventricular *rate* is 60 to 100.

2. *Rhythm* is sinus if PR and RR intervals are regular, P waves precede each QRS in a 1:1 ratio, and P waves are upright in the inferior leads.

3. Normal *axis* is between –30° and 110°. The axis is normal if leads I and II or I and aVF are positive.

4. Normal *intervals*: PR 200, QRS 120, QTc 300 to 450 milliseconds (i.e., QT roughly half the visualized RR).

5. *Chambers.* Atrial enlargement is suggested by large and or wide P waves in II and or V1.

Table 24.1 Left and right atrial enlargement

Leads	LA enlargement	RA enlargement
II	>120 ms	>2.5 mm
V1	>40 ms or >1 mm deep	>1.5 mm

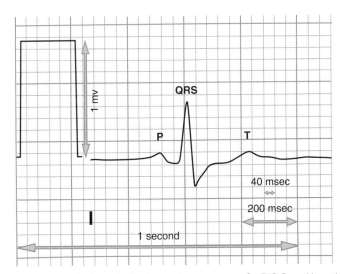

Figure 24.1 Grid, standardization, and measurements for EKG. From: Vacanti et al., 2011, p. 173.

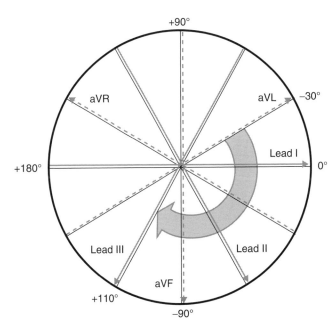

Figure 24.2 Frontal plane axis. The standard and augmented limb leads are shown on a plot of the frontal plane axis. The curved arrow indicates the range of normal axis, from –30° to 110°. From: Vacanti et al., 2011, p. 173.

Essential Clinical Anesthesia Review: Keywords, Questions and Answers for the Boards, ed. Linda S. Aglio, Robert W. Lekowski, and Richard D. Urman. Published by Cambridge University Press. © Cambridge University Press 2015.

Left Atrial Enlargement

Right Atrial Enlargement

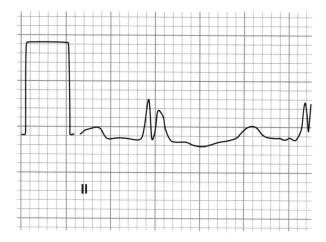
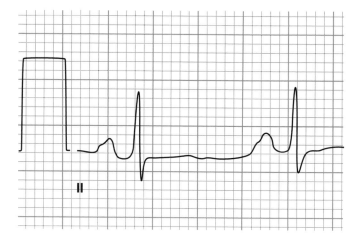
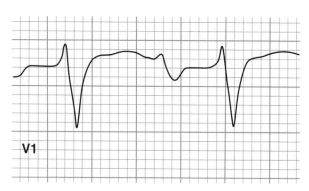
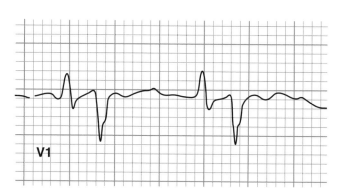

Figure 24.3 Atrial enlargement. From: Vacanti et al., 2011, p. 180.

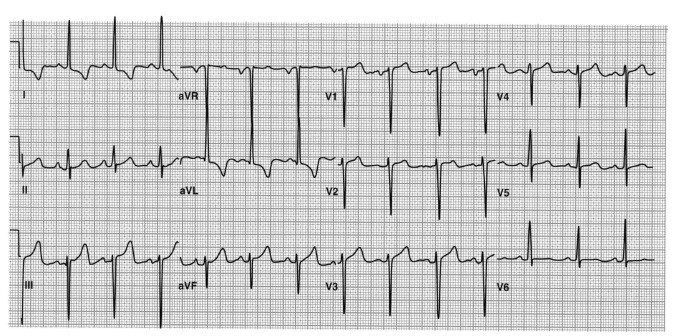

Figure 24.4 Left ventricular hypertrophy. From: Vacanti et al., 2011, p. 181.

LVH: an R wave in a VL >11 mm, and/or a sum of the deepest S plus the tallest R in the precordial leads >35 mm, is suggestive. RVH:R > S in V1 is suggestive.

6. *Ischemia*: pathologic Q waves (>30 ms or >25% the height of the R wave), particularly in a vascular distribution, suggest prior ischemia, as in the old LAD infarct (seen in Figure 24.7).

ST depression can represent ischemia but also repolarization abnormalities (i.e., LBBB, LVH), electrolyte disturbances (i.e., hypokalemia), or drug effects (i.e., downsloping ST segment seen in digitalis). Similarly, T-wave inversion may represent ischemia but can have a number of other explanations.

ST elevations are concerning for ischemia, as in the show in LAD STEMI Figure 24.8.

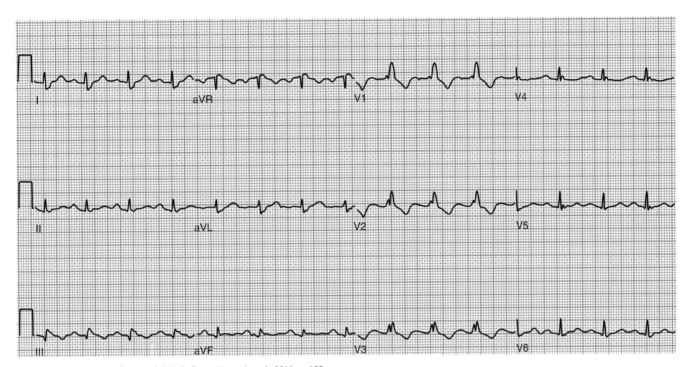

Figure 24.5 Right bundle branch block. From: Vacanti et al., 2011, p. 182.

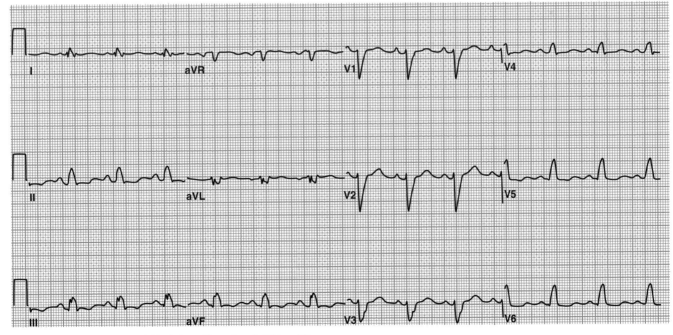

Figure 24.6 Left bundle branch block. From: Vacanti et al., 2011, p. 181.

Table 24.2 Abnormal QRS in the precordial leads can represent bundle branch block

RBBB	QRS ≥120 ms rSR' in V1, V2 Wide S in I, V6
LBBB	QRS ≥120 ms Absent Q and broad, monophasic R in lateral leads Often left axis deviation

Localization of an MI

Cardiac cycle: EKG correlation. P wave represents right atrial depolarization. Normal AV nodal conduction delay manifests

Table 24.3 Localization of an MI

Anatomy	Leads with STE	Blood supply
Septal	V1, V2	Proximal LAD
Anterior	V3, V4	LAD
Apical	V5, V6	Distal LAD or LCx, possibly RCA
Lateral	I, aVL	LCx
Inferior	II, III, aVF	RCA
RV	V1, V2	Proximal RCA
Posterior	ST depression in V1, V2, V3	RCA or LCx

as PR interval. Ventricular depolarization correlates to the QRS complex. The T wave represents ventricular repolarization.

Pacer lead placement: EKG morphology. Atrial pacing is visible on the EKG as a pacing spike followed by a P wave; if AV conduction is intact a QRS complex will follow. Ventricular pacing appears as a spike followed by a wide QRS complex as the depolarization is conducted outside the normal pathway. In dual chamber pacing a spike is followed by an often flattened P wave then a second spike is followed by a QRS complex.

EKG leads: P-wave detection. Lead II is commonly used to monitor rhythm as it best displays the P wave.

EKG loose lead effect. "Baseline wander" describes a changing isoelectric baseline. It can be caused by loosely attached EKG stickers, leads under tension, or patient movement.

Myocardial ischemia intraop Dx/Rx: leads II and V5 may detect 95% of ischemic events. Consider patient history, intraoperative events, and hemodynamic trends when evaluating ischemic changes. Cardiac enzymes can be sent but should not delay treatment and will likely not yet be elevated in an acute MI. TEE can detect subtle wall motion abnormalities that are indicative of ischemia. General treatments include 100% FiO_2, β-blockade, opioid for pain control, nitrates, blood products if indicated, aspirin and other antiplatelet agent, cardiology consult, and potential catheterization. (Note that some studies have shown association between blood transfusion and increased mortality in myocardial infarction.)

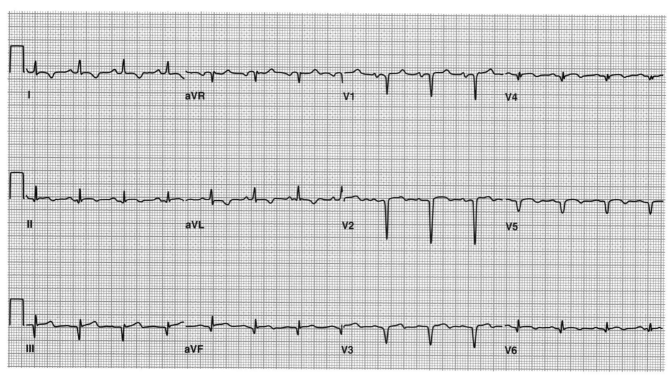

Figure 24.7 Old myocardial infarction. From: Vacanti et al., 2011, p. 183.

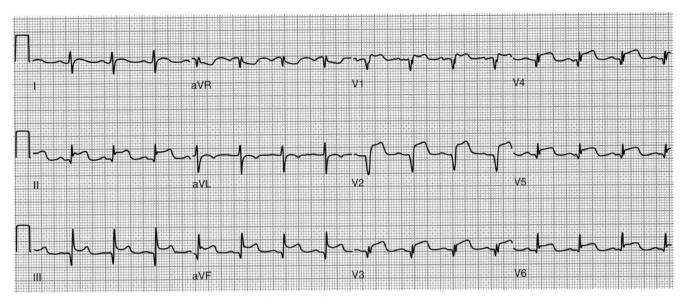

Figure 24.8 Acute myocardial infarction. From: Vacanti et al., 2011, p. 182.

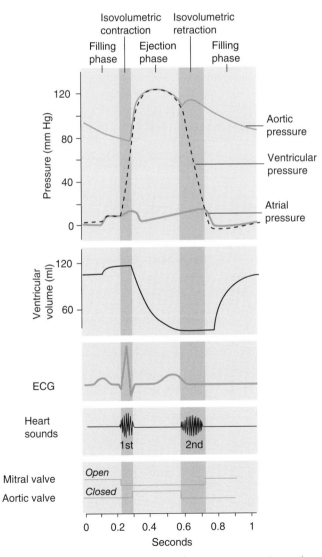

Figure 24.9 Normal cardiac cycle depicted as pressure versus time and volume versus time. From: Vacanti et al., 2011, p. 431.

Complete heart block (CHB): Rx. PR prolongation alone is called first-degree AV block. There are two types of second-degree AV block: Type 1, also known as Mobitz I or Wenckebach, involves progressive PR prolongation until there is a nonconducted P wave; Type 2, also known as Mobitz II, involves fixed PR interval with intermittent nonconducted P waves. Type 1 is a disease of the AV node, while Type 2 indicates more distal conduction system disease and predicts a higher risk of progression to third-degree AV block (CHB). The ventricular escape rhythm often has a rate below 40 bpm. The main treatment for CHB is ventricular pacing. While arranging pacing, atropine or isoproterenol can be used.

Hypocalcemia: EKG effects. Hypocalcemia results in a prolonged QT and flat T waves, and can progress to CHB. If severe, hypotension and arrhythmia may be seen, along with tetany and laryngospasm. *Hypercalcemia* results in tall T waves with a shortened QT interval; if severe the QRS can prolong in a pattern resembling that seen in hyperkalemia. In *hyperkalemia* there is a variable progression from peaked T waves to QRS prolongation (often in a BBB pattern) to a sinusoidal shape to bradycardia and VT. These arrhythmias occur when the hyperkalemia is severe (i.e., >7.0 mmol/l). *Hypokalemia* can result in flattening of the T waves to ST depression or T-wave inversion, in a pattern similar to hypocalcemia.

Subarachnoid bleed: EKG effects. SAH predisposes to many unstable arrhythmias, including supraventricular and ventricular (especially if QT prolongation) arrhythmias. A variety of changes can be seen involving the ST segment, T wave (peaked or deeply inverted), PR interval (shortened), and QTc (prolonged). U waves can also be seen.

Sinus Bradycardia

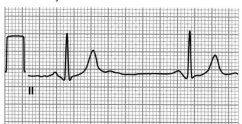

Mobitz I Block

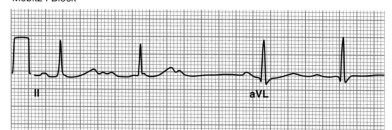

Mobitz II Block

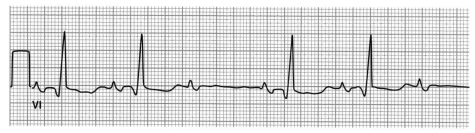

Complete Heart Block

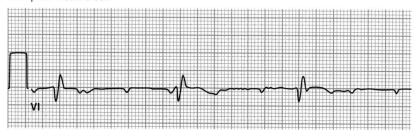

Figure 24.10 Bradycardia. From: Vacanti et al., 2011, p. 175.

Hyperkalemia

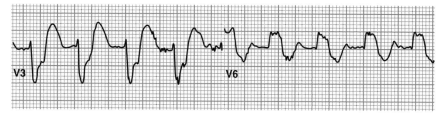

Figure 24.11 Hyperkalemia and hypocalcemia. From: Vacanti et al., 2011, p. 184.

Hypocalcemia

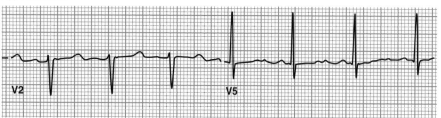

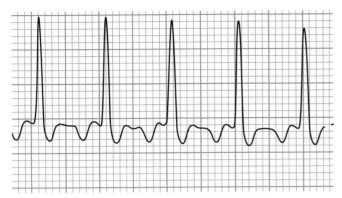

Figure 24.12 Acute ischemia. Adapted From: Vacanti et al., 2011, p. 176.

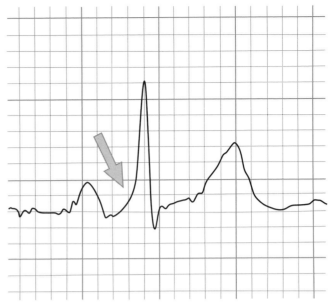

Figure 24.13 Delta wave. From: Vacanti et al., 2011. Essential Clinical Anesthesia, Cambridge University Press, p. 177.

Questions

1. A 22-year-old woman is seen preoperatively for a cosmetic surgery. ROS is positive only for occasional palpitations without lightheadedness, chest pain, or dyspnea. She denies syncope. EKG demonstrates shortened PR interval with slurred upstroke of the R wave. If the suspected diagnosis is confirmed, what is the definitive long-term management?
    a. catheter ablation
    b. flecainide
    c. sotalol
    d. verapamil

2. A 62-year-old man with longstanding hypertension becomes tachycardic with a ventricular rate of 140 during a cystoscopy procedure. The rhythm strip is seen in Figure 24.12. What is the rhythm?
    a. atrial fibrillation (AFIB)
    b. sinus tachycardia
    c. AVRT
    d. AVNRT
    e. multifocal atrial tachycardia (MAT)
    f. atrial flutter (AFL)

Answers

1. a. WPW involves an AP that can conduct directly from the atrium to the ventricle. Antegrade conduction through the AP causes early ventricular depolarization seen as the "*delta*" wave indicaated by the arrow in Figure 24.13. If the AP only allows retrograde conduction, no delta wave will be seen. The refractoriness of the AP is naturally different from the nodal pathway. Atrioventricular reentrant tachycardia (AVRT) occurs when a premature atrial beat conducts down the AV node but not the AP; by the time the impulse encounters the ventricular side of the AP, the tissue may allow conduction retrograde into the atrium, where it can reenter the ventricle via the AV node, then the atrium via the AP, and so on. This is the most common mechanism of SVT and is called *orthodromic*. *Antidromic* conduction down the AP and retrograde up the AV node is less common. Sudden cardiac death in WPW often comes in the setting of AFIB when the AP refractory period is short. In this context, rapid conduction through the pathway can result in an irregular, rapid, wide complex rhythm with possible degeneration to VF.

    AP ablation in WPW achieves over 90% success rate. Acute medical management includes nodal blockade with agents such as verapamil, β-blockers, and adenosine. Adenosine has been shown to achieve cardioversion in nearly 90% of WPW-associated narrow complex tachycardias. Antiarrhythmic drugs such as procainamide, flecainide, sotalol, and amiodarone may also be used. Calcium channel blockers are not advised in patients with AFIB as they can result in accelerated conduction through the AP with possible cardiac arrest.

2. f. Narrow complex tachycardias are often divided into regular and irregular. Atrial flutter often originates in the right atrium around the tricuspid annulus. Typical atrial rates are 260 to 300 bpm with the ventricular response most commonly 2:1. The characteristic saw-toothed flutter waves are seen occurring regularly within the RR interval. AFL often coexists with AFIB, and treatments are similar. Antiarrhythmics may enhance both the efficacy of cardioversion and the maintenance of sinus rhythm. Catheter ablation by an experienced provider is successful in eliminating flutter in >90% of patients.

Atrial Tachycardia

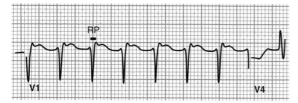

Multifocal Atrial Tachycardia

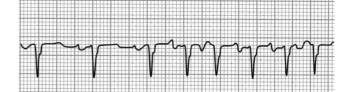

AV Node Reentrant Tachycardia

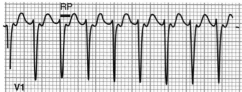

Atrial Flutter

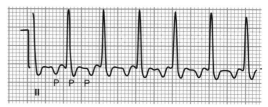

AV Reciprocating Tachycardia

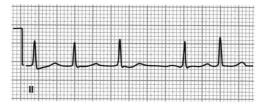

Atrial Fibrillation

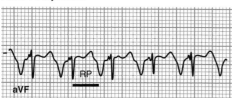

Figure 24.14 Narrow tachycardia. From: Vacanti et al., 2011, p. 176.

Further reading

Vacanti, C., Sikka, P., Urman, R., Dershwitz, M., and Segal, B. (eds) (2011). *Essential Clinical Anesthesia*. Cambridge: Cambridge University Press, Chapter 25.

Chapter

25

Pulse oximetry and capnography

Hanjo Ko and George P. Topulos

Keywords

Principles of pulse oximetry
Limitations to pulse oximetry
Normal capnogram with its relationship to inspiratory and expiratory phases
End-tidal CO_2
Abnormal capnograms

Pulse oximetry measurements (SpO_2) are based on the transmission of two wavelengths of light (red and infrared) through pulsatile tissue beds, and subsequent estimates of true arterial hemoglobin saturation (SaO_2). Pulse oximetry measures the functional saturation, the ratio of $O_2Hb/(O_2Hb$ + reduced Hb). Laboratory CO-oximeters (usually using seven or more wavelengths of light) measure the fractional saturation, the ratio of O_2Hb to total Hb.

Functional saturation = $O_2Hb/(O_2Hb$ + reduced Hb)

Fractional saturation = $O_2Hb/(O_2Hb$ + reduced Hb + Met Hb + COHb)

As a result, the SpO_2 will be falsely high, and laboratory CO-oximeter analysis is mandatory, if high levels of nonfunctional Hb are suspected (e.g., patient may have smoke inhalation from a fire). In the absence of significant levels of nonfunctional Hb, SpO_2 readings are most accurate in the range of 70% to 100% (standard error of ±2%) and less so in the range of 50% to 70% (but still with standard error of ±3%).

Pulse oximeter reading may be importantly false in the presence of:

1. Nonfunctional hemoglobins (measured correctly by laboratory CO-oximeters): SpO_2 may significantly overestimate true SaO_2:

    Significant CO present $SpO_2 \approx O_2Hb + COHb$
    High methemoglobinemia SpO2 ≈ 85% (regardless of the true oxygen saturation).

2. Low peripheral pulsatile flow (e.g., in shock).
3. Various dyes (e.g., methylene blue, indocyanine green, indigo carmine).
4. Excessive ambient light.
5. Motion artifacts (e.g., shivering).
6. Nail polish, especially black, blue, and green.

The CO_2 concentration at the end of the plateau is referred to as *end-tidal CO_2* ($PETCO_2$). Because there is always some dead space, $PaCO_2 > PETCO_2$. In healthy anesthetized patients the difference is small, ≈ 5 mm Hg. In patients with large areas of alveolar dead space (e.g., emphysema or PE), the $PaCO_2$–$PETCO_2$ difference can be very large, and using $PETCO_2$ to estimate $PaCO_2$ dangerous.

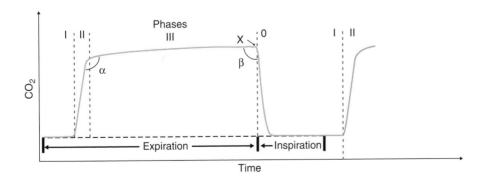

Figure 25.1 Normal capnogram: three phases of expiration. Phase I = anatomic dead space; Phase II = mixture of dead space and alveolar gas; Phase III = alveolar gas plateau. From: Vacanti et al., 2011, p. 188.

Essential Clinical Anesthesia Review: Keywords, Questions and Answers for the Boards, ed. Linda S. Aglio, Robert W. Lekowski, and Richard D. Urman. Published by Cambridge University Press. © Cambridge University Press 2015.

Table 25.1 Factors that cause increase and decrease in PETCO₂. Adapted form: Vacanti et al., 2011, p. 190.

Increase in PETCO₂	Decrease in PETCO₂

Due to an increase in CO₂ production:
  increases in metabolic rate;
  sepsis;
  malignant hyperthermia;
  shivering/seizure;
  hyperthyroidism.
	Due to a decrease in CO₂ production:
	  decreases in metabolic rate;
	  hypothermia;
	  hypothyroidism.

Due to a decrease in CO₂ elimination:
  hypoventilation;
  rebreathing;
  CO₂ absorber exhaustion.
	Due to an increase in CO₂ elimination:
	  hyperventilation.

Due to artifact:
  malfunction of CO₂ measuring system.
	Due to a decrease in alveolar CO₂ delivery:
	  hypoperfusion;
	  pulmonary embolism.

	Due to artifact:
	  gas sampling tube leak or loose connection;
	  malfunction of CO₂ measuring system.

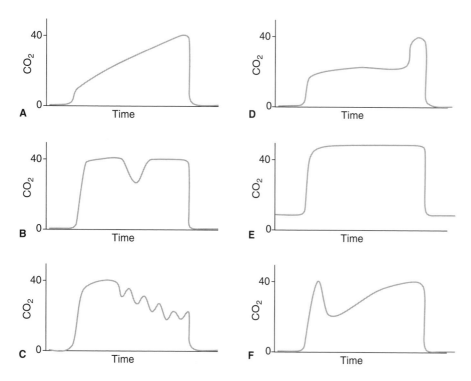

Figure 25.2 Abnormal capnograms. (A) Capnogram from a patient with severe obstructive pulmonary disease or another cause leading to increased airway resistance, such as asthma, endobronchial intubation, or endotracheal tube kinking. No plateau is reached before the next inspiration. The gradient between PETCO₂ and arterial CO₂ is increased. (B) Downward wave curing the plateau phase, indicating spontaneous respiratory effort. (C) Cardiogenic oscillations appearing as small regular, tooth-like "humps" at the latter part of the expiratory phase. The rate of the humps is identical to the patient's heart rate. (D) A leak in the sampling line during positive pressure ventilation. (E) Failure of inspired CO₂ to return to zero because of an incompetent expiratory valve or exhausted CO₂ absorbent. (F) Bifid waveform of expired CO₂ in a patient with emphysema undergoing elective surgery after unilateral lung transplantation. The initial upstroke represents gas from the normal (transplanted) lung, which is followed by gas exhaled from the remaining (emphysematous) lung. (From Vacanti et al. 2011. *Essential Clinical Anesthesia*, Cambridge University Press, p. 189.)

Questions

1. Which of the following statements regarding central venous saturation is FALSE?

   a. Central venous saturation is measured in the superior vena cava and is different from mixed venous saturation, which is measured in the pulmonary artery.

   b. Central venous saturation is slightly lower than mixed venous saturation.

   c. In patients presenting with sepsis, the goal for central venous saturation is greater than 70%.

   d. Laboratory-measured oxygen saturation is higher than oxygen saturation measured by pulse oximetry.

   e. In patients with congenital heart disease where baseline SpO₂ is much lower than normal range, the most accurate parameter is the difference between SpO_2 and venous saturation since it takes into account oxygen delivery.

2. Which of the following statements regarding capnography is FALSE?
   a. $PETCO_2$ is high during cardiac arrest.
   b. Migration of the endotracheal tube into a mainstem bronchus will decrease $PETCO_2$.
   c. A high gradient between $PETCO_2$ and $PaCO_2$ signifies worsening dead space, such as in the cases of pulmonary embolism, hypotension, and COPD.
   d. Shunt has no effect on the difference between $PETCO_2$ and $PaCO_2$.
   e. Esophageal intubation can produce CO_2 up to three tidal volumes

Answers

1. d. Oxygen saturation measured in the laboratory using a multiwavelength CO-oximeter is slightly lower than SpO_2.
2. a. During cardiac arrest, $PETCO_2$ may be helpful in evaluating the effectiveness of cardiac compressions in generating blood flow. When there is little or no blood flow, $PETCO_2$ is low because little CO_2 is delivered to the lungs, and very low pulmonary artery pressures create large areas of Zone 1, which is alveolar dead space.

Further reading

Vacanti, C., Sikka, P., Urman, R., Dershwitz, M., and Segal, B. (eds) (2011). *Essential Clinical Anesthesia*. Cambridge: Cambridge University Press, Chapter 26.

www.openanesthesia.org

Chapter

26 Monitoring of neuromuscular blockade

M. Tariq Hanifi, J. Matthew Kynes, and Joseph M. Garfield

Keywords

Peripheral nerve stimulator
Corrugator supercilii
Adductor pollicis
Single twitch
Train-of-four (TOF)
TOF ratio
Tetanus
High-frequency stimulation
Post-tetanic facilitation
Post-tetanic count (PTC)
Double-burst stimulation
Postoperative residual curarization (PORC)
Mechanomyography
Acceleromography
EMG

Muscle paralysis is often desirable during general anesthesia to improve intubating and operative conditions. There is no clinically detectable block until 75% to 85% of the receptors are occupied, owing to a margin of safety for receptor occupancy of approximately 4:1 for the most sensitive fibers (extraocular muscles) and 12:1 for the most resistant fibers (diaphragm). Complete paralysis occurs at 90% to 95% occupancy. Given this narrow therapeutic window, adequate monitoring of blockade is essential.

When monitoring neuromuscular blockade using a *peripheral nerve stimulator*, one electrode is placed over the nerve to be monitored and another is placed proximally or distally along the same nerve. Depolarizing current in the range of 60 to 80 mA is then delivered across the nerve and contractile response is assessed.

Assessing target muscle relaxation must take nerve selection into account. Muscles used clinically include *adductor pollicis* (used to describe any residual blockade before extubation/surgical relaxation for surgery of the extremities) and *corrugator supercilii* (best used to assess for airway/

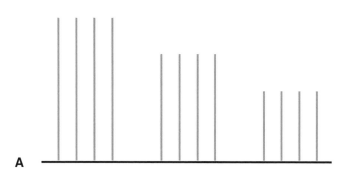

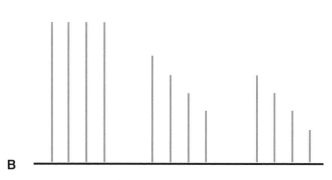

Figure 26.1 Illustration of train-of-four stimuli following administration of neuromuscular blockers. (A) With incremental doses of SCh, the twitch height decreases. All four twitches are decreased by the same height. (B) During nondepolarizing relaxation, increasing doses result in a decrease of twitch height and a lower second, third, and fourth twitch compared with the first (the twitch amplitude fades during train-of-four stimulation). (From Vacanti et al. 2011. *Essential Clinical Anesthesia*, Cambridge University Press, Figure 38.2.)

diaphragmatic relaxation/surgical relaxation for abdominal and thoracic surgery).

Several patterns of nerve stimulation by a peripheral nerve stimulator can be used to assess the degree of neuromuscular blockade. *Single twitch* can be used to assess the onset of blockade when compared to pre-blockade twitch.

Train-of-four (TOF) monitoring can distinguish the degree of blockade and readiness for reversal or extubation. In this mode, four consecutive stimuli lasting 0.2 ms each are applied at 2 Hz.

Essential Clinical Anesthesia Review: Keywords, Questions and Answers for the Boards, ed. Linda S. Aglio, Robert W. Lekowski, and Richard D. Urman. Published by Cambridge University Press. © Cambridge University Press 2015.

Disappearance of the fourth twitch corresponds to a 75% block, a third twitch an 80% block, and a second twitch corresponds to a 90% block. When progressive stimulation depletes acetylcholine stores to an appreciable amount, the degree of fade between the fourth and first contractions (T4/T1) reveals the *TOF ratio*. A TOF ratio >0.75 at the adductor pollicis correlates with recovery of diaphragm, handgrip, and five-second head lift, although current evidence indicates that a ratio >0.9 is required to achieve adequate airway protection at extubation.

Tetanus or *high-frequency stimulation* is sustained contraction that occurs during high-frequency stimulation (>50 Hz) and is more sensitive than TOF or single twitch for assessing residual blockade. Observation of fade during five-second stimulation indicates neuromuscular blockade, with increasing frequency required to cause fade at decreasing levels of blockade.

After tetanic stimulation, neuromuscular response is temporarily augmented, resulting in *post-tetanic facilitation*. The *post-tetanic count (PTC)* can be used during profound relaxation and is the number of twitches following five seconds of 50 Hz tetanus. The PTC correlates inversely with the time to spontaneous recovery. For vecuronium, a PTC of one correlates with a time of 8.5 minutes (6 to 15 minutes) before single twitch recovery.

Double-burst stimulation involves two bursts of three 0.2 ms impulses at 50 Hz separated by 0.75 s. The degree of fade with double-burst stimulation is similar to the TOF ratio but easier to detect manually or visually particularly in the range of 0.5 to 0.6.

The degree of recovery of neuromuscular function is a key component in the time to complete reversal of blockade. When zero twitches are present reversal is considered unattainable. In this situation, it is best to wait until a response to stimulation occurs before administering reversing agents. Antagonism of atracurium, vecuronium, or pancuronium blockade by neostigmine occurs in 30 minutes when two responses to the TOF are present, and in ten minutes when all four TOF responses are evident.

Postoperative residual curarization (PORC) describes residual neuromuscular blockade after extubation. Several clinical tests can be used to assess the degree of neuromuscular recovery (Table 26.1).

Objective methods of measuring neuromuscular block are also available, with *mechanomyography* being the gold standard for research purposes. This measure monitors the degree of neuromuscular block by quantifying the force of isometric contraction of the adductor pollicis muscle in response to ulnar nerve stimulation. The force is then transduced into an electric signal that is displayed on an interfaced pressure monitor and then recorded. It requires stringent preparation and precautions, is often bulky and difficult to prepare, and is not often used clinically.

The most versatile method of objective monitoring in the clinical setting is *acceleromyography*. This method is based on the rate of angular acceleration of the thumb. It is based on Newton's second law and shows that acceleration is directly proportional to force, which is inversely proportional to

Table 26.1 Clinical tests to assess recovery from neuromuscular blockade

Both legs lifted off the bed	TOF 0.6 Probably not sufficient to ensure protection of airway
Head lift >5 s	TOF 0.6 Probably not sufficient to ensure protection of airway
Normal handgrip strength	TOF 0.7
Teeth clenched to prevent removal of wooden spatula (masseter muscle strength)	TOF 0.86 Most sensitive test to ensure adequate recovery, but not all patients may be able to demonstrate

(From Vacanti et al. 2011. *Essential Clinical Anesthesia*, Cambridge University Press, Table 27.5.)

neuromuscular blockade. It has been shown to reduce the incidence of residual paralysis when used clinically.

EMG has also been used but mostly for experimental studies. The principle of *EMG* is to record the electrical response of muscle after evoked stimulation of a motor nerve by a peripheral nerve stimulator.

Questions

1. Which of the following can be used to assess recovery from neuromuscular blockade?
   a. head lift >5 seconds
   b. teeth clenched to prevent removal of wooden spatula
   c. both legs lifted off the bed
   d. all of the above

2. The following provides objective information on more than one parameter of neuromuscular blockade in the clinical setting:
   a. EMG
   b. mechanomyography
   c. acceleromyography
   d. TOF monitoring

Answers

1. d. Each of these clinical tests can give an indication of neuromuscular recovery, although none is specific for full recovery of airway reflexes. Of the choices, adequate masseter strength by testing teeth clenching of a wooden spatula correlates most closely with full return of airway reflexes.

2. c. Acceleromyography measures not only the exerting force of the thumb during stimulation but also its acceleration, while other monitors can only provide information on electrical response to stimulation (EMG), force of isometric contraction (mechanomyography), or twitch response to stimulation (TOF monitoring).

Further reading

Paton, W. D. M. and Waud, D. R. (1967). The margin of safety of neuromuscular transmission. *Journal of Physiology* 191, 59–90.

Vacanti, C., Sikka, P., Urman, R., Dershwitz, M., and Segal, B. (eds) (2011). Monitoring of neuromuscular blockade. In *Essential Clinical Anesthesia*. Cambridge: Cambridge University Press. pp. 191–197.

Fuchs-Buder, T., Schreiber, J.-U., and Meistelman, C. (2009). Monitoring neuromuscular block: an update. *Anaesthesia* 64, 82–89.

Chapter

27

Thermoregulation and temperature monitoring

Jessica Bauerle and Zhiling Xiong

Keywords

Temperature regulation during anesthesia
$CMRO_2$ and hypothermia
Temperature monitoring
Temperature regulation: infants versus adults

Table 27.1 Organ system effects of hypothermia

- Bradycardia
- CNS disturbances
- Decreased drug metabolism
- Coagulation abnormalities
- Renal vasoconstriction

(Adapted from Vacanti et al. 2011. *Essential Clinical Anesthesia*, Cambridge University Press, Table 28.2.)

Body temperature is primarily controlled by two mechanisms: autonomic control and behavioral modifications. However, the anesthetized patient loses the behavioral control when rendered unconscious, and the autonomic nervous system is altered by medications affecting vessel tone. The anterior hypothalamus is the main temperature regulator of the body. $A\delta$ and C fibers transmit temperature to the hypothalamus. Temperature is maintained tightly within 0.2°C from the hypothalamic set point, although the body varies by 1°C daily, with the lowest temperature occurring in early morning and the highest occurring approximately 12 hours later. The body produces heat through the conversion of glucose into ATP. Heat is then handled by the body with one metabolic equivalent (MET) being equal to the calorie consumption of 1 kCal/kg/h. As an estimate, two flights of stairs walked at a steady pace are equivalent to approximately four METs.

Heat exchange occurs via conduction, convection, radiation, and evaporation. The majority of heat loss in the operating room is by radiation loss (60%), followed by convection (30%). Radiation represents loss of heat in the form of electromagnetic waves and is related to the temperature of the object. Convection occurs when there is a constant contact of a substance with the body resulting in heat loss (airflow over patient). There are three stages of heat change in the anesthetized patient. In the first stage, the core body temperature decreases by 1 to 2°C, and heat is redistributed from the trunk to the extremities. To prevent this, forced air warmers should be placed prior to induction of anesthesia. The second stage proceeds over three to four hours when heat loss is greater than heat production, resulting in overall cooling. Finally, the third stage occurs when heat production equals heat loss at

approximately 33°C. Active measures should be continued to maintain core temperature above 36°C.

Hypothermia is associated with numerous complications, and is defined as a temperature <36°C. Elderly, neonates, and paraplegic patients are predisposed to the development of hypothermia. The coagulation cascade is impaired and platelet function is decreased. There is increased oxygen demand from shivering and other warming actions. Also, wound infections are more likely to occur. Additionally, the metabolism of drugs is slowed, which may result in a slow emergence from anesthesia, and should be on the differential for any patient slow to wake.

Hyperthermia is much more serious than hypothermia, and is defined as a temperature >38°C, not congruent with the hypothalamic set point (which is elevated with fever). The major complication associated with hyperthermia is injury to the central nervous system, with resultant increasing levels of neuro-excitatory transmitters and further precipitation of ischemic injury.

Multiple techniques exist for measuring temperature. The core body temperature is best reflected at the site of the pulmonary artery via a catheter thermistor. Core temperature may also be measured at the distal esophagus, tympanic membrane, and nasopharynx. Secondary sites of measurement termed "transition zone sites" include the axilla, bladder, and rectum.

Several strategies for maintaining normothermia exist, and multiple studies have been performed evaluating the different techniques. Currently, it is recommended that a

Essential Clinical Anesthesia Review: Keywords, Questions and Answers for the Boards, ed. Linda S. Aglio, Robert W. Lekowski, and Richard D. Urman. Published by Cambridge University Press. © Cambridge University Press 2015.

Table 27.2 Sites for temperature monitoring

- Core temperature sites:
  - pulmonary artery
  - nasopharynx
  - tympanic membrane
  - distal esophagus

- Transitional zone sites:
  - axillary
  - rectum
  - bladder

- Peripheral temperature monitoring:
  - skin

(Adapted from Vacanti et al. 2011. *Essential Clinical Anesthesia*, Cambridge University Press, Table 28.4.)

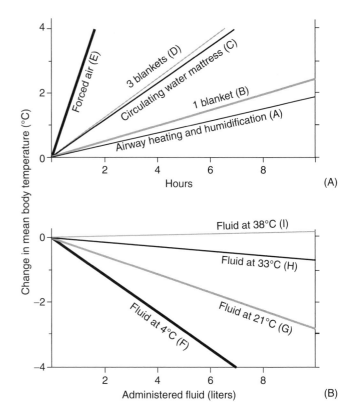

Figure 27.1 Effects of warming techniques on body temperature. (A) shows change in body temperature over elapsed time. (B) shows change in body temperature with administration of fluid at varying temperatures. (From Vacanti et al. 2011. *Essential Clinical Anesthesia*, Cambridge University Press, Figure 28.3)

forced warming blanket be used prior to induction of anesthesia and should cover at least 25% of the body surface area. Warmed fluid has little effect if only a small volume is being administered; however, with amounts above two liters, 1°C can be conserved. For the infant, a warming lamp should be used due to the higher surface area to volume ratio. It is recommended that temperature be monitored for any case >30 minutes.

For a small number of specific cases, hypothermia will be intentionally induced, such as in cardiopulmonary bypass, some neurosurgery cases, cardiac arrest outside of hospital, and circulatory arrest. In these instances, the benefits of cooling are believed to outweigh the risks, with the goal being to protect ischemic injury to tissues already damaged or at risk of further insult.

Questions

1. Which nerve fibers carry temperature sensation?
   a. C fibers
   b. Aα
   c. Aβ
   d. Aδ
   e. a and d
   f. all of the above

2. What type of heat loss is most common in the operating room?
   a. convection
   b. radiation
   c. conduction
   d. evaporation

Answers

1. e.
2. b.

Further reading

Vacanti, C., Sikka, P., Urman, R., Dershwitz, M., and Segal, B. (eds) (2011). *Essential Clinical Anesthesia*. Cambridge: Cambridge University Press, Chapter 28.

Sessler, D. I. (2010). Chapter 48. Temperature regulation and monitoring. In Miller, R. D., Eriksson, L. I., Fleisher, L. A. et al. (eds) *Miller's Anesthesia*, 7th edn. Philadelphia: Churchill-Livingstone Elsevier.

Chapter

28

Neurophysiologic monitoring

Scott W. Vaughan and Linda S. Aglio

Essential Clinical Anesthesia Review: Keywords, Questions and Answers for the Boards, ed. Linda S. Aglio, Robert W. Lekowski, and Richard D. Urman. Published by Cambridge University Press. © Cambridge University Press 2015.

Keywords

Electroencephalography (EEG)
Electrocorticography (ECoG)
Evoked potential monitoring
Visual evoked potentials (VEPs)
Motor evoked potentials (MEPs)
Brainstem auditory evoked potentials (BAEPs)
Wake-up test
Cranial nerve monitoring
Intracranial pressure (ICP) monitoring
Transcranial Doppler ultrasound (TCD)
Cerebral oxygenation/metabolism monitors

Electroencephalography (EEG): records field electrical potentials generated by the intracellular and extracellular electrical activity of the pyramidal cells in the granular cortex by scalp electrodes that are positioned using the 10–20 International Electrode System. Clinically, EEG is used to monitor for cerebral ischemia, hypoxia, and epileptiform activity.

Clinically, EEG recordings are divided into four frequency ranges based on clinical exam, pathologic states, and anesthetic depth:

Delta rhythm (0–3 Hz): deep sleep; deep anesthesia; pathologic states: brain tumors, hypoxia, metabolic encephalopathy.

Theta rhythm (4–7 Hz): sleep and anesthesia in adults; hyperventilation in awake children and young adults.

Alpha rhythm (8–13 Hz): resting, awake adult with eyes closed; predominately in occipital leads.

Beta rhythm (>13 Hz): mental activity; light anesthesia.

Physiologic factors such as:

PaO_2: hypoxia initially may produce EEG activation, followed by slowing or electrical silence.

$PaCO_2$: hypocarbia: EEG slowing; mild hypercarbia; increased frequency and amplitude.

Temperature: hypothermia: progressive slowing; electrical silence at 15 to 20°C. Temperature and sensory stimulation increase or decrease the EEG activity.

Sensory stimulation: EEG activation.

Electrocorticography (ECoG): the intraoperative cortical surface recording for localization of epileptic foci.

Evoked potential monitoring – anesthetic effects: in general concerning volatile agents, SSEPs and VEPs are sensitive, noting an *increase in latency and a decrease in amplitude* with end-tidal concentrations greater than 0.5 MAC. BAEPs are the least sensitive to volatile agents. MEPs are extremely sensitive to volatile agents. With IV agents *propofol, etomidate, thiopental,* and *pentobarbitol,* there is an *increase in latency and decrease of amplitude for SSEPs and VEPs*. With *ketamine* there is an *increase in latency and amplitude of SSEPs and an increase in latency and decrease in amplitude of VEPs*. MEPs show depression with *benzodiazepines, barbiturates,* and *propofol*. Muscle relaxants have no effect on SSEPs and VEPs, but a depressing effect on MEPs.

Visual evoked potentials (VEPs)–use: to monitor the integrity of the *visual pathway* by monitoring the wavelets that are produced in the *occipital cortex with visual stimuli*.

Motor evoked potentials (MEPs) – interpretation: depending on the study *reduction in compound muscle action potential (CMAP) amplitude (25% vs. 50% vs. 80%)* or *change in stimulation threshold* are used to signify a critical change.

Motor evoked potentials (MEPs) – moderating factors: systemic blood pressure, PaO_2, $PaCO_2$, and temperature.

Motor evoked potentials (MEPs) – pathways: the stimuli at the scalp electrode activates an action potential at the motor cortex that travels down the *corticospinal tract* activating *alpha-motor neurons at the anterior horn of the spinal cord*. From the anterior horn cells the action potential travels to the *motor end-plate* via the peripheral nerves, generating a compound muscle action potential that is recorded at the electrode overlying the muscle.

Motor evoked potentials (MEPs) – uses: monitoring for nerve injury during spinal surgery and cerebral tumor

Table 28.1 Evoked potential monitoring

Monitoring	Technique	Anesthetic considerations
SSEPs	Evaluation of functional integrity of ascending sensory pathways by somatosensory stimulation	A significant change of SSEPs is considered if the amplitude is reduced by 50% from baseline in response to surgical manipulation. TIVA may be preferred over inhalational agent anesthesia. End-tidal concentrations of 0.6 MAC of volatile agent are compatible with satisfactory readings. Nitrous oxide in combination with a volatile anesthetic produces profound depression unless total MAC <1.0.
VEPs	Evaluation of functional integrity of ascending sensory pathways by visual stimulation	TIVA may be preferred over inhalational agent anesthesia. End-tidal concentrations of 0.5 MAC volatile agent are compatible with satisfactory readings. VEPs tend to be more sensitive than SSEPs to the effect of inhalational anesthetics. Nitrous oxide in combination with a volatile anesthetic produces profound depression.
BAEPs	Evaluation of functional integrity of ascending sensory pathways by auditory stimulation at the brainstem	BAEPs are less vulnerable than SSEPs or VEPs to anesthetic influences. Most anesthetic regimens are compatible. Increase of latency with minimal amplitude effects. An increase in latency of >1 ms is considered clinically significant. Large steps of inhalational agent increases (>0.5 MAC) should be avoided during critical periods.
MEPs	Evaluation of functional integrity of descending motor pathways	MEPs are extremely sensitve to volatile agents, but less so to nitrous oxide. Benzodiazepines, barbiturates, and propofol produce marked depression of myogenic MEPs. Fentanyl, etomidate, and ketamine have little or no effect. Muscle relaxants affect the recorded EMG response by depressing myoneural transmission but may be used as a continuous infusion maintaining one or two twitches.

BAEPs, brainstem auditory evoked potentials; MAC, minimum alveolar concentration; TIVA. total intravenous anesthesia.
(Adapted from Vacanti et al. 2011. *Essential Clinical Anesthesia*, Cambridge University Press, p. 205.)

resection. Also it is useful for monitoring ischemic changes to the ventral horn cells during aortic reconstruction.

Brainstem auditory evoked potentials (BAEPs) – interpretation: an increase in the latency of greater than 1 ms over baseline is considered of clinical significance.

Wake-up test – use: to assess lower extremity motor function, which can be compromised by spinal cord ischemia that is related to intraoperative distraction of the vertebrae during scoliosis correction surgery.

Cranial nerve monitoring – procedures used in: cranial nerve monitoring is used in intracranial procedures that involve the *posterior fossa and the lower brainstem*. Both spontaneous and triggered muscle activity is monitored.

Intracranial pressure (ICP) monitoring – use: to optimize cerebral perfusion pressure in patients with head injury, large brain tumors, ruptured intracranial aneurysms, cerebrovascular occlusive disease, and hydrocephalus. It is also used to monitor for intracranial hypertension.

Transcranial Doppler ultrasound (TCD) – uses: to measure relative changes in cerebral blood flow. These changes are present in patients with vasospasm, hyperemia, emboli, stenosis, abnormal collateral flow, and inadequate CBF. During carotid endarterectomy it is used to monitor for acute thrombotic occlusion, microemboli, and for assessing postoperative hyperperfusion syndrome.

TCD interpretation: the Doppler shift is proportional to the blood flow velocity.

TCD pulsatile index: is the systolic velocity – diastolic velocity/mean viscosity and is a means of estimating the cerebral pulse pressure.

Cerebral oxygenation/metabolism monitoring methods: consists of transcranial oximetry (near-infrared spectroscopy), brain tissue oxygenation, and jugular bulb venous oximetry monitoring methods. Near-infrared spectroscopy (NIRS) is a noninvasive method to monitor regional cerebral oxygenation. It uses differences in wavelength absorption between

Table 28.2 ICP monitoring techniques

Method	Technique	Advantages	Disadvantages
Intraventricular catheters (standard)	Small scalp incision Small burr hole through skull Insertion of a soft nonreactive plastic catheter into the lateral ventricle, connection to transducer	Relatively reliable measurement of ICP Allows CSF drainage and compliance measurement	Occlusion of tubing may obliterate recording Ventricle is difficult to locate in the setting of brain swelling Brain injury is possible during passage of catheter Risk of hematoma and infection of catheter
Subdural–subarachnoid bolts or catheters	Hollow screw fixed into the skull with the tip passing through the incised dura	No brain tissue penetration or knowledge of ventricular position May be placed in any skull location with avoidance of venous sinuses	Occlusion of tubing may obliterate recording Brain tissue may obstruct the tip of the bolt Risk of infection, epidural bleeding, or focal seizures if bolt is positioned too deeply
Epidural transducers	Placement of epidural catheter with 2 pressure-sensitive membrane or a Mu mot 0 pressure switch (Ladd transducer)	Lower risk of brain infection because of extradural placement	Difficult placement in potential space Risk of bleeding No possibility for compliance testing or CSF drainage
Intraparenchymal fiberoptic devices	Fiberoptic catheter introduced within conical gray matter	Direct measurement of brain tissue pressure Easy insertion Small diameter Less disruptive of brain tissue Lower risk of infection (no fluid column) New fiberoptic ICP monitors allow measurement of local CBF, PO_2, PO_2, PCO_2, pH, and other metabolic markers	No possibility of calibration in situ No possibility of compliance testing or CSF drainage

(From Vacanti et al., 2011, p. 206.)

Table 28.3 Cerebral oxygen/metabolism monitoring techniques

Monitoring method	Technique	Anesthetic considerations
Brain tissue oxygenation	A multiparameter sensor is available for measuring brain tissue PO_2, PCO_2, pH, and temperature using a combined electrode–fiberoptic system.	The placement of the sensor requires insertion into the cortex tissue under direct visualization.
Jugular bulb venous oximetry	Measurement of $SjVO_2$ through a percutaneous retrograde cannulation of the internal jugular vein using a catheter with embedded optical fibers. Normal $SjVO_2$ is 60 to 70%.	Increases in $SjVO_2$ indicate relative hyperema as a result of reduced metabolic requirement (comatose or brain-dead patient) or excessive flow (severe hypercapnia). A value <50% reflects increased oxygen extraction and potential risk of ischemic injury. This also may be caused by increased metabolic demand (fever, seizure) or by an absolute reduction in flow. A major limitation is the inability to detect focal ischemia.
Transcranial oximetry	NIRS is a noninvasive optical method for monitoring cerebral regional oxygenation. It reflects off oxy- and deoxyhemoglobin and allows quantitative assessment of those based on the absorption of light at several wavelengths. It is used as a monitor during carotid endarterectomy. head injury, and subarachnoid hemorrhage.	Major limitations include intersubject variability, variable optical path length, potential contamination from extracranial blood, and lack of a definable threshold. It can be used only as a trend monitor. As a bilateral monitor, it is useful to detect regional ischemia during carotid endarterectomy and temporary clip application during intracranial aneurysm surgery.

(Adapted from Vacanti et al. 2011. *Essential Clinical Anesthesia*, Cambridge University Press, p. 207.)

oxyhemoglobin and deoxyhemoglobin to assess venous oxygen content. Brain tissue oxygen monitors are invasive methods to monitor local tissue PO_2, PCO_2, pH, and temperature using an electrode–fiberoptic system. Jugular venous bulb oximetry ($SjVO_2$) involves insertion of a catheter into the internal jugular vein that has optical fibers. The normal $SjVO_2$ value range is 60% to 70%. A *value greater than 70% suggests hyperemia* secondary to decreased cerebral metabolic demand (comatose or brain death) or excessive CBF (severe hypercapnea). A value less than 50% *indicates elevated $CMRO_2$ with potential risk of ischemic injury.* $SjVO_2$ is insensitive to focal ischemia.

Questions

1. Which of the following agents will NOT produce burst suppression pattern on EEG?
   a. isoflurane
   b. propofol
   c. sevoflurane
   d. midazolam

2. What effect does spinal cord ischemia have on SSEP waveform?
   a. increased amplitude and increased latency
   b. decreased amplitude and increased latency
   c. decreased amplitude and decreased latency
   d. increased amplitude and decreased latency

3. Which is the correct order of neurophysiologic monitoring techniques as relates to sensitivity to inhaled anesthetic agents from greatest to least?
   a. SSEP > VEP > BAEP
   b. VEP > SSEP > BAEP
   c. BAEP > VEP > SSEP
   d. SSEP > BAEP > VEP

Answers

1. d. Halogenated inhalation agents, thiopental, and propofol have an EEG pattern that transitions from initial loss of alpha activity and increase in frontal beta, to theta then delta to reach burst suppression. Midazolam, a benzodiazepine, is unable to produce burst suppression.

2. b. A decrease in the amplitude or an increase in the latency in the SSEP waveform from baseline may indicate ischemia.

3. b. Inhaled agents have a dose-dependent decrease in amplitude and increase in latency with VEPs being the most sensitive and BAEPs being the least.

Further reading

Vacanti, C., Sikka, P., Urman, R., Dershwitz, M., and Segal, B. (eds) (2011). *Essential Clinical Anesthesia.* Cambridge: Cambridge University Press.

Simon, M. (2010). *Intraoperative Neurophysiology: A Comprehensive Guide to Monitoring and Mapping.* Demos Medical Publishing.

Reich, D. L., Kahn, R. A., Mittnacht, A. J. C. et al. (2011). *Monitoring in Anesthesia and Perioperative Care.* Cambridge University Press.

29

Intraoperative awareness

Nantthasorn Zinboonyahgoon and Joseph M. Garfield

Keywords

Definition, incidence, and etiology
Risk factors: surgical procedure, patient characteristics,
   anesthetic management
Prevention: clinical signs, end-tidal agent, processed
   EEG monitoring

Definition, incidence, and etiology

General anesthesia is a state during which the patient is rendered unconscious, accompanied by loss of perception of pain and attenuation of reflex responses. After awakening from most general anesthetics, the patient is unable to recall any details of the surgical procedure or the administration of the anesthetic. Unfortunately, on rare occasions, inadequate anesthesia during the operative procedure may result in episodes of consciousness and postoperative recall, a complication known as intraoperative awareness with recall.

Incidence: the incidence is 0.1% to 0.2% overall, depending on design of study, anesthetic management, and patient population.

0.1% for GA without neuromuscular blocking agents
0.2% for GA with neuromuscular blocking agents
0.4% to 1% for high-risk patients (indicated below)

Etiology: (from ASA Closed Claims Database and Anesthesia Awareness Registry, published in 2010).

1. Problematic anesthetic management: inadequate anesthetic depth from issues relating to the anesthetic administration itself and operator error. Inadequate anesthetic depth can result from a number of factors, including vaporizer malfunction and undetected empty vaporizer, machine malfunction, incorrect calculation of volatile agent and IV drug administration (TIVA), failure to observe the patient for signs of awareness (sweating, attempts to communicate), failure to note inspired and end-expired concentrations of volatile agents, and incorrect interpretation of anesthesia depth monitors.

2. Hemodynamic instability: reduction of anesthetic concentrations and IV drug dosages in the face of severe hypotension and/or other signs of hemodynamic instability may result in temporary episodes of intraoperative awareness owing to inadequate anesthetic depth to ensure unconsciousness.

3. Difficult intubation: this is a common cause of awareness; it may result when the patient remains paralyzed but the hypnotic agent (propofol, etomidate, etc.) wears off during prolonged, multiple attempts at endotracheal intubation.

4. Unknown factors: these include episodes of awareness where comprehensive review of the agent doses and vital signs during the anesthetic fail to indicate anything consistent with conditions promoting the episodes.

Risk factors for awareness

1. Type of *surgical procedure*: cardiac, trauma, emergency surgical procedures, and emergency cesarean section are associated with a higher incidence of intraoperative awareness.

2. *Patient characteristics* predisposing to intraoperative awareness:

   a. substance use or abuse
   b. alcoholism
   c. chronic pain patients on high dose of opioids
   d. ASA status 4 or 5
   e. history of problems related to anesthetic administration (anticipated or history of difficult intubation, previous episode of awareness).

3. *Anesthetic management*: use neuromuscular blocking agents and reduced anesthetic concentrations/doses during paralysis, TIVA, nitrous oxide–opioid anesthesia.

Prevention

Preoperative measures: identify patients at risk.

1. Explain about risks of awareness as part of consent process.

Essential Clinical Anesthesia Review: Keywords, Questions and Answers for the Boards, ed. Linda S. Aglio, Robert W. Lekowski, and Richard D. Urman. Published by Cambridge University Press. © Cambridge University Press 2015.

2. Plan for additional monitoring and anesthesia management for high-risk patients (consider use of EEG/BIS anesthetic depth monitors).
3. Preoperative administration of benzodiazepine.
4. Check anesthetic system/drug delivery systems.

Intraoperative measures: monitor and maintain adequate depth of anesthesia.

As no single perfect tool can prevent awareness completely, multiple modalities, as follows, should be applied to assess depth of anesthesia during surgery, especially in high-risk patients:

1. *Clinical signs*: observation of movement, sweating, lacrimation, eyelash reflex, pupils, blood pressure, heart rate, respiratory rate; however, use of NMB agent may mask somatic signs (movement) and vital signs may not change in patients who receive certain medications (beta-blockers) or patients who have poor cardiac reserve.
2. *End-tidal agents*: keep end-tidal gas >0.7 MAC. Even this monitoring can decrease incidence of awareness, but awareness during agent monitoring has been reported (this conclusion is still controversial).
3. *Processed EEG monitoring*: e.g. bispectral index monitoring (BIS monitor), keep index <60.

   a. brain function monitoring may decrease incidence of awareness; however, awareness during brain monitoring has been reported (this area remains controversial)
   b. for TIVA, BIS monitoring provides feedback as to depth of anesthesia and decreases risk of awareness in TIVA patients.

Postoperative measures: early detection and management.

1. Early detection by interviewing high-risk patients or patients who had intraoperative events that predispose to recall (e.g., unanticipated difficult airway, mechanical failure of anesthetic delivery).
2. Early intervention to avoid further complications and early management of consequences.

   a. as psychological injury can range from short-term psychological stress to permanent long-term damage (i.e., post-traumatic stress disorder), a frank discussion with the patient, emphasizing that what he or she experienced was real and not a figment of their imagination, validation that the experience was disturbing and traumatic, a sincere apology if caused by a preventable event (empty vaporizer, wrong drug dose, etc.), coupled with a psychiatric consultation and follow-up

b. medico-legal implications: ASA Closed Claims analysis shows payment was made to 46% of claims, ranging from US$3,960 to US$1,016,470.

Questions

1. Under general anesthesia with inhalation agents, which operation is the LEAST likely to result in a patient experiencing awareness?
   a. emergency C/S under GA
   b. parotid mass removal with EMG monitoring
   c. CABG
   d. exploratory laparotomy for patient who had a motor vehicle accident with multiple injuries

2. Which of the following should decrease the likelihood of awareness?
   a. BIS monitoring showing index less than 60
   b. inhalational agent monitor shows end-inspired gas concentration more than 0.7 MAC
   c. TIVA
   d. administration of neuromuscular blocking agents

3. Which statement is true?
   a. BIS monitoring cannot completely prevent awareness.
   b. End-tidal agent monitoring can prevent awareness more effectively than BIS monitoring.
   c. Patients who have no hemodynamic response to surgical stimuli, should not have awareness.
   d. Consequences of awareness are not life-threatening, short, and transient.

Answers

1. b. Emergency, cardiac, and trauma cases have higher risk of awareness.
2. a. BIS monitoring index less than 60, end-expired gas concentration more than 0.7 MAC may, but not definitely, decrease risk of awareness; TIVA and administration of neuromuscular blocking agents are associated with higher risk of awareness.
3. a. Neither BIS monitoring nor end-tidal gas monitoring can completely prevent awareness. There is still not enough convincing evidence proving one monitoring is superior to another. Patients who have poor cardiac reserve might not have hemodynamic response to surgical stimuli, despite awareness. Awareness can lead to serious long-term consequences such as post-traumatic stress disorder.

Further reading

Kelly, S. D. (2011). Intraoperative awareness. In Vacanti, C. A., Sikka, P. J., Urman, R. D., Dershwitz, M., and Segal, B. S. (eds) *Essential Clinical Anesthesia*. Cambridge: Cambridge University Press.

Domino, K. B. and Cole, D. J. (2011). Awareness under anesthesia. In Miller, R. D. and Pardo, M. C. (eds) *Basics of Anesthesia*, 6th edn. Philadelphia: Elsevier Saunders.

Bowdle, T. A. (2009). Can we prevent recall during anesthesia? In Fleisher, L. A. (ed)

Evidence-based Practice of Anesthesiology, 2nd edn. Philadelphia: Elsevier Saunders.

Gallagher, T. H., Garbutt, J. M., Waterman, A. D. et al. (2006). Choosing your words carefully: how physicians would disclose harmful medical errors to patients. *Archives of Internal Medicine* 166, 1585–1593.

Chapter

30

Inhalation anesthetics

Carly C. Guthrie and Jeffrey Lu

Keywords

Halothane
Isoflurane
Sevoflurane
Compound A
Desflurane
Tec6 vaporizer
CO production
Nitrous oxide
Contraindications to nitrous oxide
Altitude changes and vaporizer output
Changing vaporizers and vapor pressure
Malignant hyperthermia

Halothane: a halogenated alkane compound that is a potent bronchodilator with very little pungency. For these reasons, it is extremely useful for inhalational inductions in children. Its MAC is 0.75 and its blood/gas partition coefficient is 2.4. It has the highest level of metabolization by the liver of any of the volatile anesthetics. The major metabolite is trifluoroacetic acid (TFA) and an immune-mediated reaction to this is the likely culprit for the hepatotoxicity that sometimes results, i.e., "halothane hepatitis."

Isoflurane: a halogenated ether with a MAC of 1.1 and a blood/gas partition coefficient of 1.4. It is highly pungent and can cause some upper airway irritation. There is some concern for use of isoflurane in patients with coronary artery disease due to its dilation of coronary arteries, potentially causing diversion of blood away from areas of myocardium with stenotic lesions and inadequate perfusion ("coronary steal syndrome"). This has yet to be shown to have clinical significance.

Sevoflurane: similar in structure to isoflurane and desflurane, with all being substituted halogenated ethers. However, like halothane, it has a low pungency and is a potent bronchodilator, so it is also commonly used for inhalational inductions in children. It is currently one of the most commonly used agents due to its potency, moderately quick onset and

elimination (MAC 2.05 and blood/gas partition coefficient of 0.65), and relative inexpensiveness.

Compound A: when sevoflurane comes into contact with soda lime contained in a CO_2 absorber, it is degraded into several breakdown products, one of which is known as *Compound A*. This compound has been shown to cause kidney disease in rat models, but has yet to be shown to cause kidney disease in humans. However, due to this theoretical concern, sevoflurane is administered with higher fresh gas flows to prevent formation of larger amounts of breakdown products and accumulation within the system. More Compound A is formed when the soda lime is at an increased temperature and when it is desiccated.

Desflurane: a halogenated ether with very low solubility in the blood and tissues (blood/gas partition coefficient 0.42) and thus a very rapid onset and elimination. However, it is less potent than the other inhaled anesthetics with a MAC of 6.0. Furthermore, desflurane has a relatively high vapor pressure of over 681 mm Hg, which means that it boils at close to room temperature and requires a special vaporizer for anesthetic delivery. Desflurane is very pungent and irritating to the upper airways and rapid rises in anesthetic concentrations can cause tachycardia as a response.

Tec6 vaporizer: desflurane is unique among the inhaled anesthetics in that its vapor pressure is so high, 681 mm Hg at 20°C, that it nearly boils at room temperature. This high volatility requires a special vaporizer to administer desflurane in the operating room environment. The *Tec6 vaporizer* works differently than the variable bypass vaporizers in that it first heats a reservoir of liquid desflurane to 39°C and creates a vapor pressure of 2 atm. Instead of the fresh gas flow passing through this chamber of vaporized desflurane, a specific amount of desflurane vapor is released from the reservoir and mixes with the fresh gas flow directly prior to leaving the vaporizer. The amount of desflurane vapor released is dependent on the concentration that the anesthesiologist selects on the control dial as well as the overall fresh gas flow.

CO production: although desflurane undergoes very minimal metabolism within the body, dry CO_2 absorbents will

Essential Clinical Anesthesia Review: Keywords, Questions and Answers for the Boards, ed. Linda S. Aglio, Robert W. Lekowski, and Richard D. Urman. Published by Cambridge University Press. © Cambridge University Press 2015.

degrade desflurane and produce carbon monoxide. This occurs primarily with desiccated absorbents, and is most common with barium hydroxide lyme (Baralyme), but can also occur with sodium and potassium hydroxide. This CO production can result in clinically significant levels of carboxyhemoglobin in the blood, requiring treatment.

Nitrous oxide (N2O): differs from the other anesthetic agents in that it is the only inorganic compound. Due to its comparatively high MAC of 105%, it is insufficient to provide adequate anesthesia on its own, thus it is most often used as an adjuvant to the other anesthetics. Its properties as an NMDA receptor antagonist and ability to provide some analgesia are also noteworthy. The blood/gas partition coefficient is 0.47, thus it has a very rapid uptake and elimination, rivaling desflurane.

Contraindications to the use of nitrous oxide: include the presence of a pneumothorax, laparoscopic abdominal surgery, concern for air embolus, neurosurgical procedures in which air may accumulate under the dura, or recent ophthalmologic procedures in which an air bubble is instilled in the eye. The common link to all of the above contraindications is that N_2O is much more soluble and more diffusible than nitrogen, thus it will enter any closed airspace more quickly than nitrogen can leave, causing that airspace to expand. For this reason, any of the above situations can become quite dangerous in the event that nitrous oxide is used and diffuses quickly into the space, increasing the volume and pressure dramatically. Other complications with the use of N_2O include bone marrow depression due to its irreversible inhibition of methionine synthase causing impaired DNA synthesis and hyperhomocysteinemia. N_2O may also cause symptoms of B_{12} deficiency including neuropathy and encephalopathy.

Changing the altitude at which a vaporizer is being utilized can have a profound effect on the delivery of the anesthetic agent due to the effect of atmospheric pressure on the principle of partial pressures. For any of the agents delivered by a variable bypass vaporizer (isoflurane, halothane, and sevoflurane), moving to a higher altitude will not have any effect on the delivered partial pressure of the agent, which determines the anesthetic effect. This is because any decrease in atmospheric pressure will be compensated for by an increased delivery of the amount of agent, resulting in a similar partial pressure. Thus no compensation is necessary on the part of the anesthesiologist. However, this concept does not hold true for the Tec6 vaporizer, which delivers desflurane. This is because the Tec6 vaporizer is pressurized internally to allow vaporization of the desflurane, thus its output is independent of the external atmospheric pressure. Thus higher elevations and decreased atmospheric pressure will result in an overall decrease in the partial pressure of desflurane delivered for a certain concentration set on the dial.

Accidentally filling a vaporizer with the wrong inhaled agent will dramatically alter the output of that agent. Each inhalational anesthetic has an inherent vapor pressure, which describes the fraction of agent that exists in vapor form above the liquid form within the vaporizer. Since variable bypass vaporizers, which are agent-specific, work by directing gas flow through a chamber and picking up a portion of the vaporized agent, the amount of agent that leaves with the fresh gas flow is directly proportional to the amount of agent that exists in vapor form. Therefore filling a vaporizer with an agent that has a higher inherent vapor pressure will result in a higher output of anesthetic agent and a potential overdose. For example, filling a sevoflurane vaporizer (sevoflurane's vapor pressure is 160) with isoflurane (vapor pressure 240) will result in a much higher percent concentration output of isoflurane than for the same dial setting of sevoflurane in its own vaporizer.

Malignant hyperthermia: an extremely dangerous syndrome that is most commonly caused by a mutation in the type 1 ryanodine receptor. This causes a hypermetabolic state, which can be triggered by the volatile anesthetics (halothane, sevoflurane, isoflurane, and desflurane) as well as succinylcholine. Symptoms include tachycardia, increasing expired CO_2 (most sensitive early sign), muscle rigidity (classically masseter spasm), respiratory and metabolic acidosis, myoglobinuria, and increasing temperature. Rapid recognition and treatment with cooling and administration of dantrolene is essential. Dantrolene lessens the loss of calcium from the sarcoplasmic reticulum, restoring the normal metabolic state.

Questions

1. What is the most reliable early sign of malignant hyperthermia?
   a. tachycardia
   b. increased CO_2
   c. masseter spasm
   d. hyperthermia
   e. myoglobinuria

2. Which of the following inhaled anesthetics would be appropriate for an inhalational induction?
   a. sevoflurane
   b. desflurane
   c. nitrous oxide
   d. isoflurane

3. Which of the following CO_2 absorbents is most concerning for production of carbon monoxide during desflurane administration?
   a. calcium hydroxide
   b. sodium hydroxide
   c. potassium hydroxide
   d. barium hydroxide

4. How will the partial pressure of desflurane released from a Tec6 vaporizer change if that vaporizer is moved from sea level in San Diego to an altitude of 5,000 ft in Denver?
   a. increase
   b. decrease
   c. stay the same

Answers

1. b. Symptoms of malignant hyperthermia include tachycardia, increasing expired CO_2 (most sensitive early sign), muscle rigidity (classically masseter spasm), respiratory and metabolic acidosis, myoglobinuria, and increasing temperature.

2. a. Sevoflurane and halothane have relatively fast onset and very low pungency and airway irritability, making them ideal for inhalational inductions.

3. d. Desflurane can interact with CO_2 absorbers to produce carbon monoxide. This reaction is most common with barium hydroxide lyme (Baralyme), but can also occur with sodium and potassium hydroxide. This CO production can result in clinically significant levels of carboxyhemoglobin in the blood, requiring treatment.

4. b. Higher elevations and decreased atmospheric pressure will result in an overall decrease in the partial pressure of desflurane delivered for a certain concentration set on the dial.

Further reading

Vacanti, C., Sikka, P., Urman, R., Dershwitz, M., and Segal, B. (eds) (2011). *Essential Clinical Anesthesia*. Cambridge: Cambridge University Press, Chapters 31–33.

Morgan, G. E., Mikhail, M. S., and Murray, M. J. (2007). *Clinical Anesthesiology*, 4th edn. McGraw-Hill Medical, Chapter 4.

Miller, R. D., Eriksson, L. I., Fleisher, L. A., et al. (eds) (2009). *Miller's Anesthesia*, 7th edn. Churchill-Livingston, Chapters 4–9.

Chapter 31

Pharmacokinetics of inhalation agents

Carly C. Guthrie and Jeffrey Lu

Keywords

Induction speed
Elevated cardiac output
Intracardiac shunts
Alveolar–venous partial pressure difference
VRG/VPG/fat/muscle groups
Alveolar tension curve
Concentration effect
Second gas effect
Meyer–Overton theory
Solubility
Elimination
Diffusion hypoxia

Induction speed: alveolar pressure (P_A) – arterial pressure (P_a) – P_{brain}, thus P_A is only an approximation of P_{brain}. Blood passes though the capillaries of the lungs and the anesthetic partial pressure equalizes between the alveolar and arterial pressure. Then, due to the movement of arterial blood throughout the body, and after a short period of equilibration, the alveolar partial pressure of the gas equals the brain partial pressure. Alveolar partial pressure can be increased by increasing minute ventilation, increasing flow rates at the level of the vaporizer, and by using a non-rebreathing circuit.

Elevated cardiac output will slow induction with inhaled anesthetics because there will be a greater removal of volatile agent from the alveoli, thus lowering the alveolar partial pressure of the agent. Since the alveolar partial pressure is taken as a surrogate for the partial pressure in the brain, the end result of a higher cardiac output will be a longer equilibration time between the alveoli and the brain, hence a longer induction time.

Intracardiac shunts can have profound effects on the speed of induction with both IV and inhaled agents, as follows. An inhalational induction in a patient with a right-to-left intracardiac shunt will be slower due to venous admixture. This will affect the rate of induction for highly soluble agents more than for poorly soluble agents, as the effect of the venous admixture will be minimal for poorly soluble agents. On the other hand, a right-to-left shunt will cause an IV induction to be more rapid for all agents because the IV anesthetic will bypass the pulmonary circulation and go directly to the systemic circulation. A left-to-right intracardiac shunt will have a negligible effect on both IV and inhalational inductions.

Alveolar–venous partial pressure difference will reflect the amount of inhaled agent taken up by the peripheral tissues as arterial blood carries the anesthetic from the lungs to the tissue compartments. A large difference is caused by an increased uptake of the agent and is generally present during induction when the tissue compartments are relatively empty of anesthetic. This large concentration gradient will help facilitate diffusion of the agent from the alveoli into the blood.

VRG/VPG/fat/muscle groups: inhaled anesthetic agent first enters the alveoli and is then transferred down the partial pressure gradient to the arterial blood via the pulmonary capillary system. The arterial blood then carries the agent to the peripheral compartments, which take up the anesthetic due to the partial pressure gradient between them and the arterial blood. This initially happens quickly due to the absence of agent in the tissue and will slow as the gradient lessens. If the alveolar-inspired concentration drops (i.e., the agent is turned off), the tissues will begin releasing the anesthetic into the venous blood as the gradient reverses. The first group to fill will be the vessel-rich group (including the brain, liver, and heart), then the muscle group, then the fat group, which can act as a large reservoir of anesthetic, then the vessel-poor group including bone.

The initial rise of the *alveolar tension curve* is formed by the rapid wash-in of inhaled anesthetic into the alveoli, before the blood begins to take it away. The alveolar plateau is then created when blood flow through the lungs

Essential Clinical Anesthesia Review: Keywords, Questions and Answers for the Boards, ed. Linda S. Aglio, Robert W. Lekowski, and Richard D. Urman. Published by Cambridge University Press. © Cambridge University Press 2015.

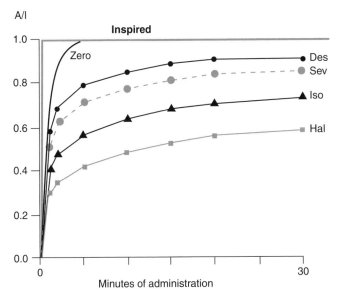

Figure 31.1 Alveolar tension curves of several anesthetics. Graphs are redrawn from the data of Yasuda, N., Lockhart, S. H., Eger, E. I. et al. 1991. Comparison of kinetics of sevoflurane and isoflurane in humans. *Anesthesia and Analgesia*, 72: 316–324. (From Vacanti et al. 2011. *Essential Clinical Anesthesia*, Cambridge University Press, p. 221.)

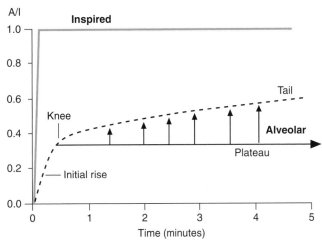

Figure 31.2 Tail of the alveolar tension curves. The rise in alveolar tension curves that transforms the plateau into a knee is produced by venous return of anesthetic-laden blood to the lungs. (From Vacanti et al. 2011. *Essential Clinical Anesthesia*, Cambridge University Press, p. 221.)

begins to remove the inhaled agent from the alveoli and is balanced by the continuous delivery of agent via ventilation. Lastly, the knee and tail of the curve result when venous blood from the tissues returns anesthetic to the alveoli, causing alveolar tension to rise. The first portion of the tail is caused by the blood from the VRG (which causes the upgoing knee), then from muscle, then finally from fat.

Concentration effect: used to describe how breathing a high concentration of gas can augment its own uptake from the lungs. When a high concentration of a gas is inspired, a large fraction of the total volume taken up from the lung is of that gas. This reduction in total alveolar volume is then offset by replacing the volume with a very concentrated volume of the initial gas. This phenomenon increases alveolar ventilation during the period of rapid gas uptake into the blood and is probably clinically useful only with nitrous oxide as this is the only agent used in very high concentrations.

Second gas effect describes the effect that occurs by combining nitrous oxide at high concentrations with a second inhaled agent. Nitrous oxide is so insoluble in blood that it is rapidly absorbed from the alveoli, leaving behind the more soluble inhaled agent. This concentrates the soluble agent remaining in the alveoli, increasing its partial pressure in the alveoli, and augmenting the speed of induction.

Meyer–Overton theory suggests that the lipid solubility of inhaled anesthetic agents is directly related to potency and the anesthetic action of these agents. However, there is proof that this is overly simplistic and specific neurotransmitters and receptors, such as the enhancement of GABA, play a role as well.

Solubility: used to describe the affinity of a gas for a specific gas, fluid, or tissue. For inhalational anesthetic purposes, solubility is usually described in terms of partition coefficients. These describe the ratio of concentration in one compartment to the concentration in a second compartment at equilibrium. For example, a higher blood/gas partition coefficient will correlate to a higher uptake of the gas into the blood and is described as a higher solubility. This will result in a slower induction time as it will take longer for the brain compartment to reach equilibrium as well.

The most important factor in determining the *elimination* of inhaled anesthetic agents is ventilation. Achievement of a decrease of 50% for the inhaled agents is rapid and should take only a few minutes. Thus the differences in emergence time between the agents will depend almost entirely on the final 20% of the elimination process.

Due to its very low solubility in blood, elimination of nitrous oxide at the end of an anesthetic can cause *diffusion hypoxia*. This occurs when nitrous oxide is turned off at the end of a case and the alveolar inspired concentration drops to zero. This causes a reversal of the concentration gradient and a rapid diffusion of nitrous oxide from the venous blood into the alveoli, thereby diluting the partial pressure of oxygen in the alveoli and creating a hypoxic mixture.

Questions

1. Which of the following partial pressures is used as a surrogate marker for the partial pressure of inhaled agent in the brain and therefore anesthetic depth?

   a. $P_{arterial}$
   b. P_{venous}
   c. $P_{capillary}$
   d. $P_{alveolar}$

2. How will a left-to-right intracardiac shunt affect the speed of induction for an inhaled agent?
   a. increase
   b. decrease
   c. no significant change

3. Elimination of inhaled anesthetic is primarily dependent on which of the following?
   a. ventilation
   b. renal metabolism
   c. hepatic metabolism
   d. redistribution

Answers

1. d. Alveolar pressure (P_A) – Arterial pressure (P_a) – P_{brain}, thus P_A is an approximation of P_{brain}. Due to the movement of arterial blood though the body, and after a short period of equilibration, the alveolar partial pressure of the gas equals the brain partial pressure.
2. c. A left-to-right intracardiac shunt will have a negligible effect on both IV and inhalational inductions.
3. a. The most important factor in determining the elimination of inhaled anesthetic agents is ventilation.

Further reading

Vacanti, C., Sikka, P., Urman, R., Dershwitz, M., and Segal, B. (eds) (2011). *Essential Clinical Anesthesia.* Cambridge: Cambridge University Press, Chapter 32.

Morgan, G. E., Mikhail, M. S., and Murray, M. J. (2007). *Clinical Anesthesiology*, 4th edn. McGraw-Hill Medical, Chapter 7.

Miller, R. D., Eriksson, L. I., Fleisher, L. A. et al. (2009). *Miller's Anesthesia*, 7th edn. Churchill-Livingstone, Chapters 4–9.

Pharmacodynamics of inhalation agents

Carly C. Guthrie and Jeffrey Lu

Keywords

Minimum alveolar concentration
Factors that change MAC
MAC changes with age
Cardiac effects of inhalation agents
Halothane and arrhythmias
Pulmonary ventilation and inhalation agents
Bronchomotor tone
Neuromuscular blocking agents
Central nervous system effects
Metabolism rates

Minimum alveolar concentration (MAC): one MAC is the level of inhaled anesthetic, reflected in the end-tidal anesthetic gas, which prevents movement to surgical stimulus in 50% of patients. MAC values are additive, meaning that 0.5 MAC of nitrous oxide and 0.5 MAC of sevoflurane will provide 1 MAC of anesthesia. MAC awake, the level of anesthetic at which the patient awakens is approximately 0.3 MAC. MAC decreases by 6% per decade of age.

Factors that change MAC

MAC changes with age: MAC is age-dependent, being lowest in newborns, reaching a peak in infants, and then decreasing progressively with increasing age. This is not true for sevoflurane, as the MAC for sevoflurane in newborns may be just slightly higher or equal to that of infants.

Cardiac effects of inhalation agents: inhaled anesthetic agents all cause a dose-dependent decrease in MAP due to decreases in SVR, although halothane's direct inhibition of cardiac contractility is its primary mechanism of decreased MAP. Inhaled anesthetics also cause increases in heart rate due to a baroreceptor response to the decrease in blood pressure, except for halothane, which blunts this response. All inhaled anesthetics prolong the QT interval and treatment with beta-blockade may be required.

Halothane can cause arrhythmias by sensitizing the heart to the arrhythmogenic effects of epinephrine; thus care should be taken when using halothane in conjunction with local anesthetics containing epinephrine.

Pulmonary ventilation: inhaled anesthetic agents cause respiratory depression by decreasing the tidal volume and increasing the respiratory rate. This leads to greater dead space ventilation and a proportional increase in PaCO2. Volatile anesthetics also blunt the ventilatory responses to both hypercapnia and hypoxia.

The inhaled anesthetics are potent bronchodilators, with the exception of desflurane, although they can also cause upper airway irritation and laryngospasm. The most irritating agents are desflurane, then isoflurane, halothane, and sevoflurane. This accounts for the use of halothane and sevoflurane in inhalational inductions. Desflurane can cause bronchospasm, especially in smokers and asthmatics.

Volatile agents potentiate neuromuscular blocking drugs via relaxation of skeletal muscles.

CNS effects: all inhalational agents decrease the cerebral metabolic rate of oxygen ($CMRO_2$) and increase cerebral blood flow (CBF) through vasodilation. At levels below 1 MAC there is more of an effect on $CMRO_2$, and at levels above 1 MAC the increase in CBF is predominant. Inhalational agents also cause increased latency and decreased amplitude of evoked potentials.

Essential Clinical Anesthesia Review: Keywords, Questions and Answers for the Boards, ed. Linda S. Aglio, Robert W. Lekowski, and Richard D. Urman. Published by Cambridge University Press. © Cambridge University Press 2015.

Table 32.1 Factors affecting MAC

Factor	Effect on MAC	Mechanism
Age	Young age (6 months): increase Increasing age: decrease	Brain development and neuron formation before and loss of neurons after age 6 months
Red hair	Increase	? Increased pheomelanin concentration caused by melanocortin-I receptor gene mutations, antagonism with opioid receptors, or influence on nociception
Body temperature	Hyperthermia: increase Hypothermia: decrease	Intrinisic properties in the brain
Blood pressure (MAP)	<40 mm Hg decrease	? Possibly impaired brain perfusion
Postpartum	Decrease by 30% immediately postpartum	Cardiovascular and hormonal changes of postpartum period
Oxygenation	PaO_2 <38 mm Hg: decrease	Attenuation of glutamate excitotoxicity
Cardiopulmonary bypass surgery	Decrease	Not known
Length of surgery	Constant or decrease	Not known
Sodium	Hypernatremia increase Hyponatremia decrease	Inhaled anesthetics inhibit synaptosomal sodium channel; amount of sodium in the body affects level of inhibition
Cyclosporine	Increase	Pharmacodynamic interaction seems to be likely, perhaps consequent to an effect of cyclosporine on ligand-gated sodium channels
Opioids	Decrease	Indirect (modulating) role but not a direct (mediating) role; provide analgesia and thus decrease MAC
Benzodiazepines	Decrease	Modulation by inhibition of GABA receptor
Ketamine	Decrease	NMDA receptor antagonism decreases temporal summation of pain stimuli
Lithium	Decrease	Not known
Lidocaine	Decrease	Modulating effect by providing analgesia
Alcohol	Acute: decrease Chronic: increase	Acute alcohol ingestion: synergistic with inhaled anesthetics; chronic alcoholism causes tolerance (?) by alteration of cytochrome P450 system

(From Vacanti et al. 2011. *Essential Clinical Anesthesia*, Cambridge University Press, p. 225.)

Questions

1. Decreases in MAP after administration of halothane are caused primarily by which factor?
   a. decreased cardiac inotropy
   b. decreased heart rate
   c. decreased SVR
   d. decreased PVR

2. Hypothyroidism will have which effect on MAC?
   a. increase
   b. decrease
   c. no change

3. Inhalational agents cause which of the follow changes in pulmonary ventilation?

   a. increased TV and increased RR
   b. decreased TV and decreased RR
   c. increased TV and decreased RR
   d. decreased TV and increased RR

Answers

1. a. Halothane's direct inhibition of cardiac contractility is its primary mechanism of decreased MAP.
2. c. Hypothyroidism and hyperthyroidism do not change MAC.
3. d. Inhaled anesthetic agents cause respiratory depression by decreasing tidal volumes and increasing respiratory rates.

Further reading

Vacanti, C., Sikka, P., Urman, R., Dershwitz, M., and Segal, B. (eds) (2011). *Essential Clinical Anesthesia*. Cambridge: Cambridge University Press, Chapter 33.

Morgan, G. E., Mikhail, M. S., and Murray, M. J. (2007). *Clinical Anesthesiology*, 4th edn. McGraw-Hill Medical, Chapter 7.

Rall, M., Gaba, D. M., Dieckmann, P., and Eich, C. (2009). Chapter 7.

Patient simulation. In Miller, R. D., Eriksson, L. I., Fleisher, L. A. et al. (eds) *Miller's Anesthesia*, 7th edn. Churchill-Livingstone.

33

Intravenous induction agents

Lisa M. Hammond and James Hardy

Keywords

Dissociative anesthesia
Synergism of IV opioids and IV induction agents
Induction modifications for the elderly
Neuroprotection of IV induction agents
Propofol allergy
Etomidate and adrenal suppression
Emetogenicity of etomidate
Induction agents and risk with porphyria
Benzodiazepine antagonism: flumazenil
Emergence delirium with ketamine

Overview

Benzodiazepines, barbiturates, etomidate, and propofol function primarily through augmentation of the γ-aminobutyric acid (GABA) neurotransmitter system.

Ketamine, in contrast, works primarily by antagonizing the N-methyl-D-aspartate (NMDA) receptor, although it also inhibits neuronal nicotinic acetylcholine receptors. Through its interaction with the NMDA receptors, it causes concurrent *depression* of the thalamocortical system and *stimulation* of the limbic system resulting in "*dissociative anesthesia.*"

IV opioids and IV induction agents are synergistic. IV opioids typically potentiate the cardiovascular and ventilator effects of IV induction agents.

Elderly patients typically require lower doses of most IV induction agents because of increased CNS sensitivity, decreased metabolic and renal clearance, and decreased plasma protein concentration resulting in increased "free" agent within the circulation.

Barbiturates

Thiopental and methohexital are short-acting barbiturates used for induction of general anesthesia.

Thiopental and methohexital both decrease the cerebral metabolic rate of oxygen consumption ($CMRO_2$), cerebral blood flow (CBF), and intracranial pressure (ICP). By decreasing cerebral metabolism, barbiturates can be *neuroprotective against ischemic injury* during periods of decreased oxygen delivery.

Thiopental at high doses produces an isoelectric EEG, and thus can be used as an anticonvulsant in status epilepticus. Methohexital in contrast has some epileptogenic activity at lower doses, useful in identifying epileptic foci, and in patients undergoing electroconvulsive therapy.

Induction doses of barbiturates can produce decreases in cardiac output, primarily through preload reduction due to venodilation and secondarily through decreases in myocardial contractility.

Low-dose barbiturates cause decreases in respiratory rate, tidal volume, and carbon dioxide responsiveness; induction-dose barbiturates commonly produce apnea; however, they do not depress laryngeal or cough reflexes as much as propofol.

All barbiturates induce δ-aminolevulinic acid (ALA) synthase, the initial enzyme in heme biosynthesis. Administration of barbiturates will result in accumulation of ALA (neurotoxic) in patients with certain types of *porphyria* (acute intermittent porphyria, hereditary coproporphyria, and variegate porphyria), and should be avoided.

Thiopental undergoes rapid redistribution, and is oxidatively metabolized by cytochrome P450 (CYP) to several metabolites, one of which is *pentobarbital*, an active and longer acting agent. This renders thiopental a suboptimal agent for repeated boluses or infusion as maintenance anesthesia.

Propofol

Like thiopental, propofol decreases $CMRO_2$, CBF, and ICP, it can be used in the treatment of status epilepticus, and appears to have a similar *neuroprotective effect*.

Propofol causes a greater decrease in systemic vascular resistance than barbiturates, but a similar degree of decrease in cardiac contractility.

Compared with barbiturates, propofol causes more blunting of airway reflexes. Induction doses universally produce apnea,

Essential Clinical Anesthesia Review: Keywords, Questions and Answers for the Boards, ed. Linda S. Aglio, Robert W. Lekowski, and Richard D. Urman. Published by Cambridge University Press. © Cambridge University Press 2015.

lower doses may cause decreases in tidal volume, minute ventilation, and carbon dioxide responsiveness.

True *allergy to propofol* is exceedingly rare. Propofol emulsion contains soybean oil and egg lecithin, but no soy protein or egg albumin. Therefore persons with soy or egg protein allergies can be given propofol safely.

Propofol undergoes rapid redistribution, and is metabolized by the liver and kidney. Even in the presence of liver and kidney disease, propofol clearance is not significantly decreased, thus it can be used as an infusion with predictable recovery.

Etomidate

Like thiopental and propofol, etomidate decreases $CMRO_2$, CBF, and ICP. It can be used in the treatment of status epilepticus, but also may increase EEG activity in epileptogenic areas.

Unlike other induction agents, which depress somatosensory evoked potentials (SSEPs), etomidate increases both the amplitude and latency of SSEPs.

Etomidate has minimal effects on cardiac contractility and vascular tone, rendering it a useful induction agent in patients with hypovolemia or significant ventricular dysfunction.

Transient apnea will occur with induction doses of etomidate, but overall it causes less ventilatory depression than propofol or thiopental.

Etomidate inhibits 11β-hydroxylase, the enzyme responsible for the final reaction in the biosynthesis of cortisol. Thus cortisol release from the *adrenal gland is suppressed* for about 12 hours following a typical induction dose of etomidate.

Etomidate is metabolized via ester hydrolysis in the liver to a water-soluble metabolite, which is excreted in the urine. Etomidate has a high hepatic extraction ratio (about 0.7), thus decreases in hepatic blood flow will decrease clearance.

Etomidate induces ALA synthase, like barbiturates, and should be avoided in patients with *porphyria*.

Etomidate is the most *emetogenic* of the IV induction agents.

Benzodiazepines

Benzodiazepines are often used for premedication to produce sedation, anxiolysis, and anterograde amnesia, with minimal ventilatory depression.

Many patients chronically maintained on benzodiazepines, may develop cross-tolerance to thiopental, propofol, or etomidate.

Benzodiazepines decrease $CMRO_2$, CBF, and ICP, and can be used in the treatment of status epilepticus; however, even with high doses they do not produce burst suppression.

Benzodiazepines produce mild decreases in systemic vascular resistance; myocardial contractility is relatively unaffected.

Given alone, benzodiazepines produce minimal ventilatory depression; when used in high doses they may cause transient apnea.

Midazolam (along with ketamine) is one of the few induction agents that can be given intramuscularly.

Most benzodiazepines are metabolized by the liver, and some of them have also been found to induce ALA synthase and thus should be avoided in certain *porphyrias*.

Benzodiazepines are the only induction agents for which there is a *specific antagonist: flumazenil*. Flumazenil may cause anxiety and panic if given alone, or may precipitate acute withdrawal including seizures if given to patients on chronic benzodiazepines.

Ketamine

Ketamine produces a cataleptic state termed "*dissociate anesthesia*" characterized by signs consistent with continued consciousness, including open eyes, nystagmus, movement, vocalization, but without the capacity to communicate, recollect events, or respond to stimuli.

Unlike other IV induction agents, ketamine increases $CMRO_2$, CBF, and ICP, and may render EEG monitoring for anesthesia depth unreliable.

Ketamine is the only IV induction agent that causes cardiovascular stimulation through centrally mediated increased sympathetic tone and increased release of adrenal catecholamines.

Table 33.1 Comparative clinical effects of IV anesthetic agents

Drug	Advantages	Disadvantages
Thiopental	Rapid onset, rapid recovery No pain on injection ↓ $CMRO_2$, CBF, ICP	↑ Airway responsiveness ↓ BP, CO ↓ Ventilatory drive
Propofol	Rapid onset, rapid recovery ↓ Airway resistance ↓$CMRO_2$, CBF, ICP ↓Nausea and vomiting	Pain on injection ↓ BP, CO ↓ Ventilatory drive
Etomidate	Minimal changes in BP, CO Rapid onset, rapid recovery ↓ $CMRO_2$, CBF, ICP	Adrenal suppression Pain on injection ↑Nausea and vomiting ↓Ventilatory drive
Midazolam	Anxiolysis, amnesia Minimal changes in BP, CO Minimal ventilatory depression Effects reversible with flumazenil ↓$CMRO_2$, CBF, ICP Effective by IM route	Longer duration than other agents
Ketamine	Minimal ventilatory depression Preservation of airway reflexes ↑HR, BP, CO Effective by IM route	Emergence delirium Longer duration than other agents ↑Ischemia risk in CAD

BP, blood pressure; CAD, coronary artery disease; CO, cardiac output; HR, heart rate. From: Vacanti et al., 2011, p. 230.

There is a transient increase in heart rate, systemic vascular resistance, pulmonary artery pressure, and cardiac output.

Ketamine does not cause significant ventilatory depression. It does, however, cause depression of airway reflexes, to a lesser degree than other IV induction agents, and an increase in salivary, tracheal, and bronchial secretions.

Ketamine may be associated with *"emergence delirium,"* characterized by confusion, impaired short-term memory, auditory and visual hallucinations, and nightmares. The incidence and intensity goes down with concurrent propofol or benzodiazepine administration.

Ketamine is metabolized by the CYP450 system, and has an active metabolite, norketamine, which is eventually renally excreted. Ketamine has a high hepatic extraction ratio like etomidate (about 0.8), and thus decreased hepatic blood flow will decrease clearance.

Questions

1. Which of the follow agents does NOT induce ALA synthase, and thus is considered safe for use in patients with porphyria?
   a. thiopental
   b. midazolam
   c. etomidate
   d. ketamine
   e. methohexital

2. Etomidate *differs* from propofol and thiopental because it does which of the following?
   a. increases CBF but decreases ICP
   b. decreases CBF and decreases ICP
   c. increases bronchial and tracheal secretions
   d. acts primarily at a different receptor
   e. causes minimal cardiovascular depression

Answers

1. d. Barbiturates, benzodiazepines, etomidate, and methohexital have all been reported to increase ALA synthase and thus should be used with caution, if at all, in patients with porphyria.
2. e. Etomidate increases CBP *and* ICP; it does not greatly increase bronchial or tracheal secretions. Etomidate acts primarily at the GABA receptor, like propofol, but is known to have less of a myocardial depressant effect.

Further reading

Dershwitz, M. and Rosow, C. E. (2008). Chapter 40. Intravenous anesthetics. In Longnecker D. E., Brown, D., Newman, M., and Zapol, W. M. (eds) *Anesthesiology*, 3rd edn. New York: McGraw-Hill.

Gooding, J. M., Weng, J. T., Smith, R. A. et al. (1979). Cardiovascular and pulmonary response following etomidate induction of anesthesia in patients with demonstrated cardiac disease. *Anesthesia and Analgesia* 58, 40–41.

Veselis, R. A., Reinsel, R. A., Freshchenko, V. A. et al. (1997). The comparative amnestic effects of midazolam, propofol, thiopental, and fentanyl at equisedative concentrations. *Anesthesiology* 87, 749–764.

Chapter

34

Mechanisms of anesthetic actions

Lisa M. Hammond and James Hardy

Keywords

Meyer–Overton correlation
Unitary theory of anesthesia
Stereoselectivity of anesthetic agents
Anesthetic "cut-off"
NMDA receptor
GABA receptor

Overview and history

Drugs with anesthetic activity include noble gases, alkanes, alcohols, ethers, and other structurally unrelated compounds.

At the end of the 19th century, the *Meyer–Overton correlation* was developed. This correlation described that potencies of general anesthetics are directly related to their lipid solubilities (Figure 34.1).

As a wide variety of structurally unrelated compounds obey the Meyer–Overton rule, it was proposed that all anesthetics were likely to act at the same molecular site, at the time thought to be lipid components of neuronal cell membranes, known as the *unitary theory of anesthesia*.

Over the past several decades four pieces of evidence have developed to argue *against* lipids as anesthetic targets.

1. Temperature mimics changes in lipid properties induced by anesthesia, but does *not* alter behavior in animals.
2. Anesthetics act *stereoselectively*, such that a compound's R-isomer and S-isomer have different capacities to produce anesthesia, a feature generally associated with protein targets.
3. An *anesthetic "cut-off"* in potency of homologous anesthetic compounds exists, such that increasing anesthetic size of homologous compounds increases anesthetic potencies, until a "cut-off" point is reached after

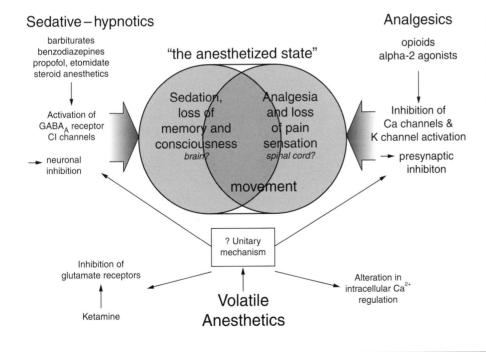

Figure 34.1 The Meyer–Overton correlator, illustrating the relationship between anesthetic potency and lipid solubility. The strong correlation between anesthetic potency and potency for luciferase inhibition demonstrates that a protein target can account for the observations of Meyer and Overton (Modified from Figure 3 in Franks, N. P. 2006. Molecular targets underlying general anesthesia. *British Journal of Pharmocology*, 147: S72–S81.)

Essential Clinical Anesthesia Review: Keywords, Questions and Answers for the Boards, ed. Linda S. Aglio, Robert W. Lekowski, and Richard D. Urman. Published by Cambridge University Press. © Cambridge University Press 2015.

which the anesthetic activity plateaus or disappears completely.

4. Some volatile compounds, which are highly lipid-soluble and therefore predicted by the Meyer–Overton correlation to be potent anesthetics, have no anesthetic activity.

Ion channels in the central nervous system

Ion channels within the central nervous system are among the most likely targets that mediate the behavior effects of anesthetic agents.

The γ-aminobutyric acid *(GABA) receptor* is a neurotransmitter-gated ion channel, such that binding of GABA produces chloride-specific ion channel opening and *hyperpolarization* of the neuronal membrane. They are the most abundantly expressed *inhibitory* receptors in the brain.

All IV induction agents, except ketamine, are proposed to augment the GABA neurotransmitter system, although the specific targets responsible for mediating behavioral effects have been difficult to elucidate.

Propofol and etomidate may specifically act at the β_3 subunit of the GABA-A receptor, as point mutations produced in "knock-in" mice at this site were highly resistant to the hypnotic, immobility, and respiratory effects of both propofol and etomidate.

Ketamine and nitrous oxide are potent inhibitors of neuronal nicotinic acetylcholine receptors (excitatory receptors), and N-methyl-D-aspartate *(NMDA) receptors*.

NMDA receptors are a subtype of glutamate receptors, which are the most widely expressed *excitatory* receptors in the brain; when bound to glutamate they cause neuronal *depolarization*.

Halogenated volatile anesthetics

Halogenated alkanes (i.e., chloroform, halothane) and ethers (i.e., isoflurane, sevoflurane, desflurane) exhibit the *least* selectivity for target proteins, include activity at GABA receptors, glutamate receptors, tandem-pore K^+ channels, neuronal nicotinic acetylcholine receptors, 5-HT3 receptors, mitochondrial adenosine triphosphate-sensitive K^+ channels, and hyperpolarization-activated cyclic nucleotide-gated channels, among others.

Anatomic site of anesthetic actions

The two measurable characteristics of inhaled anesthetics include production of *immobility* and *amnesia*.

Inhaled anesthetics produce *immobility* largely by their action on the *spinal cord*, as determined by MAC in decerebrate animals. A suggested mechanism describes activation of descending noradrenergic pathways originating in the periaqueductal gray matter brainstem, which in turn inhibits nociceptive input in the dorsal horn of the spinal cord.

Supraspinal structures are proposed to be responsible for *amnestic* effects of inhaled anesthetics. The amygdala, hippocampus, and cortex are considered highly probable targets.

Summary

It has become more evident that multiple sites and mechanisms are likely responsible for the behavioral effects of general anesthetics. These sites and mechanisms are likely different depending on the anesthetic agent (Figure 34.2).

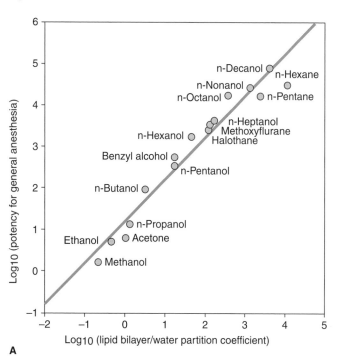

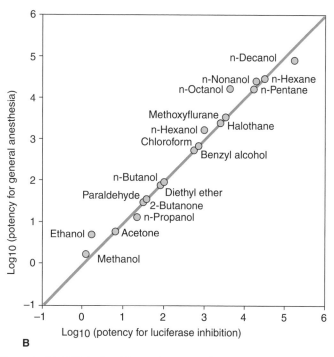

Figure 34.2 Multiple mechanisms of anesthesia. (Reproduced from Lynch, C. and Pancrazio, J. J. 1994. Snails, spiders, and stereospecificity: is there a role for calcium channels in anesthetic mechanisms? *Anesthesiology*, 81(1): 1–5.)

Questions

1. The Meyer–Overton correlation describes which relationship?
   a. Increased water solubility correlates to decreased anesthetic potency.
   b. Increased water solubility correlates to increased anesthetic potency.
   c. Increased lipid solubility correlates to increased anesthetic potency.
   d. Increased lipid solubility correlates to decreased anesthetic potency.
   e. Decreased lipid solubility correlates to increased anesthetic potency.

2. Which of the following agents does *not* augment the GABA neurotransmitter system?
   a. ketamine
   b. thiopental
   c. propofol
   d. etomidate
   e. diazepam

3. Which is most likely the anatomic site of action for anesthetic agents that produce *immobility*?
   a. amygdala
   b. hippocampus
   c. cortex
   d. muscle fiber
   e. spinal cord

Answers

1. c. The Meyer–Overton correlation describes a direct correlation between anesthetic potency and lipid solubility.
2. a. Thiopental, propofol, etomidate, and diazepam all work by augmenting the GABA receptor. Ketamine antagonizes the NMDA receptor.
3. e. The amygdala, hippocampus, and cortex are considered highly likely sites of action for the amnestic affects of anesthetics. Anesthetic action at the level of the spinal cord is likely responsible for the immobility affect of anesthetics.

Further reading

Koblin, D. D. (2010). Chapter 20. Mechanisms of action. In Miller, R. D., Eriksson, L. I., Fleisher, L. A. et al. (eds) *Miller's Anesthesia*, 7th edn. Philadelphia: Elsevier.

Lynch, C. and Pancrazio, J. J. (1994). Snails, spiders, and stereospecificity: is there a role for calcium channels in anesthetic mechanisms? *Anesthesiology* 81(1), 1–5.

Chapter

35

Pharmacokinetics of intravenous agents

Alissa Sodickson and Richard D. Urman

Drug distribution
Drug ionization
Protein binding
Elimination
Volume of distribution
Half-life
Drug clearance
Context-sensitive half-time
Effects of coexisting diseases

Drug distribution

Intravenous injection provides complete absorption and a rapid rise in plasma drug concentration. *Drugs rapidly distribute to the vessel-rich group (brain, heart, lungs, liver, kidneys).* Peripheral tissue can function as a drug reservoir. The degree to which a tissue "stores" a drug depends on the drug's solubility in that tissue, its binding to macromolecules, and tissue pH. As drug concentration in the circulation falls, redistribution to less perfused tissues, such as muscle and fat, occurs.

Drug ionization is determined by the particular drug's dissociation constant (pKa: the pH at which the drug is 50% ionized). *Non-ionized molecules have greater lipid solubility.*

The degree of *protein binding* is determined by the concentration of drug, concentration of protein, affinity of drug for protein, and number of protein binding sites. These can be affected by age, stress, liver or kidney disease, changes in tissue pH, and the presence of competing molecules for binding sites. Acidic drugs bind to albumin while basic drugs bind to α1-acid glycoprotein. *The free fraction of drug (unbound) contributes to the pharmacologic effect and ultimately undergoes metabolism and elimination.*

Elimination

Drug elimination includes both metabolism and excretion. The liver is the organ primarily involved in drug metabolism, converting lipid-soluble to water-soluble drugs for excretion in urine or bile, a process called *biotransformation*. This generally consists of two phases: phase I includes oxidation, reduction, and hydrolysis; phase II involves conjugation (glucuronic acid, sulfate, etc.).

Drug metabolism is affected by both the intrinsic ability of the liver to metabolize the drug as well as hepatic blood flow. Drugs with a high hepatic extraction ratio (ER: fraction of unbound drug cleared by the liver) are largely dependent on hepatic blood flow for clearance. Drugs with a low ER are dependent on the metabolic capacity of the liver and hence are more affected by changes in cytochrome P450 levels.

Extrahepatic metabolism is responsible for metabolism of some drugs and includes such processes as *hydrolysis by esterases and Hofmann elimination*. There is also clearance of water-soluble drugs, without metabolism, by renal excretion, the rate of which is affected by the glomerular filtration rate, protein binding, lipid solubility, and urine pH.

Volume of distribution (Vd): the volume into which a drug appears to be diluted:

$$Vd = dose/concentration = X/C$$

The three-compartment pharmacokinetic model (see Figure 35.1) divides the body into three theoretic volumes:

1. the central compartment (V1: the initial volume into which the drug is introduced)
2. rapidly equilibrating compartment (V2)
3. slowly equilibrating compartment (V3)

Drugs transfer between compartments such that the volume of distribution at a steady state includes the central and peripheral compartments:

$$V_{dss} = V1 + V2 + V3 = X/C$$

Essential Clinical Anesthesia Review: Keywords, Questions and Answers for the Boards, ed. Linda S. Aglio, Robert W. Lekowski, and Richard D. Urman. Published by Cambridge University Press. © Cambridge University Press 2015.

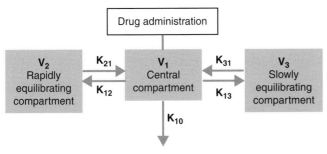

Figure 35.1 The three-compartment pharmacokinetic model. Drug is administered into a central compartment from which it is cleared by metabolism and/or elimination. Drug rapidly distributes into a peripheral compartment, and this compartment reaches equilibrium with the central compartment quickly. Drug distributes more slowly into a third compartment. The volume of distribution at stready state, v_d, equals $V_1 + V_2 + V_3$. (Redrawn with permission from Figure 52-16 in Shafer, S. L. 1998. Principles of pharmacokinetics and pharmacodynamics. In *Principles and Practice of Anesthesiology*, 2nd edn. St. Louis: Mosby)

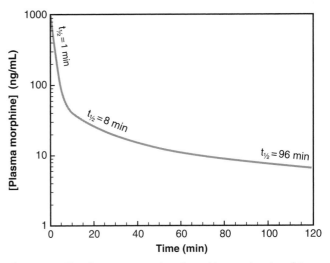

Figure 35.2 The plasma concentration of morphine as a function of time following a 10 mg bolus dose. The three phases of the disappearance curve have half-lives of 1 minute, 8 minutes, and 96 minutes, respectively. (Redrawn with permission from Figure 5 in Dershwitz, M., Walsh, J. L., Morishige, R. J. et al. 2000. Pharmacokinetics and pharmacodynamics of inhaled versus intravenous morphine in healthy volunteers. *Anesthesiology*, 93(3): 619–628.)

The three-compartment model is necessary to approximate the pharmacokinetics of lipid-soluble intravenous anesthetic agents in which the drug concentration curve appears to follow three phases.

1. The first reflects redistribution from the central to the rapidly equilibrating compartment.
2. The second reflects distribution into the slowly equilibrating compartment.
3. The third is characterized by a slow decrease resulting from metabolism and return from peripheral to the central compartment.

Drug clearance (CL) is defined as the portion of the volume of distribution from which a drug appears to be removed during a given period of time:

$$CL = k \times Vd \text{ (where k is the rate constant)}$$

Half-life ($t_{1/2}$) is the time it takes drug concentration to decrease by 50%:

$$T_{1/2} = \ln 2/k = 0.693/k$$

A pharmacokinetic process may be considered complete after five half-lives, at which point 3.125% of the original concentration is remaining. Use of terminal half-life for drug dosing fails to account for redistribution of a drug away from the central (active) compartment, such that the effect of an intravenous anesthetic agent will be terminated via redistribution long before several of its half-lives have elapsed.

Context-sensitive half-time (CSHT) is the time required for the central compartment drug concentration to fall by 50% as a function of the duration of infusion. The "context" refers to the duration of an infusion maintaining a central compartment drug concentration. The longer the duration of infusion, the more likely the rapidly and slowly equilibrating compartments approach steady state with the central compartment, and hence the decline in central drug concentration will occur more slowly. The CSHT of several intravenous anesthetic agents are displayed in Figure 35.3.

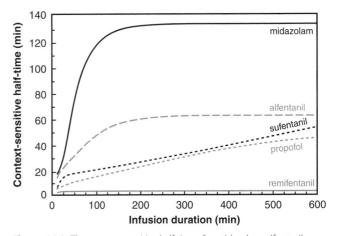

Figure 35.3 The context-sensitive half-times for midazolam, alfentanil, sufentanil, propofol, and remifentanil as a function of infusion duration. The simulations were performed using the program RECOV, written by Steven Shafer. Form: Vacanti et al., 2011, p. 239.

Effects of coexisting diseases

Effects of liver disease: typically affects phase I reactions more than phase II. *Chronic liver disease may be characterized by decreased hepatic blood flow, altered enzymatic activity, and reduced protein synthesis*, all of which can affect drug pharmacokinetics. Clearance of drugs with low hepatic ER (methadone, warfarin, thiopental, benzodiazepines) will be severely impaired in end-stage liver disease as these depend on liver function, while the clearance of drugs with high hepatic ER (fentanyl, ketamine, propofol, metoprolol) will be impaired in states of decreased hepatic blood flow (shock, CHF). The decreased production of albumin in advanced liver disease results in increased circulating free-drug concentration in drugs that are highly protein bound (warfarin, digoxin, midazolam). (See www.ccmtutorials.com/misc/albumin/page_03.htm)

Effects of renal disease: significant renal dysfunction (low creatinine clearance) *primarily affects clearance of water-soluble drugs* (atenolol, rocuronium, pancuronium) *and metabolites* (normeperidine, morphine-6-glucuronide). Accumulation of active metabolites due to reduced clearance can lead to prolonged duration of action.

Effects of age

The elderly patient will generally have a *smaller central compartment Vd* due to decreased total body water and increased percentage of body fat. There is also *decreased renal clearance* due to loss of nephrons and reduced albumin levels leading to *decreased protein binding capacity*.

Questions

1. Drug X is rapidly cleared by the liver. Prolonged duration of action may be expected:

    a. in a patient with prolonged alcohol use
    b. in a trauma victim suffering large hemorrhage
    c. in a chronically malnourished patient
    d. in a dialysis-dependent patient

2. Prolonged duration of action after a three-hour infusion may be expected with:

    a. remifentanil
    b. ketamine
    c. midazolam
    d. propofol

3. Duration of drug effect may differ from drug half-life due to:

    a. biotransformation
    b. clearance
    c. context-sensitive half-time
    d. redistribution

Answers

1. b. Drugs with high hepatic extraction ratios are dependent on hepatic blood flow for clearance. Clinical situations leading to decreased hepatic blood flow, such as in hemorrhagic shock, will lead to a prolonged duration of action.

2. c. Context-sensitive half-time relates the clearance of a drug from the central compartment to the duration of the drug infusion. Midazolam has a significantly prolonged context-sensitive half-time (see Figure 35.3) and makes this a poor choice for extended anesthetic infusions.

3. d. Most drugs exert their effect when in the central compartment. As a drug redistributes into peripheral compartments, the drug effect wanes. The time for redistribution of a drug differs from the half-life of a drug, which is dependent on drug metabolism.

Further reading

Vacanti, C., Sikka, P., Urman, R., Dershwitz, M., and Segal, B. Chapter 36. (eds) (2011). Pharmacokinetics of intravenous agents.

In *Essential Clinical Anesthesia*. Cambridge: Cambridge University Press.

Gupta, D. K. and Henthorn, T. K. (2009). Pharmacologic principles. In Barash, P.

G., Cullen, B. F., Stoelting, R. K., Cahalan, M., and Stock, S. (eds) *Clinical Anesthesia*, 6th edn. Lippincott Williams & Wilkins Chapter 7.

Alissa Sodickson and Richard D. Urman

Chapter 36

Opioids

Keywords

- Opioid receptors
- Pharmacokinetics: protein binding, lipid solubility, ionization state
- Metabolism of opioids
- Effects on nervous system
- Effects on cardiovascular system
- Effects on smooth muscle
- Tolerance and cross-tolerance
- Dependence
- Addiction
- Antagonists

Opioid receptors

Currently, four opioid receptors are identified: μ, κ, δ, nociceptin-orphanin FQ. Most clinical opioids are relatively selective μ-opioid agonists; however, multiple μ-opioid receptor subtypes exist, with different expression patterns between various tissues and among different individuals. This variability possibly accounts for the different clinical responses. Action at the κ-opioid receptor probably accounts for dysphoria and hallucinations. Opioid receptors are G protein-coupled, located in peripheral tissues, the peripheral nervous system, and the central nervous system, both presynaptic and postsynaptic. Presynaptic receptor binding inhibits voltage-sensitive calcium channels, which decreases release of neurotransmitters. Postsynaptic receptor binding increases outward K^+ flow, thereby hyperpolarizing the cell.

Pharmacokinetics

Many of the pharmacokinetic properties of various opioids are related to each drug's *lipid solubility, protein binding, and ionization state.* Lipophilic opioids rapidly distribute to the vessel-rich group, then redistribute into muscle and fat, accounting for the effects that appear and disappear rapidly. Hydrophilic opioids have slower onset and offset. *Protein binding* affects the availability of drug for diffusion across membranes and for metabolism. Opioids generally bind to α1-acid glycoprotein, the concentration of which can change as it is an acute phase reactant. *Non-ionized species are able to diffuse into the CNS.* The closer the pKa to 7.4 (most have pKa values greater than 7.4), the higher the amount of uncharged species.

Most opioids undergo *hepatic metabolism* and renal excretion. Some metabolites are active (see Table 36.1).

Effects on the nervous system

- *Analgesia*:
  - brain – antinociceptive pathways are activated via action at the periaqueductal gray matter, locus ceruleus, and raphe nuclei. Activity in the limbic system affects emotional response
  - spinal cord – acts at dorsal horn, both pre- and postsynaptic receptors
  - periphery – reduces activity in primary nociceptor during inflammation.
- *Sedation*: occurs with all opioids. Significant sedation when combined with other CNS depressants.
- *Miosis*: via stimulation of the Edinger–Westphal nucleus (cranial nerve III).
- *Antitussive effect*: via activity at the medullary cough center. Different receptor mechanism than analgesic effects.
- *Pruritis*: via activation of mu-opioid receptors in rostral medulla. Symptoms often perinasal. Reversed with opioid antagonist.
- *Nausea*: via stimulation of the chemoreceptor trigger zone on the floor of the fourth ventricle. Effect increased by input from vestibular apparatus, accounting for worsening nausea with movement.
- *Ventilatory depression*: dose-dependent depression via decreasing medullary sensitivity to hypercarbia. See rightward shift and decrease in slope of carbon dioxide response curve. Minute ventilation decreased mostly via decreased respiratory rate. Also decreased hypoxic

Essential Clinical Anesthesia Review: Keywords, Questions and Answers for the Boards, ed. Linda S. Aglio, Robert W. Lekowski, and Richard D. Urman. Published by Cambridge University Press. © Cambridge University Press 2015.

Table 36.1 Metabolism of opioids

Drug	Dose (mg)	Peak effect (min)	Duration of effect (hours)	Metabolism	Notes
Morphine	10	>30	3–4	Hepatic to 3- and 6-glucuronide, renal excretion	Morphine-6-glucuronide is active, can accumulate wth repeat doses, renal disease
Hydromorphone	1.5	10–20	2–3	Rapid hepatic metabolism	
Methadone	10	15–20	3–4	Liver and GI mucosa. Renal, small amount of biliary excretion	Significant interindividual variability in metabolism. Long terminal half-life can lead to accumulation with repeat dosing
Meperidine	80	5–7	2–3	Rapid hepatic metabolism to normeperidine, renal excretion	Normeperidine causes CNS excitation, accumulates with repeat dosing or renal insufficiency
Fentanyl	0.1	3–5	0.5–1	Hepatic and GI mucosa, renal and biliary excretion	Long context-sensitive half-time with prolonged infusions
Sufentanil	0.01	3–5	0.5–1	Hepatic and GI mucosa, renal and biliary excretion	Relatively short context-sensitive half-time
Alfentanil	0.75	1.5–2	0.2–0.3	Hepatic by CYP3A4	Longer context-sensitive half-time than sufentanil. Inhibitors of CYP3A4 (grapefruit, azoles, macrolides) reduce clearance
Remifentanil	0.1	1.5–2	0.1–0.2	Nonspecific plasma esterases	Short context-sensitive half-time (4 minutes)

ventilatory drive. Higher risk in advanced age, morbid obesity, OSA, or with other CNS depressants. All opioids produce equivalent ventilatory depression at equi-analgesic doses.

- *Muscle rigidity*: skeletal muscle hypertonus can occur with moderate to large doses. Etiology is mu-opioid receptor-mediated inhibition of GABAergic neurons in the striatum. Can make mask ventilation difficult via laryngeal muscle constriction and chest wall rigidity.
- *Cerebral blood flow/intracranial pressure*: ICP may rise with ventilatory depression and concomitant hypercarbia resulting in cerebral vasodilation. Opioids are useful in blunting the increased ICP seen in response to laryngoscopy and intubation.
- *Other effects*: can see myoclonus with high doses without evidence of seizure on EEG. No EEG suppression seen even with high doses.

Effects on cardiovascular system

Opioids cause *peripheral vasodilation* via depression of medullary vasomotor centers, causing a reduction in sympathetic activity. Baroreceptor reflexes remain intact. Little blood pressure effect in normovolemic patients, but may see hemodynamic effects in patients dependent on high sympathetic tone (hypovolemia, CHF) or when opioids are combined with other sedatives. There is a *dose-dependent decrease in heart rate* via

stimulation of the central vagal nuclei but *no significant direct myocardial depression.*

Effects on smooth muscle

Opioids cause a *reduction in propulsion throughout the GI system* via both central and peripheral effects. See *delayed gastric emptying, constipation.* In the biliary system, there is an increase *in tone in biliary tree and sphincter of Oddi*, which can occasionally lead to epigastric pain or biliary colic. Biliary spasm pain can be relieved with nitroglycerin. Opioids can lead to *urinary retention* due to decreased detrusor muscle contraction and increase in tone of the involuntary sphincter. More common in males and with neuraxial opioids.

Tolerance is a phenomenon in which the response to a drug's effect diminishes over time. That is, to attain the same effect, the dose of the drug needs to be increased. This occurs as a result of receptor uncoupling and receptor downregulation. Tolerance to opioids includes tolerance to most opioid effects, but not constipation or miosis.

Tolerance to one opioid leads to tolerance of a different opioid, a phenomenon called *cross-tolerance*. This is generally incomplete and hence switching to a different opioid will often provide additional relief.

Dependence is defined by the occurrence of a specific withdrawal syndrome when the drug is stopped abruptly, the dose is significantly reduced, or an antagonist is given. Symptoms of

Table 36.2 Agonist–antagonist opioid receptor effects and equianalgesic doses

Drug	μ-opioid receptor	κ-opioid receptor	Analgesic dose, mg[a]
Buprenorphine	Partial agonist	Antagonist	0.3
Butorphanol	Antagonist	Partial agonist	2
Nalbuphine	Antagonist	Partial agonist	10

[a] Equivalent to morphine, 10 mg.
(From: Vacanti et al., 2011, p. 248.)

withdrawal are terminated rapidly with IV opioid administration. Physical dependence differs from psychological dependence and *addiction*, which is a multifactorial, neurobiological disease characterized by drug-seeking behaviors, continued use despite negative social and physiologic effects, and impaired control over use.

Agonist–antagonists

Bind to both μ-opioid and κ-opioid receptors with different effects (see Table 36.2) and produce a ceiling effect for both analgesic and ventilatory-depressant effects. Buprenophine produces similar subjective effects as morphine, while the κ-opioid effects of nalbuphine and butorphanol cause a lack of mood elevation, thought to be related to decreased abuse potential. Mixed agonist–antagonist cause less constipation and minimal effects on the smooth muscle of the bladder and intestine. Note that they can precipitate withdrawal if given to an opioid-dependent patient.

Antagonists

- *Naloxone*: reversible, competitive antagonist at all opioid receptors with greatest affinity for μ-opioid receptors. Rapid onset, followed by rapid redistribution, leading to a duration of effect often shorter than the opioid it is being used to antagonize. For example, a dose of 0.4 mg will antagonize morphine for less than one hour. Opioid reversal can lead to increases in systemic pressure, heart rate, and plasma catecholamines, possibly related to the onset of pain but also seen in the absence of painful stimuli.
- *Naltrexone*: competitive antagonist used to block the euphoriant effects of opioids and drug cravings in the treatment of opioid addiction and alcoholism. Effects can be overcome with high doses of opioids.

Questions

1. The rapid onset of fentanyl as compared to morphine is related to:
   a. higher degree of protein binding of morphine
   b. higher lipid solubility of fentanyl
   c. higher pKa of fentanyl
   d. larger dose of morphine used clinically

2. You are called to see a patient in the PACU for hypopnea. The patient is status postexploratory laparotomy and bowel resection and has received 2 mg of IV hydromorphone. The patient's vital signs are as follows: HR: 84; BP: 114/62; RR: 6; SpO_2: 93%. The patient is arousable to moderate stimulation. What is the MOST appropriate management plan at this time?
   a. Administer naloxone, 0.04 mg at a time, titrated to respiratory rate.
   b. Administer buprenorphine to antagonize the respiratory depression but preserve some analgesia.
   c. Administer supplemental O_2 by nasal cannula, withhold further opioid, and continue to monitor.
   d. Prepare for intubation for hypercarbia and need for airway protection.

3. The MOST likely effect of parenteral opioids given to an otherwise healthy patient include:
   a. decrease in systolic blood pressure due to peripheral vasodilation and blunted baroreceptor reflex
   b. decrease in minute ventilation due to significant reduction in tidal volume and moderate decrease in respiratory rate
   c. mild pruritis, which can be controlled with diphenhydramine
   d. nausea due to stimulation of the chemoreceptor trigger zone in the fourth ventricle

Answers

1. b. The onset of a particular opioid's effect is largely related to the drug's lipid solubility. The more lipid soluble, the more rapidly the drug passes the blood–brain barrier to reach the effect-site.
2. c. Side effects of opioids include sedation and respiratory depression. There is a rightward shift in the CO_2 response curve, meaning a higher $PaCO_2$ is required to stimulate ventilation. Generally there is a decrease in rate, with the patient showing slow, deep breaths. If the patient remains arousable, it is reasonable to support

the patient with supplemental O_2 and allow the opioid effect to wane. If the patient's clinical status becomes non-reassuring, naloxone can be carefully given; however, a plan for analgesia will be necessary in the postoperative patient. Intubation always remains as a rescue measure.

3. d. Opioids often cause nausea due to stimulation of the chemoreceptor trigger zone in the CNS. Other side effects include pruritis, which is not generally relieved by antihistamines, decreased minute ventilation due mostly to a decrease in respiratory rate, and decreased systolic blood pressure though baroreceptor reflexes remain intact.

Further reading

Vacanti, C., Sikka, P., Urman, R., Dershwitz, M., and Segal, B. (eds) (2011). Chapter 37. Opioids. In *Essential Clinical Anesthesia*. Cambridge: Cambridge University Press.

Fukuda, K. (2009). Chapter 27. Opioids. In Miller, R. D., Eriksson, L. I., Fleisher, L. A. et al. (eds) *Miller's Anesthesia*, 7th edn. Philadelphia: Churchill-Livingstone.

37

Muscle relaxants

M. Tariq Hanifi and Michael Nguyen

Muscle relaxants (depolarizing, nondepolarizing)
Phase I/II blockade
Malignant hyperthermia and succinylcholine
Laudanosine
Mechanism of action
Pharmacokinetics and pharmacodynamics, abnormal
   responses
Prolongation of action; synergism
Metabolism and excretion
Side effects and toxicity
Indications and contraindications
Antagonism of blockade
Drug interactions (antibiotics, antiepileptics, lithium,
   magnesium, inhalational anesthetics)
Interactions with disease states

Muscle relaxant is the term given to medications used to provide skeletal muscle relaxation at the neuromuscular junction (NMJ). Some functions of these medications are thought to facilitate a wide variety of actions; some of which include mechanical ventilation, tracheal intubation, and optimal surgical conditions. The *mechanism of action* of neuromuscular blockers is at the NMJ and they have been conveniently divided into two subgroups corresponding to their action at the NMJ: *depolarizing and nondepolarizing muscle relaxants*.

The NMJ consists of a presynaptic neuron, a postsynaptic motor end-plate, and postsynaptic muscle fiber. Between the presynaptic neuron and the postsynaptic end-plate is the synaptic cleft. The neurotransmitter, acetylcholine (ACh) is stored in the presynaptic neuron in special organelles. Opposite to the nerve terminal is the postsynaptic motor end-plate, which contains nicotinic acetylcholine receptors (AChR) and acetylcholinesterase, which degrades ACh. Acetylcholine receptors can also be located *extrajunctionally* in the skeletal muscle membrane and may be overexpressed in pathologic states such as muscle denervation, inactivity, sepsis, burn injury, and trauma. In response to nerve stimulation, an action potential

is propagated causing ACh vesicles to fuse with the presynaptic cell membrane. This in turn causes ACh to be released into the presynaptic cleft and binding of ACh to postsynaptic nicotinic AChR, further propagating the action potential and causing skeletal muscle contraction.

Depolarizing NMBD are ACh agonists at the nicotinic AChR. They act similarly to ACh by binding to the postsynaptic AChR to cause skeletal muscle contractions. The persistent end-plate depolarization prevents further muscle contraction and therefore muscle relaxation.

Succinylcholine (SCh) is the only clinically used *depolarizing NMBD*. It is an agent whose chemical structure consists of two acetylcholine molecules linked by a methyl group. It has a fast onset (30 to 60 seconds) and fast offset (5 to 10 minutes) and is most commonly used for rapid tracheal intubation. Initial dosing of SCh is 0.5–1.5 mg/kg, at this dosage *phase I blockade* typically occurs. At higher doses or *repeated doses phase II blockade occurs. Phase I blockade* is a normal response to SCh administration. It shows a decreased height with *no* fade on TOF testing. *In phase II blockade*, the administration of SCh resembles that of NDNMB and will show no change in height but *will* show fade on TOF.

SCh is degraded by plasma cholinesterase (e.g., butyrylcholinesterase/pseudocholinesterase). *Plasma cholinesterase* can be decreased in pathologic states such as burns and chronic liver disease. It is also possible to have a genetic deficiency in which patients may have *atypical pseudocholinesterase*. In such cases, history of prolonged paralysis after general anesthesia or family history of atypical pseudocholinesterase should be noted. To test for atypical pseudocholinesterase, an in vitro assay is performed with *dibucaine* (an amide local anesthetic with 80% inhibition of pseudocholinesterase). *Dibucaine number* of 80 corresponds to a normal 80% inhibition of pseudocholinesterase. Heterozygous atypical pseudocholinesterase correlates with a dibucaine number that is between 30 and 65, and homozygous atypical pseudocholinesterase correlates with a dibucaine number of 20. Other agents such as MAOIs, organophosphates, and anticholinesterase may also inhibit pseudocholinesterase.

Essential Clinical Anesthesia Review: Keywords, Questions and Answers for the Boards, ed. Linda S. Aglio, Robert W. Lekowski, and Richard D. Urman. Published by Cambridge University Press. © Cambridge University Press 2015.

Although SCh has beneficial uses throughout the hospital, it also has many undesirable and lethal side effects. *Hyperkalemia* can occur after the administration of SCh, a rise of 0.5 to 1 meq/l in normal individuals may occur. However, in diseased states such as chemical denervation, muscle trauma, thermal injury, and sepsis, life-threatening hyperkalemia can occur. Increase in potassium release is thought to be due to the proliferation of extrajunctional AChR in diseased states. Aside from hyperkalemia, other problems may also arise from SCh administration, including sinus bradycardia, sinus arrest in children, junctional rhythms, elevated intracranial pressures, and increased intraocular pressures. Succinylcholine is a known trigger for *malignant hyperthermia* and should therefore be avoided in patients with the disease. It is also recommended that SCh should not be administered to young children as it has caused cardiac arrest in young boys with undiagnosed muscular dystrophy.

Nondepolarizing neuromuscular blockades are agents that are antagonists to ACh at the NMJ. They are divided into two subgroups, the *aminosteroids* and the *benzylisoquinolones*. Pancuronium, rocuronium, and vecuronium are aminosteroids while cis-atracurium, atracurium, and mivacurium are benzylisoquinolones. Note that when drugs from different subgroups are combined they act *synergistically* and prolong the duration of action. Alternatively, when drugs of the same group are combined their effect will be additive.

Pancuronium is a bisquaternary aminosteroid, which tends to be the longest acting NMBD. Its long action is thought to be attributed to the parent compound and an active metabolite produced in the liver, the 3-hydroxypancuronium. The dosing of this agent is 0.06 to 0.1 mg/kg and re-dosing is 0.01 mg/kg every 25 to 60 minutes. Pancuronium is a selective muscarinic AChR antagonist and has strong vagolytic properties that cause increase in HR, CO, and MAP. It should therefore be avoided in patients with CAD. It is usually eliminated from the body via urine and conversion to bile. Because of the prolonged neuromuscular effect of pancuronium, residual paralysis may occur. Therefore the use of pancuronium should be reserved for patients on prolonged ventilation.

Vecuronium is an intermediate acting aminosteroid. Similar to pancuronium, the intubating dose is 0.1 mg/kg (3-minute onset and lasting 25 to 40 minutes) with a maintenance dose of 0.01 to 0.015 mg/kg. It is not vagolytic and is eliminated both hepatically and renally.

Rocuronium is an analog of vecuronium with lower potency and a rate of onset proportional to dose. It can be used in place of SCh to facilitate rapid sequence intubation within 60 seconds at a dose of >1 mg/kg. Larger doses of rocuronium prolong the duration of action. Dosing maintenance is 0.1 mg/kg with duration intervals of 25 to 40 minutes. 70% of rocuronium is eliminated hepatically and 30% is eliminated renally. It has mild vagolytic effects.

Benzylisoquinolones are known to cause *transient histamine* release when administered rapidly. The histamine release

Table 37.1 Pathologic states affecting neuromuscular block

Conditions that antagonize NMB	Conditions that potentiate NMB
Alkalosis	Hyponatremia
Hypercalcemia	Hypocalcemia
Demyelinating lesions	Hypokalemia
Peripheral neuropathies	Hypermagnesemia
Denervation states	Certain neuromuscular diseases
Infection	Acidosis
Immobilization	Acute intermittent porphyria
Muscle trauma	Eaton–Lambert syndrome
	Myasthenia gravis
	Renal failure
	Hepatic failure

(From Vacanti et al. 2011. *Essential Clinical Anesthesia*, Cambridge University Press, p. 255.)

manifests as transient flushing and hypotension that resolves in two to three minutes.

Atracurium is an intermediate-acting benzylisoquinolone made up of ten stereoisomers. The intubating dose is 0.4 to 0.5 mg/kg with onset in two to three minutes. It is degraded by *Hoffman elimination* and *ester hydrolysis*. One of its metabolites, *laudanosine*, is a known CNS stimulant with epileptogenic effects and can cross the blood–brain barrier (BBB); however, this is very unlikely. Laudanosine is eliminated by the liver and the kidneys.

Cis-atracurium is also an intermediate-acting benzylisoquinolone but does not produce histamine release. It is an isomer of atracurium and two to three times as potent. Intubating doses for cis-atracurium is 0.15 to 0.2 mg/kg with onset in two to three minutes. It also undergoes Hoffman elimination but produces less laudanosine than atracurium. It is not affected by renal or hepatic metabolism or action.

Pathologic states affecting NMB

Renal disease can potentiate NMB if drugs that require elimination by the kidneys are used (e.g., pancuronium). Although not seen with a single dose, multiple bolus doses or a continuous infusion in patients with renal disease may prolong the action of the NMB agent. Drugs that undergo Hoffman elimination are independent of renal function.

Hepatic disease can lead to impaired metabolism and elimination of certain NMB. In fluid attention associated with liver dysfunction, larger doses of NMB agent may be needed given the *larger volume of distribution*. In patients with *severe hepatic dysfunction*, degradation of succinylcholine by pseudocholinesterase may be abnormal, thus prolonging NMB by SCh action.

Table 37.2 Effect of various medications on the neuromuscular junction

Decreases synthesis of ACh	Impairs release of ACh by block of presynaptic calcium channels	Postsynaptic block of the AChR (by allosteric binding)
Furosemide	Volatile anesthetics	Volatile anesthetics
	Magnesium	Aminoglycoside antibiotics
	Calcium channel blockers	Quinidine
	Aminoglycoside antibiotics	Tricyclic antidepressants
		Ketamine
		Midazolam
		Barbiturates

(From Vacanti et al. 2011. *Essential Clinical Anesthesia*, Cambridge University Press, p. 254.)

Patients with *myasthenia gravis* may show increased sensitivity to NDNMB and decreased sensitivity to depolarizing NMB. Patients with *LEMS (Eaton-Lambert syndrome)* show increased sensitivity to both depolarizing and nondepolarizing NMB.

Severe infection and *immobilization* can cause resistance to NMBD due to upregulation of AChRs. Certain drugs such as *CYP inducers* and *CYP inhibitors* can also alter pharmacokinetics of NMB. For instance, vecuronium elimination was increased with CYP inducers such as anticonvulsants, and vecuronium action was prolonged with CYP inhibitors. Other mechanisms that can affect NMBD function are: altered ACh release at the NMJ, decreased synthesis of ACh, and allosteric blocking of the AChR.

It is also important to note that the effects of NMB may be prolonged in patients on chronic *glucocorticoid therapy*.

Questions

1. An elderly patient is brought to the operating room for an emergent exploratory laparotomy. The patient has been in a skilled nursing facility for the last six weeks after having a stroke. He is currently being treated for a urinary tract infection with gentamicin. You elect to perform a rapid sequence induction (RSI) given that the patient has a history of dysphagia and uncontrolled acid reflux. You decide to use rocuronium as your NMB. Which of the following statements is not correct?

   a. In patients with immobility, doses of neuromuscular blockade may need to be increased.
   b. Rocuronium has vagolytic effects.
   c. Rocuronium is eliminated by Hoffman degradation.
   d. Rocuronium is a suitable agent used for RSI.

2. A patient is in the operating room undergoing a coronary artery bypass graft procedure. The anesthesiologist used vecuronium to facilitate tracheal intubation and has been re-dosing the medication approximately every 45 minutes to TOF of 2. The perfusionist runs a blood sample and hands you the following: ABG: pH: 7.1; PCO_2: 78; base excess: -9; ionized calcium: 1.01. Which of the following statements is correct?

   a. Alkalosis can potentiate NMB.
   b. Acidosis can potentiate NMB.
   c. Vecuronium is degraded by Hoffman elimination.
   d. Hypercalcemia can potentiate NMB.

Answers

1. c. Benzylisoquinolinium compounds lack any vagolytic effects but are more likely to release histamine. Rocuronium has no direct sympathomimetic effects but, in high doses, has mild vagolytic properties. In patients who are critically ill, NMB dosage may need to be increased due to extrajunctional AChR upregulation.

2. b. Vecuronium is not eliminated by Hoffman degradation. Hypercalcemia and alkalosis do not potentiate neuromuscular blockade, whereas acidosis can potentiate neuromuscular blockade.

Further reading

Naguib, M. and Lien, C. A. (2009). Chapter 29. Pharmacology of muscle relaxants and their antagonists. In Miller, R. D., Eriksson, L. I., Fleisher, L. A. et al. (eds) *Miller's Anesthesia*, 7th edn. Philadelphia: Churchill-Livingstone.

Breslin, D. S., Jiao, K., Habib, A. S., Schultz, J., and Gan, T. J. (2004). Pharmacodynamic interactions between cisatracurium and rocuronium. *Anesthesia and Analgesia* 98(1), 107–110.

Reversal of neuromuscular blockade

M. Tariq Hanifi and Michael Nguyen

Keywords

Acetylcholinesterase inhibitors: muscarinic effects
Acetylcholinesterase inhibitors: side effects
Acetylcholinesterase: pharmacodynamics
NMR reversal: atropine vs. glycopyrrolate
Pseudocholinesterase activity
TOF monitoring
Sugammadex
NMB potentiation

Neuromuscular blockade reversal is often performed when the blockade is no longer needed. The blockade is essential for protecting the airway during intubation and maintaining spontaneous ventilation.

Depolarizing neuromuscular blockade

Succinylcholine (SCh) is the most rapidly metabolized NMB. The majority of the agent is metabolized by *pseudocholinesterase* before it reaches the NMJ. In patients with normal levels of the enzyme, complete resolution may be obtained in as little as four to ten minutes. This may be prolonged in patients with abnormal levels of *pseudocholinesterase* (heterozygote or homozygote pseudocholinesterase gene carriers). Certain medications have also been shown to inhibit the function of pseudocholinesterase, therefore prolonging the neuromuscular blockade and increasing the time to muscle relaxation.

Table 38.1 Agents that decrease pseudocholinesterase activity

Agent
Metoclopramide
Oral contraceptives (OCPs)
Esmolol
Monoamine oxidase inhibitors (MAOIs)
Echothiophate
Cytotoxic agents

Nondepolarizing neuromuscular blockade

These are the agents that are targeted in NMB reversal. Nondepolarizing neuromuscular blockades (NDNMB) are *competitive antagonists* of ACh at the NMJ. ACh binding to the ACh receptor on the postsynaptic cleft is a necessary step for proper muscle excitation and contraction. The reversal of NMB is dependent on four key factors:

1. ACh concentration in the NMJ
2. NMB concentration at the AChR
3. NMB removal from the NMJ
4. Metabolism and/or elimination of NMB from the body

The actions of *NMB can be potentiated* by:

1. volatile agents
2. acidosis
3. hypothermia
4. aminoglycosides
5. polypeptide antibiotics
6. hypokalemia and hypermagnesemia

The majority of NMB are removed from the synaptic cleft via *passive diffusion*. This is driven by a concentration gradient formed by hepatic metabolism.

Prior to reversal, one must assess the level of NMB. The most common clinical assessment is *TOF monitoring*. A single twitch can roughly estimate that 90% of the AChR are occupied by the NDNMB, while four twitches can estimate that less than 25% of the AChR are occupied. As a safe practice, there must be at least two twitches before NMB reversal is given. Other methods to assess for the success of reversal include sustained tetanus at 100 Hz without fade, double-burst stimulus without fade, and clinical findings such as leg lift, grip strength, tidal volumes of 3 to 5 cc/kg, and maximum inspiratory force of –20 mm Hg. Even though a patient may pass all of these tests there is still a chance of neuromuscular blockade. This is why many anesthesiologists may choose to reverse neuromuscular blockade in anyone that has received an NMB.

Essential Clinical Anesthesia Review: Keywords, Questions and Answers for the Boards, ed. Linda S. Aglio, Robert W. Lekowski, and Richard D. Urman. Published by Cambridge University Press. © Cambridge University Press 2015.

Table 38.2 Anthicholinesterase agents

Agent	Details
Neostigmine	Dose: 0.04–0.07 mg/kg. Most potent and widely used agent. Similar pharmacokinetics of NDNMB makes it a favorable agent. Onset in five minutes and duration is one to two hours.
Pyridostigmine	Dose: 0.2 to 0.35 mg/kg. Slower in onset compared to neostigmine. Longer in duration. Used in reversal of deep neuromuscular blockade.
Edrophonium	Dose: 0.5 to 1.0 mg/kg. More rapid in onset to neostigmine (two minutes) and shorter duration (<1 hour). Less likely to cause cholinergic syndrome.
Physostigmine	Tertiary ammonium compound. Only anticholinesterase agent with BBB permeability. Can be used to treat scopolamine and atropine toxicity.

Anticholinesterase agents are all metabolized in the liver and excreted via urine. These agents do not need to be dose adjusted in patients with hepatic or renal dysfunction as the majority of NDNMB are also eliminated via these pathways. All are *quaternary ammonium compounds* with the exception of physostigmine, which is a *tertiary ammonium compound*. These agents may cause pronounced bradycardia in heart transplant patients. They also may potentiate nondepolarizing neuromuscular blockade in overdose or if given to a patient with SCh (may prolong action by decreasing pseudocholinesterase activity).

Side effects of anticholinesterase agents are due to increased ACh at nicotinic and muscarinic receptors at the NMJ, autonomic ganglia, and parasympathetically innervated organs. The increase in ACh can cause bradycardia, hypersalivation, and bronchoconstriction, as well as the cholinergic syndrome. Effects of anticholinergic agents on various organ systems is shown in Table 38.3.

Anticholinergic agents

Given to counteract the cholinergic effects of anthicholinesterase agents. Can act as antisialagogue and inhibit perspiration.

Combinations of acetycholinesterase inhibitors and vagolytic agents are shown in Table 38.5.

Sugammadex

A cyclodextrin used to encapsulate vecuronium/rocuronium. Not as active against pancuronium. Can produce a TOF ratio of 0.9 within one minute at a dose of 8 mg/kg. It has a wide therapeutic range and patients who received a ten-fold overdose tolerated the drug without side effects. It may be used in a subset of patients who are "can't ventilate, can't intubate" and may be used as an alternative to SCh. The agent has not been granted approval in the United States by the FDA as there is a concern that it has a high incidence of hypersensitivity reactions.

Table 38.3 Effects of anticholinergic agents on various organ systems

Anti-sialagogue effect	Drying of secretions, rise in body temperature
Cardiovascular[a]	Tachycardia, shortening of PR interval
CNS[b]	Sedation, amnesia, stimulation/depression
Respiratory	Inhibition of secretion of respiratory mucosa, bronchodilation
Gastrointestinal	Decreased intestinal motility, increased risk of aspiration as lower esophageal sphincter tone is decreased
Renal	Urinary retention
Ophthalmic	Pupillary dilation and cycloplegia[c]

[a] Atropine produces the highest cardiovascular effects and scopolamine the least.
[b] Glycopyrrolate does not cross the blood–brain barrier and does not produce CNS effects. Scopolamine produces the most CNS effects.
[c] Cycloplegia is the inability to accommodate to near vision.
(From Vacanti et al. 2011. *Essential Clinical Anesthesia*, Cambridge University Press, p. 259.)

Table 38.4 Anticholinergic agents

Agent	Details
Glycopyrrolate	Quaternary amine does not cross the BBB. Duration one to two hours, slower onset. Used well in conjunction with neostigmine.
Atropine	Tertiary amine, can cross the BBB. May cause paradoxical bradycardia in doses <0.5 mg. May cause central anticholinergic syndrome (excitation, delirium, hyperpyrexia)
Scopolamine	Tertiary amine, can cross the BBB. May cause central anticholinergic syndrome (excitation, delirium, hyperpyrexia)

Table 38.5 Typical combinations of acetylcholinesterase inhibitors and vagolytic agents

Combination	Dose, mg/kg
Neostigmine/glycopyrrolate	Neostigmine, 0.04–0.07 Glycopyrrolate, 0.005–0.01
Edrophonium/atropine	Edrophonium, 0.5–1 Atropine, 0.01
Pyridostigmine/glycopyrrolate	Pyridostigmine, 0.2–0.35 Glycopyrrolate, 0.005–0.01

(From Vacanti et al. 2011. *Essential Clinical Anesthesia*, Cambridge University Press, p. 259.)

Questions

1. Which of the following anticholinergic agents *cannot* cross the blood–brain barrier?

    a. scopolamine
    b. atropine
    c. glycopyrrolate
    d. none of the above

2. An elderly patient is brought to the operating room for an emergent exploratory laparotomy. The patient has been in a skilled nursing facility for the last six weeks after having a stroke. He is currently being treated for a urinary tract infection with gentamicin. You elect to perform a rapid sequence induction given that the patient has a history of dysphagia and uncontrolled acid reflux. You decide to use rocuronium as your NMB. Which of the following statements is not correct.

    a. The actions of NMB can be potentiated by aminoglycosides and polypeptide antibiotics.
    b. Rocuronium can be reversed with a combination of neostigmine and atropine.
    c. Atropine use can cause an increased risk of aspiration due to its effect on lower esophageal sphincter tone.
    d. A single twitch on TOF monitoring can roughly estimate that only 25% of receptors are bound.

Answers

1. c. Of the agents listed, scopolamine and atropine are both able to cross the blood–brain barrier and therefore must be used with caution in the elderly and those with cognitive deficits.
2. d. Usually a single twitch can roughly estimate that 90% of the AChR are occupied by the NDNMB, while four twitches can estimate that less than 25% of the AChR are occupied.

Further reading

Naguib, M. and Lien, C. A. (2009). Chapter 29. Pharmacology of muscle relaxants and their antagonists. In Miller, R. D., Eriksson, L. I., Fleisher, L. A. et al. (eds) *Miller's Anesthesia*, 7th edn. Philadelphia: Churchill-Livingstone.

Viby-Mogensen, J. (2009). Chapter 47. Neuromuscular monitoring. In Miller, R. D., Eriksson, L. I., Fleisher, L. A. et al. (eds) *Miller's Anesthesia*, 7th edn. Philadelphia: Churchill-Livingstone.

Miller, R. D. and Ward, T. A. (2010). Monitoring and pharmacologic reversal of a nondepolarizing neuromuscular blockade should be routine. *Anesthesia and Analgesia* 111(1): 3–5.

Chapter 39

Perioperative pulmonary aspiration prophylaxis

Emily L. Wang and Jeffrey Lu

Keywords

Pulmonary aspiration
Acidity of aspirated material
Volume of aspiration
Occurrence of aspiration in the perioperative period
Risk factors for pulmonary aspiration
ASA NPO guidelines for fasting
Induction techniques to reduce aspiration risk
Pharmacologic approaches to reduce aspiration risk
Antacids
Histamine H2 antagonists
Proton pump inhibitors
Metoclopramide
Signs and symptoms of aspiration
Management of perioperative pulmonary aspiration

Pulmonary aspiration: the regurgitation of gastric contents with subsequent entry into the respiratory tract, which can cause acute lung injury. Particulate matter in the aspirated contents may lead to a focal inflammatory and foreign-body reaction. Pulmonary injury includes aspiration pneumonitis, which can later evolve into aspiration pneumonia, respiratory failure, or acute respiratory distress syndrome (ARDS).

Acidity of aspirated material: the acidic nature (low pH) of the aspirated contents is one of the most important factors determining the severity of aspiration pneumonitis. Aspiration of contents with pH <2.5 is associated with pulmonary morbidity (as compared to more alkaline material, which causes little to no injury). In general, the greater the acidity, the greater the damage to tracheal mucosa and lung parenchyma.

Volume of aspiration: volume aspirated also affects the severity of lung parenchymal damage. The volume of aspirate to cause injury is controversial, and is likely in the range 0.4 to 1.0 ml/kg (or approximately 25 to 70 ml in a 70 kg adult).

Occurrence of aspiration in the perioperative period: pulmonary aspiration is an infrequent perioperative event. While the incidence during general anesthesia is one to five in 10,000 procedures, the impact on individual patients can be devastating.

Table 39.1 Risk factors for perioperative pulmonary aspiration

Increased gastric volume	Increased gastric regurgitation	Decreased laryngeal competence
Delayed gastric emptying	Gastroesophageal reflux disease	General anesthesia
Diabetic gastroparesis	Decreased lower esophageal sphincter tone	Depressed level of consciousness
Labor	Esophageal obstruction	Head injury
Pain/stress	Zenker's diverticulum	Stroke
Gastric hypersecretion	Achalasia	Neuromuscular disorders
Overfeeding	Extremes of age	Muscular dystrophies
Recent meal	Esophageal/upper abdominal surgery	
	Esophagectomy	
	Increased intra-abdominal pressure	

(From Vacanti et al. 2011. *Essential Clinical Anesthesia*, Cambridge University Press, p. 261.)

Although the incidence is slightly greater in the obstetric and pediatric populations, the overall morbidity and mortality do not seem to be increased in comparison. In general, children have less overall mortality rate from pulmonary aspiration. Trauma patients have a much higher incidence of aspiration.

Fortunately, not all patients who aspirate develop respiratory consequences. Approximately 25% of patients who have perioperative aspiration develop significant respiratory complications. Patients who appear to have the greatest risk of severe pulmonary morbidity or death after aspiration are those who are ASA Class 3 or greater, and the elderly.

Aspiration can occur at any time in the perioperative period, although it is most common during tracheal intubation or extubation. This can be associated with inadequate muscle relaxation during intubation (where laryngoscopy can cause gagging and vomiting), or being too weak or unresponsive

Essential Clinical Anesthesia Review: Keywords, Questions and Answers for the Boards, ed. Linda S. Aglio, Robert W. Lekowski, and Richard D. Urman. Published by Cambridge University Press. © Cambridge University Press 2015.

(i.e., depressed level of consciousness with impaired upper airway protective reflexes) during extubation.

Risk factors for pulmonary aspiration: it is important to identify those patients who are at increased risk for aspiration in order to help prevent it.

ASA NPO guidelines for fasting: patients are required to be nil per os (NPO) prior to undergoing general anesthesia to minimize the risk of aspiration. If the guidelines (shown in Chapter 1, Table 1.1) are not met, the patient is considered to be at an increased aspiration risk.

Induction techniques to reduce aspiration risk: if a general anesthetic is administered to a patient at risk for aspiration, protection of the airway with a cuffed endotracheal tube is necessary. However, modern high-volume, low-pressure cuffs (which are inflated to 25 cm H_2O) do not provide complete protection against aspiration.

Proposed techniques for high-risk patients include rapid sequence intubation, and application of cricoid pressure with Sellick's maneuver during induction until the airway is secured. Notably, neither has been shown to reduce the incidence of aspiration, or decrease the morbidity or mortality from pulmonary aspiration. Regardless, such techniques are considered to be the standard of care for patients at increased risk for aspiration.

Pharmacologic approaches to reduce aspiration risk: preoperative administration of medications that can help reduce aspiration risk include antacids (non particulate), histamine (H_2) antagonists, proton pump inhibitors (PPIs), and prokinetic agents.

1. *Antacids*: increase gastric pH because of gastric-acid neutralizing effect. Nonparticulate or soluble antacids are preferable to the particulate antacids because the solution mixes more effectively with gastric contents. Antacids consist of aluminum, magnesium, and calcium salts that neutralize hydrochloric acid. Aspiration of soluble antacids is associated with faster recovery and is less likely to cause a foreign-body reaction. The most commonly used solutions are sodium citrate or citric acid. (Bicitra® contains sodium citrate and citric acid, and Polycitra® contains sodium citrate, potassium citrate, and citric acid.) They are administered immediately preoperatively since they have a very rapid onset of action and a relatively short duration.

2. *Histamine H2 antagonists*: increase gastric pH by limiting histamine-induced secretion of acid by gastric parietal cells. Specifically, they antagonize the action of histamine on gastric parietal cells via competitive inhibition. Onset of action is slower than antacids, but duration is longer.

   - Famotidine (Pepcid®) is one of the most potent and highly competitive H_2 antagonists available, and has the longest duration of action. It can be given orally or parenterally. After an oral dose of 40 mg, peak plasma concentrations occur in two hours, with a plasma half-life of 3 to 3.5 hours; 60% to 70% is excreted unchanged in the urine.

Table 39.2 Suggested aspiration prophylaxis drugs, doses, and routes of administration

Drug	Dose	Route of administration
Citric acid/sodium citrate	30 ml	PO
Metoclopramide	5–15 mg	PO/IV/IM
Rabeprazole	20 mg	PO/IV
Omeprazole	20–40 mg	PO/IV
Pantoprazole	40–120 mg	PO/IV
Lansoprazole	15–30 mg	PO/IV
Esomeprazole	20–40 mg	PO/IV
Nizatidine	150–300 mg	PO/IV/IM
Famotidine	20–40 mg	PO/IV/IM
Cimetidine	400–800 mg	PO/IV/IM
Ranitidine	75–150 mg	PO/IV/IM

IM, intramuscular; IV, intravenous; PO, oral.
(From Vacanti et al. 2011. *Essential Clinical Anesthesia*, Cambridge University Press, p. 262.)

- Cimetidine (Tagamet®) is used to treat or prevent peptic ulcer disease, especially when associated with excess gastric acid secretion. It can be administered intramuscularly (IM), intravenously (IV), or orally. After an oral dose, peak plasma concentrations occur in 60 to 90 minutes. After an IV dose, it takes 45 to 60 minutes to take effect. Therapeutic effects last four to seven hours regardless of the administration route. Cimetidine can produce a large number of side effects, which include: (1) inhibiting cytochrome P450 enzyme function and decreasing the clearance of many drugs that undergo oxidative degradation; (2) central nervous system dysfunction that can be manifested as agitation, confusion, convulsions, coma, and delayed anesthesia wakening; (3) cardiovascular changes such as hypotension from peripheral vasodilation, bradycardia, heart block, and cardiac arrest after rapid IV administration; and (4) pulmonary effects such as bronchoconstriction.

- Ranitidine (Zantac®) is four to eight times more potent than cimetidine in blocking acid secretion. Can be given orally or parenterally. After an oral dose of 150 mg, peak plasma concentrations occur in 30 to 60 minutes, and duration of action is 8 to 12 hours. Approximately 25% undergoes hepatic metabolism, and 50% is excreted unchanged in the kidneys. Elimination half-life is two to three hours. Ranitidine is less likely than cimetidine to produce side effects, especially central nervous system dysfunction (because of poor permeability through the blood–brain barrier) and changes in metabolism of the cytochrome P450 system.

3. *Proton pump inhibitors* (PPIs): increase gastric pH by limiting parietal cell acid secretion. Specifically, they inhibit the action of H^+, K^+-ATPase pump on the parietal cells. PPIs consist of a family of substituted benzimidazoles, including omeprazole (Prilosec®) and lansoprazole (Prevacid®). Onset of action is slower than antacids, but has longer duration. Omeprazole 20 mg can be given orally two to four hours before surgery, and the effects can last up to 24 hours.

4. *Metoclopramide*: dopamine receptor antagonist that has prokinetic properties (due to peripheral cholinergic agonism). Effects include increased gastric contractions and speeding gastric emptying time, increased small bowel peristalsis, and relaxation of the pyloric sphincter. As it increases gastric emptying, it theoretically can reduce the risk of pulmonary aspiration by decreasing the gastric volume. It can be given orally or parenterally. Onset of action after an oral dose of 10 mg is within 30 to 60 minutes, and peak plasma concentrations occur in 40 to 120 minutes. Onset time after IV administration is approximately 20 minutes. When administered for emergency procedures, it may help reduce the risk of aspiration at extubation, even if it has no significant effect at the time of induction. Rapid IV administration can produce abdominal cramping, which can be prevented by giving it over three to five minutes. Elimination half-life is two to four hours, and about 85% of the drug excretion is in the urine. Possible side effects include extrapyramidal symptoms, sedation, dysphoria, rash, and dry mouth. Metoclopramide should be avoided in patients with bowel obstruction, pheochromocytoma, and patients taking MAOIs, TCAs, or other drugs that may cause extrapyramidal symptoms.

Although the above mentioned agents increase gastric pH and reduce gastric volume, no data has specifically proven that their use reduces the morbidity and mortality from perioperative pulmonary aspiration. It is not recommended to provide routine prophylaxis with these agents for all patients. The above measures are useful for those patients who are considered high risk for aspiration events, and for those in whom an aspiration event would be poorly tolerated.

Signs and symptoms of aspiration include bronchospasm (often associated with high airway pressures), coughing, laryngospasm, dyspnea, hypoxemia, tachypnea, tachycardia, presence of foreign material in the mouth or posterior pharynx, chest wall retraction, cyanosis, and hypotension. Typically has rapid onset.

Management of perioperative pulmonary aspiration: patients who aspirate require supportive care, including likely respiratory support. As the severity and consequences of pulmonary aspiration can vary greatly depending on the volume and acidity of the aspirate, careful suctioning is useful to help decrease the volume of aspirated material in the lungs. It is not recommended to lavage with saline as it may cause spread of the aspirate. Bronchoscopy should be performed if particulate material is present to help prevent bronchial obstruction. Approximately 25% of patients who have perioperative aspiration require intensive care support. Approximately 10% of these patients require mechanical ventilation for greater than 24 hours. The use of prophylactic antibiotics and/or steroids is not effective to reduce the incidence of pulmonary inflammation or pneumonia, or improve outcomes.

Questions

1. Which of the following statements is false?
   a. Both the pH and the amount of aspirated material determine the morbidity and mortality after gastric acid aspiration.
   b. The incidence of aspiration is higher in certain patient populations, such as obstetric, pediatric, and trauma patients.
   c. Current guidelines suggest that to reduce the risk of aspiration after eating a hamburger, a patient should be NPO for at least eight hours.
   d. Both cimetidine and omeprazole work to increase gastric pH by limiting parietal cell acid secretion.
   e. Metoclopramide is a dopamine receptor agonist that works by increasing bowel motility.

2. A trauma patient with a femur fracture underwent general anesthesia for an emergent open reduction internal fixation of his lower extremity. On emergence, the endotracheal tube is removed, and the patient is then noted to become dyspneic and cyanotic. High airway pressures are needed to provide supplemental oxygen by bag-mask ventilation. Wheezing is present on auscultation, and the patient's blood pressure decreases from 115/75 to 65/40. What is the most likely etiology of the patient's presentation?
   a. pneumothorax
   b. venous air embolism
   c. fat embolism
   d. aspiration
   e. large mucous plug

3. During induction of general anesthesia in the operating room, tracheal intubation is attempted with direct laryngoscopy. The patients begins to cough and food particles are noted in the posterior pharynx. Appropriate management and treatment of this patient may consist of the following except for:
   a. supplemental oxygen with positive pressure ventilation
   b. suctioning of the airway
   c. prophylactic administration of antibiotics
   d. bronchoscopy
   e. mechanical ventilation

Answers

1. e. Metoclopramide is a dopamine receptor antagonist that has prokinetic properties. The effects of metoclopramide include increasing gastric emptying time by promoting gastric contractions and bowel peristalsis.

2. d. Signs and symptoms of aspiration typically have a rapid onset, and include bronchospasm (which is often associated with high airway pressures and wheezing), dyspnea, hypoxemia, cyanosis, coughing, and hypotension.

3. c. Management of pulmonary aspiration requires supportive care. Respiratory support may include supplemental oxygen, as well as mechanical ventilation. Careful suctioning may be useful to help decrease the volume of aspirated material in the lungs. Bronchoscopy may be useful if particulate material is causing obstruction. The use of prophylactic antibiotics has not been shown to reduce the incidence of pneumonia or improve outcomes.

Further reading

American Society of Anesthesiologists Committee on Standards and Practice Parameters. (2011). Practice guidelines for preoperative fasting and the use of pharmacologic agents to reduce the risk of pulmonary aspiration: application to healthy patients undergoing elective procedures. *Anesthesiology* 114, 495–511.

Faust, R. J. (2002). *Anesthesiology Review*, 3rd edn. Philadelphia: W.B. Saunders Company, pp. 169–171; pp. 564–5.

Manchikanti, L., Grow, J. B., Colliver, J. A., Hadley, C. H., and Hohlbein, L. J. (1985). Bicitra (sodium citrate) and metoclopramide in outpatient anesthesia for prophylaxis against aspiration penumonitis. *Anesthesiology* 63, 378–84.

Vacanti, C., Sikka, P., Urman, R., Dershwitz, M., and Segal, B. (eds) (2011). *Essential Clinical Anesthesia*. Cambridge: Cambridge University Press, pp. 261–262.

Warner, M. A., Warner, M. E., and Weber, J. G. (1993). Clinical significance of pulmonary aspiration during the perioperative period. *Anesthesiology* 78, 56–62.

Chapter

40

Perioperative antiemetic therapies

Iuliu Fat and Devon Flaherty

Keywords

- Preemptive therapy
- Rescue therapy
- Selective serotonin receptor antagonists
- Glucocorticoids
- Dopaminergic antagonists
- Anticholinergic agents
- Antihistamines
- Neurokinin-receptor antagonist

Preemptive therapy is the prophylactic administration of antiemetics to prevent or mitigate the development of postoperative nausea and vomiting (PONV).

Rescue therapy involves the treatment of PONV in a patient who was not given prophylaxis or who develops PONV in spite of prophylactic therapy.

There are several classes of drugs available for the prophylaxis and rescue treatment of PONV, including: *serotonin receptor antagonists, corticosteroids, anticholinergic agents, butyrophenones, antihistamines,* and *neurokinin-receptor antagonists.*

Selective serotonin receptor (5-HT3) antagonists (e.g., ondansetron, dolasetron, and granisetron) can be used prophylactically or for the rescue treatment of PONV. These agents, which act by blocking serotonin peripherally at vagal afferents and centrally in the chemoreceptor trigger zone (CTZ), are most effective when given at the end of the surgical procedure. Despite their favorable side effect profile, potentially fatal cardiac arrhythmias have been reported in association with QTc prolongation after using serotonin receptor antagonists. Ondansetron should be avoided in patients with congenital long-QT syndrome, and EKG monitoring is warranted in certain patients, such as those with hypokalemia or hypomagnesemia, heart failure, bradyarrhythmias, and in patients taking other medications that increase the risk of QTc prolongation.

Glucocorticoids (e.g., dexamethasone) can also be used prophylactically to control PONV. The exact mechanism by which they prevent PONV is unclear, but likely involves their

Table 40.1 Suggested PONV prophylaxis drugs, doses, and times of administration

Drug	Dose	Time of administration[a]
Dexamethasone	4–5 mg IV	Induction of anesthesia
Dimenhydrinate	1 mg/kg IV; 25–50 mg PO	Undetermined
Dolasetron	12.5 mg IV	End of surgery
Droperidol	0.625–1.250 mg IV	End of surgery
Granisetron	0.35–1.50 mg IV	End of surgery
Haloperidol	0.5–2.0 mg IM/IV	? / End of surgery
Prochlorperazine	5–10 mg IM/IV	End of surgery
Promethazine	6.25–25 mg IV	Induction of anesthesia
Ondansetron	4 mg IV	End of surgery
Scopolamine	Transdermal patch	Preoperatively
Aprepitant	40 mg PO	Preoperatively

[a] The stated times of administration are based on the best currently available evidence; however, significant controversy remains regarding the optimal timing of perioperative antiemetic administration.
IM, intramuscularly; IV, intravenously; PO, orally.
(Data from Gan, T., Meyers, T., and Apfel, C. 2003. Consensus guidelines for managing postoperative nausea and vomiting. *Anesthesia and Analgesia* 97: 62–71; From Vacanti et al. 2011. *Essential Clinical Anesthesia,* Cambridge University Press, p. 264.)

anti-inflammatory action. To optimize PONV prophylaxis, dexamethasone should be administered relatively early in the perioperative period. The standard prophylactic dose of dexamethasone is 4 mg intravenously given immediately after the induction of anesthesia.

Dopaminergic antagonists

Butyrophenones are a class of *dopaminergic antagonists* that includes droperidol and haloperidol. They act by antagonizing the D2 receptors in the CTZ located in the area postrema of

Essential Clinical Anesthesia Review: Keywords, Questions and Answers for the Boards, ed. Linda S. Aglio, Robert W. Lekowski, and Richard D. Urman. Published by Cambridge University Press. © Cambridge University Press 2015.

the brain. Doses as low as 0.625 mg of droperidol can be effective for PONV prophylaxis. However, doses between 1.0 and 2.5 mg improve antiemetic efficacy. In 2001, the FDA issued a "black box" warning for droperidol due to the potential for QT prolongation, torsades de pointes, and sudden cardiac death. Continuous cardiac rhythm monitoring for two to three hours is recommended for any patient receiving droperidol at the approved (labeled) dose of ≥2.5 mg. Although cardiac morbidity is a well-documented effect seen with high doses of droperidol, it is unclear whether the same risk exists at the much lower doses (0.625 to 1.25 mg) used for PONV prophylaxis and treatment.

Another class of dopaminergic antagonists with antiemetic properties is the phenothiazine group. They exert antiemetic effects via antagonism of the dopamine D2 receptor in the CTZ and also through antagonism of histamine H1 receptors. Prochlorperazine, an agent in this class of medications, has been shown to be an effective antiemetic when administered at the end of surgical procedures. Caution should be taken when using prochlorperazine in the perioperative period because of its profound antagonism of alpha-adrenoceptors.

Anticholinergic agents, specifically transdermal scopolamine, are more commonly used for prophylaxis of PONV than for rescue therapy due to a slow onset of action. The exact mechanism by which scopolamine prevents PONV is uncertain. Common side effects of transdermal scopolamine include sedation, visual disturbances, dry mouth, and dizziness. The drug should be avoided in patients with narrow angle glaucoma. The transdermal patch should be applied behind the ear four or more hours prior to the end of the procedure, or it can be applied the night before surgery. It is standard practice to apply the patch no sooner than one hour before cesarean section to reduce the exposure of the newborn to the drug. The time to onset of action is slow (two to four hours), but the effect is prolonged. A scopolamine patch is typically removed 24 hours after the end of surgery.

Antihistamines exert an antiemetic effect by antagonizing histamine H1 and muscarinic receptors in the vestibular system. The most effective and frequently used antihistamines in anesthetic practice are members of the ethanolamine, piperazine, and phenothiazine families. Dimenhydrinate, an ethanolamine, appears to have antiemetic efficacy similar to that of the 5-HT3 receptor antagonists, dexamethasone and droperidol. Cyclizine and hydroxyzine are the most used antiemetic antihistamines in the piperazine family. Hydroxyzine is a favorable option because its produces anxiolysis and potentiates the effect of opioids. Promethazine exerts most of its antiemetic effects

via histamine H1 and muscarinic receptor antagonism. Antihistamines share a similar side effect profile, which tends to be the limiting factor in their perioperative use. These side effects include sedation, dry mouth, constipation, confusion, blurred vision, delirium, urinary retention, and tachycardia.

Neurokinin is a naturally occurring pro-emetic substance. *Neurokinin-receptor antagonists*, such as aprepitant, are effective prophylactic agents for PONV. In studies comparing ondansetron to aprepitant, the latter was superior in preventing vomiting up to 48 hours postoperatively, and equivalent in reducing the incidence of nausea and need for rescue antiemetics in the first 24 hours postoperatively. Aprepitant 40 mg orally may be administered within three hours before induction of anesthesia. Aprepitant is only available in an oral form, has a long onset of action, and is costly. Therefore it is typically reserved for patients in whom PONV would cause serious clinical problems.

Other treatments: randomized trials support the use of alternative therapies such as the more liberal use of IV fluids and acupuncture/stimulation therapy to reduce the incidence of PONV.

Questions

1. All of the following statements are true regarding the use of transdermal scopolamine EXCEPT:
   a. It should be avoided in patients with narrow angle glaucoma.
   b. It has a fast onset and is used as rescue therapy.
   c. Side effects include sedation, visual disturbances, and dry mouth.
   d. It has a prolonged effect.

2. Which statement about the use of dexamethasone as an antiemetic is TRUE:
   a. It is most effective when administered at the end of the surgery.
   b. It should be avoided in diabetes mellitus.
   c. The standard dose for prevention of PONV is 8 mg.
   d. It can cause QT prolongation.

Answers

1. b. The scopolamine patch has a slow onset of action and is best used for PONV prophylaxis rather than as a rescue therapy. Its mydriatic effects preclude its use in patients with narrow angle glaucoma.
2. b. The administration of dexamethasone can lead to hyperglycemia, thus should be avoided in diabetes mellitus.

Further reading

Domino, K. B., Anderson, E. A., Polissar, N. L., and Posner, K. L.(1997). Comparative efficacy and safety of ondansetron, droperidol, and metoclopramide for preventing postoperative nausea and vomiting:

a meta-analysis. *Anesthesia and Analgesia* 88, 1370–1379.

Gan, T., Meyers, T., and Apfel, C. (2003). Consensus guidelines for managing postoperative nausea and vomiting. *Anesthesia and Analgesia* 97, 62–71.

Wilhelm, S. M., Dehoorne-Smith, M. L., and Kale-Pradhan, P. B. (2007). Prevention of postoperative nausea and vomiting. *Annals of Pharmacotherapy* 41, 68–78.

COX inhibitors and alpha2-adrenergic agonists

Iuliu Fat and Devon Flaherty

Cyclooxygenase (COX) inhibitors

COX inhibitors act by blocking the enzyme cyclooxygenase (COX), which prevents the formation of prostaglandins, prostacyclins, and thromboxane from arachidonic acid. Most NSAIDs are nonselective, inhibiting both cyclooxygenase-1 and cyclooxygenase-2. They exhibit antipyretic and analgesic properties and, with the exception of acetaminophen, they also reduce inflammation. Common agents in this class include, but are not limited to, aspirin, ibuprofen, ketorolac, and acetaminophen. The advantages of using COX inhibitors over other pain relievers, such as opioids, are that they do not cause sedation, respiratory depression, or tolerance.

Ketorolac

Ketorolac is an NSAID indicated for the short-term management of moderate to severe acute pain. It is not indicated for chronic pain conditions. Ketorolac is contraindicated during labor and delivery and for nursing mothers, and is not indicated for use in children. It is available in oral, intramuscular (IM), and intravenous (IV) formulations. The recommended dosage for postoperative pain management is 30 mg IM or IV every six hours, with a maximum daily dose of 120 mg. The dose should be decreased by half in persons over 65 years of age, in persons with renal insufficiency, or in adults weighing less than 50 kg. The onset of analgesia is slow, occurring about 30 minutes following IV administration and 60 minutes following IM administration. The duration of therapy should not exceed five days. Ketorolac is metabolized by the liver into metabolites that are excreted primarily in the urine. About 40% of an administered dose is metabolized, whereas the

Table 41.1 Doses of COX inhibitors

Drug	Dose, mg	Interval, h	Maximum daily dose, mg
Ketorolac	30 IV/IM	6	120
	10 PO	6	40
Acetaminophen	500–1,000	4–6	4,000
Aspirin	500–1,000	4–6	4,000
Ibuprofen	200–800	4–6	2,400
Naproxen	500 initially, then 250	6–8	1,500
Celecoxib	200–400 initially, then 100–200	12–24	400

IM, intramuscularly; IV, intravenously; PO, orally.
(From Vacanti et al. 2011. *Essential Clinical Anesthesia*, Cambridge University Press)

remainder is excreted unchanged. The comparative doses of ketorolac and other COX inhibitors are shown in Table 41.1.

Although potency ratios are difficult to measure, a 30 mg dose of ketorolac is approximately equipotent to 4 mg of morphine. Ketorolac has become particularly popular in ambulatory surgery because its use may permit faster patient recovery and shorter discharge times.

Alpha2-adrenoceptor agonists

Alpha2-adrenoceptor agonists are important adjuncts to anesthesia practice. Dexmedetomidine and clonidine are among the most commonly used alpha2-adrenoceptor agonists in anesthesia practice. Though they do not reliably produce amnesia or general anesthesia, they are effective sedatives and do exhibit analgesic properties. Their primary effect is to decrease sympathetic outflow from the central nervous system (CNS), leading to a decrease in heart rate, blood pressure, and cardiac output. However, a bolus of dexmedetomidine may lead to a paradoxical increase in blood pressure thought to be a

Essential Clinical Anesthesia Review: Keywords, Questions and Answers for the Boards, ed. Linda S. Aglio, Robert W. Lekowski, and Richard D. Urman. Published by Cambridge University Press. © Cambridge University Press 2015.

result of agonist effects at vascular alpha1-adrenoceptors. The main advantage of using these agents is the lack of respiratory depression associated with their use. Dexmedetomidine is approved for short-term sedation in the ICU setting and for procedural sedation, such as awake fiberoptic intubation. The usual loading dose is 1.0 µg/kg given over ten minutes. Maintenance doses are typically 0.1 to 1.0 µg/kg/h. Clonidine is commonly used in neuraxial blocks and also in peripheral nerve blocks with varying results. Some studies have suggested improved onset and quality of the block, whereas others have documented prolongation of the block. The mechanism of action is unknown.

Questions

1. Ketorolac is contraindicated in which of the following?
   a. labor
   b. severe pain
   c. cancer pain
   d. elderly patients

2. The primary effect of alpha2-adrenoceptor agonists is:
   a. NMDA antagonism
   b. decrease in the sympathetic outflow
   c. increase in the sympathetic outflow
   d. GABA receptor agonism

Answers

1. a. Ketorolac is contraindicated during labor and delivery as it inhibits prostaglandin synthesis and may decrease uterine blood flow and contractions. Ketorolac is also excreted in breast milk.

2. b. The primary effect of alpha2-adrenoceptor agonists is to decrease sympathetic outflow from the CNS.

Further reading

American Pain Society (2003). *Principles of Analgesic Use in the Treatment of Acute Pain and Cancer Pain*, 5th edn. Glenview, IL: American Pain Society.

Barash, P. G., Cullen, B. F., and Stoelting, R. K. (2006). *Clinical Anesthesia*, 5th edn.

Philadelphia: Lippincott Williams & Wilkins.

Morgan, G. E., Mikhail, M. S., and Murray, M. J. (2006). *Clinical Anesthesiology*, 4th edn. New York: Lange Medical Books.

Tollison, C. D., and Satterthwaite, J. (2002). *Practical Pain Management*, 3rd edn.

Philadelphia: Lippincott Williams & Wilkins.

Watcha, M. F., Issioui, T., Klein, K. W., and White, P. F. (2003). Costs and effectiveness of rofecoxib, celecoxib, and acetaminophen for preventing pain after ambulatory otolaryngologic surgery. *Anesthesia and Analgesia* 96, 987.

Diuretics

42

Iuliu Fat and Devon Flaherty

Keywords

Loop diuretics
Thiazide diuretics
Potassium-sparing diuretics
Carbonic anhydrase inhibitors
Osmotic diuretics

Diuretics are generally divided into five major classes, which are distinguished by the site at which they impair sodium reabsorption.

1. Loop diuretics act on the thick ascending limb of the loop of Henle.
2. Thiazide-type diuretics act on both the distal tubule and connecting segment.
3. Potassium-sparing diuretics act on the aldosterone-sensitive principal cells in the cortical collecting duct.
4. Acetazolamide acts on the proximal tubule.
5. Mannitol acts primarily at the loop of Henle.

The site of action of a diuretic within the nephron is a major determinant of its potency. Roughly 60% to 65% of the filtered sodium is reabsorbed in the proximal tubule and about 20% in the loop of Henle. As a result, it might be expected that a proximally acting diuretic, such as the carbonic anhydrase inhibitor acetazolamide, could induce relatively large losses of sodium and water. However, this does not occur since almost all of the excess fluid delivered out of the proximal tubule can be reabsorbed more distally.

Loop diuretics block the Na-K-2Cl carriers in the ascending loop of Henle, thereby diminishing the net reabsorption of sodium. When administered at maximum dosage, up to 20% to 25% of filtered sodium can be excreted. The loop of Henle is also the primary site for reabsorption of Ca^{++} and Mg^{++}, whose reabsorption is inhibited by excess luminal Na^+. Therefore Ca^{++} (as in the treatment of hypercalcemia) and Mg^{++} are excreted along with Na^+, K^+, and water. Because of their potency, loop diuretics may cause significant electrolyte loss. Consequently, hypokalemia and other electrolyte deficiencies

are common with their use. Loop diuretics are often used in neurosurgical settings as a means to lower intracranial pressure. Commonly used loop diuretics include furosemide, bumetanide, torsemide, and ethacrynic acid.

The *thiazide diuretics* primarily inhibit sodium transport in the thick ascending loop and the distal tubule. These segments reabsorb a smaller proportion of the filtered load than the loop of Henle. As a result, the thiazide-type diuretics have a smaller natriuretic effect than loop diuretics. When they are administered at their maximum dosage, they inhibit the reabsorption of at most 3% to 5% of filtered sodium. The thiazides inhibit NaCl reabsorption by competing for the chloride site on the transporters. Adverse effects related to their use include dehydration, metabolic alkalosis, hyponatremia, hypokalemia, hypercalcemia, hyperuricemia, hyperlipidemia, and impaired glucose tolerance.

The *potassium-sparing diuretics* include amiloride, triamterene, spironolactone, and eplerenone. They act on the principal cells in the cortical collecting duct to inhibit Na^+ reabsorption and K^+ secretion by closing sodium channels. Their diuretic effects are weak because more than 90% of the filtered load is reabsorbed prior to the distal tubule and only a small amount of Na^+ is reabsorbed in the terminal distal tubule and collecting duct. Spironolactone inhibits the effects of aldosterone by competing for mineralocorticoid receptors in the cortical collecting duct. The oral formulation is commonly used to treat ascites and heart failure. However, it does have an antiandrogen effect that may result in gynecomastia and menstrual irregularities. In contrast to spironolactone, amiloride and triamterene are noncompetitive inhibitors of aldosterone. With all potassium-sparing diuretics, hyperkalemia and metabolic acidosis may result in patients with renal insufficiency or in those taking angiotensin-converting enzyme (ACE) inhibitors.

The proximal convoluted tubule is the primary site of action for Na^+ reabsorption and seems a likely site for effective diuretic action. However, the large number of downstream reabsorption sites limits the effectiveness of any diuretic targeting this region. While *carbonic anhydrase inhibitors*

Essential Clinical Anesthesia Review: Keywords, Questions and Answers for the Boards, ed. Linda S. Aglio, Robert W. Lekowski, and Richard D. Urman. Published by Cambridge University Press. © Cambridge University Press 2015.

target this region of the nephron, they are rarely used as diuretics. They act by inhibiting the enzyme carbonic anhydrase, which decreases bicarbonate ion (HCO_3^-) reabsorption and leads to a metabolic acidosis. To maintain electrochemical neutrality, Na^+ (the most abundant cation) accompanies HCO_3^- out of the proximal tubule. The thick ascending limb of the loop of Henle is capable of reabsorbing increased loads of NaCl. As a result, a large amount of the Na^+ is reabsorbed there, accounting for the relatively weak diuretic effect of acetazolamide. In the distal tubule, Na^+ is exchanged for potassium (K^+), with a net result of a small increase in the excretion of HCO_3^-, K^+, and water. Acetazolamide is occasionally used for the treatment of glaucoma, as it inhibits the production of aqueous humor by the ciliary body, resulting in decreased intraocular pressure. It is also used for the treatment of acute mountain sickness (AMS). Although the exact mechanism by which it ameliorates the symptoms of AMS is unclear, it is presumed to counter the hyperventilation-induced respiratory alkalosis that results from exposure to the hypoxic atmosphere of high altitudes.

Osmotic diuretics act primarily at the loop of Henle. Examples of osmotic diuretics include mannitol, glycerin, and, occasionally, glucose. Mannitol and glycerin are freely filtered into the tubular fluid but are inert and not reabsorbed from the filtrate. In the proximal tubule, Na^+ is reabsorbed, resulting in an increased filtrate osmolality due to the increasing concentration of mannitol. The increased oncotic pressure opposes water reabsorption from the filtrate and results in increased excretion of water as well as Na^+. Osmotic diuretics also increase the serum osmolarity following their administration, which results in net water extraction from the extravascular to the intravascular compartment. This effect is commonly observed when osmotic diuretics are administered to decrease intracranial volume and pressure. Although the increase in intravascular volume is transient, it may cause

congestive cardiac failure in a minority of patients. Mannitol is the most rapidly acting and commonly used osmotic diuretic. Although the evidence is mixed, some research suggests that mannitol exerts renal protective effects by causing renal vasodilation. Glucose is also freely filtered, but it undergoes significant reabsorption by proximal tubular sodium–glucose transport proteins. Excess glucose due to severe hyperglycemia that exceeds the capacity of proximal tubular reabsorption, can result in an osmotic diuresis. This leads to dehydration and can be seen in diabetics with poor glucose control.

Questions

1. At which part of the nephron do the loop diuretics act?
   a. proximal convoluted tubule
   b. loop of Henle
   c. distal convoluted tubule
   d. collecting duct

2. Side effects of thiazide diuretics include which of the following?
   a. hyponatremia, hyperglycemia, and hypocalcemia
   b. hypernatremia, hypoglycemia, and hypercalcemia
   c. hyponatremia, hyperglycemia, and hypercalcemia
   d. hyponatremia, hypoglycemia, and hypocalcemia

Answers

1. b. The site of action of the loop diuretics is the thick ascending limb of the loop of Henle where it blocks the type 2Na-H-Cl cotransporter.
2. c. Adverse effects of thiazide diuretics include metabolic alkalosis, hyponatremia, hypokalemia, hypercalcemia, hyperuricemia, hyperlipidemia, and impaired glucose tolerance.

Further reading

Ellison, D. H. (1991). The physiologic basis of diuretic synergism: its role in treating diuretic resistance. *Annals of Internal Medicine* 114 (10), 886–894.

Hardman, J. G., Limbird, L. E., and Gilman, A. G. (eds) (2005). *Goodman and Gilman's: The Pharmacologic Basis of Therapeutics*, 11th edn. New York: McGraw-Hill.

Stanton, B. and Kaissling, B. (1988). Adaptation of distal tubule and collecting duct to increased sodium delivery. II. Sodium and potassium transport. *American Journal of Physiology* 255, F1269–F1275.

Thenuwara, K., Todd, M., and Brian, J. (2002). Effect of mannitol and furosemide on plasma osmolality and brain water. *Anesthesiology* 96 (2), 416–421.

Drug interactions

Iuliu Fat and Devon Flaherty

Keywords

Pharmaceutical interactions
Pharmacokinetic interactions
Absorption
Distribution
Metabolism
Elimination
Pharmacodynamic interactions

A *pharmaceutical interaction* is a chemical or physical interaction that occurs between drugs before they are administered or absorbed systemically. An example of this type of interaction is the precipitation that occurs when bicarbonate is added to a solution of bupivacaine.

A *pharmacokinetic interaction* occurs when one drug alters the absorption, distribution, metabolism, or elimination of another drug. Pharmacokinetic interactions are a common source of adverse effects in anesthesia.

Absorption occurs when a substance enters the vascular circulation. Drug absorption can be altered by the presence of other drugs. This can occur via a direct chemical interaction between drugs or one drug can alter the physiology of the absorption of the other drug. An example of the latter is the decrease in the rate of absorption of local anesthetics produced by epinephrine.

Distribution refers to the movement of drug molecules to various tissue sites after the chemical enters the circulatory system. Variations in hemodynamics, drug ionization, lipid solubility, and plasma protein binding can alter the distribution of drugs. In addition, the presence of one drug can change the distribution of another drug. An example of this is the decrease in cardiac output caused by intravenous and volatile anesthetics, which increases the concentration and the effects of other drugs in both the cardiovascular and central nervous systems.

Metabolism involves the biochemical transformation of pharmaceutical substances. There are several processes by which drugs are metabolized, including oxidation, reduction, hydrolysis, and glucuronidation. The metabolism of one drug can be altered by the presence of another drug. For example, the administration of an acetylcholinesterase inhibitor, such as neostigmine, will prolong the effects of succinylcholine due to its inhibition of plasma butyrylcholinesterase. Oxidative metabolism by one of the isoforms of cytochrome P450 (CYP) is a common mechanism for the metabolism of anesthetic drugs. A wide range of chemical compounds can interact with CYP, resulting in either an increase or decrease in its activity. This will directly impact the metabolism of anesthetic agents that undergo CYP metabolism. The list of potential drug interactions due to the induction or inhibition of CYP is extensive. Some examples of inducers of CYP are phenobarbital, phenytoin, rifampin, carbamazepine, and ethanol. Inhibitors of CYP include cimetidine, antifungal agents, macrolide antibiotics, antiretroviral protease inhibitors, verapamil, and grapefruit juice.

Elimination is the removal of substances from the body. Changes in renal clearance or in pulmonary excretion can significantly alter the elimination of drugs. At certain cellular barriers, such as the stomach, placenta, or renal tubules, the pH on either side of the barrier is very different. Since only the non-ionized fraction of drug diffuses across these membranes, drugs that are weak acids or bases will be partially ionized at physiologic pH. Therefore small changes in pH can have a large effect on the degree of ionization and the rate of transport across these membranes. An example of this phenomenon is the decrease in renal tubule reabsorption of drugs such as aspirin or phenobarbital in the presence of alkaline urine.

A *pharmacodynamic interaction* occurs when one drug alters the sensitivity of a target receptor or tissue to the effects of another drug. These interactions can be classified as additive, antagonistic, or synergistic. Additive interactions occur when drugs with the same mechanism of action are administered concurrently. An example of an additive interaction is the administration of both rocuronium and vecuronium, two aminosteroid nondepolarizing muscle relaxants. A drug–drug interaction that is antagonistic causes a decrease in the effects of one or both of the drugs. For example, the concomitant

Essential Clinical Anesthesia Review: Keywords, Questions and Answers for the Boards, ed. Linda S. Aglio, Robert W. Lekowski, and Richard D. Urman. Published by Cambridge University Press. © Cambridge University Press 2015.

Table 43.1 Claimed effects and potential toxic effects of herbal preparations

Name	Common use	Potential toxicity
Ephedra	Energy building, weight loss, antitussive, bacteriostatic	Hypertension, tachycardia, dysrhythmias; stroke, seizure Effects potentiated by agents with MAOI activity
Echinacea	Respiratory and urinary infections, promote wound and burn healing	Hepatotoxicity Decreased glucocorticoid effects Macrophage and natural killer cell activation
Garlic	Hyperlipidemia, hypertension, antiplatelet, antioxidant, and antibiotic effects	Increased risk of perioperative bleeding, potentiation of anticoagulant effects; risk of interactions with cardiovascular medications, MAOIs, hypoglycemics
Ginger	Antinausea, antispasmodic; respiratory ailments; motion sickness	Increased risk of perioperative bleeding, potentiation of anticoagulant effects; hyperglycemia
Ginkgo	Circulatory stimulant; dementia, Alzheimer's disease; asthma, angina	Increased risk of perioperative bleeding, potentiation of anticoagulant effects; neurotoxicity, decreased seizure threshold, decreased efficacy of anticonvulsants; interaction with MAOIs
Ginseng	Energy building	Elevates digoxin concentration by 75%; interaction with MAOIs
Goldenseal	Diuretic, antiinflammatory, laxative, hemostatic	Oxytocic, paralysis, edema, hypertension
Kava	Anxiolytic	Hepatotoxicity; potentiates barbiturate and benzodiazepine effects
Licorice	Peptic ulcer disease, respiratory infections	Hypertension, hypokalemia, edema; reduction in ADH, aldosterone and plasma renin activity
St. John's Wort	Depression, anxiety, insomnia	Decreased digoxin concentrations; prolonged general anesthesia, sedation; induction of CYP and P-glycoprotein (i.e., numerous drug interactions)
Valerian	Sedative, anxiolytic	Potentiates barbiturate and benzodiazepine effects
Vitamin E	Antiaging; prevention of stroke, blood clots, and atherosclerosis; promotes wound healing	Increased risk of perioperative bleeding, potentiation of anticoagulant effects

ADH, antidiuretic hormone.
(From Vacanti et al. 2011. *Essential Clinical Anesthesia*, Cambridge University Press, p. 276.)

administration of PPIs can decrease the effectiveness of platelet inhibition by Plavix®.

Herbal preparations and drug interactions

The consumption of herbal supplements, vitamins, and other over-the-counter preparations has become increasingly popular. Though these preparations may have some health benefits, adverse effects can occur with their use. Many of these substances are not prescribed by a physician and, as a result, patients may fail to report their use during medication reconciliation. Therefore patients should be questioned diligently about all substances they consume, whether they are over-the-counter or prescribed medications. The potential beneficial and toxic effects of common herbal preparations are listed in Table 43.1.

Questions

1. Side effects of ginger include which of the following?
   a. hypertension
   b. bleeding
   c. constipation
   d. nausea

2. Which of the following herbal preparations has sedative effects?
   a. St. John's Wort
   e. ephedra
   c. licorice
   d. echinacea

Answers

1. b. Potential side effects of ginger include an increased risk of perioperative bleeding and hyperglycemia.
2. a. St. John's Wort has sedative effects and can prolong the duration of general anesthesia and sedative medications.

Further reading

Bovill, J. G. (1997). Adverse drug interactions in anesthesia. *Journal of Clinical Anesthesia* 9, 3S–13S.

Cheng, B., Hung, C. T., and Chiu, W. (2002). Herbal medicine and anesthesia. *Hong Kong Medical Journal* 8, 123–130.

Hodges, P. J. and Kam, P. C. A. (2002). The peri-operative implications of herbal medicines. *Anesthesia* 57, 889–899.

Kam, P. C. A. and Liew, S. (2002). Traditional Chinese herbal medicine and anesthesia. *Anesthesia* 57, 1083–1089.

Barash, P., Cullen, B., and Stoelting, R. (eds) (2006). *Clinical Anesthesia*, 5th edn. Philadelphia: Lippincott Williams & Wilkins.

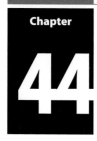

Chapter

44

Allergic reactions

Iuliu Fat and Devon Flaherty

An *allergic* or *hypersensitivity reaction* is an immunologic response caused by the exposure to an antigen. The four types of allergic reactions are listed in Table 44.1.

Anaphylaxis is an acute, potentially lethal, multisystem syndrome resulting from the sudden release of mast cell- and basophil-derived mediators into the bloodstream. The onset of symptoms after parental administration is usually immediate, but it can be delayed up to three hours. Dermatologic manifestations include urticaria, itching, rash, and facial swelling. Conscious patients may complain of dizziness, chest tightness, difficulty breathing, or coughing. In addition, wheezing, tachypnea, and laryngeal stridor can occur with upper airway edema and acute respiratory distress in severe cases. In an anesthetized patient, the first sign of an anaphylactic reaction may be cardiovascular collapse due to profound hypotension or severe bronchospasm.

There are many agents used in the perioperative environment that can elicit allergic reactions. The most allergenic agents used in anesthesia include muscle relaxants, latex, and antibiotics. In addition, patients can have reactions to local anesthetics, opioids, and hypnotic agents, such as propofol, colloids, and blood products.

Table 44.1 Four types of allergic reactions

Type	Alternative names	Associated disorders	Mediators
I	Allergy (immediate)	• Atopy • Anaphylaxis • Asthma	• IgE
II	Cytotoxic, antibody-dependent	• Autoimmune hemolytic anemia • Thrombocytopenia • Erythroblastosis fetalis • Goodpasture's syndrome • Membranous nephropathy • Graves' disease	• IgM or IgG • (Complement)
III	Immune complex disease	• Serum sickness • Arthus reaction • Rheumatoid arthritis • Post-streptococcal glomerulonephritis • Lupus nephritis • Systemic lupus erythematosus (SLE) • Extrinsic allergic alveolitis (Hypersensitivity pneumonitis)	• IgG • (Complement)
IV	Delayed-type hypersensitivity, cell-mediated immune memory response, antibody-independent	• Contact dermatitis • Mantoux test • Chronic transplant rejection • Multiple sclerosis	• T cells

Essential Clinical Anesthesia Review: Keywords, Questions and Answers for the Boards, ed. Linda S. Aglio, Robert W. Lekowski, and Richard D. Urman. Published by Cambridge University Press. © Cambridge University Press 2015.

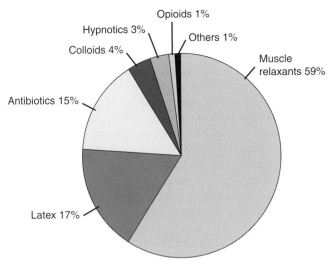

Figure 44.1 Incidence of allergic reactions by agent. (From Vacanti et al. 2011. *Essential Clinical Anesthesia*, Cambridge University Press, p. 278.)

Muscle relaxants

The administration of muscle relaxants is the leading cause of intraoperative anaphylaxis. Rocuronium (43%) has a higher incidence than succinylcholine (23%) and females are more likely than males to develop an allergic reaction to these agents. Cross-reactivity between these agents is observed in 75% of cases of anaphylaxis; antibodies to neuromuscular blocking agents can persist for years.

Latex

Latex allergy is the second most common cause of anaphylaxis in surgical suites (17% of cases). Health care workers, who come in contact with latex in the form of gloves or other latex-containing medical equipment may become sensitized to latex. Other high-risk groups include nonhealth care workers with occupational exposure to latex, patients with an atopic background, and children with spina bifida or genitourinary abnormalities who have undergone multiple surgeries. In addition, certain fruits, such as bananas, avocados, and kiwis, contain proteins that cross-react with latex. The most common latex-mediated reaction is irritant-contact dermatitis, but allergic-contact dermatitis (type IV) and type I IgE-mediated hypersensitivity reactions (i.e., anaphylaxis) are also possible. There is no data to support the use of pharmacologic prophylaxis (e.g., histamine H1 or H2 antagonists, steroids) prior to a surgical procedure.

Antibiotics

In the general population, antibiotics, particularly beta-lactams, are the most common drugs that cause anaphylaxis. Antibiotics that share the beta-lactam ring include penicillins, cephalosporins, carbapenems, and monobactams. Although cross-reactivity between cephalosporins and penicillins has an incidence of 8% to 10%, recent data suggest the actual incidence is lower. A detailed history of the specific reaction to penicillin will eliminate those reactions due to nonimmunologic processes. Patients who have a definite allergic reaction to a specific antibiotic are more likely to develop anaphylaxis upon exposure to any other antibiotic. Earlier generations of cephalosporins contained trace amounts of penicillin and were more likely to cause an anaphylactic reaction in penicillin-allergic patients. More recently, the side-chain structure attached to the beta-lactam ring has been identified as an important component in determining the allergenicity of the molecule. Because first-generation cephalosporins and cefamandole share a similar side chain with penicillin and amoxicillin, a higher incidence of allergic reactions to first-generation cephalosporins and cefamandole is likely to occur in those with a history of penicillin allergy. In contrast, second- and third-generation cephalosporins have different side chains from penicillin and amoxicillin and are unlikely to cross-react with penicillin.

Local anesthetics

The most common immune-mediated reaction to local anesthetics is a delayed hypersensitivity (type IV) reaction or contact dermatitis. Paraaminobenzoic acid (PABA) is the key metabolite of ester local anesthetics implicated in causing allergic reactions. Practitioners should be aware that preservatives such as methylparaben, propylparaben (both metabolized to PABA), and metabisulfite are often added to multiple-dose vials of local anesthetics. Cross-reactivity exists among the ester local anesthetics and is unusual among amides. There is no cross-reactivity between amide and ester local anesthetics. It is also important to distinguish between a true allergic reaction and reactions due to anxiety or epinephrine.

Opioids

The incidence of allergic reactions to opioids is one in every 100,000 to 200,000 anesthetics. Some opioids (e.g., morphine, meperidine) cause a direct release of histamine, leading to dermatologic manifestations such as urticaria, itching, and vasodilation. Studies looking at the effects of large doses of morphine used during cardiac anesthesia did not show an increased incidence of bronchospasm or angioedema. Anaphylactoid reactions to codeine and morphine have been reported. However, skin tests were negative when affected patients were tested.

Hypnotics

Propofol is currently formulated in a lipid-emulsion vehicle containing 10% soybean oil, 1.2% egg lecithin, and 2.25% glycerol. Most cases of allergic reactions to propofol are IgE mediated and are related to its two isopropyl groups. Current evidence suggests that patients who are allergic to eggs are at low risk for developing anaphylaxis if exposed to propofol. The

Table 44.2 Treatment of anaphylaxis

Withdrawal of agent
Assessment of airway, breathing, circulation
Early administration of epinephrine
Oxygen supplementation
Intravenous fluids
Histamine H1 and H2 antagonists, bronchodilators, hydrocortisone

(From Vacanti et al. 2011. *Essential Clinical Anesthesia*, Cambridge University Press, p. 282.)

egg lecithin component of the lipid vehicle for propofol is highly purified egg yolk. Ovalbumin, the principal protein of eggs and common source of allergic reactions, is present in the egg white.

Colloids

Colloids are another source of allergic reactions. Gelatins and dextrans are more likely than albumin or hetastarch to cause an allergic reaction. Hetastarch is less allergenic as compared to albumin. The presence of IgE antibodies and positive intradermal tests against gelatins has proved that an IgE-mediated anaphylactic reaction occurs. A documented egg allergy is not a contraindication to the use of albumin because the principal egg protein, ovalbumin (45 kDa), is different from human serum albumin (67 kDa).

Blood products

Urticarial reactions are seen in 0.5% of all transfusions with frozen plasma. A small amount of plasma is present in all blood products and can cause allergic reactions when units of red blood cells or platelets are transfused. It is recommended that patients with a history of a reaction be transfused with saline-washed red cells. True anaphylactic reactions to blood products are infrequent, except in patients with IgA deficiency, who were likely sensitized by a prior transfusion or pregnancy.

Treatment

The mainstay of treating anaphylaxis is the immediate discontinuation of the offending agent and the administration of epinephrine. An immediate assessment of the airway, breathing, and circulation (ABC) is imperative to avoid airway compromise and cardiovascular collapse. In addition, it is important to decrease or discontinue anesthetic agents likely to cause vasodilation, such as inhalational agents, as well as any medications with negative inotropic effects. Other important steps include the administration of 100% oxygen, IV crystalloid replacement, and the administration of histamine H1 and H2 antagonists, bronchodilators, and steroids to decrease airway swelling and prevent recurrence of symptoms.

Questions

1. Which of these substances is most commonly associated with an allergic reaction under anesthesia?
    a. latex
    b. antibiotics
    c. neuromuscular muscle blocking agents
    d. opioids

2. Which of these substances is the first-line treatment for anaphylaxis?
    a. steroids
    b. epinephrine
    c. H1 blocker
    d. IV fluids

Answers

1. c. Neuromuscular muscle blocking agents are the most common cause of an allergic reaction during anesthesia, with an incidence of 59% of all agents.
2. b. Administration of epinephrine is the treatment of choice with IV fluids, antihistamines, and steroids used as adjuncts.

Further reading

Dewachter, P., Mouton-Faivre, C., and Emala, C. W. (2009). Anaphylaxis and anesthesia: controversies and new insights. *Anesthesiology* 111: 1141–1150.

Hepner, D. L. and Castells, M. C. (2003). Anaphylaxis during the perioperative period. *Anesthesia and Analgesia* 97: 1381–1395.

Lieberman, P., Nicklas, R. A., Oppenheimer, J. et al. (2010). The diagnosis and management of anaphylaxis practice parameter: 2010 update. *Journal of Allergy and Clinical Immunology* 126, 477–480.

Chapter

45

Pharmacology of local anesthetics: mechanism of action and pharmacokinetics

Jessica Bauerle and Zhiling Xiong

Keywords

Local anesthetics
Local anesthetics: mechanism of action
Local anesthetics: metabolism
Local anesthetics: toxicity
Local anesthesia potency: lipid solubility

Local anesthetics result in loss of sensation in the targeted area by stopping propagation of nerve impulses. In 1884, cocaine was the first local anesthetic discovered, but given its addictive and dependent properties, it was not a reasonable and routine clinical option. Procaine was then introduced in 1905, and lidocaine in 1944.

Local anesthetics are made up of a lipophilic benzene ring and a hydrophilic tertiary amine, with either an ester or amide bond. The amino-amide local anesthetics are more stable, longer acting, and associated with fewer allergic reactions than the ester local anesthetics.

Myelination and axon size determine the speed of transmission of an action potential. The types of nerve fibers include Aα, Aβ, Aδ, Aγ, B, and C. All types include myelin except for the C fibers. Impulses travel rapidly from one unmyelinated area (termed node of Ranvier) to the next. This mechanism of transit is termed saltatory conduction. Sodium channels are in high concentration within the nodes of Ranvier.

Nerve impulse conduction is determined by sodium entering into the nerve cell through the voltage-gated sodium channels. Local anesthetics reversibly bind to the interior of the sodium channel receptor to prevent impulse conduction. Despite controversy, traditional texts often state that small-diameter axons (such as C fibers) are more sensitive to local anesthetics than are large-diameter A-type fibers. Therefore pain, temperature, and touch are the first sensations to be lost from local anesthetic effect. Local anesthetics exhibit different specificities for fiber-type blockade. For instance, the favorable sensory to motor differential blockade profile of bupivacaine

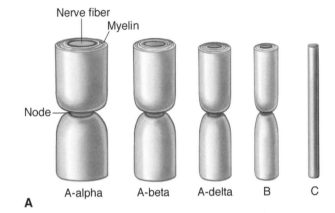

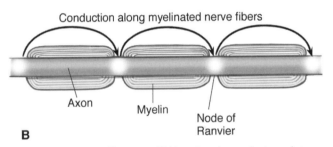

Figure 45.1 (A) Nerve fiber types. (B) Nerve impulse conduction, saltatory conduction. (From Vacanti et al. 2011. *Essential Clinical Anesthesia*, Cambridge University Press, Figure 46.1.)

makes it a popular choice in the obstetric population where preservation of motor function is essential. However, if any local anesthetic is given in high enough concentration, all fiber types will be blocked.

Local anesthetics are weak bases (uncharged) and therefore pass easily through the cellular phospholipid membrane. Once inside the cell, they bind to the sodium ion channel and are protonated, thereby inactivating the sodium channel. The pKa is the pH at which 50% of the local anesthetic is uncharged, as determined by the Henderson–Hasselbach

Essential Clinical Anesthesia Review: Keywords, Questions and Answers for the Boards, ed. Linda S. Aglio, Robert W. Lekowski, and Richard D. Urman. Published by Cambridge University Press. © Cambridge University Press 2015.

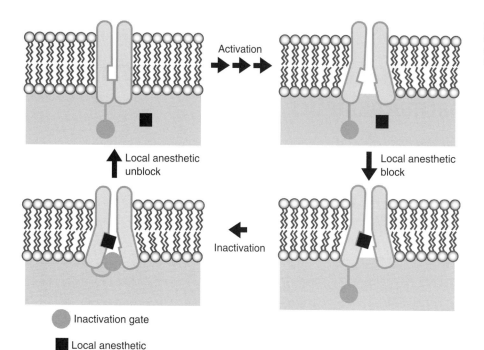

Figure 45.2 Voltage-gated Na$^+$ channel activation and inactivation with local anesthetic. (From Vacanti et al. 2011. *Essential Clinical Anesthesia*, Cambridge University Press, Figure 46.3.)

Activation

Local anesthetic unblock

Local anesthetic block

Inactivation

- Inactivation gate
- Local anesthetic

equation: pH $= \text{pKa} + \log_{10}$ [B]/[BH$^+$]. The closer the pKa is to the physiologic pH, the faster the onset for amide anesthetics. *Lipid solubility* of the local anesthetic is directly proportional to potency, whereas protein binding (albumin, α1-acid glycoprotein) is related to duration of action.

Systemic administration of local anesthetics is often performed with lidocaine infusions given for chronic or refractory pain syndromes. The *mechanism of action* is unclear, but it is believed to target sodium channels in the central and peripheral nervous system.

Local anesthetics have the potential to result in significant systemic *toxicity* when administered to an undesired area or when administered in too high concentrations. The injection sites most likely to result in high systemic levels include from highest to lowest: intravenous > tracheal > intercostal > caudal > epidural > brachial plexus > sciatic > subcutaneous.

Metabolism of local anesthetics is dependent on the classification type. Amide local anesthetics are metabolized by the liver through hydroxylation and N-dealkylation by microsomal cytochrome P450. Any disease state affecting the liver may result in impaired metabolism of the local anesthetics. Prilocaine and benzocaine metabolites can result in methemaglobinemia. Ester local anesthetics are metabolized by plasma pseudocholinesterases to alkaline and paraaminobenzoic acid (PABA), which represents a potential allergen for some patients.

Questions

1. Which injection site of local anesthetics is most likely to result in local anesthetic-induced toxicity?
   a. intercostal
   b. epidural
   c. intravenous
   d. intrathecal

2. What determines the potency of local anesthetics?
   a. lipid solubility
   b. pH
   c. pKa
   d. local anesthetic class

Answers

1. c.
2. a.

Further reading

Vacanti, C., Sikka, P., Urman, R., Dershwitz, M., and Segal, B. (eds) (2011). *Essential Clinical Anesthesia*. Cambridge: Cambridge University Press, Chapter 46.

Berde, C. B. and Strichartz, G. R. (2009). Chapter 30: Local anesthetics. In Miller, R. D., Eriksson, L. I., Fleisher, L. A. et al. (eds) *Miller's Anesthesia*, 7th edn. Philadelphia: Churchill-Livingstone.

Clinical applications of local anesthetics

46

Julia Serber and Evan Blaney

Amino-amides
Amino-esters
Local anesthetic onset time
Local anesthetic potency
Local anesthetic duration of action
Cauda equina syndrome
Transient neurologic symptoms (TNS)
Intralipid
Lidocaine
Prilocaine
Mepivacaine
Bupivacaine
Levobupivacaine
Ropivacaine
Procaine
Chloroprocaine
Tetracaine
Cocaine
Benzocaine
EMLA cream
Lidocaine patch

Table 46.1 Maximum recommended doses of local anesthetics

Drug	Onset	Maximum dose for plain solution, mg/kg	Maximum dose with epinephrine[a], mg/kg
Lidocaine	Rapid	5	7
Mepivacaine	Rapid	5	7
Chloroprocaine	Rapid	10	15
Prilocaine	Rapid	7	8
Ropivacaine	Slow	3	3
Bupivacaine	Slow	2	2.5
Levobupivacaine	Slow	2.5	3
Procaine	Slow	8	10

[a] Epinephrine is a potent vasoconstrictor. It thus reduces systemic absorption of local anesthetics.
(From Vacanti et al. 2011. *Essential Clinical Anesthesia*, Cambridge University Press, p. 288.)

All local anesthetics are weak bases and are classified as either amino-amides or esters. Examples of *amino-amides* include: lidocaine, mepivacaine, prilocaine, bupivacaine, levobupivacaine, and ropivacaine. Examples of *amino-esters* include: procaine, chloroprocaine, tetracaine, and cocaine.

Amides are broken down in the liver, while esters are hydrolyzed by pseudocholinesterase enzymes in the plasma. An exception is cocaine, which is an ester metabolized predominantly by the liver.

Allergies to local anesthetics are rare. However, para-aminobenzoic acid (PABA), a metabolite of esters, can cause allergic reactions.

Local anesthetics work by blocking the transmission of the action potential. This occurs by inhibition of voltage-gated sodium channels.

Local anesthetic onset time is determined by the degree of ionization. The closer the pKa of the local anesthetic is to the tissue pH, the quicker the onset time. (pKa = the pH at which the un-ionized and ionized forms are present in equal concentrations.)

Local anesthetic potency is determined by solubility. Local anesthetics with a higher solubility are more potent.

Local anesthetic duration of action is determined by protein binding. The more the local anesthetic binds to proteins, the longer its duration of action will be.

Local anesthetic toxicity

Direct local toxicity (direct neurotoxicity and nerve degeneration) may occur at doses used in clinical practice. *Cauda equina syndrome* is an acute loss of function of lumbar plexus nerve roots below the termination of the spinal cord. It is characterized by incontinence, impotence, and paresthesias in

Essential Clinical Anesthesia Review: Keywords, Questions and Answers for the Boards, ed. Linda S. Aglio, Robert W. Lekowski, and Richard D. Urman. Published by Cambridge University Press. © Cambridge University Press 2015.

the buttocks as well as the perineal area and legs. Characteristics of *transient neurologic symptoms* (TNS) include a burning pain in the back, lower extremities, and buttocks. Symptoms usually resolve over a time span of three to five days. This is seen most commonly when lidocaine is used for spinal anesthesia.

Systemic toxicity may be due to vascular absorption or inadvertent intravascular injection of the local anesthetic. Both cardiovascular and CNS symptoms are seen. CNS manifestations are usually seen first and include lightheadedness, tinnitus, perioral numbness, and confusion. Later signs of CNS toxicity include seizures, unconsciousness, and respiratory arrest. Cardiotoxicity is less common but can be fatal. Manifestations include HTN, tachycardia, decreased cardiac output and contractility, hypotension, bradycardia, cardiac arrhythmias, and circulatory arrest.

Intravenous *intralipid* solution ("lipid rescue") should be used when local anesthetic toxicity is suspected. A bolus of 1.5 ml/kg should be infused over one minute followed by a continuous infusion of 0.25 ml/kg/min. Parenteral administration of 20% intralipid solution has been shown to improve the survival of animals with bupivacaine-induced asystole.

Clinically used local anesthetics
Amino-amide local anesethetics

Lidocaine has a rapid onset of action and a moderate duration of action. Its use in spinal anesthesia has declined due to concerns about neurotoxicity and transient neurologic symptoms. Lidocaine can be used topically or nebulized as an aerosol in order to anesthetize the upper airway. Intravenous injections of lidocaine are used to cause systemic analgesia and can be used as an infusion to treat chronic neuropathic pain. Because lidocaine causes vasodilation, the addition of epinephrine can significantly reduce the intravascular absorption of lidocaine, thus prolonging its effect.

Prilocaine is also an amino-amide with a similar clinical profile to that of lidocaine. However, it causes significantly less vasodilation than does lidocaine. Prilocaine causes the least amount of systemic toxicity when compared to all of the amide local anesthetics. However, it is not widely used because it causes methemoglobinemia at higher rates than other agents.

Mepivacaine: duration of action is slightly longer than that of lidocaine. The toxicity of mepivacaine appears to be less than that of lidocaine but the metabolism is prolonged in the fetus and newborn. Therefore it is not utilized for obstetric anesthesia.

Bupivacaine provides a prolonged and dense sensory analgesia, which often outlasts the motor block. Bupivacaine has been associated with cardiac arrest, especially in higher concentrations.

Levobupivacaine is the S-enantiomer of bupivacaine. Bupivacaine is a racemic mixture, which contains equal amounts of the R-and S-enantiomers. The toxicity profile of levobupivacaine is much less than that of bupivacaine, which allows a larger dose to be given.

Ropivacaine was developed following concerns about cardiotoxicity associated with bupivacaine.

Amino-ester local anesthetics

Procaine has low potency, slow onset, and short duration. Allergic reactions are possible because the metabolite PABA is produced.

Chloroprocaine has low potency and extremely low toxicity. The low toxicity allows relatively high concentrations to be used. Chloroprocaine has a very short plasma half-life due to the rapid metabolism by cholinesterase. It is thought to have the lowest CNS and cardiovascular toxicity rates of all agents that are used today. There is also close to no transmission of this agent to the fetus when used in obstetric anesthesia.

Cocaine is the only local anesthetic used clinically that occurs in nature. It is also the only local anesthetic that causes intense vasoconstriction. It is used as a topical anesthetic. It inhibits neuronal reuptake of catecholamines and therefore can lead to hypertension, tachycardia, dysrhythmias, and other serious cardiac effects.

Benzocaine has a slow onset, short duration of action, is minimally potent, and minimally toxic. Its clinical use is limited to the topicalization of mucous membranes. If used in excess, it is associated with methemoglobinemia.

Topical local anesthetics

Eutectic mixture of local anesthetic (EMLA) cream: a mixture of lidocaine and prilocaine.

Lidocaine patch (5%): a topical delivery system. The goal is to deliver low doses of lidocaine to superficially damaged or dysfunctional nociceptors.

Questions

1. Which of the following local anesthetics has the fastest onset of action?
   a. mepivacaine 1%
   b. chloroprocaine 3%
   c. ropivacaine
   d. bupivacaine 0.25%

2. You have just placed a peripheral nerve block with a catheter and given a bolus of bupivacaine. You leave to see your next patient and hear a stat page for anesthesia to your first patient's bedside. You look up at the monitor and see that the patient is in asystole. You immediately:
   a. give propofol
   b. give intralipid
   c. call for help, ask for the code cart and start CPR
   d. give atropine

3. Which is the maximum recommended dose of mepivacaine for a 70 kg patient?
   a. 560 mg
   b. 140 mg
   c. 490 mg
   d. 210 mg

Answers

1. b. The onset of action of local anesthetics is determined by the pKa of the local anesthetic. The closer the pKa is to physiologic pH, the more rapid the onset. The caveat here is that chloroprocaine is 3%. Because of the high percentage, it will have the fastest onset of action.

2. c. In this situation, it is likely that the bupivacaine has been given intravascularly. As with any code situation, you should call for help and have everything you need for a code. Then intralipid should be started.

3. c. The maximum recommended dose of mepivacaine with epinephrine is 7 mg/kg (without epinephrine, the maximum recommended dose of mepivacaine is 3.5 mg/kg). Therefore the maximum recommended dose of mepivacaine with epinephrine for a 70 kg patient would be 70 kg × 7 mg/kg, which is equal to 490 mg.

Further reading

Modak, R. (2008). *Anesthesiology Keywords Review. Local Anesthetic Toxicity: Management*. Philadelphia: Lippincott Williams & Wilkins, pp. 264–265.

Morgan et al. (1996). Chapter 14. Local anesthetics. In *Lange Clinical Anesthesiology*, 4th edn. New York: McGraw-Hill.

Vacanti, C., Sikka, P., Urman, R., Dershwitz, M., and Segal, B. (eds) (2011). Chapter 47. Clinical applications of local anesthetics. In *Essential Clinical Anesthesia*. Cambridge: Cambridge University Press.

Chapter

47 Administration of general anesthesia

Carly C. Guthrie and Jeffrey Lu

Preoperative preparation should include evaluating the patient with a history and physical, any necessary laboratory tests, inquiring about the NPO status of the patient, examining the airway, and determining the appropriate anesthetic plan. Discussing the anesthetic plan along with the risks and benefits of the anesthesia, as well as any procedures specific to the anesthetic, is essential for patient satisfaction, anxiety reduction, and for obtaining informed consent.

Preoperative preparation in the emergent setting is by necessity a streamlined process. Time for preparation may be limited, so the crucial pieces of information to ascertain include the immediate problem, relevant comorbidities, medication list, allergies, NPO status, and heart, lung, and airway examinations. Occasionally, there may not be time for informed consent or discussion of the anesthetic with the patient, and this should be clearly documented in the chart.

ASA guidelines for preoperative fasting include the following guidelines for *NPO (nothing by mouth) status* prior to elective regional or general anesthesia and monitored anesthesia care:

- There should be at least two hours for clear liquids, which include water, fruit juices without pulp, carbonated beverages, clear tea, and black coffee, but do not include alcohol.
- There should be a period of at least four hours for breast milk, and six hours for infant formula or nonhuman milk.

- There should also be six hours or more fasting from the intake of a light meal and at least eight hours or more fasting after the intake of a larger meal or one that consists of fried foods, fatty foods, or meat. (American Society of Anesthesiology. 1999. Practice guidelines.)

Airway exam: as part of every anesthesiology preoperative evaluation there should be a comprehensive airway exam. The size and length of the neck, range of motion present, and presence of a cervical collar should be noted. Furthermore, the thyromental distance, ability to prognath the jaw, and compliance of the mandibular space should be assessed. Finally, on inspection of the mouth, the shape of the palate, Mallampati score, inter incisor distance, length of upper incisors, tongue size, and presence of an overbite should be evaluated.

Predictors of difficult intubation include some general nonreassuring findings on a patient's airway exam as well as some specific disease processes or syndromes. Generally, concerning findings include a thick neck, decreased range of motion at the neck (especially extension), beard or facial abnormalities, small mouth opening (<4 cm), large upper incisors, inability to prognath, high-arched palate, large tongue, or small thyromental distance (<3 finger breadths). Specific concerns may include a trauma patient with a C-collar, rheumatoid arthritis patients with atlanto-axial instability, neck or facial tumors or masses, facial fractures, pregnancy, or a number of pediatric congenital syndromes. Airway evaluations should be made with close attention to detail, and preparation for alternative airway strategies is always prudent.

Difficulty with mask ventilation can be predicted by the presence of a BMI >26 kg/m^2, age >55, neck circumference >40 cm, obstructive sleep apnea or history of snoring, or presence of a beard.

Stages and signs of anesthesia

Rapid sequence induction is utilized to induce the patient quickly and secure the airway in the event that there is concern for aspiration. This is generally achieved by IV induction

---

Essential Clinical Anesthesia Review: Keywords, Questions and Answers for the Boards, ed. Linda S. Aglio, Robert W. Lekowski, and Richard D. Urman. Published by Cambridge University Press. © Cambridge University Press 2015.

Table 47.1 Guedel's stages of general anesthesia with ether as the sole agent

Stage	General description	Guedel's clinical criteria, simplified				
		Respiratory pattern	Eyeball activity	Pupil size	Eyelid reflex	Risk of vomiting, laryngospasm
I	Analgesia	Slow, regular	Baseline	Baseline	Present	
II	Delirium Excitement Unconsciousness	Irregular	Markedly increased	Reactive to light, may be dilated	Present, starts to disappear	Increased
III	Surgical anesthesia	Regular, then progresses to complete paralysis	Decreases progressively, then ceases	Gradual dilation	None	
IV	Respiratory paralysis Cardiovascular collapse	Complete paralysis	None	Complete dilation	None	

(From Vacanti et al. 2011. *Essential Clinical Anesthesia*, Cambridge University Press, p. 297.)

followed by the immediate administration of a drug to produce rapid onset of paralysis (i.e., succinylcholine or rocuronium). Furthermore, mask ventilation is generally avoided and cricoid pressure is applied until the airway is secured.

Emergence and extubation: prior to awakening and extubation, a plan for emergence should be crafted and should include reversal of any paralytic agents and discontinuation of all anesthetic agents. Before the endotracheal tube is removed, the patient should meet the following criteria for extubation: stable vital signs, reversal of paralysis shown by 4/4 TOF and sustained tetany, proven muscular strength (tested by sustained head lift for five to ten seconds), adequate tidal volume and respiratory rate, and an awake and cooperative patient.

Questions

1. How many hours must a patient be NPO prior to a procedure after having a light meal?
   a. two hours
   b. four hours
   c. six hours
   d. eight hours

2. Which stage of general anesthesia is associated with excitement, irregular respirations, and an increased risk of vomiting and laryngospasm?
   a. Stage 1
   b. Stage 2
   c. Stage 3
   d. Stage 4

Answers

1. c. There should also be six hours or more fasting from the intake of a light meal and at least eight hours or more fasting after the intake of a larger meal or one that consists of fried foods, fatty foods, or meat.

2. b. Stage 2 of anesthesia can consist of delirium, excitement, increased pupil size, increased eye movements, and an increased risk of laryngospasm.

Further reading

Vacanti, C., Sikka, P., Urman, R., Dershwitz, M., and Segal, B. (eds) (2011). *Essential Clinical Anesthesia*. Cambridge: Cambridge University Press, Chapter 48.

Morgan, G. E., Mikhail, M. S., and Murray, M. J. (2007). *Clinical Anesthesiology*, 4th edn. McGraw-Hill Medical, Chapters 1 and 5.

American Society of Anesthesiology. (1999). Practice guidelines for preoperative fasting and the use of pharmacologic agents to reduce the risk of pulmonary aspiration: application to healthy patients undergoing elective procedures: a report by the American Society of Anesthesiologists Task Force on Preoperative Fasting. *Anesthesiology* 90, 896–905.

Chapter
48

Total intravenous anesthesia

Alissa Sodickson and Richard D. Urman

Keywords

Hypnotic drugs for infusion
Analgesics for TIVA
Context-sensitive half-time
Manual-controlled versus target-controlled infusion systems
Advantages and limitations of TIVA

Total intravenous anesthesia (TIVA) generally consists of a combination of hypnotic and analgesic drugs. The technique is relatively new to anesthesia practice due to the need for an infusion delivery system and drugs with appropriate pharmacokinetic profiles (fast onset, short recovery).

Intravenous hypnotic drugs

- Ideally we want an easily titratable drug with a *short context-sensitive half-time* (decrease in plasma concentration by 50% as a function of the duration of infusion).
- Propofol is the drug of choice due to short context-sensitive half-time and reduced incidence of postoperative nausea and vomiting (PONV).
- Thiopental (no longer available) and midazolam are poor choices for maintenance due to prolonged context-sensitive half-time.
- Etomidate has multiple side effects including PONV, phlebitis, excitatory movements, and adrenal cortical suppression.
- Ketamine is a dissociative anesthetic with a favorable pharmacokinetic profile and offers analgesic effects, but has neuro-excitatory effects, rendering depth-of-anesthesia monitors inaccurate.
- Dexmedetomidine infusion, when used as an adjunct to propofol, further reduces PONV and enhances sedation, amnesia, anxiolysis, and analgesia via its sympatholytic effects.

Table 48.1 Suggested dosages for anesthetic agents used in general anesthesia

Agent	Loading dose, mg/kg	Maintenance infusion rate
Midazolam	0.15–0.35	–
Propofol	1–3	50–200 µg/kg/min
Thiopental	3–6	–
Etomidate	0.2–0.4	–
Ketamine	1–2	5–10 µg/kg/min
Dexmedetomidine	1 µg/kg	0.2–1.0 µg/kg/h

(From Vacanti et al. 2011. *Essential Clinical Anesthesia*, Cambridge University Press, p. 305.)

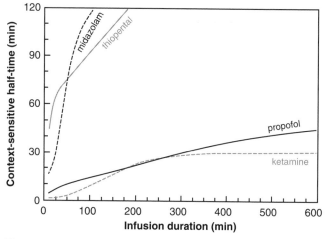

Figure 48.1 Context-sensitive half-time values of hypnotic drugs, shown as a function of infusion duration. (From Vacanti et al. 2011. *Essential Clinical Anesthesia*, Cambridge University Press, p. 306.)

Analgesics for TIVA

- Opioids: fentanyl offers fast onset and good postoperative analgesia but has significant context-sensitive half-time,

Essential Clinical Anesthesia Review: Keywords, Questions and Answers for the Boards, ed. Linda S. Aglio, Robert W. Lekowski, and Richard D. Urman. Published by Cambridge University Press. © Cambridge University Press 2015.

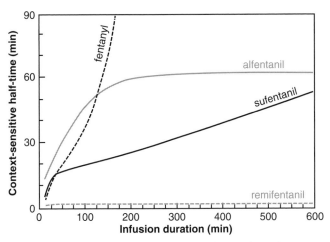

Figure 48.2 Context-sensitive half-time values of opioid drugs, shown as a function of infusion duration. Among the opioids, remifentanil is associated with the most rapid return to consciousness. (From Vacanti et al. 2011. *Essential Clinical Anesthesia*, Cambridge University Press, p. 306.)

Table 48.2 Suggested opioid dosages for TIVA

Agent	Loading dose, μg/kg	Maintenance infusion rate	Additional boluses
Alfentanil	25–100	0.5–2 μg/kg/min	5–10 μg/kg
Sufentanil	0.25–2	0.005–0.025 μg/kg/min	2.5–10 μg
Fentanyl	4–20	0.03–0.17 μg/kg/min	25–100 μg
Remifentanil	1–2	0.025–1 μg/kg/min	0.1–1.0 μg/kg

(From Vacanti et al. 2011. *Essential Clinical Anesthesia*, Cambridge University Press, p. 306.)

which can delay awakening. Alfentanil and sufentanil are good choices for TIVA. Remifentanil offers the advantages of a very short onset time and a short half-life, which is independent of hepatic/renal function as well as duration of infusion. It does not provide postoperative analgesia, which requires longer acting analgesics.

- Ketamine: can be used as an adjunct to reduce opioid requirement.
- Local anesthetics: may be sufficient in some procedures.

Infusion delivery systems

Currently in the United States, the only pump system is a *manual-controlled infusion (MCI)*, in which there is continuous IV infusion via a pump programmed for the particular drug and delivered at a rate set by the anesthesiologist. Elsewhere in the world, there are *target-controlled infusion (TCI)* systems in use. These devices deliver drug to achieve and maintain the set target blood concentration based on data entered by the anesthesiologist, including patient age and weight. The anesthesiologist can then adjust the set point up or down to achieve the desired depth of anesthesia. A Cochrane review in 2008 comparing MCI and TCI did not demonstrate an advantage of either system in clinical practice. "Closed-loop" TCI systems are in development. These will measure various feedback signals from the patient (for example, BIS index or evoked potentials) and adjust the target drug concentration automatically.

Advantages

TIVA offers a few distinct advantages including the absence of operating room pollution by inhalational agents, less

PONV, possibly less recovery room time, and the avoidance of triggering anesthetics in patients with personal or family history of malignant hyperthermia.

Disadvantages

The disadvantages of using a TIVA include the inability to measure drug concentration and the difficulty establishing a relationship between infusion rate and effect-site concentration across the population. There is also the possibility of significant overdose and prolonged awakening if no depth-of-anesthesia monitor is used. Controversy exits as to whether there is an increased incidence of awareness with a TIVA technique. The most common reasons for awareness are related to pump malfunctions or disconnections.

Questions

1. Which of the following is not useful in a TIVA technique due to prolonged context-sensitive half-time?
   a. alfentanil
   b. sufentanil
   c. ketamine
   d. midazolam

2. Which of the following is a FALSE statement concerning TIVA?
   a. It may be associated with less PONV.
   b. It avoids malignant hyperthermia triggering anesthetics.
   c. It is associated with a higher incidence of awareness.
   d. Target-controlled infusion systems are currently in clinical use.

Answers

1. d. In looking at Figure 48.1, it is apparent that midazolam has a significantly prolonged context-sensitive half-time, thereby limiting its utility in a TIVA technique.

2. c. The incidence of awareness in TIVA appears to be equivalent to inhalational techniques. Most cases of awareness are related to equipment malfunction that may be overlooked by the clinician, hence vigilance remains important. Target-controlled infusion systems, while not in use in the United States, are in use elsewhere in the world.

Further reading

Vacanti, C., Sikka, P., Urman, R., Dershwitz, M., and Segal, B. (eds) (2011). Chapter 49. Total intravenous anesthesia. In *Essential* *Clinical Anesthesia*. Cambridge: Cambridge University Press.

Elkaas, H. and Raeder, J. (2009). Total intravenous anaesthesia techniques for ambulatory surgery. *Current Opinion in Anaesthesiology* 22 (6), 725–729.

Chapter

49

Monitored anesthesia care

Lisa M. Hammond and James Hardy

Keywords

ASA definition of MAC
ASA practice guidelines: four levels of sedation
"Conscious sedation"
Basic anesthetic monitoring standards
Titration to effect technique
Benzodiazepine and opioid reversal agents

Overview

Monitored anesthesia care (MAC) is an anesthetic technique used in an estimated 10% to 30% of all surgical procedures in the operating room.

The American Society of Anesthesiologists (ASA) definition of MAC is a procedure in which an anesthetic provider is requested or required to provide anesthetic services, which include preoperative evaluation, care during the procedure, and management after the procedure. These responsibilities include:

1. Diagnosis and treatment of clinical problems during the procedure.
2. Support of vital functions.
3. Administration of sedatives, analgesics, hypnotics, anesthetic drugs, or other medications as necessary for patient safety; sometimes the anesthesiologist may not need to administer any medications at all.
4. Psychological support and physical comfort.
5. Provision of other services as needed to complete the procedure safely.

Only an anesthesiologist, anesthesia resident, or fully trained nurse anesthetist can deliver a MAC anesthetic technique.

Levels of sedation

The ASA practice guidelines define four states of sedation on a continuum: "minimal sedation," moderate sedation (aka "*conscious sedation*"), "deep sedation," and finally "general anesthesia" (see Table 49.1).

"*Conscious sedation*"/ moderate sedation is a controlled state of depressed consciousness that allows protective reflexes to be maintained, and an intact capacity to respond to verbal and physical stimulation.

"*Conscious sedation*" is delivered *or* supervised by the provider performing the procedure; in contrast, MAC is provided by a trained anesthesia care provider who has no direct role in performing the procedure.

Any sedation with propofol is classified as "deep sedation" by the ASA practice guidelines.

Preoperative/preprocedure

Choosing MAC as the anesthetic technique over regional or general anesthesia depends on many factors, including: type of procedure, the patient's medical condition including mental status, specific positioning requirements during the procedure, and the surgeon's and patient's preference.

As a MAC technique may need to be converted to a general endotracheal anesthetic at a moment's notice, careful preoperative airway assessment is emphasized, and preprocedure assessment of rescue airway equipment is paramount.

ASA fasting guidelines should be used for MAC and are the same as those for a general anesthetic.

Intraoperative/intraprocedure

Anesthesia monitoring standards for MAC are no different than those for regional or general anesthesia. The anesthetic provider must meet *basic anesthetic monitoring standards* as defined by the ASA, which includes continuous monitoring of oxygenation, ventilation (capnography), circulation, and body temperature.

Various techniques have been used from intermittent boluses, to multiple concurrent, continuous infusions of drugs to achieve the goals of providing sedation and analgesia. The most important principle in this setting is "*titration to effect*," which involves delivering a drug and waiting for peak effect prior to re-dosing, in order to best match drug delivery with the level of stimulation from the procedure.

Essential Clinical Anesthesia Review: Keywords, Questions and Answers for the Boards, ed. Linda S. Aglio, Robert W. Lekowski, and Richard D. Urman. Published by Cambridge University Press. © Cambridge University Press 2015.

Table 49.1 Continuum of depth-of-sedation definitions

Parameter	Minimal sedation (anxiolysis)	Moderate sedation/analgesia (conscious sedation)	Deep sedation/analgesia	General anesthesia
Responsiveness	Normal response to verbal stimulation	Purposeful response to verbal or tactile stimulation[a]	Purposeful response following repeated or painful stimulation[a]	Unarousable even with painful stimulus
Airway	Unaffected	No intervention required	Intervention may be required	Intervention often required
Spontaneous ventilation	Unaffected	Adequate	May be inadequate	Frequently inadequate
Cardiovascular function	Unaffected	Usually maintained	Usually maintained	May be impaired

[a] Reflex withdrawal from a painful stimulus is *not* considered a purposeful response.
From ASA. Continuum of depth of sedation definition of general anesthesia and levels of sedation/analgesia. (Approved by ASA House of Delegates on October 13, 1999 and amended on October 27, 2004.)

Table 49.2 Commonly used intravenous agents in MAC

Desired end point	Drug group	Commonly used agents
Sedation	Benzodiazepines α_2-agonists	Midazolam Dexmedetomidine
Hypnosis	Hypnotics	Propofol
Analgesia	Opioids	Fentanyl

(Adapted from: Vacanti et al., 2011, p. 311.)

Benzodiazepines and opioids can be reversed with *flumazenil* and *naloxone*, respectively. A list of common anesthetic dosing regimens for MAC and respective reversal/antagonism approaches are shown in Tables 49.2 and 49.3.

Postoperative/postprocedure

Patients who have undergone MAC must be provided the same standard of postoperative/postprocedure care given to patients who underwent a regional or general anesthetic.

Discharge criteria include: return to baseline mental status, minimal pain, vital signs within 20% of preprocedure values, control of nausea and vomiting.

A reasonable adult must be available to escort the patient home and observe the patient for any unexpected events in the postprocedure period.

Questions

1. In "deep sedation," spontaneous ventilation is?
   a. unaffected
   b. adequate
   c. may become inadequate
   d. usually inadequate
   e. guaranteed inadequate

Table 49.3 Benzodiazepine and opioid antagonists

Factor	Flumazenil	Naloxone
Antagonist	Benzodiazepines	Opioids
Dose	0.2 mg IV Repeat 0.2 mg every 1 min maximum 1 mg IV	40 µg IV Repeat to effect every 1–2 min
Duration of action	30–60 min	30–45 min
Side effects	Seizures Agitation/confusion Acute anxiety Sweating or shivering Blurred vision Headache	Reversal of analgesia Nausea and vomiting[a] Hypertension, tachycardia, ventricular dysrhythmias Pulmonary edema

[a] Dependent upon the prior dose of opioid and the dose of naloxone; an antagonist such as naloxone might be very effective in treating opioid-induced nausea and vomiting.
(From: Vacanti et al., 2011, p. 311.)

2. Which of the following is *not* necessary to meet the ASA standard definition of MAC?
   a. diagnosis of a clinical problem during the procedure
   b. psychological support of patient
   c. support of vital functions
   d. administration of at least one medication
   e. preoperative assessment of patient

3. Which of the following is not considered part of the basic anesthetic monitoring standards?
   a. oxygenation
   b. ventilation
   c. urine output
   d. body temperature
   e. circulation

Answers

1. c. Spontaneous ventilation is unaffected in minimal sedation, adequate in moderate sedation, may be inadequate in deep sedation, and is frequently inadequate in general anesthesia.

2. d. The ASA standard definition of MAC requires perioperative patient assessment, support of vital signs, provision as needed to complete the procedure safely, including diagnosis and treatment of problems during the procedure – this may or *may not* include administration of medications.

3. c. While urine output monitoring may be a helpful surrogate for hemodynamics, circulation, and end-organ perfusion, it is *not* considered part of the basic anesthetic monitoring standards.

Further reading

Kaur, S. (2011). Chapter 50. Monitored anesthesia care. In Vacanti, C. A., Sikka, P. J., Urman, R. D., Dershwitz, M., and Segal, B. S. (eds) *Essential Clinical Anesthesia*. Cambridge: Cambridge University Press.

ASA Newsletter. (2004). Definitions of monitored anesthesia care. 68, 6.

Patient positioning and common nerve injuries

50

J. Matthew Kynes and Joseph M. Garfield

Keywords

Patient positioning: risk factors
Supine position
Ulnar neuropathy
Trendelenburg position
Prone position
Retinal ischemia
Lateral decubitus position
Brachial plexus injury
Lithotomy position
Common peroneal nerve injury
Sitting position

Nerve injury during anesthesia can occur by several mechanisms, including direct trauma, burns, compression, or stretch. Significant *risk factors* for nerve injury due to positioning include: *preexisting neurologic symptoms, body habitus, diabetes mellitus, peripheral vascular disease, alcohol dependency,* and *arthritis.*

General practices to help prevent nerve injury due to position include cushioning all pressure points and supporting vulnerable joints. Certain procedures and positions have specific indications for positioning to prevent common nerve injuries.

In the *supine position,* areas at increased risk of injury include the heel, lumbar area, ulnar nerve, and radial nerve. Arms may be abducted or at the side; however, arm abduction beyond 90° is associated with brachial plexus injury and, if at all possible, the degree of abduction should be less than 90°.

Ulnar neuropathy is the most common position-associated nerve injury during surgery and may be more common with the arm in a nonsupinated position and when not properly padded. Radial nerve injury can also occur, often from external compression of the lower third of the humerus.

Trendelenburg ("head-down") position is a modification of the supine position and can cause physiologic changes including baroreceptor activation and decreased cardiac output, decreased lung capacity and increased ventilation/perfusion mismatch, and increased intracranial pressure. Additionally, gravitational effects from the Trendelenburg position can increase abduction of outstretched arms. This should be monitored closely and corrected to avoid prolonged hyperextension of the upper limbs.

The *prone position* can cause pressure to toes, knee, male genitalia, breast, and, face including the eyes. Often a chest roll is placed to allow for diaphragmatic excursion. To prevent exacerbation of underlying cervical spine pathology the head must be placed in a neutral position using specialized padding. Prolonged pressure on the eyes can cause *retinal ischemia.* The arms may be placed at the sides or flexed at the elbow and shoulder and placed along the patient's head. Again, adequate padding around the ulnar nerve is essential.

The *lateral decubitus position,* often used for orthopedic and intrathoracic procedures, can cause pressure points at the malleolus, medial and lateral epicondyles, greater trochanter, ileum, ribs, acromion process, and ear. *Brachial plexus injury* is of particular concern in this position both from direct compression by the humeral head in the dependent arm and by stretch of the plexus in the elevated arm. An axillary roll is often placed to relieve pressure on the brachial plexus in the dependent arm. Proper head support in a neutral position is also important to prevent strain of the cervical facet joints.

Several lower extremity nerves are exposed to injury in the *lithotomy position,* including the femoral, common peroneal, sciatic, saphenous, and obturator nerves. External compression by braces can cause significant injury at these sites that can be prevented by proper padding. The most evident sign of *common peroneal nerve injury,* caused by compression as it crosses the fibular head, is foot drop. In supine and lithotomy positions, the Trendelenberg ("head-down") position is often utilized but can cause brachial plexus injury if shoulder restraints are employed.

The *sitting position* can cause pressure points at the ischial tuberosity, posterior knee, calcaneus, and scapula. Nerve complications encountered in this position can include spinal cord ischemia from excessive neck flexion and sciatic nerve injury from extreme lower extremity extension. Physiologic complications in the sitting position include pooling of blood

Essential Clinical Anesthesia Review: Keywords, Questions and Answers for the Boards, ed. Linda S. Aglio, Robert W. Lekowski, and Richard D. Urman. Published by Cambridge University Press. © Cambridge University Press 2015.

in the lower extremities leading to decreased cardiac output and decreased cerebral blood flow.

Diagnosis of nerve injuries involves a detailed history and neurologic examination followed by formal neurologic consultation if nerve injury is suspected after initial evaluation. Electromyography (EMG) may be normal within two weeks of an acute injury and can help distinguish new-onset neuropathy from a chronic and preexisting condition. In the case of acute neuropathy, most symptoms resolve within six weeks and 80% of patients have complete resolution of all symptoms within six months.

Questions

1. A patient postoperative day one from laparoscopic hysterectomy is found to have new-onset foot drop. Which peripheral nerve is MOST likely associated with this finding?
   a. tibial nerve
   b. sural nerve
   c. common peroneal nerve
   d. saphenous nerve
   e. sciatic nerve

2. The most common positioning-related peripheral nerve injury involves which nerve?

   a. ulnar nerve
   b. radial nerve
   c. femoral nerve
   d. common peroneal nerve
   e. saphenous nerve

Answers

1. c. Common peroneal nerve. Signs of common peroneal nerve injury include paresthesia or decreased sensation of the anterior and lateral lower leg or dorsum of the foot and impaired dorsiflexion of the foot. The sural nerve provides sensation to the lateral foot, the saphenous nerve provides sensation to the medial foot, the tibial nerve provides sensation to the plantar surface of the foot as well as flexion of the digits. Sciatic injury would cause decreased dorsiflexion but would be less likely than peroneal nerve injury.

2. a. Ulnar nerve. A closed claims analysis of 4,100 claims showed that ulnar nerve injury was the most frequent nerve injury (28% of nerve injuries). Other sites of injury in the analysis included brachial plexus (20%), lumbosacral nerve root (16%), and spinal cord (13%). Ulnar nerve injuries were more likely to have occurred with general anesthesia.

Further reading

Vacanti, C., Sikka, P., Urman, R., Dershwitz, M., and Segal, B. (eds) (2011). Patient positioning and common nerve injuries. In *Essential Clinical Anesthesia*. Cambridge: Cambridge University Press, pp. 313–316.

Chaney, F. W., Domino, K. B., Caplan, R. A., and Posner, K. L. (1999). Nerve injury associated with anesthesia: a closed claims analysis. *Anesthesiology* 90(4),1062–1069.

Sawyer, R. J., Richmond, M. N., Hickey, J.D., and Jarrratt, J. A. (2000). Peripheral nerve injuries associated with anaesthesia. *Anaesthesia* 55(10), 980–991.

Chapter

51

Emergence from anesthesia

Pete Pelletier and Galina Davidyuk

Keywords

Delayed emergence
Respiratory failure
Extubation
Airway obstruction
Laryngospasm
Bronchospasm
Pulmonary aspiration
Pulmonary edema
Hypoventilation
Emergence delirium

Delayed emergence is common after prolonged anesthesia, and can be the result of residual drug effect, respiratory failure (hypercarbia and decreased oxygen delivery), cardiovascular complications, metabolic derangements, or neurologic complications.

Residual drug effects are the most frequent cause of *delayed emergence*. The speed of emergence from volatile anesthetics depends primarily on the duration of the anesthetic, the patient's alveolar ventilation (hypoventilation slows emergence), and the anesthetic's blood/gas solubility (more soluble agents, such as isoflurane, are eliminated much slower than less soluble agents such as desflurane). Elimination of IV and PO medications that may have sedative effects (opioids, benzodiazepines, gabapentin) is often dependent on renal and liver function.

Respiratory failure resulting in hypoxia and hypercarbia can contribute to increased sedation and *delayed emergence*. When respiratory failure is suspected, a blood gas analysis may be helpful in its diagnosis and treatment.

Electrolyte disturbances as well as hypo- and hyperglycemia are common contributors to *delayed emergence*. Hypoglycemia is most common in infants and patients with hepatic failure, but can also occur in patients taking insulin and oral hypoglycemics. Additionally, hyperglycemia can be an additional cause that is more commonly seen in diabetic patients in the form of diabetic ketoacidosis or coma.

Neurologic complications such as increased ICP, cerebral hemorrhage, and air or fat embolism can be causes of *delayed emergence*. Consider neurology consultation and head CT if these complications are suspected. Patient may be re-intubated or remain intubated for airway protection until the evaluation is complete.

Extubation criteria: prior to extubation patients should be hemodynamically stable, relatively normothermic, able to perform simple actions on command, have a regular respiratory pattern, be able to cough and clear secretions, and meet the following criteria:

- respiratory rate <30 bpm
- tidal volumes $\geq$5 ml/kg
- PEEP $\leq$5 cm H_2O
- negative inspiratory force $\geq$–20 cm H_2O
- $PaCO_2$ <50 mm Hg
- PaO_2 65–70 mm Hg on FiO_2 <40%

Airway obstruction may occur secondary to secretions, glottic edema, and foreign bodies, with the most common cause being the posteriorly displaced tongue. Common signs and symptoms include snoring, intercostal and suprasternal retractions, and paradoxical respirations. The obstruction is often relieved by stimulating the patient, repositioning the head, applying jaw thrust, applying the "head tilt, chin lift" technique, inserting nasal or oral airway devices, or utilizing noninvasive ventilation. Other rare but very important causes of *airway obstruction* include extrinsic airway compression from an expanding neck hematoma, and vocal cord paralysis caused by recurrent laryngeal nerve injury.

Laryngospasm occurs when stimulation of the superior laryngeal nerve results in spontaneous prolonged closure of the vocal cords. Treatment consists of suctioning the oropharynx, applying positive pressure ventilation with 100% oxygen, maintaining PEEP, deepening the level of anesthesia (often with IV anesthetics), and if the above maneuvers fail, treating with succinylcholine may be necessary. The dose of succinylcholine used to treat *laryngospasm* in an adult is 10 to 20 mg IV.

Essential Clinical Anesthesia Review: Keywords, Questions and Answers for the Boards, ed. Linda S. Aglio, Robert W. Lekowski, and Richard D. Urman. Published by Cambridge University Press. © Cambridge University Press 2015.

Bronchospasm is caused by increased bronchial smooth muscle tone that results in closure of the small airways. Patients with reactive airway disease and smokers are at greater risk than others and may need to be treated prior to induction and emergence with a bronchodilator such as the ß$_2$-agonist albuterol. If the *bronchospasm* is life-threatening, epinephrine may be administered IV or endotracheally.

Pulmonary aspiration upon emergence often results in severe hypoxemia and bronchospasm, and may lead to chemical pneumonitis, pneumonia, and even ARDS. After ensuring airway patency, it should be treated by administering supplemental oxygen, administration of bronchodilators, and supporting hemodynamics if needed. Antibiotics should be initiated only in response to culture-proven pneumonia. Bronchoscopy can be performed to suction particulate matter from the airways, but lavage is not recommend.

Pulmonary edema is characterized by engorgement of the perivascular and peribronchial interstitial tissues as well as alveolar edema. Negative pressure *pulmonary edema* can develop when a patient develops a large negative pressure within the thoracic cavity, most often secondary to attempting to take a breath against an obstructed airway. Cardiogenic *pulmonary edema* may also manifest during emergence and extubation. Neurogenic *pulmonary edema* may result from an acute increase in ICP. The treatment of pulmonary edema is supportive and often begins with supplemental oxygen therapy, administration of diuretics, and fluid restriction. Additionally, noninvasive ventilation or re-intubation may be necessary.

Hypoventilation is a common finding after general anesthesia and is often defined as a $PaCO_2$ >45 mm Hg, although it is often only clinically apparent when the $PaCO_2$ is >60 mm Hg. Causes of hypoventilation include decreased respiratory drive (most commonly due to opioids), inadequate ventilation secondary to pain from surgery, inadequate reversal of paralytics, or neuromuscular disease resulting in weakness. Treatment is aimed at correcting the underlying cause (i.e., naloxone for opioid overdose, reversal of neuromuscular blockade), and maintaining adequate ventilation either through noninvasive ventilation or re-intubation if needed.

Emergence delirium is characterized by a disturbance of consciousness with reduced ability to focus, a change in cognition (such as memory deficit, disorientation, language disturbance) that is not better accounted for by a preexisting or evolving dementia. It may be caused by a number of physiologic and pharmacologic factors (Table 51.1). It occurs commonly in extremes of age. Because *emergence delirium* is a diagnosis of exclusion, evaluation and treatment of other etiologies of agitation is the first step in its management. Pharmacologic agents are not the first line; however, they may be necessary when agitation puts the patient and/or caregiver at risk. Drug of choice remains haloperidol. Atypical antipsychotics and benzodiazepines may also be considered.

Table 51.1 Common causes of emergence delirium

Physiologic		Pharmacologic
Hypoxemia	Gastric dilation	Ketamine
Hypercapnia	Bladder distention	Benzodiazepines
Electrolyte imbalance	Pain	Metoclopramide
Alcohol withdrawal	Hypothermia	Atropine, scopolamine
Intracranial injury	Sensory overload	Inhalational anesthetics
Sepsis	Sensory deprivation	

(From Vacanti et al. 2011. *Essential Clinical Anesthesia*, Cambridge University Press, Table 52.5.)

Questions

1. What is the dose of IV succinylcholine recommended to treat laryngospasm in adult patients?
   a. 5–10 mg
   b. 10–20 mg
   c. 25–50 mg
   d. 50–75 mg
   e. 50–100 mg

2. True or false? A 55-year-old, 100 kg male who underwent laparoscopic hernia repair is being evaluated for extubation at the end of the case. He has had neuromuscular blockade reversed, and will raise his head for five seconds when asked. He is currently on spontaneous ventilation with a PEEP of 5 cm H_2O, has a regular respiratory pattern with a rate of 16, an end-tidal CO_2 of 35, SpO_2 of 100%, and is taking tidal volumes of 750 ml. He meets the criteria for extubation at this time.
   a. true
   b. false

3. Which of the following patients is most likely to develop emergence delirium?
   a. 43-year-old female following laparascopic lysis of adhesions
   b. 84-year-old male following cystoscopy
   c. 29-year-old male following partial thyroidectomy
   d. 37-year-old female following total abdominal hysterectomy

Answers

1. b. Laryngospasm is a life-threatening event, which can occur in the perioperative environment. It is important to remember that when jaw thrust, positive pressure ventilation, and deepening the level

of anesthesia fail, it can be treated with 10 to 20 mg of IV succinylcholine.

2. a. This patient meets all of the criteria for extubation, and his tidal volume of 750 ml is equivalent to 7.5 ml/kg, which is $\geq$5 ml/kg.

3. b. Emergence delirium is most common in the extremes of age, and therefore the 84-year-old patient in this question would be at a greater risk than any of the other patients presented.

Further reading

Miller, K. A., Harkin, C. P., and Bailey, P. L. (1995). Postoperative tracheal extubation. *Anesthesia and Analgesia* 80, 149–172.

Forman, S. (2002). Administration of general anesthesia. In Hurford, W. E. (ed) *Clinical Anesthesia Procedures of the Massachusetts General Hospital*, 6th edn. New York: Lippincott Williams & Wilkins, pp. 210–213.

Chapter

52

Postoperative complications in the post-anesthesia care unit

Pete Pelletier and Galina Davidyuk

Keywords

Hypoxemia
Hypotension
Hypertension
Oliguria
Urinary retention
Hypothermia
Hemorrhage

Hypoxemia is defined as a PaO$_2$ of 60 mm Hg or less on room air, and is most frequently the result of hypoventilation and atelectasis. Hypoventilation may be secondary to decreased ventilatory drive (from residual anesthetics, benzodiazepines, or opioids), exacerbation of pulmonary disease, or muscle weakness. It can result in carbon dioxide retention, respiratory acidosis, and *hypoxemia*. Other causes of hypoxia include inadequate analgesia, gastric distention, restrictive surgical dressings, cerebral vascular accidents, aspiration, pulmonary edema, pulmonary embolism, pneumothorax, and obesity.

Hypotension is a common postoperative complication that may result from intravascular volume depletion, decreased cardiac output, or decreased vascular tone. Identifying the underlying cause is the initial step in managing patients with hypotension. Treatment should be directed at optimizing the patient's fluid status by administering blood products as clinically indicated and supporting blood pressure with vasoactive medications when necessary.

Hypertension is a common postoperative problem, frequently observed in patients who did not receive their regular antihypertensive medications preoperatively. If uncontrolled, postoperative hypertension may potentially precipitate surgical bleeding.

Reversible causes of hypertension, such as pain, anxiety, hypoxemia, and hypercarbia, should be treated before antihypertensive treatment is initiated. The decision to treat hypertension should take into consideration the patient's baseline blood pressure, coexisting diseases, and perceived risk of complications. Short-term treatment in the PACU is achieved using IV agents such as ß-blockers (e.g., metoprolol, labetalol) and vasodilators (e.g., hydralazine, nitroglycerine). For persistent or refractory hypertension, continuous infusion of a vasodilator such as nitroglycerin or nitroprusside may be needed.

Oliguria is defined as urine output less than 0.5 ml/kg/h, and may be a sign of acute renal failure. It may be classified as prerenal, renal, or postrenal, with the former being the most common. Prerenal *oliguria* is the result of decreased renal perfusion commonly related to hypovolemia, and usually resolves after IV fluid administration. *Oliguria* may also be due to *urinary retention* in the setting of obstruction of urinary outflow (postrenal). Acute tubular necrosis in the setting of nephrotoxic medications or prolonged renal ischemia is an example of perioperative renal *oliguria*.

Hypothermia remains a common problem in the postoperative period, and is associated with adverse postoperative complications, including myocardial ischemia, arrhythmias, coagulopathy, and wound infection. Warm blankets usually are sufficient therapy for patients with mild *hypothermia*, although forced-air warming devices are more efficient. Pharmacologic control of shivering may sometimes be achieved with a small dose of meperidine (e.g., 12.5–25 mg IV).

Postoperative *hemorrhage* requires rapid evaluation to differentiate poor surgical hemostasis from a diffuse coagulopathy. Surgical and nonsurgical bleeding often coexist.

Saturated dressings, increased drain output, decrease in hemoglobin level, *hypotension*, tachycardia, or decreased urine output can guide the clinician in assessing the bleeding patient. Unfortunately, internal bleeding is not always obvious and may not be identified until the patient is severely compromised. Coordination among the surgical and anesthesia teams, the operating room staff, and the blood bank is essential. Adequate IV access should be established immediately and the availability of appropriate blood products ensured. Thrombocytopenia, hypothermia, and loss/consumption of coagulation factors are common causes of coagulopathy in postoperative patients. Preexisting medical conditions, such as liver failure and bone marrow suppression, and specific

Essential Clinical Anesthesia Review: Keywords, Questions and Answers for the Boards, ed. Linda S. Aglio, Robert W. Lekowski, and Richard D. Urman. Published by Cambridge University Press. © Cambridge University Press 2015.

surgical or nonsurgical complications, such as disseminated intravascular coagulation and consumptive coagulopathy, also should be considered.

Questions

1. True or false? Hypothermia is associated with postoperative complications including myocardial ischemia, arrhythmias, coagulopathy, and wound infection.

    a. true

    b. false

2. You are called to evaluate a patient in the PACU for hypertension following uncomplicated hernia repair on a 33-year-old male. Past medical history is significant for mild anxiety and childhood asthma. Vital signs upon your arrival include a heart rate of 95 beats per minute, blood pressure of 185/90, respiratory rate 25, SpO_2 100% on 2LNC. The patient rates his pain at 9/10. What is the most appropriate initial intervention?

    a. labetolol IV

    b. hydralazine IV

    c. lorazepam IV

    d. hydromorphone IV

    e. nitroglycerine IV

Answers

1. a. True. Hypothermia is something that can easily occur in the perioperative environment, but should not be taken lightly. Even mild hypothermia is associated with numerous postoperative complications including myocardial ischemia, arrhythmias, coagulopathy, and wound infection.

2. d. The most likely etiology of this patient's hypertension is postoperative pain, and it is most appropriately treated with IV opioids such as hydromorphone. If this were related to anxiety, then lorazepam would be the agent of choice, and options (a), (b), and (e) could be indicated if pain and anxiety were ruled out or if the hypertension persisted following adequate control of pain and anxiety.

Further reading

Lepouse, C., Lautner, C. A., Liu, L. et al. (2006). Emergence delirium in adults in the post-anesthesia care unit. *British Journal of Anaesthesia* 96, 747–753.

Bittner, E. A., Grecu, L., and George, E. (2008) Postoperative complications. In D. E. Longnecker et al. (eds) *Anesthesiology*. New York: McGraw-Hill.

Management of postoperative nausea and vomiting

M. Tariq Hanifi and Michael Nguyen

Keywords

Postoperative nausea and vomiting (PONV)
PONV mechanism
PONV etiology
PONV risk factors
PONV incidence
PONV preventive strategies
PONV medications
PONV management

Postoperative nausea and vomiting (PONV) is a significant problem in the general surgical population, with 20% to 30% prevalence. PONV can lead to patient distress as well as staggering health care costs. The degree of PONV can vary between individuals and its cause can be multifactorial.

PONV is classified as either early (six hours postprocedure) or late (24 hours postprocedure). The *mechanism of PONV is* still not clearly understood. It is a *multifactorial* problem associated with alteration of chemical signals sent via *neurotransmitters as well as activation/stimulation* of several nerves. As a result altering these *neurotransmitters* can treat PONV.

PONV can be managed in several ways. The steps are outlined below.

1. The patient's risk must be assessed preoperatively. The anesthetic regimen may need to be tailored to the individual.
2. Intraoperative prophylaxis for PONV should be administered.
3. Treatment of PONV may be given postoperatively in the post-anesthesia care unit.

Risk factors for PONV include prior PONV, use of perioperative opioids, and the type and duration of surgery. Additionally, PONV is more prevalent in women. Using these risk factors, patients can be separated into three categories. *Low risk* is classified as having zero to one risk factors, *moderate*

Table 53.1 Neurotransmitters and nerves associated with PONV

Neurotransmitters involved with PONV	Nerves associated with PONV
Histamine	Vestibular-cochlear nerves
Acetylcholine	Vagus nerve
Muscarinic	Glossopharyngeal nerve
Neurokinin-1	
Serotonin	
Dopamine	

Table 53.2 Medications used to treat PONV

Medication	Mechanism
Ondansetron	5-HT3 antagonist
Dexamethasone	Steroid agonist
Metoclopramide/ prochlorperazine/haldol	Dopamine 2 antagonist
Scopolamine	AChR antagonist
Promethazine/hydroxyzine	Histamine 1 antagonist
Aprepitant	Neurokinin-1 antagonist
Droperidol	Unknown

risk as having two risk factors, and *high risk* as having three or more risk factors.

Risk reduction strategies include giving medications to reduce the risk of PONV. However, even the most effective medications can only reduce the risk of PONV in one out of four to five patients treated. Medications that can be used to treat PONV are outlined in Table 53.2.

In patients with low risk for PONV, no medication prophylaxis is necessary. In patients with moderate risk, therapy with one to two drugs is recommended. For patients at high risk, a combination of three or more drugs may be required.

Treatment of *PONV* may extend into the post-anesthesia care unit (*PACU*) where a multiple drug therapy may be required. In addition to common prophylactic agents, drugs

Essential Clinical Anesthesia Review: Keywords, Questions and Answers for the Boards, ed. Linda S. Aglio, Robert W. Lekowski, and Richard D. Urman. Published by Cambridge University Press. © Cambridge University Press 2015.

such as haloperidol and promethazine can be used in treating refractory PONV.

Anesthetic technique may also influence risk for PONV. Volatile agents and nitrous oxide are widely thought to increase PONV. It was found in a meta-analysis of 24 trials that omitting N_2O reduced the risk of PONV by 27% in 13 patients. This effect was highly dependent on the patient's underlying risk for PONV. In patients with low risk for PONV, omitting N_2O was not statistically significant. However, in patients with high risk for PONV, omitting N_2O was shown to decrease the risk of PONV. One caveat in this meta-analysis was that omitting N_2O led to more episodes of intraoperative awareness.

Conversely, propofol may help prevent PONV. In one meta-analysis, the effects of propofol with and without N_2O are compared to the effects of volatile agents with and without N_2O. Propofol was shown to contribute to early prevention (0–6 hours) of PONV. TIVA with propofol compared to general anesthesia with N_2O had an NNT of 6. In some high-risk patients, alternative anesthetic choices such as total intravenous anesthetic or regional may be preferred. It is important to choose the safest and most appropriate anesthetic to reduce significant morbidity and patient dissatisfaction.

Questions

1. Which of the following agents used for PONV prophylaxis has been shown to alter serotonin transmission?

   a. dexamethasone
   b. aprepitant
   c. dilaudid
   d. ondansetron

2. Which of the following is a risk factor for developing PONV?

   a. female gender
   b. use of morphine during the procedure
   c. ten-hour-long facial reconstruction
   d. all of the above

Answers

1. d. Ondanestron works by inhibiting serotonin at the 5-HT3 receptor.
2. d. Risk factors for PONV include: female gender, use of perioperative opiods, type of surgery, and duration of surgery.

Further reading

Apfel, C. (2009). Chapter 86. Postoperative nausea and vomiting. In Miller, R. D., Eriksson, L. I., Fleisher, L. A. et al. (eds) *Miller's Anesthesia*, 7th edn. Philadelphia: Churchill-Livingstone.

Tramer, M. R. (2003). Treatment of postoperative nausea and vomiting. *British Medical Journal* 327, 762–3.

Chapter

54

Cognitive changes after surgery and anesthesia

Allison Clark and Lisa Crossley

Keywords

Delirium: Dx
Delirium: risk factors
Postoperative cognitive dysfunction: Dx
Postoperative cognitive dysfunction: risk factors

Postoperative delirium places patients at risk for injury, increased length of stay, discharge to skilled nursing facility, and one-year mortality.

Delirium is a *clinical diagnosis* of an acute alteration in consciousness and cognition that waxes and wanes. The Confusion Assessment Method (CAM) is a bedside tool used to make the diagnosis. This requires presence of (1) an acute or fluctuating course and (2) inattention, associated with either (3) disorganized thinking or (4) altered level of consciousness.

Risk factors for delirium are shown in Table 54.1 and include age, physiologic derangements, and pain.

Postoperative cognitive dysfunction (POCD) is diagnosed through *neurophysiological testing* and is defined as long-term impairment of cognitive function following anesthesia and surgery.

Risk factors are shown in Table 54.2 and include age, history of stroke, and prolonged hospitalization. Type of anesthesia (regional vs. general) does not alter risk of POCD.

Questions

1. The diagnosis of delirium requires which of the following?

   a. disorganized thinking
   b. altered level of consciousness
   c. inattention
   d. neurophysiological testing

Table 54.1 Risk factors for delirium

Nonmodifiable factors[a]	Modifiable factors
Age >70 years	Metabolic/physiologic derangements
Preexisting cognitive impairment	Hypoxemia
History of delirium	Hypercarbia
History of depression	Hypoglycemia
Multiple comorbidities	Hypoalbuminemia[b]
Poor functional status	Perioperative anemia[b]
Genetic factors – apo E4	Electrolyte disturbances
Type of surgery	Hypothermia
Major orthopedic	Occult infection
Cardiac	Occult cerebrovascular event
Thoracic	Iatrogenic causes[c]
Vascular	Pain
Emergency	Acute systemic disturbances Urinary retention, fecal impaction

[a] Patients with any of the nonmodifiable factors demonstrate an increased risk for the development of delirium postoperatively and should be identified during the preoperative assessment. Patients who develop delirium after surgery should be evaluated for any of the modified factors and treated accordingly.
[b] Linked to the development of postoperative delirium, although perioperative correction has not been demonstrated to improve the clinical course of delirium.
[c] Anticholinergics (with the exception of glycopyrrolate), benzodiazepines, and anti-dopaminergic agents are the most commonly implicated agents.
(From: Vacanti et al., 2011, p.330.)

Essential Clinical Anesthesia Review: Keywords, Questions and Answers for the Boards, ed. Linda S. Aglio, Robert W. Lekowski, and Richard D. Urman. Published by Cambridge University Press. © Cambridge University Press 2015.

Table 54.2 Risk factors for POCD[a]

| Age >70 years |
| Low educational level |
| History of cognitive impairment |
| Type of surgery |
| Duration of anesthesia |
| Prolonged hospital course |
| Postoperative infection |
| Postoperative respiratory complications |
| ? Genetic predisposition[b] |

[a] Patients with any of these risk factors demonstrate an increased incidence of POCD.
[b] Currently under investigation.
(From: Vacanti et al., 2011, p.332.)

2. Risk factors for POCD include all of the following except for which?
   a. prior stroke
   b. low educational level
   c. ambulatory surgery
   d. general anesthesia

Answers

1. c. Delirium is a clinical diagnosis, requiring an acute or fluctuating course, inattention, and either disorganized thinking or an altered level of consciousness.
2. d. Anesthesia type does not alter risk for POCD. See Table 54.2 for POCD risk factors.

Further reading

Vacanti, J., Crosby, G., and Culley, D. (2011). Cognitive changes after surgery and anesthesia. In Vacanti, C. A., Sikka, P. J., Urman, R. D., Dershwitz, M., and Segal, B. S. (eds) *Essential Clinical Anesthesia*. Cambridge: Cambridge University Press, pp. 330–333.

Chapter

55

Anatomy of the vertebral column and spinal cord

Jennifer Oliver and Jose Luis Zeballos

Keywords

Cervical, thoracic, and lumbar spinal anatomy
Functions of the vertebral column
Cervical and lumbar lordosis
Thoracic kyphosis
Vertebral body
Vertebral arch
Pedicles
Lamina
Vertebral foramen
Zygapophyseal joint
Atlas
Axis
Transverse cervical ligament instability
Vertebral prominans
Joints of Lushka
Costovertebral ligament
Costotransverse joint
Anterior longitudinal ligament
Posterior longitudinal ligament
Supraspinous ligament
Interspinous ligament
Ligmentum flavum
Sacral hiatus
Annulus fibrosis
Nucleus pulposus
Conus medularis
Filum terminale
Cauda equina
Dural layers
Spinal cord blood supply
Artery of Adamkiewicz
Anterior spinal artery syndrome
Batson's plexus
Azygous vein
Spinal cord tracts

The spinal column

The spinal column is comprised of the spinal cord and the vertebral column. There are seven cervical, twelve thoracic, five lumbar, five fused sacral, and four fused coccygeal, giving a total of 33 vertebrae.

Functions of the bony vertebral column include protection of the enclosed spinal cord and nerve roots; support of the head, shoulders, and chest; mobility of the upper body via flexion, extension, and rotation; and an attachment place for ligaments, tendons, and muscles.

The natural curvature of the spinal column influences the spread of medications injected into the intrathecal space. The *cervical and lumbar regions are lordotic*, while the *thoracic region is kyphotic*. Each vertebra is composed of a *verterbral body* anteriorly and a *vertebral arch* posteriorly. The two *pedicles* fuse the vertebral arch to the vertebral body and serve to attach the transverse process. The *vertebral foramen* (spinal canal) is found within these structures. Each *vertebral arch* consists of two lamimane, two pedicles, and supports one spinous process, two transverse and four articular processes (two superior and two inferior). The articular processes form the synovial joints (facet or *zygapophyseal joints)*, while the pedicles establish the *intervertebral foramina* through which the spinal nerves pass as they exit the spinal column.

Cervical vertebrae

Cervical vertebrae are the smallest vertebrae and have horizontal spinous processes allowing a midline approach for neuraxial block. Each transverse process contains a foramen transversarium that allows for passage of the vertebral artery, vein, and sympathetic nerve plexus. *The atlas* (first cervical vertebra) lacks both a body and a spinous process. The spinous process of the axis is short and bifid. The ring of the atlas is divided into an anterior and posterior portion by the *transverse cervical ligament*. The anterior portion houses the odontoid process of *the axis* (the second cervical vertebra) and

Essential Clinical Anesthesia Review: Keywords, Questions and Answers for the Boards, ed. Linda S. Aglio, Robert W. Lekowski, and Richard D. Urman. Published by Cambridge University Press. © Cambridge University Press 2015.

the posterior portion houses the spinal cord. The atlanto-occipital joint is a condyloid joint between the atlas and the occiput of the skull. Patients with rheumatoid arthritis, diabetes mellitus, ankylosing spondylitis, or trisomy 21 may have inflammatory changes in the transverse cervical ligament, which predisposes them to *atlanto-axial instability* during intubation. The *joints of Luschka* are formed from the articulation of each cervical vertebral body with the one immediately below it. C7 has a prominent spinous process known as the *vertebral prominans*.

Thoracic vertebrae

The thoracic vertebrae increase in size from cephalad to caudad and have facets that articulate with the tubercles of the ribs (except for T11 and T12). The two components of the *costotransverse ligament* attach the neck of the rib to the transverse process of the vertebra above. The articulation of the rib with the transverse process with associated ligaments forms the *costovertebral joint*. The spinous processes are directed inferiorly and overlap with each other such that a paramedian approach to neuraxial anesthesia may be preferred.

Lumbar vertebrae

The lumbar vertebrae differ in that they have wider pedicles, horizontal spinous processes, and square vertebral bodies compared to other regions of the vertebral column.

Sacrum

The sacrum is triangular in shape and composed of the five fused sacral vertebra that lack pedicles, laminae, and spinous processes. The *sacral hiatus* is formed from the lamina of S4 and S5.

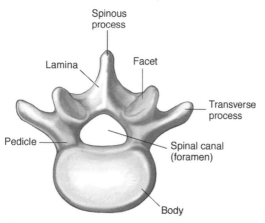

Figure 55.1 A typical lumbar vertebra. From: Vacanti et al., 2011, p. 336.

Intervertebral disc

The disc is composed of the strong avascular *annulus fibrosis*, *nucleus pulposus*, and cartilaginous end-plate. The outer layer is a frequent source of chronic back pain due to its rich innervations.

Ligaments

The *anterior longitudinal ligament* adheres to the anterior surface of the vertebral bodies and the annulus fibrosis, while the *posterior longitudinal ligament* runs along the posterior surface. The *supraspinous ligament* connects the tips of the spinous processes, while the *interspinous ligament* connects the bases. The *ligamentum flavum* runs from the base of the skull to the pelvis, it is made up of two fused ligaments joined in the middle. The distance from the skin to the ligamentum flavum is variable. The thickness of the ligamentum flavum is 1.5 mm at the cervical level to 6.0 mm in the lumbar area.

Spinal cord

The spinal cord extends from the foramen magnum to L1 in adults and L3 in children. There are *31 spinal nerves* comprised of both sensory and motor nerve roots: *eight cervical, twelve thoracic, five lumbar, five sacral, and one coccygeal*. The C1–C7 nerves emerge above their respective vertebra while the C8 nerve emerges between C7 and T1. The spinal cord terminates as the *conus medullaris*, which is attached to the coccyx by the *filum terminale* surrounded by the lumbar and sacral nerve roots, which form the *cauda equina*.

Three layers of meninges cover the spinal cord. The outermost layer is the *dura mater*, which is a tough, fibrous sheath closely connected to the bones surrounding the spinal canal. The dura often touches, but does not attach to, the periosteum, unless inflammation has occurred. The *epidural space* is the space between the dura and the bone. The *arachnoid mater* is closely applied to the dura and consists of a network of thin trabeculae. Beneath the arachnoid mater and closely attached to the spinal cord is the *pia mater*, the innermost meningeal layer. CSF is contained between the arachnoid and pia mater. The pia mater continues caudally as the *filum terminale* that emerges through the dural sac and attaches to the coccyx.

Arterial and venous supply

The spinal cord is supplied by a single *anterior spinal artery* and two *posterior spinal arteries*. The anterior spinal artery supplies the anterior two-thirds of the spinal cord and the posterior spinal arteries supply the posterior one-third. The *artery of Adamkiewicz* is the largest segmental radicular artery and originates between T9 and T12. It is usually on the left, and supplies the lower one-third of the spinal cord. Injury to this artery may result in *anterior spinal artery syndrome* or Beck's syndrome and can present as loss of temperature and pain sensation below the level of the injury,

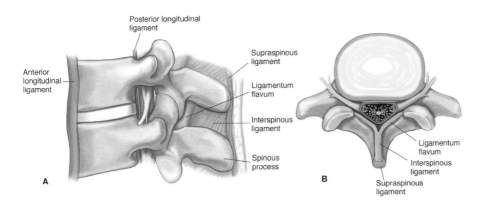

Figure 55.2 Ligaments of the spinal column. (A) Lateral view. (B) Transverse view. From: Vacanti et al., 2011, p. 337.

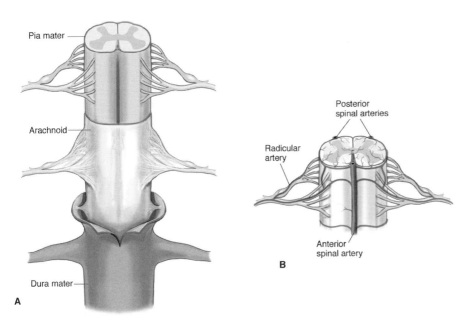

Figure 55.3 Spinal cord anatomy. (A) Coverings of the spinal cord. (B) Arterial supply of the spinal cord. From: Vacanti et al., 2011, p. 337.

weakness, urinary and fecal incontinence, with sparing of vibration and position sensation.

Batson's plexus (internal vertebral venous plexus) is found in the epidural space, comprised of four interconnecting longitudinal vessels: two anterior and two posterior. Increased intra-abdominal pressure, pregnancy, or obstruction of the IVC distends the epidural venous plexus. The epidural veins drain to the *azygous vein*, which enables inadvertently injected intravascular local anesthetics to potentially travel to the heart.

Ascending tracts of the spinal cord

The dorsal column/medial lemniscus provides propiception, vibration, and tactile sensation. The first-order neurons can be found in dorsal root ganglia (DRG), travel on the same side of the ganglia, and decussate in the brainstem.

The lateral spinothalamic tracts is responsible for the sensation of pain and temperature. It decussates across the anterior white commissure in the spinal cord and ascends contralateral to the DRG.

Descending tracts of the spinal cord

The corticospinal tract (ventral and lateral) descends in the spinal cord and crosses over the motor (pyramidal) decussation to provide voluntary motor movement.

The hypothalamospinal tract overlaps with the lateral corticospinal tract. It projects from the hypothalamus to the intermedialateral nucleus.

Questions

1. Beck's syndrome is characterized by which findings below the level of injury?
   a. loss of propioception and pain sensation
   b. loss of temperature and pain sensation
   c. loss of propioception and temperature
   d. loss of vibration and position sensation

2. Which of the following lists the correct order of structures pierced during placement of a spinal anesthetic?
   a. supraspinous ligament, intraspinous ligament, posterior longitudinal ligament, epidural space

b. supraspinous ligament, intraspinous ligament, ligmentum flavum, epidural space
c. ligmentum flavum, epidural space, dura, pia mater
d. supraspinous ligament, intraspinous ligament, posterior longitudinal ligament, ligmentum flavum

Answers
1. b.
2. b. See Figure 55.2.

Further reading

Vacanti, C., Sikka, P., Urman, R., Dershwitz, M., and Segal, B. (eds) (2011). *Essential Clinical Anesthesia.* Cambridge: Cambridge University Press.

Morgan, G. (2013). *Lange Clinical Anesthesiology*, 5th edn. New York, McGraw-Hill.

Urman, R. (2013). *Pocket Anesthesia.* Philadelphia, PA: Lippincott Williams & Wilkins.

Gray, H. (2008). *Anatomy of the Human Body*, 40th edn. Elsevier.

www.openanesthesia.org/ABA: Spinal_cord_anatomy [Accessed May 2014].

Chapter

56

Spinal anesthesia

Jennifer Oliver and Jose Luis Zeballos

Keywords

Contraindications to neuraxial anesthesia
Disadvantages of spinal anesthesia
Postdural puncture headache (PDPH)
Order of nerve blockade
Sympathetic outflow versus parasympathetic outflow
Cardiovascular effects of spinal anesthesia
Respiratory effects of spinal anesthesia
Gastrointestinal effects of spinal anesthesia
Thermoregulatory effects of spinal anesthesia
High spinal
Choice of local anesthetic agents
Transient neurologic symptoms (TNS)
Bupivacaine toxicity
Adverse neurologic effects of spinal anesthesia
Anticoagulation guidelines for neuraxial anesthesia

Table 56.1 Advantages and disadvantages of spinal anesthesia.

Advantages	Disadvantages
Cost-effectiveness	Difficult needle placement
High patient satisfaction	Inability to obtain CSF
Preserved protective reflexes	Hypotension
Decreased risk of aspiration	PDPH
Less bleeding	Urinary retention
Rapid return of bowel function	Infection
Decreased incidence of DVT	Possible conversion to general
Less incidence of nausea	anesthesia
Decreased postoperative	Failed spinal
pain	
Lower incidence of cognitive	
impairment	

(From: Vacanti et al., 2011, p. 341.)

Spinal anesthesia is most often indicated for surgeries below the level of the umbilicus. *Absolute contraindications* to spinal anesthesia include patient refusal and allergy to local anesthetics, while *relative contraindications* include bacteremia, anticoagulation, infection at the site of needle puncture, preexisting neurologic deficit, spinal column deformities, coagulopathy, elevated ICP, severe uncorrected hypovolemia, and stenotic valvular lesions. *Controversial contraindications* include chronic back pain, severe headache, severe anatomic abnormality, neurologic disease (such as multiple sclerosis), back surgery with instrumentation, and complex or prolonged surgery. Advantages and disadvantages are listed in Table 56.1.

The *order of nerve blockade* after exposure to local anesthetics is: small sympathetic C fibers, small sensory A-delta fibers (pain and temperature), larger sensory A-beta fibers (proprioception and touch), and large motor fibers. The level of sympathectomy is approximately two levels above the level of sensory loss. Benefits of spinal anesthesia are listed in Table 56.1.

Cardiovascular effects of spinal anesthesia

Sympathetic outflow from the spinal cord occurs from T1 to L2, while *parasympathetic outflow* is craniosacral. *Sympathetic cardioaccelerator fibers* from T1 to T4 increase the heart rate. Blockade of these fibers from a high spinal anesthetic can cause bradycardia and decreased cardiac output. Hypotension results from decreased systemic vascular resistance through dilation of arteries and venous capacitance vessels. The incidence of hypotension following spinal anesthesia is 10% to 40%.

Cardiac arrest is a rare, but serious complication. *Risk factors for bradycardia* include a baseline heart rate less than 60 bpm, age less than 50, ASA class I patients, use of β-blockers, a high spinal, and a prolonged PR interval. Hypotension and bradycardia should be treated with IV fluids and pharmacologic agents (anticholinergics and alpha/beta-agonists).

Respiratory effects of spinal anesthesia

The intercostal and abdominal muscles may be paralyzed leading to decreased ability to cough. Caution should be used

Essential Clinical Anesthesia Review: Keywords, Questions and Answers for the Boards, ed. Linda S. Aglio, Robert W. Lekowski, and Richard D. Urman. Published by Cambridge University Press. © Cambridge University Press 2015.

in patients with a preexisting pulmonary disease as they are most likely to experience respiratory distress from loss of these muscles. The sensation of dyspnea results from the loss of intercostal muscle, proprioception and the inability to sense chest wall movement.

Other well known effects

Spinal anesthesia also impairs thermoregulation due to peripheral vasodilatation from sympathectomy. Unopposed parasympathetic activity to the viscera may lead to nausea and vomiting. Decrease in hepatic flow secondary to a decrease in the mean arterial pressure has been described. Additionally, the inflammatory response to surgical trauma mediated by the neuroendocrine system is attenuated.

Choice of local anesthetic agents

The most common anesthetic agents for spinal anesthesia are bupivicaine, lidocaine, and tetracaine. Other local anesthetics such as ropivacaine and mepivicaine are frequently used in epidurals and peripheral nerve blocks. Bupivicaine is considerably more cardiotoxic than other local anesthestics and may cause refractory cardiovascular collapse with intravascular injection. Chloroprocaine is not approved for spinal anesthesia in the United States and was formerly thought to be neurotoxic. It is rapidly hydrolyzed in the bloodstream and therefore has decreased risk of systemic toxicity and decreased risk of fetal toxicity in obstetrics. Clearance may be prolonged in patients with liver disease.

Premedication

Anxiolytics and opioids are commonly used as premedication prior to spinal. Intravenous preloading with 500 to 1,000 ml crystalloids mitigates the impact of sympathectomy.

Equipment

The *Whitacre and Sprotte needles* are pencil-point tipped. The *Quincke needle* is the traditional cutting needle. Smaller gauge needles (25–27G) and pencil-point needles have a lower incidence of PDPH than larger gauge and cutting needles.

Monitoring

Standard ASA monitors should be placed prior to initiation of procedure as hypotension may occur precipitously.

Factors affecting spinal block

Baricity, patient posture, and total dose of local anesthetic have the greatest effect on the spinal block. Isobaric solutions have a more even distribution; hyperbaric solutions move to dependent areas while hypobaric solutions move opposite the dependent areas. In the supine position the mid-thoracic (T5–T8) region is the most dependent point of the spine.

Adverse neurologic effects of spinal anesthesia

The incidence of adverse neurologic effects from spinal anesthesia is one per 20,000. Aseptic meningitis presents within 24 hours following spinal anesthesia. Nuchal rigidity, photophobia, and fever are the most common symptoms. Aseptic meningitis is usually benign and resolves with symptomatic treatment but must be distinguished from infectious meningitis, especially in the presence of fever.

Meningitis may be due to a breach in sterile technique or in the presence of severe untreated bacteremia. Oral commensal microorganisms have been detected in some cases, implying a lack of face mask use by personnel or inadequate sterile technique. Replacing or removing epidural catheters within five days of placement may reduce the risk of epidural abscess or meningitis.

Postdural puncture headache (PDPH) is caused by CSF leak through the dural puncture site. Young female patients are at higher risk for PDPH than older male patients. Pregnancy, the use of large gauge or cutting spinal needles, and parallel orientation of the needle bevel along the long access of the body are also risk factors.

Transient neurologic symptoms (TNS) or transient radicular irritation presents with low back, buttock, thigh, or calf pain without motor or sensory deficit five to ten days after uncomplicated spinal anesthesia. Somatosensory evoked potentials, electromyography, and nerve conduction studies do not show any abnormalities. TNS is more common with the use of lidocaine, after surgery in the lithotomy position, in obese patients, and in ambulatory surgery. Pregnancy may be protective. There is no association with patient age, difficulty of placement of the spinal anesthetic, paresthesia during needle placement, gender, or needle type. COX inhibitors are the first-line treatment followed by opioids.

Epidural or spinal hematoma is a devastating complication that may result in permanent neurologic deficits. Risk factors include coagulopathy, therapeutic anticoagulation, multiple placement attempts, and traumatic needle placement. Presentation may include an unresolving spinal block, persistent back pain, and neurologic deficits that may range from limited sensory deficits to frank paraplegia. MRI is the gold standard for diagnosis. Delays in surgical decompression longer than six to eight hours are associated with poorer outcomes.

High or total spinal is a serious complication caused by high cephalad spread of local anesthetic. It may present with tingling of the fingers, nausea, hypotension, bradycardia, difficulty breathing, and respiratory depression. Treatment is supportive.

Urinary retention is common after spinal anesthesia due to blockade of the S2–S4 nerve roots and may lead to bladder distension requiring catheterization. Severe bladder distension may be associated with tachycardia, bradycardia, and hypertension.

Anticoagulation guidelines

Table 56.2 Current recommendations for spinal/epidural anesthesia and anticoagulants

Classification	Medications	Recommendations	Laboratory
Antiplatelets	Aspirin/NSAIDS Ticlopidine Clopidogrel	None Discontinue 14 days before Discontinue 7 days before	
Anticoagulants	Warfarin	Discontinue 4–5 days before Monitor patient for 24 hours post removal of catheter	PT/INR should be <1.5 prior to needle placement or catheter removal
Heparin	SubQ heparin IV heparin	Delay until after block Delay until 1 hour after needle placement; remove catheter after evaluation of coagulation status, 1 hour before next dose, and 2–4 hours after last dose	>4 days check platelet count Measure PTT
LMWH	Dalteparin Enoxaparin	High (therapeutic) dose: may place neuraxial block >24 hours after last dose Remove catheter >24 hours after last dose Catheters are contradicated with this dosing Initiate therapy >2 hours after catheter removal Low (prophylactic) dose: may place neuraxial block 12 hours after last dose Initiate therapy >2 hours after catheter removal	

Questions

1. Which of the following is LEAST likely true regarding the benefits of neuraxial anesthesia?

   a. decreased surgical blood loss
   b. decreased time to postoperative ambulation
   c. decreased postoperative illeus
   d. decreased incidence of postoperative renal insufficiency

2. To which levels will a spinal anesthetic most likely travel if the patient is immediately placed in the supine position after injection of a hyperbaric solution of local anesthetic?

   a. T5–T8
   b. L1–L3
   c. C3–C5
   d. S1–S3

3. A patient has a spinal anesthetic with lidocaine for a D&C in the lithotomy position. She then experiences numbness and tingling in the buttock with no loss of motor function or sensory deficits. How do you respond?

   a. COX inhibitors are the first line of treatment.
   b. The patient needs an urgent MRI.
   c. This is more common during pregnancy.
   d. An epidural blood patch is the definitive treatment.

Answers

1. d. See Table 56.2.
2. a.
3. a. COX inhibitors are the first-line treatment for TNS.

Further reading

Vacanti, C., Sikka, P., Urman, R., Dershwitz, M., and Segal, B. (eds) (2011). *Essential Clinical Anesthesia*. Cambridge: Cambridge University Press.

Morgan, G. (2013). *Lange Clinical Anesthesiology*, 5th edn. New York: McGraw-Hill.

Urman, R. (2013). *Pocket Anesthesia*. Philadelphia, PA: Lippincott Williams & Wilkins.

Section 10 · Regional anesthesia

Chapter 57 · Epidural anesthesia

Jennifer Oliver and Jose Luis Zeballos

Keywords

Benefits of neuraxial versus general anesthesia
Contraindications to epidural anesthesia
Test dose
Clonidine
Anatomy of epidural space
Anatomical changes during pregnancy
Local anesthetic spread
Substantia gelatinosa
Substance P
Cardiorespiratory effects
Postdural puncture headache (PDPH)
Epidural hematoma
Epidural blood patch
Local anesthetic spread
Management of retained catheter

The benefits of neuraxial versus general anesthesia include: reduced stress response to surgery, less intraoperative blood loss, fewer thromboembolic events, fewer postoperative pulmonary complications, earlier return of gastrointestinal function, earlier ambulation, earlier hospital discharge, and less perioperative mortality.

Contraindications to epidural anesthesia are the same as for spinal anesthesia (see Chapter 56).

Equipment: the most commonly used epidural needle is the 17-gauge 3.5 inch *Tuohy* needle. A modification of this needle is named the Weiss needle. It has a winged hub with a blunt curved tip similar to the Touhy needle. This needle penetrates through the *skin, supraspinous ligament, interspinous ligament, and ligamentum flavum to reach the epidural space*. Using a syringe for loss of resistance, the epidural space can be found either via the midline approach or the paramedian approach. Once reached a single dose of local can be injected or a 19- or 20-gauge nonstimulating catheter can be left there for continuous infusion. Some catheters have multiple orifices and others have a single orifice for infusion of local anesthetics. Studies indicate that there are fewer "patchy" or incomplete blocks with the multi-orifice catheter. Catheters

that are stiffer are associated with higher frequency of paresthesia and intravascular placement. During the procedure supplemental oxygen, suction, and bag-valve mask and resuscitation drugs should be available.

The most common *test dose* of local anesthetic is 3 ml of 1.5% lidocaine with 1:200,000 epinephrine (5 μg/ml). Intrathecal administration of this test dose will result in rapid spinal block with motor weakness, whereas intravascular injection will result in an increased blood pressure, and increase in heart rate greater than 30 bpm within 45 seconds in a patient not taking β-blockers.

Blood vessels are located primarily laterally and anteriorly within the epidural space and may become engorged during pregnancy or in disease states with increased intra-abdominal pressure. This can result in a higher risk of inadvertent intravascular injection, which can cause CNS toxicity, cardiovascular toxicity, and, ultimately, cardiovascular collapse. To prevent these complications, epidural catheters should be aspirated prior to injection of test dose and prior to the start of infusion and bolus of local anesthetic.

The total volume of local anesthetic injected into the epidural space determines *the spread of the local anesthetic* block, while the concentration of the local anesthetic determines the density of the block. As with any block the speed of onset is determined by: the local anesthetic agent, the fraction of the agent in non-ionized form, and the concentration of agent. Duration of action correlates with degree of protein binding and lipid solubility. Epidural fat sequestration can prolong epidural action by acting as a drug reservoir. Adrenergic agonists can prolong the action by causing local vasoconstriction and decreased clearance from the epidural space. Older patients have increased caudal and cephalad spread of local anesthetics due to age-related anatomic changes.

Opioids used in the epidural space provide analgesia by binding to the pre- and postsynaptic receptors in the *substantia gelatinosa of the dorsal horn of the spinal cord* and to opioid receptors in the brainstem. This results in inhibition of the release of neuromediators such as *Substance P*. Early respiratory depression for activation of *μ2 receptors* may occur from epidural opioid use. Late respiratory depression

Essential Clinical Anesthesia Review: Keywords, Questions and Answers for the Boards, ed. Linda S. Aglio, Robert W. Lekowski, and Richard D. Urman. Published by CAMBRIDGE UNIVERSITY PRESS. © Cambridge University Press 2015.

up to 24 hours after administration may occur. It is believed that neuraxial morphine is associated with reactivation of the *varicella zoster virus* associated with shingles.

Clonidine is an α-2 agonist with an analgesic and sedative effect that results from activation of receptors in the dorsal horn, which mimics descending norepinephrine inhibitory pathways.

Serious complications such as *cardiac arrest* are rare and occur more commonly with spinal rather than epidural anesthesia. Minor complications such as back pain, urinary retention, pruritus, nausea, and vomiting are more frequent.

Postdural puncture headache (PDPH) may result from inadvertent dural puncture or wet tap. The headache occurs due to increased traction on intracranial structures and compressed or stretched nerves. It is characterized by severe bilateral fronto-occipital positional headache that occurs 12 to 48 hours after the procedure. Pain is aggravated by sitting up or standing and relieved by lying supine. The headache often persists for three to seven days and may be relieved by conservative management including IV fluids, bed rest, caffeine, theophylline, or analgesics. If conservative management fails, an *epidural blood patch* provides rapid and complete improvement in 70% to 98% of cases. An epidural blood patch involves injecting 15 to 25 ml of autologous blood into the epidural space one level below the dural puncture to compress and block the defect in the dura.

An epidural hematoma can occur spontaneously, during the placement of epidural and during removal of a catheter. Incidence is one in 150,000 for epidural and one in 220,000 for spinal anesthesia. The increase in use of perioperative anticoagulation may be a factor.

Questions

1. A 38-year-old patient is undergoing an abdominal exploratory laparotomy. The epidural placement prior to the surgery was uneventful. During the surgery the patient has been hemodynamically stable and the surgeon is starting to close. You decide to bolus 6 ml of bupivacaine 0.5%. Soon after, the patient becomes unstable and starts to develop arrhythmias and develops PEA arrest. What is the most likely cause?
   a. surgical complication
   b. pulmonary embolism
   c. inadvertent IV injection of local
   d. allergic reaction

2. A 40-year-old woman is being worked up for a headache. The medical team is concerned for meningitis. A lumbar puncture is performed and 12 hours later her headache is worse. What is the most appropriate way to differentiate the headache?
   a. obtain the results from the LP
   b. obtain an MRI
   c. clinical exam
   d. perform an epidural blood patch

3. Which of the following is consistent with the ASRA 2010 guidelines regarding neuraxial anesthesia and enoxaparin?

   a. The epidural catheters can be removed 12 hours after the last dose of once-daily enoxaparin; may restart enoxaparin 2 hours after catheter removal.
   b. The epidural catheters can be removed 12 hours after the last dose of once-daily enoxaparin, restarting enoxaparin 12 hours after catheter removal.
   c. Placement of a spinal anesthetic 12 hours after the last dose of once-daily enoxaparin, restarting enoxaparin 12 hours after spinal placement.
   d. Placement of a spinal anesthetic 12 hours after the last dose of once-daily enoxaparin, restarting enoxaparin 2 hours after spinal placement.

4. Which of the following anticoagulants is correctly paired with the minimum time it should be discontinued prior to a neuraxial anesthetic according to the ARSA guidelines?
   a. heparin prophyalactic dosing: 4 hours
   b. clopidagril: 5 days
   c. dibigatran: 5 days
   d. abiximab: 2 days

5. In a patient with severe aortic stenosis, which of the following anesthetic techniques is LEAST preferred?
   a. propofol induction
   b. etomidate induction
   c. spinal anesthetic with 15 mg bupivicaine
   d. Epidural anesthesia with 2% lidocaine

Answers

1. c. The highest incidence on LAST is related to unintentional intravascular injection of local anesthetic. The best approach is to administer a test dose with epinephrine followed by a local in small divided doses.
2. c. This headache presents 12–48 hours after the procedure. The pain is related to the position. Laying flat relives the headache, while sitting up worsens the headache.
3. a. See Vacanti et al. 2011. *Essential Clinical Anesthesia,* Table 57-1A, p. 346 for additional guidelines.
4. d. See Vacanti et al. 2011. *Essential Clinical Anesthesia,* Table 57-1A, p. 346 for additional guidelines.
5. c. Blockade of sympathetic fibers from a high spinal anesthetic causes decreased heart rate, decreased contractility, and decreased cardiac output. Spinal anesthetics also cause decreased systemic vascular resistance through dilation of arteries and venous capacitance vessels, leading to decreased venous return and hypotension. In severe aortic stenosis, changes in cardiac output are poorly tolerated.

Further reading

Vacanti, C., Sikka, P., Urman, R., Dershwitz, M., and Segal, B. (eds) (2011). *Essential Clinical Anesthesia.* Cambridge: Cambridge University Press.

Morgan, G. (2013). *Lange Clinical Anesthesiology,* 5th edn. New York: McGraw-Hill.

Urman, R. (2013). *Pocket Anesthesia.* Philadelphia, PA: Lippincott Williams & Wilkins.

Chapter

58

Principles of ultrasound-guided nerve blocks

Rejean Gareau and Kamen Vlassakov

Keywords

Ultrasound physics
Transducer properties
Techniques of ultrasonography
Structure appearances under ultrasound
Peripheral equipment

The ultrasound *transducer* emits ultrasound waves (sound waves with a frequency above 20 kHz) and then acts as a *receiver* for the reflected signal. The ultrasound waves interact with the tissues and after attenuation, reflection, refraction, and scattering, the received sound signal is transformed into an electrical signal, which is processed to generate an image.

Ultrasound frequencies used in regional anesthesia range from 4 to 17 MHz. Structures appear differently depending on their *echogenicity*.

Hyperechoic "bright"-appearing images are obtained from structures that have a lower water content and reflect the ultrasound waves – examples would include fascias, distal nerves, tendons, and bone, as well as from areas where the acoustic impedance mismatch (difference in propagation of sound waves) between adjacent tissues is larger.

Hypoechoic structures appear dark and allow waves through with little reflection – examples include patent blood vessels, cysts, effusions, and, to some extent, fat.

US transducers ("probes") are usually *"broad-band"* and emit/receive *low- (4–7 MHz) or high-frequency (10–15 MHz)* ultrasound waves. They can also be linear (flat) or curvilinear (convex). Low-frequency ultrasound penetrates deeper into tissues but produces a lower resolution image than high-frequency ultrasound. Therefore superficial structures, such as the brachial plexus (in the axilla, the supraclavicular fossa, the interscalene groove) are usually visualized better with high-frequency US probes, while low-frequency transducers are recommended for the neuraxial and the proximal sciatic nerve blocks (often also for infraclavicular and paravertebral, and sometimes for TAP blocks).

Structures can be viewed in *short axis (cross-section) or long axis (longitudinal)*.

An *in-plane (IP)* technique involves entry of the needle along the path of imaging toward the target (Figure 59.1).

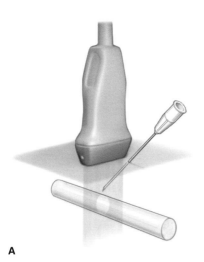

A

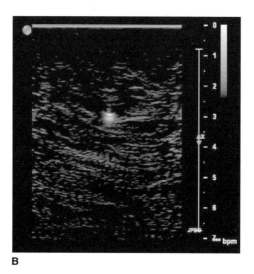

B

Figure 58.1 Short- or transverse-axis IP technique (A) and needle appearance on ultrasound (B). (From Vacanti et al. 2011. *Essential Clinical Anesthesia*, Cambridge University Press, p. 257.)

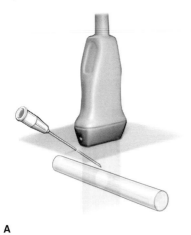

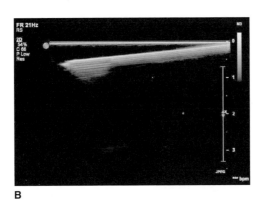

Figure 58.2 Short- or transverse-axis OOP technique (A) and needle tip appearance on ultrasound (B). (From Vacanti et al. 2011. *Essential Clinical Anesthesia*, Cambridge University Press, p. 258.)

A

B

An *out-of-plane (OOP)* technique involves entry of the needle into the path of the ultrasound image from outside the plane of vision and using tissue deflection to ensure accurate needle placement (Figure 58.2).

Peripheral equipment includes *sterile equipment (drapes, local anesthetic, nerve catheters, probe covers, echogenic needles, gel) and cleaning supplies.*

Questions

> a = 1,2,3
> b = 1,3
> c = 2,4
> d = only 4 is correct
> e = all are correct

1. A hypoechoic structure:
   1. appears bright under ultrasound
   2. blocks the transmission of ultrasound waves
   3. has a low water content
   4. may be a blood vessel

2. When performing ultrasound-guided nerve blocks:
   1. nerves are always hyperechoic
   2. bones are always hyperechoic
   3. blood vessels are always avoided
   4. nerves and tendons have similar echogenicity

One best answer:

3. When performing a nerve block under ultrasound guidance, which is NOT TRUE?
   a. Large blood vessels are easily identified.
   b. Bone structures transmit ultrasound well.
   c. The pleural interface appears hyperechoic.
   d. When using the in-plane approach, the entire needle may be visualized.
   e. Nerves are usually easier to visualize than blood vessels.

Answers

1. d. A hypoechoic structure appears dark under ultrasound imaging, transmits ultrasound waves more easily than denser structures, and may have a high water content.
2. c. Under ultrasound guidance, nerves may appear hyperechoic or hypoechoic; tendons have similar hyperechoic image "texture"; bones are hyperechoic, because of enhanced reflection. Blood vessels may be encountered either accidentally or on purpose with use of the ultrasound.
3. e. Nerves are usually more difficult to visualize than blood vessels and they often have similar echogenicity to tendons; the pleural interface appears hyperechoic because of the pronounced impedance mismatch; bone has good US transmission, but high reflection and attenuation.

Further reading

Vacanti, C., Sikka, P., Urman, R., Dershwitz, M., and Segal, B. (eds) (2011). *Essential Clinical Anesthesia.* Cambridge: Cambridge University Press, Chapter 59.

Tsui, B. (2007). *Atlas of Ultrasound and Nerve Stimulation-Guided Regional Anesthesia.* New York: Springer Science+Business Media, LLC, Chapters 3 and 4.

Pollard, B. and Chan, V. (2009). *An Introductory Curriculum for Ultrasound-Guided Regional Anesthesia.* Toronto: UTPPRINT.

Bigeleisen, P. et al. (2010). *Ultrasound-Guided Regional Anesthesia and Pain Medicine.* Philadelphia: Lippincott Williams & Wilkins.

Upper extremity nerve blocks

Rejean Gareau and Kamen Vlassakov

Keywords

Brachial plexus
Interscalene block
Supraclavicular block
Infraclavicular block
Axillary block
Distal nerve blocks

Aide memoire: **Remember To Drink Coffee Black** – **R**oots, **T**runks, **D**ivisions, **C**ords, **B**ranches.

The *brachial plexus* (Figure 59.1) is formed by the primary anterior rami of spinal nerves C5 through T1, known as the "nerve *roots*." Varying contributions from C4 and/or T2 are common. Three *trunks* (superior: C5–6; middle: C7; and inferior: C8, T1) are formed by the nerve roots. Anterior and posterior *divisions* are derived from each trunk and then combine to form three *cords* (lateral, medial, and posterior). While several proximal nerves are derived directly from the trunks and divisions (e.g., the suprascapular nerve), the majority of the peripheral nerves (brachial plexus *branches*) arise from the cords with the most common configuration, as follows:

Lateral cord: **musculocutaneous** nerve, the lateral part of the **median** nerve, lateral pectoral nerve.
Medial cord: **ulnar** nerve, the medial part of the **median** nerve, medial cutaneous nerves of the arm and forearm, medial pectoral nerve.
Posterior cord: **radial** nerve, **axillary** nerve, and subscapular nerves.

Different brachial plexus block approaches are used to anesthetize the upper extremity (the most common are briefly described below). The choice of approach is based on surgical site, individual patient anatomy, and specific coexisting morbidity. To achieve complete anesthesia/analgesia of the upper limb, a separate **intercostal nerve** block (T2–3: supplying cutaneous innervation to the axilla, proximal medial arm, and anterior shoulder) and **cervical plexus** block (C2–4: supplying sensory innervation to the top of the shoulder, supraclavicular fossa, and proximal clavicle) are usually necessary.

It is also important to remember that the sensory innervation of the skin (Figure 59.2.) often does not match that of the underlying tissues, including muscles and bones, as presented by peripheral nerve or spinal "root" supply. Both nerve formation/location and innervation patterns may also vary significantly inter- and intra-individually (left from right side), adding challenges and need for profound anatomy knowledge and expert ultrasound imaging skills.

Interscalene block

Level: roots and proximal trunks
Blocks: shoulder and arm
Not covered (usually): C8, T1, and respective innervation – medial cord (ulnar, medial antebrachial cutaneous, medial brachial cutaneous nerves), medial head of the median nerve, parts of the radial nerve
Location: interscalene groove between anterior and middle scalene muscles at level of C6 (cricoid cartilage line)
Complications: pneumothorax, neural injury, local anesthetic toxicity
Expected side effects: phrenic nerve block (~100%), Horner's syndrome (sympathetic block), voice change (possible recurrent laryngeal nerve block), partial cervical plexus block

Supraclavicular block

Level: trunks and divisions
Blocks: arm, elbow, forearm
Not covered: the dorsal scapular, long thoracic, and sometimes the suprascapular (shoulder joint) nerves are missed; at times complete block of the inferior trunk or T1 root might be difficult to obtain

---

Essential Clinical Anesthesia Review: Keywords, Questions and Answers for the Boards, ed. Linda S. Aglio, Robert W. Lekowski, and Richard D. Urman. Published by Cambridge University Press. © Cambridge University Press 2015.

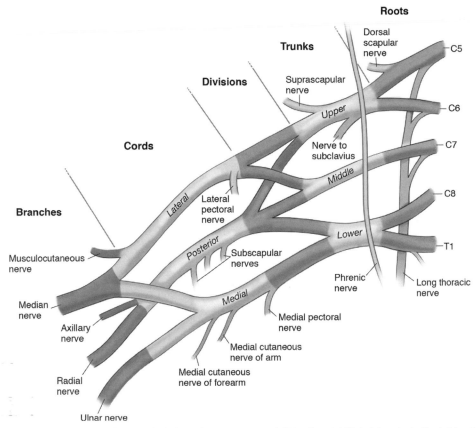

Figure 59.1 Diagram of the brachial plexus. (From Vacanti et al. 2011. *Essential Clinical Anesthesia*, Cambridge University Press, p. 362.)

Location: posterior, lateral, and cephalad to subclavian artery

Complications: pneumothorax (up to 6% before ultrasound-guidance), vascular puncture, chylothorax on left-sided blocks, neural injury, local anesthetic toxicity

Expected side effects: phrenic nerve block (25–60%), Horner's syndrome (sympathetic block)

Infraclavicular block

Level: cords

Blocks: elbow, forearm, hand

Not covered (usually): proximal plexus branches (long thoracic, dorsal scapular, suprascapular, and lateral pectoral nerves)

Location: around subclavian/axillary artery, under the pectoral muscles

Complications: hematoma, neural injury, vascular puncture, chylothorax on left-sided blocks, pneumothorax

Axillary block

Level: branches

Blocks: arm, forearm, hand

Not covered: proximal plexus branches (long thoracic, dorsal scapular, suprascapular, axillary, medial and lateral pectoral nerves)

Location: within the axillary sheath, median nerve anterior and lateral to axillary artery, ulnar nerve posterior and medial to artery, and radial nerve posterior and lateral to artery. Musculocutaneous nerve is found and blocked lateral to the sheath, often with a separate needle pass

Complications: vascular puncture, hematoma, systemic toxicity, and nerve injury*:

Radial nerve: at lateral epicondyle of the humerus, posteromedial to the profunda brachii artery

Median nerve: at antecubital fossa medial to brachial artery

Musculocutaneous nerve: at axillary level lateral to axillary sheath or midhumeral level deep within coracobrachialis muscle

Ulnar nerve: at the midforearm near ulnar artery

Distal nerve blocks can be used for supplementation of incomplete blocks or if there are contraindications to other upper extremity blocks.

Bier block

Used for short procedures (<1.5 hours)

Exsanguination of arm using Esmarch bandage

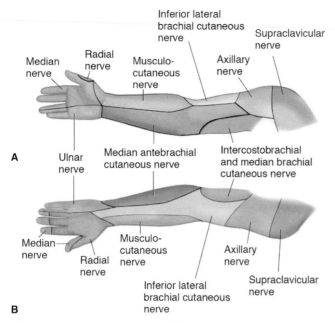

Figure 59.2 Cutaneous innervation of the upper extremity. (A) Arm supinated. (B) Arm prone. (From Vacanti et al. 2011. *Essential Clinical Anesthesia*, Cambridge University Press, p. 362.)

Double-cuff tourniquet with cuff pressure 1.5 times above systolic pressure
Local anesthetic solution injected intravenously
Onset 5 to 10 minutes
Limitations: time, tourniquet pain, local anesthetic toxicity risk (need to use high-volume, low-concentration local anesthetics, e.g., lidocaine 0.5% 30–50 ml for average adult)

Questions

a = 1,2,3
b = 1,3
c = 2,4
d = only 4 is correct
e = all are correct

1. The lateral cord:
   1. is involved in arm abduction
   2. is responsible for elbow flexion
   3. includes the musculocutaneous and radial nerves
   4. provides partial movement in forearm pronation and wrist flexion

2. The ulnar nerve:
   1. originates from C8 and T1
   2. allows 5th finger flexion and opposition
   3. is derived from the medial cord
   4. is often missed or incompletely blocked with supraclavicular blocks

One best answer:

3. Which statement about the brachial plexus is CORRECT?
   a. The intercostobrachial nerve is a proximal branch of the brachial plexus.
   b. The brachial plexus is formed by the C2 to C8 spinal nerves.
   c. The trunks of the brachial plexus are formed and travel with the subclavian artery.
   d. The brachial plexus cords are found in the proximal supraclavicular fossa.
   e. All brachial plexus blocks are associated with moderate to high risk of pneumothorax.

4. When performing a supraclavicular nerve block with ultrasound guidance:
   a. Continuous aspiration is not necessary.
   b. The nerves of the brachial plexus are usually visualized surrounding the subclavian artery.
   c. Phrenic nerve block is very rare at less than 1%.
   d. The first rib is usually easy to identify.
   e. The musculocutaneous nerve is easy to visualize and block.

Answers

1. c. The lateral cord includes the musculocutaneous nerve and part of the median nerve, which allows for elbow flexion, forearm pronation, and wrist flexion.
2. e. All answers are correct.
3. c. The intercostobrachial nerve is a distal branch of the brachial plexus. The brachial plexus is formed by C5 to T1 spinal nerves with the occasional contributions from C4 and T2. The brachial plexus cords can be found below the clavicle (infraclavicular). Brachial plexus blocks are associated with a small risk of pneumothorax, especially when using ultrasound guidance.
4. d. Continuous aspiration aids in assessment of entry into vessels including the subclavian artery and helps to avoid unanticipated intravascular injection. The nerves of the brachial plexus are located lateral to the subclavian artery. Phrenic nerve block is seen in approximately 60% of supraclavicular blocks. The musculocutaneous nerve can be identified in the axillary block but not in the supraclavicular block.

Further reading

Vacanti, C., Sikka, P., Urman, R., Dershwitz, M., and Segal, B. (eds) (2011). *Essential Clinical Anesthesia*. Cambridge: Cambridge University Press, Chapter 60.

Tsui, B. (2007). *Atlas of Ultrasound and Nerve Stimulation-Guided Regional Anesthesia*. New York: Springer Science +Business Media, LLC, Chapters 5, 6, 7, 8, 9, and 10.

Lower extremity nerve blocks

Rejean Gareau and Kamen Vlassakov

Keywords

Lumbar plexus
Femoral nerve block
Lateral femoral cutaneous nerve block
Obturator nerve block
Sciatic nerve block
Popliteal nerve block
Ankle block

The *lumbar plexus* is formed by the anterior rami of spinal nerves L1–4. Occasionally, T12 and L5 contribute.

L1 (T12) forms the *iliohypogastric and ilioinguinal nerves*.
L1 and L2 form the *genitofemoral nerve*.
L2–L4 form the **obturator** *nerve* (anterior divisions) and the *lateral femoral cutaneous and femoral nerves* (posterior divisions).

Lumbar plexus (psoas compartment) block

Origin: L1–4
Supplies: lower extremity
Location: psoas compartment, 4 to 5 cm from midline at level of iliac crest
Complications: hematoma, nerve injury, vascular puncture, local anesthetic toxicity, spread of local anesthetic to epidural or subarachnoid space

Femoral nerve block

Origin: L2–4
Supplies: anterior thigh, knee, medial thigh and leg, sartorius, pectineus and quadriceps muscles, medial ankle
Location: lateral to femoral vessels, covered by fascia iliaca
Complications: vascular puncture, hematoma, neural injury, local anesthetic toxicity

Lateral femoral cutaneous nerve block

Origin: L2–3
Supplies: lateral thigh

Location: distal to the inguinal ligament, it is found below fascia lata, between the sartorius and iliacus muscles, medial to the tensor fasciae latae muscle, and superficial to the fascia iliaca
Complications: hematoma, neural injury, local anesthetic toxicity

Obturator nerve block

Origin: L2–4
Supplies: sensory – medial thigh and hip joint; motor – thigh adductors
Location: deep and medial to femoral vessels; between the adductor muscles
Complications: hematoma, vascular puncture, neural injury, local anesthetic toxicity

"3 in 1" block and fascia iliaca block (FIB)

These are techniques **designed to block the femoral, lateral femoral cutaneous, and obturator nerves with one high-volume injection** (20–45 ml in adult patients) of local anesthetics, by localizing either the femoral nerve ("3 in 1") or the tissue plane immediately beneath the fascia iliaca (FIB). These techniques are easy to perform, useful, and widely popular.

However, it is important to remember that **while the femoral and lateral femoral cutaneous nerves are blocked very consistently, complete block of the obturator nerve is rarely achieved** (in about 50% or less).

Sciatic nerve block

Origin: L4–S3. Consists of tibial (medial) and common peroneal (lateral) nerves, which separate in the popliteal fossa
Supplies: posterior thigh and knee, lateral leg, ankle, superior and inferior foot
Locations/approaches:

posterior: 4 cm distal to midline between posterior superior iliac spine and greater trochanter

---

Essential Clinical Anesthesia Review: Keywords, Questions and Answers for the Boards, ed. Linda S. Aglio, Robert W. Lekowski, and Richard D. Urman. Published by Cambridge University Press. © Cambridge University Press 2015.

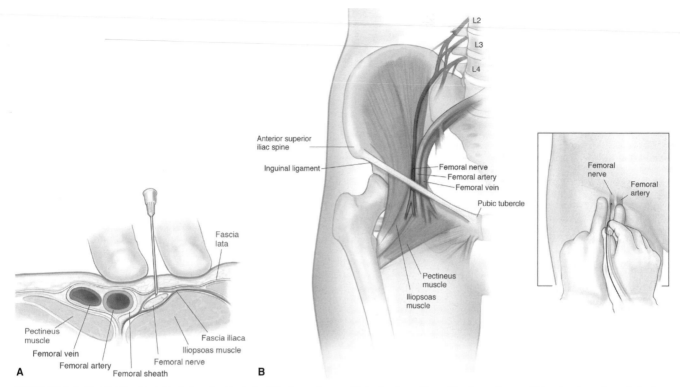

Figure 60.1 Surface landmarks and technique for blockade of the femoral nerve. (A) Anatomic position of the femoral nerve. (B) Landmarks and needle for femoral nerve block. From: Vacanti et al., 2011. *Essential Clinical Anesthesia*, Cambridge University Press, p. 373.

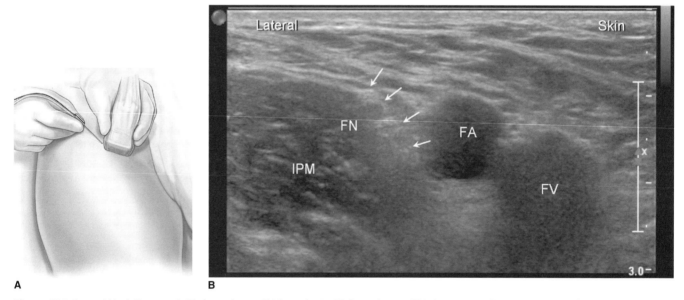

Figure 60.2 Femoral block IP approach. FA, femoral artery; FV, femoral vein; FN, femoral nerve; IPM, iliopsoas muscle. From: Vacanti et al., 2011. *Essential Clinical Anesthesia*, Cambridge University Press, p. 374.

subgluteal: 4 cm caudal to midline between greater trochanter and ischial tuberosity
Franco: 10 cm lateral to intergluteal sulcus
popliteal fossa: between biceps femoris (laterally) and semimembranosus and semitendinosus (medially)

muscles. Under ultrasound guidance, the sciatic nerve is usually blocked above the bifurcation of the nerve into tibial and common peroneal components

Complications: hematoma, vascular puncture, neural injury, local anesthetic toxicity

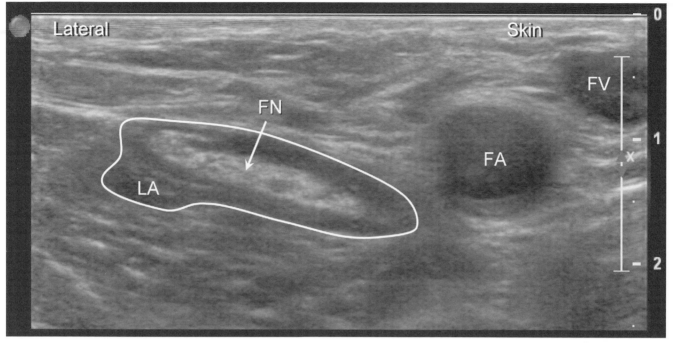

Figure 60.3 Femoral nerve post injection. FA, femoral artery; FV, femoral vein; FN, femoral nerve; LA, local anesthetic. (From: Vacanti et al. 2011. *Essential Clinical Anesthesia*, Cambridge University Press, p. 375.)

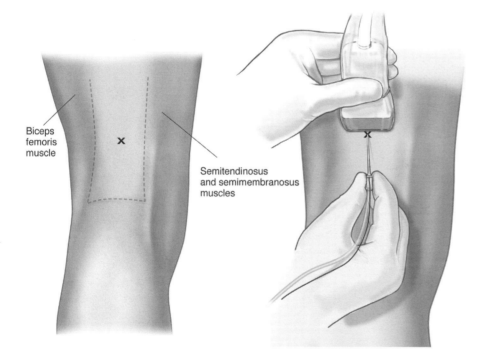

Figure 60.4 Popliteal block OOP approach; X, needle insertion site. (From: Vacanti et al. 2011. *Essential Clinical Anesthesia*, Cambridge University Press, p. 378.)

Ankle block

There are five nerves to block:
Deep nerves:

- *posterior tibial (posterior to medial malleolus)*
- *deep peroneal (between the extensor hallucis longus tendon medially and extensor digitorum longus tendon laterally)*

Superficial nerves:

- *superficial peroneal (subcutaneous injection over lateral foot)*
- *sural (posterior to lateral malleolus)*
- *saphenous (subcutaneous injection over medial ankle)*

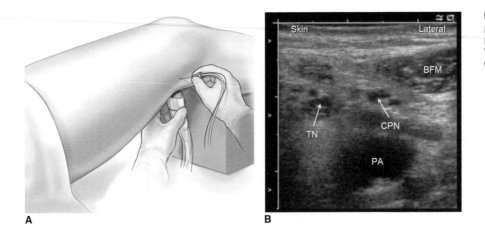

A   B

Figure 60.5 Popliteal block IP approach. PA popliteal artery; TN, tibial nerve; CPN, common peroneal nerve; BFM, biceps femoris muscle. (From: Vacanti et al. 2011. *Essential Clinical Anesthesia*, Cambridge University Press, p. 378.)

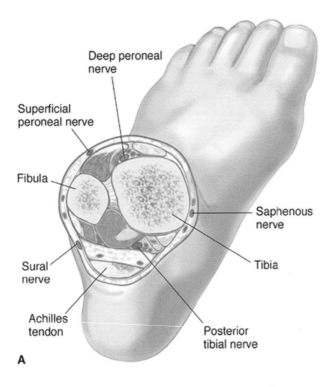

A

Figure 60.6 Innervation of the foot. (A) Anatomy of the five nerves innervating the foot. (B) Cutaneous distribution of the nerves of the foot. (From Vacanti et al. 2011. *Essential Clinical Anesthesia*, Cambridge University Press, p. 380.)

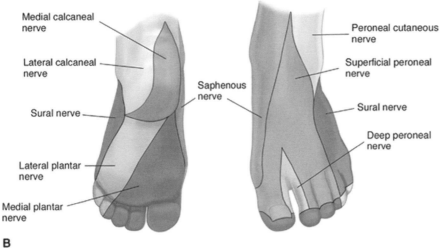

B

Questions

A = 1,2,3
B = 1,3
C = 2,4
D = only 4 is correct
E = all are correct

1. The femoral nerve:
   1. lies above the iliacus muscle
   2. arises from the lumbar plexus levels L2, 3, 4
   3. is responsible for knee extension
   4. causes a patellar twitch when stimulated

2. Sciatic nerve:
   1. stimulation causes foot dorsiflexion
   2. stimulation causes foot plantar flexion
   3. stimulation causes foot eversion
   4. stimulation causes knee extension

One best CORRECT answer:

3. The femoral nerve:
   a. travels antero-medially to the psoas muscle
   b. is found between the fascia lata and fascia iliaca
   c. is usually located 4 to 6 cm lateral from the femoral artery at the inguinal crease
   d. is usually blocked with the fascia iliaca compartment block
   e. is located very close to the obturator and lateral femoral cutaneous nerves at the inguinal crease

4. The femoral nerve block:
   a. is sufficient to provide anesthesia for major knee surgery
   b. is often performed with the "paresthesia technique"
   c. is never associated with local anesthetic toxicity
   d. should never be performed on patients on antiplatelet medications
   e. may be performed both in-plane and out-of-plane under ultrasound guidance

5. Which ONE of the following statements is NOT correct:
   a. When performing a femoral nerve block with nerve stimulation, the goal is to elicit patellar movement.
   b. When performing a femoral nerve block with a nerve stimulator, intraneural injection is impossible.
   c. When performing a femoral nerve block, the needle is always inserted lateral to the femoral artery pulsation.
   d. When performing a femoral nerve block with ultrasound guidance, continuous aspiration during needle advancement is mandatory.
   e. A femoral nerve block does not always produce adductor muscle weakness.

Answers

1. e. All answers are correct.
2. a. Knee extension is facilitated by the femoral nerve.
3. d. The femoral nerve travels between the psoas muscle and iliacus muscle underneath (covered by) fascia iliaca. It is also deep to the fascia lata and is located approximately 1 cm lateral to the femoral artery. The fascia iliaca block is performed in the same plane as the femoral nerve is located and it is, subsequently, often blocked during the procedure.
4. e. The femoral nerve does not supply the posterior compartment of the knee and its blockade is therefore not sufficient for surgical anesthesia. It is most often performed with either ultrasound guidance, nerve stimulation, or both. It can be performed in patients taking antiplatelet medications, as it is in a compressible area of the body should hematoma form. Local anesthetic toxicity is a complication that can occur with any nerve blockade.
5. b. Intraneural injection is possible even under ultrasound guidance.

Further reading

Vacanti, C., Sikka, P., Urman, R., Dershwitz, M., and Segal, B. (eds) (2011). *Essential Clinical Anesthesia*. Cambridge: Cambridge University Press, Chapter 61.

Tsui, B. (2007). *Atlas of Ultrasound and Nerve Stimulation-Guided Regional Anesthesia*. New York: Springer Science +Business Media, LLC, Chapters 11, 12, 13, 14, 15.

Fluid replacement

Pingping Song and Gyorgy Frendl

Keywords

Body fluid distribution
Clinical evaluation of fluid status
Body compensation for hypovolemia
Perioperative fluid deficit
Perioperative fluid replacement
Advantages and disadvantages of crystalloid colloid
  versus crystalloid resuscitation

Fluid compartments and body fluid distribution

Body fluid distribution

Total body water ranges from 50% (in females) to 60% (in males) of body mass and is distributed differentially among body tissues (Table 61.1).

Fluid shift between body compartments

The movement of body fluid across the capillary membrane is defined by the Ernest Starling equation:

$$J_v = K_f ([P_c - P_i] - \sigma[\pi_c - \pi_i])$$

where J_v is the net fluid movement across the capillary membrane; K_f is the filtration coefficient, which is a constant; P_c is the capillary hydrostatic pressure; P_i is the interstitial hydrostatic pressure; π_c is the capillary oncotic pressure; π_i is the interstitial oncotic pressure; σ is the reflection coefficient, describing the permeability of a substance through a specific capillary membrane.

The major protein responsible for the oncotic pressure is albumin. Crystalloid decreases the oncotic pressure of plasma, driving fluid movement from capillary to interstitium, causing edema formation.

Clinical evaluation of fluid status

- **History:** NPO status; nausea/vomiting; diarrhea; bowel preparation; diuresis; trauma; burns; infection; pleural effusion; ascites; fever; hyperventilation.
- **Physical exam:**
  - *signs of intravascular volume depletion*:

    dry mucous membrane; poor skin turgor; tented skin tone; flat neck veins
    orthostatic signs
    tachycardia with a weak, thready pulse
    dark and concentrated urine
  - *signs of volume overload*:

    pitting edema; tachycardia; pulmonary crackles; wheezing; cyanosis.
- **Lab indicators** of intravascular volume depletion:
  - increased HCT, plasma sodium or base deficit; high serum osmolarity; low mixed venous oxygenation saturation
  - **prerenal azotemia:** serum BUN/creatinine ratio >20
  - urine analysis: low urine sodium (<20 mEq/L); Fe Na <1%; high urine specific gravity (>1.025 in adults); high urine osmolarity (>800 mOsm/kg).
- **Invasive monitors:** stroke volume variation (SVV), CVP, PCWP:
  - SVV: stroke volume variation. Dynamic indicator for fluid responsiveness in patients on mechanical ventilation and in normal sinus rhythm. SVV >10–15

Table 61.1 Body fluid distribution

	Total body weight
Total body water (TBW)	60%
Intracellular fluid (ICF)	40%
Extracellular fluid (ECF)	20%
Lymph and interstitial fluid	15%
Plasma	5%

Essential Clinical Anesthesia Review: Keywords, Questions and Answers for the Boards, ed. Linda S. Aglio, Robert W. Lekowski, and Richard D. Urman. Published by Cambridge University Press. © Cambridge University Press 2015.

indicates fluid responsiveness (administrating fluid will increase stroke volume)

$$SVV = (SV_{max} - SV_{min})/SVmean$$

.   PCWP: static indicator. Together with values of cardiac output (CO), systemic vascular resistance (SVR), and pulmonary vascular resistance (PVR), pulmonary arterial catheter (PAC) will provide valuable information on patient's volume status; but high risks associated with PA catheter insertion

.   CVP: static indicator. The trend of CVP is more informative than the absolute value. CVP can not accurately predict left-side filling pressure in the presence of RV dysfunction, COPD, cor pulmonale, or pulmonic/tricuspid valve pathology.

Body compensation for hypovolemia

1. Activation of sympathetic nervous system: increased sympathetic tone, peripheral vasoconstriction.
2. Activation of renin–angiotensin–aldosterone and ADH system: increased levels of angiotensin I, angiotensin II, and aldosterone; increased level of ADH (vasopressin).
3. Decreased levels of atrial natriuretic peptide.

Perioperative fluid deficit

1. Preexisting fluid deficit:

   ● NPO status
   ● vomiting, diarrhea, diuresis; hemodialysis
   ● drainage of body cavity fluid accumulation: pleural effusion, pericardial effusion, or ascites
   ● insensible loss due to burns, fever, hyperventilation.

2. Maintenance requirement for each kg of body weight:

   ● 1–10 kg: 4 ml/kg/h
   ● 10–20 kg: 40 ml/h + 2 ml/kg/h
   ● 20 kg and above: 60 ml/h + 1 ml/kg/h.

3. Surgical loss: blood loss and "third space" redistribution:

● blood loss: 1:3 ratio supplement by crystalloid; 1:1 ratio supplement by colloid or blood product
● estimate blood loss from surgical sponges: fully soaked sponge (4 × 4) holds 10 ml of blood; fully soaked laparotomy pads "laps" hold 100–150 ml of blood
● "third space" redistribution: surgical trauma and inflammation create extracellular fluid sequestration into a "third space" not in equilibrium with the interstitial or plasma compartments (Table 61.2). Fluid in the "third space" cannot be readily mobilized into the intravascular space until days later.

Perioperative fluid replacement

● Goal: achieve euvolemia, optimize cardiac output, ensure adequate tissue oxygenation, and correct coagulopathy.
● Types of fluid replacement: crystalloid or colloid (Table 61.3).

Advantages and disadvantages of crystalloid

● Decreases plasma oncotic pressure, causing fluid to shift from intravascular space to interstitium.
● Interstitial rather than intravascular volume expansion: 80% of crystalloid will leave the intravascular space about 30 minutes after administration.
● Inexpensive.
● Low risk of allergic reaction.

Table 61.2 "Third space" fluid deficit classification

Scale of surgical stress	Estimated "third space" deficit
Minimal (herniorrhaphy)	1–2 ml/kg/h
Moderate (appendectomy)	2–4 ml/kg/h
Severe (colectomy)	4–8 ml/kg/h

(Adapted from: Vacanti et al., 2011, p. 385.)

Table 61.3 Composition of replacement fluids

Fluid	Electrolytes (mEq/l)					Osmolarity(mOsm/l)	pH	Buffers (mEq/l)
	Na	Cl	K	Ca	Mg			
Plasma	141	103	4–5	5	2	289	7.4	Bicarbonate (26)
0.9% sodium chloride	154	154				308	5.7	—
Lactated Ringer's solution	130	109	4	3		273	6.4	Lactate(28)
Normosol or plasma-lyte	140	98	5		3	295	7.4	Acetate (27) Gluconate (23)
5% albumin	145 ± 15	<2.5				330	7.4	—
Hetastarch	154					310	5.9	—

(Adapted from *Miller's Anesthesia*, 7th edn. and Stapczynski, J. S. et al. 1994. *Emerg Med Reports*, 15:245.)

Table 61.4 Degree and duration of volume expansion

Fluid	Volume infused (ml)	Plasma volume expansion (ml)	Time in plasma
NS or LR	1,000	250	2–3 h
5% albumin	500	375	Half-life 16 h
25% albumin	100	450	Half-life 16 h
Hetastarch	500	650	12–48 h

(Contributed by Dr. Gyorgy Frendl.)

Characteristics of different types of crystalloid

- Normal saline (0.9% NaCl): isotonic and iso-osmotic, but contains more chloride than plasma:
  - large volume resuscitation will cause non-anion gap hyperchloremic metabolic acidosis
  - preferred in conditions of brain injury, hypochloremic metabolic alkalosis, or hyponatremia.
- Lactate Ringer's solution: balanced salt solution, mildly hypo-osmotic compared to plasma:
  - no concerns of causing acidosis
  - contains potassium, use with caution in patients with hyperkalemia or renal failure
  - contains calcium, avoid mixing with blood products
  - may worsen cerebral edema.

Advantages and disadvantages of colloid

- Larger molecular weight, more rapid volume expansion, remains in the intravascular space for longer (Table 61.4).
- Colloid eventually also enters the interstitial space. Removal of colloids requires longer periods than crystalloids.
- Clinically used colloids include natural colloid (albumin) and synthetic hetastarch:
  - albumin: available in 5% and 25% solutions; most expensive of all fluids; low incidence of allergic reaction; theoretical risk of infection:

    - there is no difference in mortality and major outcome when administrating albumin compared to normal saline in critically ill patients
    - albumin is associated with higher rate of mortality in patients with traumatic brain injury.
  - hetastarch: three preparations are available in the United States – Hespan: 6% HES 450/0.7; Hextend: 6% HES 670/0.7; Voluven: 6% HES 130/0.4:
    - affect on coagulation: reduces levels of factor VIII and vWF, with prolongation of the partial thromboplastin time; interferes with platelet adhesion and clot formation. Maximal dose for hespan is 20 ml/kg/day
    - Voluven (6% HES 130/0.4) has an improved safety profile compared to Hespan due to lower molecular size. But recent studies have shown increased mortality and renal failure in severe septic patients.

In conclusion, there is no "ideal" fluid for resuscitation currently; edema is the consequence of fluid resuscitation, regardless of the type of fluid chosen.

Question

1. Fluid resuscitation during major abdominal surgery with which of the following agents is associated with the best survival data?
   a. 5% albumin
   b. 6% hydroxyethyl starch
   c. dextran 70
   d. hypertonic saline
   e. none of the above

Answer

1. e. None of the listed agents has been shown to have clear advantages over the others.

Further reading

Chappell, D., Jacob, M., Hofmann-Kiefer, K., et al. (2008). A rational approach to perioperative fluid management. *Anesthesiology* 109, 723–740.

SAFE Study Investigators: Finfer, S., Bellomo, R., Boyce, N., et al. (2004). A comparison of albumin and saline for fluid resuscitation in the intensive care unit. *New England Journal of Medicine* 350, 2247–2256.

SAFE Study Investigators (2007). Saline or albumin for fluid resuscitation in patients with traumatic brain injury. *New England Journal of Medicine* 357, 874–884.

Perner, A., Haase, N., Guttormsen, A. B. et al. (2012). Hydroxyethyl starch 130/0.42 versus Ringer's acetate in severe sepsis. *New England Journal of Medicine* 367, 124–134.

Vacanti, C. A., Sikka, P. K., Urman, R. D., Dershwitz, M., and Scott Segal, B. (2011). *Essential Clinical Anesthesia*, 1st edn. Cambridge University Press.

Miller, D. (2011). *Miller's Basics of Anesthesia*, 6th edn. Saunders.

Frendl, G. and Urman, R. (2012). *Pocket ICU*, 1st edn. Lippincott Williams & Wilkins.

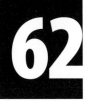

Chapter 62

Acid–base balance in anesthesia and intensive care medicine

Pingping Song and Gyorgy Frendl

Normal values used for interpretation of acid–base disorders

pH: 7.36–7.44
$PaCO_2$: 40 mm Hg
HCO_3^-: 24 mEq/l
H^+: 40 nmol/l

Definitions

- acidemia: blood pH <7.36
- alkalemia: blood pH >7.44
- acidosis: a process causing acid (proton) accumulation (not necessarily implying an abnormal pH)
- alkalosis: a process causing alkali accumulation (not necessarily implying an abnormal pH)

Body buffering system

- Bicarbonate/carbonic acid:

$$CO_2 + H_2O \rightleftharpoons H_2CO_3 \rightleftharpoons HCO_3^- + H^+$$

The equilibrium is catalyzed by the enzyme carbonic anhydrase, which is most active in the kidneys, red blood cells, and liver.

- Phosphate
- Serum protein: albumin
- Serum hemoglobin

Bicarbonate is the most important buffering system of all.

Body compensation to pH abnormalities

- Respiratory compensation: fast response via central and peripheral chemoreceptors:
  - central chemoreceptors: in medulla, respond to changes of pH in cerebrospinal fluid. Most sensitive to hydrogen ions
  - peripheral chemoreceptors: carotid bodies at the bifurcation of common carotid arteries, respond to changes of pH, PaO_2, and $PaCO_2$ in blood. Most sensitive to PaO_2.
- Renal compensation: slow onset and takes up to five days to achieve maximal response. Three mechanisms: (1) reabsorption of the filtered HCO_3^-; (2) excretion of hydrogen ions; (3) production of ammonia.

Interpreting acid–base disorders

Rule of thumb:

1. pH determines the leading acidemia or alkalemia disorder.
2. Changes in $PaCO_2$ cause serum HCO_3^- changes in the same direction; changes in $PaCO_2$ cause serum pH changes in the opposite direction, and vice versa.
3. Body never overcompensates. The compensating mechanisms can only lead pH toward (but not to) normal; they can not overcorrect pH to the opposite of the primary acid–base imbalance.
4. If actual HCO_3^- or $PaCO_2$ values are different from predicted values, a mixed acid–base disorder exists.

Key concepts in acid–base physiology
Henderson–Hasselbalch equation

Calculate the pH of blood to constituents of the bicarbonate buffering system.

$$pH = pK_{a\ H_2CO_3} + \log\left(\frac{HCO_3^-}{H_2CO_3}\right)$$

Essential Clinical Anesthesia Review: Keywords, Questions and Answers for the Boards, ed. Linda S. Aglio, Robert W. Lekowski, and Richard D. Urman. Published by Cambridge University Press. © Cambridge University Press 2015.

Table 62.1 Primary acid–base disturbance

Primary disorder	Changes in PaCO₂ (mm Hg)	Changes in HCO₃⁻ (mEq/l)	Changes in pH
Acute respiratory acidosis	10	1	0.08
Acute respiratory alkalosis	10	2	0.08
Chronic respiratory acidosis	10	4	0.03
Chronic respiratory alkalosis	10	5	0.03
Primary disorder	**Changes in HCO₃⁻ (mEq/l)**	**Changes in PaCO₂ (mm Hg)**	**Formulas**
Metabolic acidosis	1	1	$PaCO_2 = 1.5 \times HCO_3^- + 8 \, +/-2$
Metabolic alkalosis	10	7	$PaCO_2 = 0.9 \times HCO_3^- + 16$

(Frendl, G. and Urman, R. 2012. *Pocket ICU*, 1st edn. Lippincott Williams & Wilkins, p. 7-1.)

- $pK_{a\ H_2CO_3}$ is the pH at which 50% of the carbonic acid is ionized in the blood. It is equal to 6.1.
- $[HCO_3^-]$ is the concentration of bicarbonate in the blood.
- $[H_2CO_3]$ is the concentration of carbonic acid in the blood.

Components of normal plasma in acid–base physiology

- Weak ions: incompletely dissociated at physiological pH. They include bicarbonate (HCO_3^-), charged albumin (Alb^-), and inorganic phosphate (P_i^-).
- Strong ions: completely dissociated (>99.9%) at all physiological pH levels. They include Na^+, K^+, Ca^{2+}, Mg^{2+}, Cl^-, organic acids (lactic acid, keto acids, sulfate, methanol, aspirin, ethylene glycol, etc.).
- Water and its dissociation products. Water is present in a very high concentration and only slightly dissociated.

Stewart hypothesis

Three independent variables determining acid–base balance:
1. $PaCO_2$
2. concentration of weak anions: albumin and inorganic phosphate
3. strong ion difference (SID) = $[Na^+ + K^+ + Ca^{2+} + Mg^{2+}]$ – Cl^- – lactic acid

Anion gap and base excess

- anion gap (AG) = $Na^+ - (HCO_3^- + Cl^-)$
- normal value: 8–12 mEq/l
- base excess (BE): +/–2 mEq/l

Both AG and BE need to be corrected for abnormal serum albumin level ([Albumin] g/dl).

$AG_{corrected} = AG_{observed} + 2.5 \times$ ([normal albumin] – [measured albumin])

$BE_{corrected} = BE_{observed} + 3.7 \times$ ([normal albumin] – [measured albumin])

Determining the underlying cause of the acid–base imbalance is key to the successful care of the patient.

Systemic effects of acidemia

- Cardiovascular system: arrhythmia; arterial vasodilation; decrease cardiac output; decrease responses to vasopressors and catecholamines.
- Respiratory: respiratory muscle fatigue; pulmonary vasoconstriction.
- Cerebral: vasodilation.
- Metabolic: hyperkalemia; insulin resistance; decreased ATP synthesis.

Treatment of severe acidemia

- Correct underlying causes.
- Intravenous $NaHCO_3$ until pH $\geq$7.2 and HCO_3^- reaches 8–10 mEq/l. Although no benefit has been proven for the use of $NaHCO_3$, it is administered when pH <7.2 to maintain the activity of body enzymes and body responses to vasopressors.
  - For intubated patients: need to increase minute ventilation prior to $NaHCO_3$ administration.
  - For patients with poor pulmonary reserve or undergoing CPR, rapid $NaHCO_3$ infusion will cause acute increase of $PaCO_2$, and paradoxical intracellular or even extracellular acidosis may occur.
- Hemodialysis can rapidly correct acidemia.

Systemic effects of alkalemia

- Cardiovascular system: arrhythmia; arterial vasoconstriction; angina.
- Respiratory: decreases ventilation, may cause hypoxemia; reverses hypoxemic pulmonary vasoconstriction, worsens V/Q mismatch; respiratory alkalosis may also cause bronchospasm and direct lung injury.
- Cerebral: vasoconstriction; seizure, delirium, tetany.
- Metabolic: hypokalemia; decreases serum calcium, magnesium and phosphate levels; increases anaerobic glycolysis, increases lactate and ketones.

Treatment of severe alkalemia

- Correct underlying causes.
- Goal: HCO_3^- <40 mEq/l, pH <7.55.
- Hemodialysis can rapidly correct alkalemia.
- In metabolic alkalosis, measure urinary chloride concentration:
  . if urine $[Cl^-]$ <20 mmol/l, the alkalosis is chloride sensitive and can be corrected with normal saline
  . if urine $[Cl^-]$ >20 mmol/l (except if patient is on diuretics), the alkalosis is chloride resistant, aggressively correct with KCl
  . if patient is hypervolemic, give acetazolamide (e.g., contraction alkalosis with CHF).

Causes of metabolic acidosis

Calculate anion gap (AG) with correction of serum albumin.

- Non-AG metabolic acidosis: bicarbonate loss from GI tract or excretion from renal proximal tubules; impaired H^+ excretion from renal collecting tubules:
  . GI loss: ostomy loss (colostomy, ureterosigmoidostomy, etc.); diarrhea; pancreatic fistula
  . renal causes: renal tubular acidosis; early renal failure
  . iatrogenic: carbonic anhydrase inhibitors; large volume saline resuscitation; TPN (excessive chloride compared to acetate); amino acids.
- AG metabolic acidosis ("KUSMALE"). Unmeasured anions: ketones, lactate, phosphates, sulfates, etc. conjugate H^+ and contribute to metabolic acidosis:
  . ketones: beta-hydroxybutyrate and acetoacetate. diabetic ketoacidosis; alcoholic ketoacidosis; starvation ketoacidosis
  . uremia: accumulation of phosphates, sulfates
  . salicylates: metabolic acidosis from lactate and ketones; respiratory alkalosis from CNS stimulation
  . methanol: formate accumulation
  . alcohol: ethanol, isopropyl alcohol
  . lactate: overproduction by anaerobic metabolism. Sepsis, bowel ischemia, carbon monoxide toxicity, seizure; liver failure, thiamine deficiency, metformin, linezolid
  . ethylene glycol: anti-freeze intoxication.
- Osmolar gap (OG): OG = measured osmolarity – calculated osmolarity:
  . Calculated osmolarity= $2 \times Na + Glucose/18 + BUN/2.8 + EtOH/4.6$
  . If OG >10, suspect ingestion of toxins, such as methanol, ethylene glycol.

Causes of metabolic alkalosis

- Saline responsive: urine Cl^- <20 mEq/l.
- Volume depletion: vomiting, nasogastric tube suction, diuresis.

- Saline resistant: urine Cl^- >20 mEq/l:
  . hypertensive: hyperaldosteronism; Cushing's syndrome; exogenous mineralocorticoids
  . normotensive: profound hypokalemia; exogenous alkali administration (milk alkali syndrome, acetate in TPN, citrate in blood products); Bartter's/Gitelman's syndrome (genetic mutation of the ion channel protein at the loop of renal tubules); refeeding syndrome.

Causes of respiratory acidosis

$PaCO_2$ reflects the balance between CO_2 production and alveolar ventilation.

- Increased CO_2 production:
  . malignant hyperthermia
  . hyperthyroidism
  . sepsis
  . overfeeding
- Decreased CO_2 elimination:
  . intrinsic pulmonary disease (pneumonia, acute respiratory distress syndrome [ARDS], fibrosis, pulmonary edema)
  . upper airway obstruction (laryngospasm, foreign body, obstructive sleep apnea [OSA])
  . lower airway obstruction (asthma, chronic obstructive pulmonary disease [COPD])
  . chest wall restriction (obesity, scoliosis, burns, flail chest, pleural effusion or fibrosis, pneumothorax)
  . CNS depression (anesthetics, opioids, CNS lesions)
  . decreased skeletal muscle strength (residual effects of neuromuscular blocking drugs, myopathy, neuropathy, hypophosphatemia)
- Increased rebreathing or absorption:
  . exhausted soda lime
  . incompetent one-way valve
  . laparoscopic surgery

Causes of respiratory alkalosis

- Increased minute ventilation:
  . hypoxia (high altitude, low FiO_2, severe anemia)
  . iatrogenic (mechanical ventilation)
  . anxiety and pain
  . CNS disease (tumor, infection, trauma)
  . fever, sepsis
  . drugs (salicylates, progesterone, doxapram, beta-agonists)
  . liver disease
  . pregnancy
  . restrictive lung disease
  . pulmonary embolism (can also cause increased $PaCO_2$ with massive PE due to largely increased dead space)

- Decreased production:
  - hypothermia
  - skeletal muscle paralysis

Questions

1. An acute increase in $PaCO_2$ of 10 mm Hg will result in a decrease in pH of:
   a. 0.01 pH units
   b. 0.02 pH units
   c. 0.04 pH units
   d. 0.08 pH units

2. A 44-year-old patient is hyperventilated to a $PaCO_2$ of 24 mm Hg for 48 hours. What $[HCO_3^-]$ level do you expect?
   a. 10 mEq/l
   b. 12 mEq/l
   c. 14 mEq/l
   d. 16 mEq/l

Answers

1. d. In acute respiratory acidosis, an increase of $PaCO_2$ of 10 mm Hg will result in a decrease of pH of approximately 0.08 pH units.

2. b. Total body deficit of $[HCO_3^-]$ can be estimated as follows: total body weight (kg) $\times$ (24 − serum $[HCO_3^-]$ level) $\times$ 0.3.

Further reading

Vacanti, C. A., Sikka, P. K., Urman, R. D., Dershwitz, M., and Scott Segal, B. (2011). *Essential Clinical Anesthesia*, 1st edn. Cambridge University Press.

Miller, R. D. (2011). *Miller's Basics of Anesthesia*, 6th edn. Saunders.

Frendl, G. and Urman, R. (2012). *Pocket ICU*, 1st edn. Lippincott Williams & Wilkins.

Chapter

Ion balance

63

Pingping Song and Gyorgy Frendl

Keywords

Hypernatremia
Hyponatremia
Hyperkalemia
Hypokalemia
Calcium and phosphate balance
Magnesium balance

Table 63.1 Electrolyte composition in body fluids (normal)

Electrolyte	Plasma (mEq/l)	Interstitial fluid (mEq/l)	Intracellular fluid (mEq/l)
Na^+	142	145	10
K^+	4	4	159
Mg^{2+}	2	2	40
Ca^{2+}	5	3	1
Cl^-	103	117	10
HCO_3^-	25	27	7

(Adapted from Campbell, I. 2006. Physiology of fluid balance. *Anaesthesia and Intensive Care Medicine*, 7:462–465.)

Hypernatremia

Total body sodium determines clinical volume status, as sodium draws water wherever it is concentrated. Sodium is also essential for generation of action potentials in various tissues of the body. Sodium is regulated mainly by aldosterone, antidiuretic hormone (ADH), and atrial natriuretic peptide (ANP). The normal range of plasma sodium is 135 to 145 mEq/l, and the adult requirement of daily sodium is 1 to 2 mEq/kg/day.

Hypernatremia is defined as plasma sodium >145 mEq/l. It reflects a deficit of total body free water.

Causes of hypernatremia

Depending on patient's volume status:

- Hypovolemic patient:
  - extrarenal loss: urine osmolarity >600 and urine [Na^+] <20 mEq/l; inadequate access to free water; diarrhea; burns
  - renal loss: urine [Na^+] >20 mEq/l; diuretics use; osmotic diuresis (DKA); adrenal insufficiency; postobstructive nephropathy; recovery phase of acute tubular necrosis.
- Euvolemic patient:
  - diabetic insipidus (DI); lack of ADH resulting in excessive loss of free water
  - central DI: brain pathology, surgery, trauma, tumor etc.
  - nephrogenic DI:
    - drugs: lithium, amphotericin, ifosfamide

- metabolic: severe hypercalcemia or hypokalemia
- autoimmune diseases: sarcoidosis, Sjogren's syndrome.

- Hypervolemic patient:
  - increased mineralocorticoids: Conn's syndrome (primary hyperaldosteronism); Cushing's syndrome
  - iatrogenic: infusion of hypertonic saline or sodium bicarbonate
  - high salt diet.

Clinical manifestation of hypernatremia

Caused by loss of cell volume, and loss of brain volume. Symptoms are more likely to occur when there are rapid changes in sodium concentration.

Symptoms include irritability, spasticity, and tremulousness. A decrease in brain volume causes lethargy, weakness, and headache. If sodium levels rise above 158 mEq/l, severe symptoms may emerge, such as seizures, coma, and eventually death.

Treatment of hypernatremia

Rule of thumb: correct underlying causes; target decreasing serum [Na^+] no more than 0.5 mEq/l/h to avoid cerebral edema.

Essential Clinical Anesthesia Review: Keywords, Questions and Answers for the Boards, ed. Linda S. Aglio, Robert W. Lekowski, and Richard D. Urman. Published by Cambridge University Press. © Cambridge University Press 2015.

- Hypovolemic patients: use isotonic saline initially for volume repletion; followed by hypotonic crystalloid solutions, such as 0.45% normal saline.
- Euvolemic patients: replacement of free water.
  - central DI: administer DDAVP
  - nephrogenic DI: treat underlying causes; restrict sodium and protein; diuretics (distal tubule diuretics, thiazide, amiloride); NSAIDs.
- Hypervolemic patients: removal of the excess sodium (e.g., thiazide or loop diuretics) while replacing water. Intravenous infusions should be hypotonic compared with the urine.

Free water deficit

Free water deficit = Total body water $\times$ (140 – serum $[Na^+]$)/140.
- In females: total body water = $0.5 \times$ total body weight
- In males: total body water = $0.6 \times$ total body weight

One-half of the calculated water deficit can be administered either enterally or parenterally during the first 24 hours and the rest over the following one to two days.

Hyponatremia

Plasma $[Na^+]$ <135 mEq/l. It reflects total body water overload.

Causes of hyponatremia

Depending on urine osmolarity and urine sodium level:
- Isotonic hyponatremia (pseudohyponatremia): isotonic urine. Due to hyperlipidemia or hyperproteinemia (e.g., multiple myeloma). *No need to treat.*
- Hypertonic hyponatremia: hypertonic urine >100 mOsm. Due to hyperglycemia (corrected serum $[Na^+]$ = measured $[Na^+]$ + 0.016 $\times$ (serum glucose [mg/dl] – 100)); hypertonic infusions, such as mannitol, TPN, etc. *Goal of treatment is to remove the osmotically active substance and to restore euvolemia.*
- Hypotonic hyponatremia: hypotonic urine <100 mOsm. Depending on patient's volume status and urine $[Na^+]$:
  - hypovolemic hypotonic hyponatremia: urine $[Na^+]$ <20 mEq/l
    Renal loss (diruetics, postobstructive nephropathy); GI loss (vomiting, diarrhea); adrenal insufficiency; burns
  - euvolemic hypotonic hyponatremia: urine $[Na^+]$ >20 mEq/l
    SIADH (inappropriate ADH level increases caused by pulmonary or brain pathology); thiazide, water intoxication (TURP, psychogenic polydipsia); hypothyroidism; cortisol deficiency
  - hypervolemic hypotonic hyponatremia: urine $[Na^+]$ <20 mEq/l
    CHF; cirrhosis; renal failure; nephrotic syndrome.

Clinical manifestation

Symptoms are often vague and nonspecific, including malaise, nausea, confusion, and lethargy. When serum $[Na^+]$ falls below 120 mEq/l, more severe symptoms develop (headache, obtundation, seizures, coma, and death).

Treatment of hypotonic hyponatremia

Maximum rate of sodium correction should not exceed 3 mEq/h to avoid central pontine myelinolysis.
- Hypovolemic hypotonic hyponatremia: sodium is lost in greater proportion than water. Replace volume depletion with normal saline.
- Euvolemic hypotonic hyponatremia: free water restriction; hypertonic saline (use if patient is severely symptomatic or free water restriction fails to raise serum $[Na^+]$; goal is to increase serum $[Na^+]$ by 8 to 12 mEq/l in the first 24 h); normal saline + loop diuretics; demeclocycline.
- Hypervolemic hypotonic hyponatremia: fluid and salt restriction; proximal and loop diuretics.

Hyperkalemia
Causes of hyperkalemia

Serum potassium >5.5 mEq/l.
- Decreased renal excretion:
  - renal insufficiency or renal failure
  - mineralocorticoid deficiency
  - drugs: ACE inhibitors; angiotensin receptor blockers; K^+ sparing diuretics (spironolactone, triamterene; amiloride); succinylcholine; cyclosporine, tacrolimus.
- Increased intake: blood transfusion.
- Redistribution from intracellular space: acidosis; burn; rhabdomyolysis; vigorous exercise; infection.
- Pseudohyperkalemia: leukocytosis (WBC >100,000/mm^3); thrombocytosis (PLT >1,000,000/mm3); hemolysis.

Clinical manifestation of hyperkalemia

- EKG changes: atrial and ventricular ectopy, decreased QT interval, peaked T waves, loss of P waves, widening of the QRS complex (QRS widening and merging with T wave, "sinusoidal waves"), can progress to ventricular fibrillation or asystole.
- Neuromuscular weakness: muscular and respiratory paralysis.

Treatment of hyperkalemia

Regardless of the cause, therapy to lower serum potassium should be initiated immediately if K^+ >5.5 mEq/l or EKG shows signs of conduction abnormalities. Initially membrane

Table 63.2 Treatment options for hyperkalemia

Mechanism	Medication	Dose	Onset	Comment
Membrane stabilizer	Calcium chloride; calcium gluconate	1 amp of 10 ml 10% solution IV; 3 amp of 10 ml 10% solution IV	<5 min	Transient effect, lasts 15–30 min
Driving K into cells	Insulin	Regular insulin 10 units + glucose (D50 50 ml) IV	10–20 min	Lasts 2–3 h
	Bicarbonate	50–100 mEq IV	15–30 min	Use only if metabolic acidosis exists
	Beta$_2$ agonist	Albuterol 10–20 mg via inhaler over 10 min	20–30 min	Lasts 2–3 h
Increase K excretion	Cation exchange resin	Kayexalate (sodium polystyrene) 30–90 g po/PR	1–2 h	From sorbitol, risk of intestinal necrosis
	Loop diuretics	Furosemide 40 mg or more IV	30 min	
	Renal replacement therapy	Hemodialysis		

(Frendl, G. and Urman, R. 2012. *Pocket ICU*, 1st edn. Lippincott Williams & Wilkins p. 1–1.)

stabilizers are used to protect normal function of the myocardium. Ultimately measures to increase potassium excretion are needed (Table 63.2).

Hypokalemia
Causes of hypokalemia

Serum [K$^+$] <3.5 mEq/l.

- Increased excretion: vomiting, diarrhea; loop and thiazide diuretics; renal tubular acidosis; mineralocorticoid excess (primary hyperaldosteronism).
- Intracellular shift: alkalosis; insulin; beta$_2$-agonist (bronchodilators; tocolytics, theophylline, caffeine, epinephrine); barium; hyperthyroidism; hypothermia.

Clinical manifestation of hypokalemia

- EKG changes: flattened T wave, prominent U wave; ventricular ectopy; ventricular fibrillation.
- Neuromuscular weakness: fatigue and muscle cramps; flaccid paralysis, hyporeflexia; hypoventilation, tetany, and rhabdomyolysis may be seen with severe hypokalemia (<2.5 mEq/l).

Treatment of hypokalemia

Replace K$^+$ at 0.2 to 0.5 mEq/kg/h if urine output is adequate.

- Enteral supplement: in the setting of normal renal function and mild to moderate diuretic dosage, 20 mEq/day of oral potassium is generally sufficient to prevent hypokalemia, whereas 40 to 100 mEq/day is needed to treat hypokalemia when it occurs.
- Parenteral supplement: intravenous potassium replacement is indicated for patients with severe hypokalemia and for those who cannot take oral supplementation. From a peripheral IV line, the potassium concentration should not exceed 40 mEq/l and the rate should not exceed 10 mEq/h because of its local and systemic toxicity. When a central line is present, it should be the route of choice to

administer IV potassium. Rates of 10 to 20 mEq/h require continuous EKG monitoring. Daily potassium replacement should not exceed 240 mEq.

Calcium balance

Normal range: normal total plasma calcium concentration is 8.5 to 10.5 mg/dl. Ionized calcium (4.4 to 5.3 mg/dl) is the physiologically active calcium.

Physiological function: calcium is necessary for almost every function in the human body, including muscle contraction, nerve function, and blood coagulation.

Regulation: calcium is regulated primarily by parathyroid hormone (PTH) and vitamin D. Albumin levels do not affect ionized calcium levels; but the total calcium increases or decreases with a decrease or an increase in albumin levels, respectively. An albumin level decrease of 1 g/dl increases the calcium level by 0.8 mg/dl. Metabolic acidosis increases ionized calcium levels.

Causes of hypercalcemia

Hypercalcemia (total plasma calcium >10.5 mg/dl and ionized calcium >1.3 mmol/l).

- Malignancy: local osteolytic hypercalcemia; PTH-related peptide releasing tumor.
- Endocrine disorders: hyperparathyroidism; thyrotoxicosis; pheochromocytoma; granulomatous disease.
- Drug-induced: vitamin D, vitamin A; thiazide; lithium; estrogen, androgens.
- Others: immobilization; TPN; renal insufficiency.

Clinical manifestation

- GI: nausea, vomiting, abdominal pain, constipation.
- CNS: muscle weakness, ataxia, and confusion.
- Renal: nephrogenic diabetic insipidus; renal failure with volume depletion.
- CVS: hypertension; shortened QT interval on EKG.

Treatment of hypercalcemia

Until the primary disease is controlled, renal excretion of calcium should be promoted. Serial measurements of potassium and magnesium should also be done while the calcium is being corrected.

- Volume repletion: maintain euvolemia with normal saline.
- Diuretics: loop diuretics. Saline (250–500 ml/h) with furosemide (20–40 mg every 2 hours IV) is the common practice.
- Bisphosphonates (pamidronate) or calcitonin: treatment for hypercalcemia of malignancy.
- Hemodialysis: when other measures fail.

Causes of hypocalcemia

Hypocalcemia (total plasma calcium <8.6 mg/dl and ionized calcium <1.12 mmol/l).

- Rule out hypoalbuminemia.
- Decreased intake: vitamin D deficiency; hypomagnesemia.
- Increased loss: diuretics; chronic renal insufficiency; alcoholism; citrate infusion or massive transfusion of blood and plasma.
- Endocrine disorders: hypoparathyroidism; pancreatitis; following hyperphosphatemia caused by rhabdomyolysis, tumor lysis syndrome.
- Sepsis.

Clinical manifestation

- Neuromuscular: extensive spasm of skeletal muscle may cause weakness, cramps, tetany, and eventually, laryngospasm with stridor. Seizure, paresthesias of the lips and extremities, and abdominal pain may occur.
- Trousseau's sign: inflate a blood pressure cuff above the systolic pressure for three minutes and watch for spasm of the outstretched hand.
- Chvostek's sign: tap on the facial nerve near the temporal mandibular joint and watch for grimacing caused by spasm of the facial muscles.
- CVS: hypotension and prolongation of the QT interval on EKG; ventricular arrhythmias.

Treatment of hypocalcemia

- Symptomatic patients: intravenous calcium. Calcium gluconate 10% (10–20 ml) administered IV over 10 to 15 minutes.
- Asymptomatic hypocalcemia: oral calcium and vitamin D. Vitamin D will increase the amount of calcium being absorbed.
- Hypomagnesemia: needs to be corrected concomitantly.
- Drug modification: consider switching from loop diuretics to thiazides.

Magnesium physiology

Normal plasma magnesium ranges between 1.5 and 2.5 mEq/l. Mg^{2+} promotes intracellular enzyme reactions, helps in the production of adenosine triphosphate (ATP), and plays a role in neuromuscular activity, coagulation, and platelet aggregation.

Causes of hypermagnesemia

Hypermagnesemia (plasma magnesium >2.5 mEq/l).

- Increased intake, such as magnesium-containing antacids and laxatives; treatment of preeclampsia (therapeutic dose is 4–6 mEq/l).
- Decreased excretion: renal insufficiency.

Clinical manifestation

- Somnolence.
- EKG changes: occur at 5 to 10 mEq/l.
- Skeletal muscle weakness, hyporeflexia: occurs at 10 mEq/l.
- Hypoventilation and respiratory paralysis: occurs at 15 mEq/l.
- Vasodilation, bradycardia, hypotension.
- Cardiac arrest: occurs at 20 mEq/l.
- Drug interaction: potentiates the action of both depolarizing and nondepolarizing neuromuscular blocking agents. No fasciculation after succinylcholine.

Treatment

- stop magnesium intake
- calcium
- diuretics
- hemodialysis

Causes of hypomagnesemia

Hypomagnesemia (plasma magnesium <1.5 mEq/l).

- Decreased intake: alcoholism; starvation.
- Increased excretion: diuretics; DKA.
- Often associated with hypocalcemia and hypokalemia.

Clinical manifestation

- Increased neuromuscular irritability, hyperreflexia, confusion, and seizures may occur.
- EKG changes: prolonged PR and QT intervals, widened QRS complexes, ST depression, and T wave inversion. Atrial fibrillation may also occur.

Treatment of hypomagnesemia

- Oral or IV supplement magnesium.
- Serious manifestations of hypomagnesemia (seizures) should be corrected by IV replacement (2–4 g infusion over

30–60 min). Avoid an IV bolus of magnesium sulfate, as it may cause cardiac arrhythmias.

Phosphorus physiology

In plasma, phosphate is present mainly as a very small inorganic fraction (PO_4, normal range 2.5–4.5 mg/dl). About 85% of phosphorus is stored in the bone. It is used to form ATP, nucleic acids, 2,3-diphosphoglycerate (2,3-DPG, offloading oxygen from hemoglobin) and cyclic adenosine monophosphate (cAMP).

Causes of hyperphosphatemia

Plasma phosphate >4.5 mg/dl. Renal failure; tumor lysis syndrome; rhabdomyolysis; malignant hyperthermia; hypomagnesemia; vitamin D; hypoparathyroidism.

Clinical manifestation

Clinical signs of hyperphosphatemia are related primarily to the development of hypocalcemia and ectopic calcification.

Treatment

- Chronic hyperphosphatemia: low phosphate diet; phosphate binder.
- Acute hyperphosphatemia: saline and diuresis (acetazolamide); dialysis for patients with renal failure.

Causes of hypophosphatemia

Plasma phosphate <2.5 mg/dl. Chronic alcoholism; TPN with inadequate phosphate; refeeding syndrome in malnourished patients.

Clinical manifestation

In the presence of severe hypophosphatemia (PO_4 <1 mg/dl), decreased levels of 2,3–DPG will result in an increased affinity of hemoglobin for oxygen, which impairs tissue oxygenation.

- Muscle weakness, rhabdomyolysis, paresthesia.
- Encephalopathy: irritability, confusion, or seizures.
- Platelet and leukocyte dysfunction.

- Respiratory failure.
- Myocardial dysfunction.

Treatment

The best treatment is prophylaxis, by including phosphate in repletion and maintenance fluids (total parenteral nutrition).

- Oral replacement: preferred, as rapid correction may cause hypocalcemia.
- Intravenous supplement: for moderate hypophosphatemia (1.25–2.5 mg/dl), 0.08 to 0.24 mmol/kg phosphate can be given over 6 h (maximal total dose 30 mmol); for severe hypophosphatemia (<1.25 mg/dl), 0.25 to 0.5 mmol/kg phosphate can be given over 8 to 12 h (maximal total dose 80 mmol).

Questions

1. Which of the following is the first manifestation of hyperkalemia?
   a. ST depression
   b. prolonged PR interval
   c. symmetrically peaked T wave
   d. widened QRS

2. A 100 kg male patient has a measured serum sodium concentration of 105 mEq/l. How much sodium would be needed to bring the serum sodium to 120 mEq/l?
   a. 600 mEq
   b. 900 mEq
   c. 1,200 mEq
   d. 2,400 mEq
   e. 3,600 mEq

Answers

1. c. EKG changes progress in order from symmetrically peaked T waves, to widening of the QRS complex, to prolongation of the PR interval, to loss of P wave, to loss of R wave amplitude, ST depression, then to a sine wave, ventricular fibrillation, and asystole.
2. b. Dose of $[Na^+]$ = body weight × 0.6 × (desired $[Na^+]$ level – current $[Na^+]$ level).

Further reading

Vacanti, C. A., Sikka, P. K., Urman, R. D., Dershwitz, M., and Scott Segal, B. (2011). *Essential Clinical Anesthesia*, 1st edn. Cambridge University Press.

Miller, R. D. (2011). *Miller's Basics of Anesthesia*, 6th edn. Saunders.

Frendl, G. and Urman, R. (2012). *Pocket ICU*, 1st edn. Lippincott Williams & Wilkins.

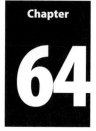

Total parenteral nutrition

Pingping Song and Gyorgy Frendl

Keywords

Enteral and parenteral nutrition
Assessment of nutritional status
Initiation of total parenteral nutrition (TPN)
Nutritional composition of TPN
Metabolic monitoring
Complications of TPN
Perioperative management of TPN

Enteral and parenteral nutrition

- Enteral nutrition, if possible, should always be the preferred route of nutrient administration. Enteral feeding maintains the integrity of absorptive villi of the gastrointestinal tract, and decreases translocation of pathological organisms across the gastrointestinal mucosa and into the blood stream. Patients on enteral feeding have decreased infectious complications, and fewer ventilator and intensive care unit days.
- Intravenous feeding (total parenteral nutrition, or TPN) is required when the gastrointestinal tract is not functional.

Assessment of nutritional status

Nutritional status can be evaluated by body weight, subjective global assessment (SGA), and certain biochemical markers.

Body weight

Malnutrition may be present when there is weight loss of 10% to 20% over a short time, or weight is less than 90% of ideal body weight, or BMI is less than 18.5. Nutritional assessments in critically ill patients by body weight are often inaccurate due to significant amount of fluid shift in the disease state.

Subjective global assessment (SGA)

The SGA is a clinical method to evaluate the nutritional status of a patient. See Table 64.1 for detailed components of SGA.

Table 64.1 Subjective global assessment

Medical history	Physical examination
Weight change	**Muscle wasting**
No change; change	biceps
	triceps
% Weight loss	quadriceps
<5%; 5–10%; >10%	temple
Weight change in past two weeks	**Subcutaneous fat wasting**
Increase; no change; decrease	eyes
Dietary intake	perioral
Reduction	palmar
Unintentional; intentional	
Overall change	**Edema**
Change	upper extremities
No change	sacral
Increase or decrease	lower extremities
Gastrointestinal symptoms	
None; nausea; diarrhea; vomiting	
Dysphagia; anorexia	
Functional impairment	
Overall impairment	
None; mild; severe	
Duration	
Days; weeks; months	

(From Vacanti et al. 2011. *Essential Clinical Anesthesia*, Cambridge University Press, p. 402.)

Biochemical markers of malnutrition and metabolic stress

- Pre-albumin: level decreases acutely. Half-life 2 days.

Essential Clinical Anesthesia Review: Keywords, Questions and Answers for the Boards, ed. Linda S. Aglio, Robert W. Lekowski, and Richard D. Urman. Published by Cambridge University Press. © Cambridge University Press 2015.

- Transferrin: level decreases at later stage of malnutrition. Half-life 8–10 days.
- Albumin: poor marker for nutritional status, may be affected by many other pathological status. Half-life 20 days.
- C-reactive protein: acute phase reactant. Level decreases in malnutrition. Half-life 19 hours.

Initiation of TPN

Indication

TPN is initiated if patient cannot tolerate enteral nutrition and if duration of nutritional support is anticipated to be >7 days.

Route of TPN administration

- Peripheral access: use only if central access is not available and lipid concentration <20% and glucose concentration <10%.
- Central access: for long-term use.
    - location: tip of catheter needs to be confirmed in the vena cava before administration of TPN
    - insertion site: internal jugular vein or subclavian vein (short-term access), PICC (peripherally inserted central catheter, mid-term access), or tunneled catheters (long-term access); femoral vein is not preferred due to higher risk of infection
    - a dedicated port is required for TPN infusion, to decrease risk of infection.

Contraindications to TPN

Severe hyperglycemia (serum glucose >250 mg/dl); lipid nephrosis; egg allergy; acute pancreatitis, bacteremia or fungemia (relative contraindications).

Nutrient composition of the TPN mixture

The base solution is commonly 500 ml of 10% amino acids and 500 ml of 50% dextrose.

Additives: electrolytes, vitamins, minerals, trace elements, insulin, H_2 blockers, etc. The following steps are used to determine the composition of the TPN mixture:

Table 64.2 Major components of TPN

TPN mixture	Percentage of total calories provided	Calorie yield per gram (kcal/g)
Glucose (dextrose)	30–70%	3.4
Fat (lipid)	20–30%; maximum 2.5 g/kg/day	9.4
Protein (amino acids)	5–20%	4.1

1. Determine total volume.
    - Holliday–Segar method: the total daily fluid needs can be estimated as follows: 100 ml/kg for the first 10 kg; 50 ml/kg for the second 10 kg; 20 ml/kg for each additional kg.
    - The final volume is usually 2 to 2.5 l/day for an average adult patient.
2. Determine caloric and protein needs.
    - Total caloric needs = 25 (kcal/kg) × body weight (kg).
    - Total protein needs = [0.8–1.0] (g/day) × body weight (kg).
    - For patients on renal replacement therapy, 1.5 to 2.5 g/kg/day of protein is required to maintain a positive nitrogen balance.
3. Determine volume of lipid.
    - Calories provided by lipid: 20% to 30% of total caloric intake.
    - Volume of lipid: 1.1 kcal/ml of 10% lipid emulsions or 2 kcal/ml of 20% lipid emulsions.
4. Goal rate: initiate with 1 liter on day one, advancing 20–50 ml/h.
5. Determine additives.
    - Sodium and potassium are added as chlorides or acetates, with the ratio of acetates to chlorides increased in patients with hyperchloremia or acidosis. Sodium bicarbonate is incompatible with the nutrient solution; therefore acetate is used.

Metabolic monitoring

Daily weight

Persistent weight loss with fluid balance taken account of indicates additional calories (500–1,000 kcal/day) are needed to maintain lean body mass.

Nitrogen balance

$$N_{in} - N_{out} = [\text{protein (g)}/6.25] - [24 \text{ h UNN (urine urea nitrogen, g)} + 4]$$

- Positive nitrogen balance: indicative of anabolism. Desired to maintain lean body mass.
- Negative nitrogen balance: indicative of catabolism.

Respiratory quotient (RQ)

Ratio of CO_2 production and O_2 consumption. Can be measured using indirect calorimetry in a closed ventilator system.

- RQ ≥1: excessive calorie intake; indicating need to decrease glucose or lipids.
- RQ <0.82: inadequate calorie intake.

Complications of TPN

- Complications related to central venous access: pneumothorax, thrombosis, infection, etc. The most common organism of infection is staphylococcus, followed by enterococcus.

- Metabolic complications:
  - hyperglycemia: monitor glucose at least every 2 h
  - fatty liver
  - increased CO_2 production, acidosis, and respiratory failure.
- Refeeding syndrome: rapid refeeding causes an insulin surge, which increases intracellular uptake of potassium and phosphate from the extracellular space.
  - decreased serum concentration of potassium, phosphorus, and magnesium
  - respiratory failure: decreased vital capacity, tidal volume, respiratory rate; difficult to wean from mechanical ventilation; increased CO_2 production, respiratory acidosis
  - cardiac failure: increased fluid retention, increased cardiac workload and oxygen consumption.
- To prevent refeeding syndrome, gradually increase the calories per day, and closely monitor serum electrolytes level as well as patient's fluid status.

Perioperative management of TPN

- TPN should always be continued in the perioperative period, to minimize risk of hypoglycemia and maximize the nutritional benefit.

- When TPN is discontinued, to prevent hypoglycemia: place patient on dextrose 10% infusion at the same rate the TPN was infused. Monitor glucose frequently.

Question

1. Potential complications associated with TPN include all of the following except which?
   a. ketoacidosis
   b. hyperglycemia
   c. hypoglycemia
   d. hypophosphatemia
   e. increased work of breathing

Answers

1. a. Acidosis in patients receiving TPN is hyperchloremic nonketone acidosis, resulting from formation of HCl during metabolism of amino acids. Other electrolyte abnormalities include hypomagnesemia and hypocalcemia.

Further reading

Vacanti, C. A., Sikka, P. K., Urman, R. D., Dershwitz, M., and Scott Segal, B. (2011). *Essential Clinical Anesthesia*, 1st edn. Cambridge University Press.

Miller, R. D. (2011). *Miller's Basics of Anesthesia*, 6th edn. Saunders.

Frendl, G. and Urman, R. (2012). *Pocket ICU*, 1st edn. Lippincott Williams & Wilkins.

Chapter

65

Blood products

Hanjo Ko and Robert W. Lekowski

Keywords

CPDA
Leukocyte-reduced red blood cells
Washed red blood cells
Apheresis platelet
Cryoprecipitate components
Irradiated blood products
Transfusion-associated GVHD
Type and screen
Cross-match

One donated unit of whole blood can be processed to produce one RBC unit, one platelet concentrate, and one unit of fresh frozen plasma (FFP).

Red blood cells (RBC)

- with citrate phosphate dextrose solution (CPD): ~250 cc, Hct 70–80%, up to 21 days storage
- with *CPDA-1* (CPD plus adenosine): up to 35 days
- with CPDA-1 and additive solutions: ~300 cc, Hct 55–65%, up to 42 days, stored at 4°C, expect to see 3% increase in Hct
- if irradiated, then storage time is shortened to 28 days

Leukocyte-reduced RBC

- used in patients with:
    - febrile non-hemolytic transfusion reactions
    - need for cytomegalovirus-negative blood
    - risk for HLA alloimmunization
    - need for exchange transfusion
- does not prevent graft-versus-host disease (GVHD)
- cryoprecipitate and FFP do not need leukoreduction since they do not contain significant numbers of leukocytes

Washed RBC

- used in patients with:
    - history of anaphylactoid reaction
    - patients who are IgA-immunized
    - sometimes washed RBC is not sufficient to prevent hypersensitivity reactions in IgA-immunized patients so blood collected from IgA-deficient donor may be necessary

Platelets

- 50 cc per concentrate.
- 300 cc per pool ("six-pack").
- Stored at 20–24°C.
- 30,000–60,000 increase in platelet count per each pool, up to five days.
- If posttransfusion platelet count is lower than expected, this can represent a refractory state secondary to many etiologies (fever, sepsis, DIC, etc). In certain cases, refractoriness is due to HLA alloimmunization and the patient may respond to HLA-matched or simply cross-matched platelets:
    - *low numbers of RBCs are present in platelet concentrates so Rh sensitization may be induced if an Rh-positive platelet unit is transfused to an Rh-negative recipient*
    - transfusing ABO-compatible platelets is not required.

Apheresis platelets

- Harvested from a single donor and contain four to eight whole-blood-derived platelet concentrates.
- Apheresis platelets can also be labeled as leukocyte-reduced, since they contain very few leukocytes.

Essential Clinical Anesthesia Review: Keywords, Questions and Answers for the Boards, ed. Linda S. Aglio, Robert W. Lekowski, and Richard D. Urman. Published by Cambridge University Press. © Cambridge University Press 2015.

FFP

- 200–250 cc per unit, stored at –18°C within eight hours of collection, up to one year.
- Transfusing ABO-compatible FFP is *not* required.
- FFP should be transfused within 24 hours of thawing.

Cryoprecipitate

- 15 cc, *contains factor VII, von Willebrand factor, fibrinogen, fibronectin, factor XIII.*
- Transfusing ABO-compatible cryoprecipitate is *not* necessary, although in infants, ABO compatibility is typically achieved due to their small blood volume.
- Cryoprecipitate can also be used to treat uremic bleeding, abruptio placentae, HELLP syndrome, and factor XIII deficiency.

Transfusion-associated GVHD (TA-GVHD)

- Lymphocytes present in RBC and platelets can respond to host antigens and cause *TA-GVHD* – especially in immunocompromised recipients.
- TA-GVHD is fatal but can be prevented by *irradiated blood products.*
- Cryoprecipitate and FFP have not been associated with TA-GVHD and do not require irradiation.
- Some institutions are moving toward "universal" irradiation of blood products due to the dire consequences of TA-GVHD.
- Absolute indications for irradiated blood products include:
  - bone marrow transplant recipients
  - T-cell immunodeficiency
  - intrauterine transfusions
  - HLA-matched platelet transfusions
  - transfusions from any family members
  - lymphomas/leukemia
  - neuroblastoma and glioblastoma
  - patients receiving fludarabine as part of their chemotherapy.

Type and screen

- Takes about 55 minutes if no unexpected antibodies are discovered.
- Type refers to ABO-Rh testing while screen refers to the detection of the presence of most common antibodies in serum (also known as indirect Coombs test).
- Cross-match refers to the process of securing a unit of RBC where the compatibility between the unit of RBC and the patient's serum is achieved.
- RBC can be physically available within ten minutes if no unexpected antibodies were found during the initial type

and screen process but may take considerable time if antibodies were discovered.
- FFP, platelets, and cryoprecipitate do *not* require compatibility testing with the caveat that Rh sensitization can be induced with platelets (see above).

Questions

1. Which of the following statements is FALSE regarding cryoprecipitate?
   a. It contains factor VIII, factor XIII, von Willebrand factor, fibrinogen, and fibronectin.
   b. It is indicated in patients with hemophilia when factor concentrates are not available.
   c. It is the first-line agent for patients with von Willebrand's disease.
   d. It is indicated in patients with hypofibrinogenemia.

2. What is the storage life of whole blood stored with citrate phosphate dextrose (CPD)?
   a. 14 days
   b. 21 days
   c. 35 days
   d. 42 days

3. A 65-year-old, non-immunocompromised male develops a fever during transfusion of one unit of RBC. The cross-match is confirmed as accurate, and the storage time of the donor unit is determined to be seven days. Which of the following is the most likely cause of a febrile transfusion reaction in this patient?
   a. bacterial sepsis
   b. cytomegalovirus
   c. hemolysis
   d. donor lymphocytes

Answers

1. c. In patients with von Willebrand's disease, the first agent of choice is DDAVP, followed by factor concentrates.
2. b. See above.
3. d. The most likely cause of a febrile non-hemolytic transfusion reaction is a reaction to donor lymphocytes or cytokines in banked blood, which can occur during the transfusion or up to six hours following the transfusion. Such reaction can be eliminated by leukoreduction.

Further reading

Vacanti, C. A., Sikka, P. K., Urman, R. U., Dershwitz, M., and Segal, B. S. (2011). *Essential Clinical Anesthesia*, 1st edn. Cambridge University Press, Chapter 66.

www.openanesthesia.org keywords

Chapter

66

Blood transfusion

Hanjo Ko and Robert W. Lekowski

Keywords

Universal donor
Hemolytic transfusion reaction
Febrile non-hemolytic transfusion reaction
Transfusion-related acute lung injury
Transfusion-associated circulatory overload
Transfusion-associated graft-versus-host disease
Citrate toxicity
Transfusion-related immunomodulation
Transfusion triggers

- For RBCs, type O blood lacks A and B antigen and therefore is the *universal donor.*
- When transfusing plasma products (FFP and platelets), preformed anti-ABO antibodies in the donor plasma are the limiting factor, so type AB plasma is the universal donor for FFP and platelets.
- Type O negative RBCs can be used as universal donor blood without waiting for further typing or cross-matching.
- For male patients, it is permissible to transfuse type O positive RBCs.

Hemolytic transfusion reaction

Diagnosis:

- visual hemolysis (pink or red discoloration) of the recipient plasma
- direct antiglobulin test (i.e., direct Coomb's test)
- acute due to ABO-incompatible RBC or FFP; presents with fever, hypotension, red urine, and coagulopathy seen as diffuse bleeding at the surgical site
- delayed – happens three or more days after RBC transfusion; may be asymptomatic or present with jaundice and anemia

Table 66.1 Management of a suspected acute hemolytic transfusion reaction

Stop the transfusion, save the remaining blood product for testing. Check for an obvious error in patient identity or blood product match. Support the patient's circulation, treat hypovolemia and hypotension. If immediate transfusion is needed, give type O negative blood and AB+ FFP if needed.
Send a new blood sample for cross-match to the blood bank, along with the remainder of the suspect unit for testing.
Support the patient's renal function with fluids and diuretics, starting with furosemide and then mannitol if needed.
Monitor the coagulation system for signs or laboratory values suggestive of disseminated intravascular coagulation, and treat if needed.
Send the patient's blood for a direct antiglobulin test, free hemoglobin, and haptoglobin; send urine for free hemoglobin.

(From *Essential Clinical Anesthesia*, Chapter 67, p. 413. Modified from Table 34-2 in *Clinical Anesthesia Procedures of the Massachusetts General Hospital*, 7th edn., 2007, p. 612.)

Febrile non-hemolytic transfusion reaction

- Defined as temperature rise >1°C without other etiology.
- Can be treated with acetaminophen and/or meperidine if patient also presents with rigors.
- Consider using leukocyte-reduced RBC if further transfusion is needed.

Transfusion-related acute lung injury

- Syndrome of dyspnea, hypoxia, and bilateral chest radiograph abnormalities within six hours of blood product transfusion.
- One of the leading causes of transfusion-related mortality.
- Seen with FFP > platelets > RBC.

Essential Clinical Anesthesia Review: Keywords, Questions and Answers for the Boards, ed. Linda S. Aglio, Robert W. Lekowski, and Richard D. Urman. Published by Cambridge University Press. © Cambridge University Press 2015.

Transfusion-associated circulatory overload

- Congestive heart failure from intravascular volume expansion following blood product transfusion.

Transfusion-associated graft-versus-host disease

- Caused by donor lymphocytes attaching recipient tissues. Fatal condition but can be prevented by irradiated blood products.

Patients taking angiotensin-converting enzyme inhibitors (ACE-Is)

- At risk for hypotension during RBC transfusion since these patients cannot metabolize bradykinin.
- ACE-Is block the metabolism of bradykinin in addition to blocking the conversion of angiotensin.
- Cessation of ACE-Is prevents recurrence of this reaction.

Citrate toxicity

- Citrate chelates extracellular calcium in order to prevent clotting during the storage of blood products.
- Citrate typically is quickly metabolized by the liver.
- During massive transfusion, liver transplant, or hypothermia, the addition of citrate can lead to hypocalcemia and metabolic alkalosis.
- Treatment: calcium chloride (calcium gluconate is not as effective).

Transfusion-related immunomodulation

- Unclear etiology but there appears to be a dose–response relationship between perioperative transfusion and postoperative infections, as well as rate of cancer recurrence.

Transfusion trigger

- Hemoglobin that optimizes both oxygen-carrying capacity and viscosity = 10 g/dl.
- Healthy volunteers have impaired cognition when hemoglobin is <5 g/dl.
- Postoperative mortality increases when hemoglobin is <6 g/dl.
- Normal hemostasis is achieved when:
  - coagulation factors are >30% of their normal value
  - fibrinogen is >50% of its normal 200 to 400 mg/dl value.
- Thrombocytopenia without platelet dysfunction should only affect hemostasis when platelet count is <50,000/mm^3.
- In neurosurgical or ophthalmologic procedures, platelet transfusion threshold of 80,000 or 100,000/mm^3 might be desired.

Table 66.2 Current risks of infection from test-negative blood

Components	Risk
HIV-1	1 in 1,525,000–2,135,000
Hepatitis C virus	1 in 1,935,000
Hepatitis B virus	1 in 205,000–488,000
West Nile virus	Approaching zero

(From *Essential Clinical Anesthesia*, Chapter 67, Table 67.4, p. 415. Adapted from Stramer, S. L. 2007. Infectious risk from blood transfusion. *Arch Pathol Lab Med*, 131: 703)

Questions

1. Which of the following transfusion strategies is MOST likely to reduce the risk of non-hemolytic febrile transfusion reaction?
   a. Administration of RBCs collected using a leukocyte reduction filter.
   b. Administration of fresh whole blood (less than 24 hours old).
   c. Administration of cytomegalovirus-negative RBCs.
   d. Use of a blood warmer.

2. Which statement about the application of leukocyte filters for donated blood is MOST likely true?
   a. It is most effective when done at the time of donation.
   b. It is most effective when done at the blood bank.
   c. It is most effective when done during transfusion at the bedside.
   d. Leukocyte filtration is not effective in reducing febrile transfusion reactions.

3. Which of the following statements regarding citrate toxicity is FALSE?
   a. Signs and symptoms of citrate toxicity include hypotension, arrhythmias, tetany, Chvostek and Trousseau signs.
   b. Citrate toxicity is very rare but is more likely in the setting of hyperthermia.
   c. EKG findings in citrate toxicity include prolonged QT and possible heart block.
   d. FFP and platelets have higher citrate content when compared to RBCs.

Answers

1. a. Febrile non-hemolytic transfusion reactions occur more commonly with administration of platelets than RBCs. The increased risk of such reaction has been attributed to leukocyte activation and cytokine accumulation, which are more likely to occur at room temperature.

2. a. It is most effective when performed pre-storage, when the filter is incorporated into the collection bag at the blood center. Early filtration also avoids the fragmentation of white blood cells that occurs during storage, making these cells more difficult to filter.

3. b. Citrate toxicity is more likely in the setting of hypothermia since metabolism is decreased. It is also more likely in patients who hyperventilate since hyperventilation leads to respiratory alkalosis.

Further reading

Vacanti, C. A., Sikka, P. K., Urman, R. U., Dershwitz, M., and Segal, B. S. (2011). *Essential Clinical Anesthesia*, 1st edn. Cambridge University Press, Chapter 67.

www.openanesthesia.org: keywords

Chapter

67

Massive transfusion

Hanjo Ko and Robert W. Lekowski

Keywords

Massive transfusion
Hemodilution
Hypothermia
Metabolic acidosis
Coagulopathy of trauma

Massive transfusion: definition

- 8 to 10 units of blood transfused within 12 hours.
- Replacement of one blood volume within 24 hours.
- Replacement of half of blood volume in three hours.
- Transfusion of ≥ 4 units of RBC within one hour and at risk of ongoing need for further transfusion.

Hemodilution

- Occurs frequently in both trauma patients and patients undergoing elective surgery since the initial resuscitation typically starts with crystalloids or colloids.
- Leads to dilutional coagulopathy itself.
- Some synthetic colloid solutions may also play a role in platelet inhibition.
- RBCs also contribute to hemostasis since RBCs help activate platelets by releasing adenosine diphosphate and activate platelet cyclooxygenase.
- As a result, some suggest relative high hematocrits (such as 35%) may be required during massive transfusion.

Hypothermia

- Defined as a core temperature $<35°C$.
- Detrimental during massive transfusion.
- Slows the activity of enzymatic processes.
- Reduces the synthesis of coagulation factors.
- Increases fibrinolysis.
- Inhibits platelet function.

- Hypothermia combined with trauma is associated with a worse prognosis and should be actively treated.

Metabolic acidosis

- Observed during massive blood loss due to hemorrhagic shock leading to anaerobic metabolism and acidosis.
- pH <7.10 is associated with coagulopathy.

Coagulopathy of trauma

- May occur in the setting of depleted coagulation factors or even in the setting of normal coagulation factor levels but dysfunctional coagulation factors.
- Four risk factors were identified:
  - pH <7.10
  - core temperature $<34°C$
  - mean injury severity score >25
  - systolic pressure <70.
- Many experts suggest early administration of platelets and FFP (a ratio of 1:1:1 = RBC: FFP: platelets) to help prevent coagulopathy.

No hard evidence or transfusion triggers exist for patients undergoing elective surgery with massive blood loss; however, the following guidelines have been proposed to guide transfusion:

- RBCs should be given when hemoglobin is <6 g/dl and are usually not necessary when hemoglobin is >10 g/dl.
- Platelets should be administered when platelet count is $<50,000$/dl.
- FFP transfusion is indicated for the prothrombin time >1.5 times normal or for an activated partial thromboplastin time >2 times normal.
- Cryoprecipitate is to be administered when the fibrinogen level is $<80–100$ mg/dl.

Essential Clinical Anesthesia Review: Keywords, Questions and Answers for the Boards, ed. Linda S. Aglio, Robert W. Lekowski, and Richard D. Urman. Published by Cambridge University Press. © Cambridge University Press 2015.

Questions

1. A 50-year-old patient with chronic kidney disease is admitted to the ICU with altered mental status, fever, tachycardia, and hypoxemia. CXR reveals an RLL infiltrate. Prolonged bleeding from venipuncture sites and bleeding from the nasal mucosa after NGT placement are also noted. Platelet count is 100,000/dl; PT 11.5 s; PTT 35 s; BUN 150 mg/dL; creatine is 10. Which of the following treatments is MOST likely to result in rapid improvement in the bleeding diathesis?

   a. platelet transfusion
   b. hemodialysis
   c. conjugated estrogens
   d. cryoprecipitate
   e. desmopressin acetate

2. A 22-year-old patient suffered blunt trauma in a motor vehicle collision. After exploratory laparotomy with a splenectomy, he required transfusion of four units of RBCs. Postoperatively, he had diffuse oozing at the site of the incision. His labs preoperatively revealed platelet count of 210,000/dl; PT of 12.8 s; and PTT of 44 s.

Which of the following is the MOST likely etiology of his bleeding?

   a. DIC
   b. hypothermia
   c. von Willebrand's disease
   d. salicylate use
   e. citrate toxicity

Answers

1. e. DDAVP is the first line of treatment in patients who present with bleeding secondary to uremia.
2. c. This patient has isolated PTT preoperatively, which should raise suspicion of von Willebrand's disease in a young patient.

Further reading

Vacanti, C. A., Sikka, P. K., Urman, R. U., Dershwitz, M., and Segal, B. S. (2011). *Essential Clinical Anesthesia*, 1st edn. Cambridge University Press, Chapter 68.

www.openanesthesia.org: keywords

Chapter

68 Normovolemic hemodilution, perioperative blood salvage, and autologous blood donation

Hanjo Ko and Robert W. Lekowski

Keywords

Acute normovolemic hemodilution
Intraoperative blood salvage
Autologous blood donation

Acute normovolemic hemodilution

- Anemia is iatrogenically induced by harvesting a patient's whole blood and returning an acellular substitute to maintain normovolemia.
- Harvested blood is reinfused after the major blood loss has occurred (or sooner if deemed clinically necessary).
- Benefits of normovolemic hemodilution are greatest when the starting hemoglobin is high, the target hemoglobin is low, and the blood loss is high.
- Harvested blood may contain drugs circulating from the time when it was obtained (e.g., opioids and muscle relaxants).

Intraoperative blood salvage

- Known as cell saver.
- Blood is drawn from the operative field, taken to the centrifuge bowl, and returned to the patient.
- Bowl fill rate and size determine the hematocrit and volume of the washed blood.
- Typically, the hematocrit is 50–70%.
- Controversies exist for cell saver, such as obstetric procedures (for the fear of amniotic fluid embolus), oncological procedures, and bowel procedures (including trauma).

Autologous blood donation

- Patients undergoing elective procedures with high likelihood of transfusion.
- Parturients at risk of peripartum hemorrhage.
- Patients with multiple antibodies or rare blood types.

- Patients' hemoglobin must be ≥ 11 g/dl and all donations are to occur >72 hours prior to surgery.
- The blood is typically stored as whole blood and can be refrigerated for up to 35 days.
- Oral iron supplementation should be started prior to initial donation.
- Autologous units are generally donated at one-week intervals.
- Limiting factors for harvest of additional units are mostly inadequate hemoglobin level and the limited time frames available to collect the blood units.
- Autologous blood is not allowed to enter the general pool for allogeneic blood.
- The oldest unit of blood should be transfused first to prolong the fixed shelf life of other collected autologous units.

Questions

1. When anemia develops, which of the following physiological changes is NOT usually seen?
   a. increased cardiac output
   b. increased oxygen extraction
   c. decreased oxygen-carrying capacity
   d. decreased tissue oxygen consumption

Answers

1. d. When anemia occurs, oxygen-carrying capacity is reduced but the body maintains adequate oxygen delivery to the tissues by compensatory mechanisms, including an increase in cardiac output and oxygen extraction.

Further reading

Vacanti, C. A., Sikka, P. K., Urman, R. U., Dershwitz, M., and Segal, B. S. (2011). *Essential Clinical Anesthesia*, 1st edn. Cambridge University Press, Chapter 69.

www.openanesthesia.org: keywords

Essential Clinical Anesthesia Review: Keywords, Questions and Answers for the Boards, ed. Linda S. Aglio, Robert W. Lekowski, and Richard D. Urman. Published by Cambridge University Press. © Cambridge University Press 2015.

Cardiac physiology

Erich N. Marks and Lauren J. Cornella

Keywords

Normal anatomy of heart and major vessels
Coronary circulation
Coronary perfusion pressure
Cardiac conduction system and innervation
Cardiac cycle: control of heart rate
Cardiac cycle: normal EKG
Cardiac cycle: electrophysiology, ion channels, and
    currents
Cardiac cycle: synchronicity of pressure, flow, EKG,
    sounds, valve action
Ventricular function: Frank–Starling law, preload,
    afterload
Blood pressures: intracardiac, pulmonary, venous
Ventricular function: cardiac output determinants
Ventricular function: myocardial oxygen utilization,
    regulation of coronary blood flow
Ventricular function: systolic and diastolic function
Laplace's law

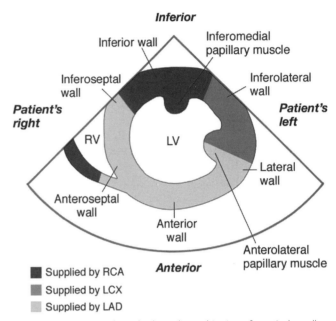

Figure 69.1 Transesophageal echocardiographic view of ventricular walls and coronary blood supply in a right dominant heart. From: Vacanti et al., 2011. *Essential Clinical Anesthesia*, Cambridge University Press, p. 428.

The *normal cardiac anatomy* consists of four chambers – two atria and two ventricles – divided into two separate circulatory pumps: the right heart, which pumps deoxygenated blood to the lungs, and the left heart, which pumps oxygenated blood to the body.

Coronary circulation

Coronary arterial blood is supplied by the left and right coronary arteries, which arise from the aortic root. Blood flows from the epicardium to the endocardium.

The *left main coronary artery* divides into the *left anterior descending artery (LAD)* and the *circumflex artery (LCX)*. The LAD supplies diagonal branches. The LCX supplies obtuse marginal branches.

The *right coronary artery* (RCA) supplies the posterior descending artery (PDA) in 70% of people (*"right dominant"* circulation). The LCX supplies the PDA in 10%

of people (*"left dominant"* circulation). Both the RCA and the LCX supply the PDA in 20% of people (*"codominant"* circulation).

The arterial blood supply for the sino-atrial (SA) node comes from the RCA in 60% of people and the LAD in 40% of people.

The atrioventricular (AV) node generally receives arterial blood from the PDA and thus follows the dominance of the circulation. In a codominant circulation the AV node is supplied by the RCA 75% of the time.

The posteromedial papillary muscle is more susceptible to ischemic dysfunction and postinfarct rupture due to its single blood supply (PDA). The coronary blood supply of a right dominant heart, as seen by transesophageal echocardiography, is shown in Figure 69.1.

Essential Clinical Anesthesia Review: Keywords, Questions and Answers for the Boards, ed. Linda S. Aglio, Robert W. Lekowski, and Richard D. Urman. Published by Cambridge University Press. © Cambridge University Press 2015.

Myocardial perfusion pressure

Perfusion of the left ventricular myocardium occurs only during diastole, when intramyocardial pressure is low. *Coronary perfusion pressure* (CPP) to the left heart is aortic diastolic blood pressure (AoDBP) minus left ventricular end-diastolic pressure (LVEDP):

$$CPP = AoDBP - LVEDP$$

The right ventricle is perfused during both systole and diastole because its intramyocardial pressures are low.

The cardiac conduction system

The cardiac conduction system consists of pacemaker cells that independently stimulate electrical activity and coordinate stimulation of the myocardium.

The cardiac cycle is initiated in the SA node. The impulse then travels through the atria to the AV node. The AV node delays electrical transmission to the ventricles, allowing for ventricular filling.

The impulse then travels to the bundle of His in the interventricular septum. The His bundle divides into left and right branches that rapidly depolarize both ventricles.

The heart is *innervated* by sympathetic and parasympathetic nerve fibers. Central control of the heart originates in the medulla.

The normal EKG

The *P wave* corresponds to atrial depolarization.
The *PR interval* indicates the delay in conduction through the AV node.
The *QRS wave* corresponds to ventricular depolarization.
The *T wave* corresponds to ventricular repolarization.

Cardiac cycle: control of heart rate, synchronicity of pressure, flow, and heart sounds

The sympathetic *cardioacceleratory center* sends signals via T1–4 to the SA and AV nodes, as well as the myocardium. Norepinephrine release leads to increased chronotropy (faster heart rate) and inotropy (stronger contraction).

The parasympathetic *cardioinhibitory center* sends signals via the vagus nerve to the SA and AV nodes. Stimulation of muscarinic receptors by acetylcholine causes negative chronotropy and inotropy.

The *integration of the entire cardiac cycle*, including EKG correlation, atrial and ventricular pressure waveforms, valve opening and closing, and heart sounds is summarized in Figure 69.2.

The cardiac cycle: pressure–volume loops

The **cardiac cycle** can be understood by charting pressure vs. volume throughout the cycle, which demonstrates several physiologic variables.

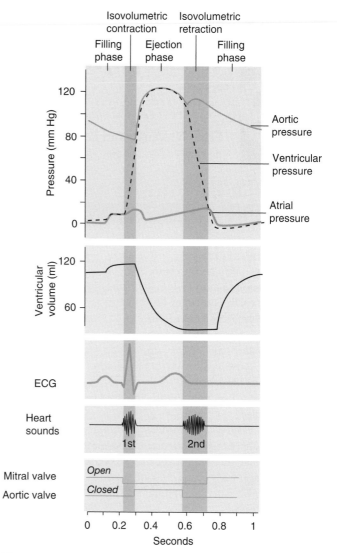

Figure 69.2 Normal cardiac cycle depicted as pressure versus time and volume versus time. From: Vacanti et al., 2011. *Essential Clinical Anesthesia*, Cambridge University Press, p. 431.

Stroke volume is end-diastolic volume (EDV) minus end-systolic volume (ESV):

$$SV = EDV - ESV$$

Ejection fraction is the percentage of EDV ejected with each systole:

$$EF (\%) = (SV/EDV) \times 100$$

Ventricular performance

Ventricular performance can be described by *cardiac output (CO)* and *cardiac index (CI)*. Cardiac index is cardiac output normalized to body surface area:

$$CO = HR \times SV \text{ (normal 4–6 l/min)}$$
$$CI = CO/BSA \text{ (normal 2.5–4 l/min/m}^2)$$

Stroke volume is determined by: (1) ventricular preload, (2) ventricular afterload, and (3) contractility.

Ventricular preload

Preload is determined by EDV. Ventricular filling is affected by venous vascular tone and venous return. Changes in circulating blood volume, HR and rhythm, intrathoracic pressure, and ventricular compliance will also affect venous return. Filling of the left ventricle can be affected by pulmonary hypertension, right heart dysfunction, or mitral valve disease.

The *Frank–Starling law* describes the relationship between ventricular EDV and cardiac output. As EDV increases and HR remains constant, SV and CO increase. This holds true until the muscle fibers reach maximal distention, beyond which further increases in EDV impair contractility and CO decreases. Increased SV according to the Frank–Starling law is depicted in Figure 69.4.

Central venous pressure (CVP) can be used to estimate left-sided filling pressures in the absence of right ventricular dysfunction or pulmonary disease. Pulmonary capillary wedge pressure (PCWP) can estimate LVEDP, which correlates to LVEDV in the absence of abnormal ventricular compliance. Approximation of LVEDV using PCWP requires insignificant intrathoracic end-expiratory pressure and the absence of mitral stenosis.

Ventricular afterload

Afterload is the tension that the ventricle must generate during systole to eject a stroke volume. For a spherical object, wall tension is described by *Laplace's law*:

$$\text{Wall tension} = (P \times R)/2h$$

Where P = pressure in the chamber (EDP)

R = radius of the chamber

h = the wall thickness of the chamber

In the absence of aortic stenosis, LV afterload is determined by *systemic vascular resistance* (SVR):

$$\text{SVR} = [(\text{MAP} - \text{CVP})/\text{CO}] \times 80 \ (\text{normal } 900 - 1,500 \text{ dyne s cm}^{-5})$$

Where MAP = mean arterial pressure

In the absence of pulmonic stenosis, *pulmonary vascular resistance* (PVR) determines right ventricular afterload:

$$\text{PVR} = [(\text{PAP}_{\text{mean}} - \text{LAP})/\text{CO}] \times 80 \ (\text{normal } 50 - 150 \text{ dyne s cm}^{-5})$$

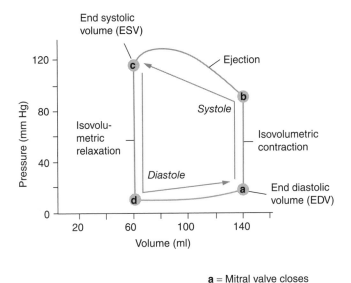

a = Mitral valve closes
b = Aortic valve opens
c = Aortic valve closes
d = Mitral valve opens

Figure 69.3 Normal cardiac cycle depicted as pressure versus volume.

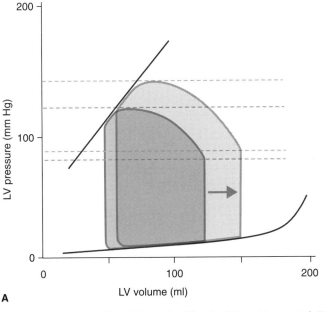

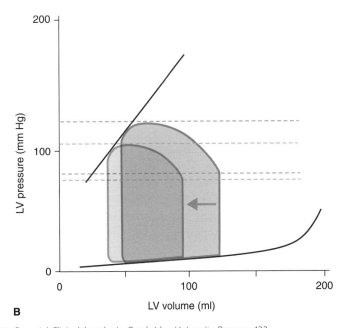

Figure 69.4 Increasing (A) and decreasing (B) preload. From: Vacanti et al., 2011. *Essential Clinical Anesthesia*, Cambridge University Press, p. 433.

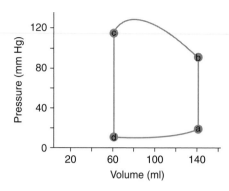

Figure 69.5 Normal cardiac cycle depicted as pressure vs. volume. (Modified from Vacanti et al. 2011. *Essential Clinical Anesthesia,* Cambridge University Press, Figure 70.6.)

Where PAP_{mean} = mean pulmonary artery pressure

LAP = left atrial pressure

Ventricular contractility

Myocardial contraction relies on the calcium-dependent interaction of actin and myosin. Myocardial contractility is directly related to the amount of Ca^{2+} released from the sarcoplasmic reticulum via cyclic AMP pathways. Increased contractility leads to increased SV and increased systemic blood pressure. Factors affecting contractility are listed in the Table 69.1.

Myocardial oxygen utilization

Between perfusion pressures of 50 and 120 mm Hg, coronary blood flow is *autoregulated* to match *myocardial oxygen demand.* Sympathetic stimulation through β_2 receptors causes vasodilation in intramyocardial vessels, increasing myocardial blood flow. Local myocardial hypoxia releases adenosine, leading to local vasodilation.

Myocardial oxygen consumption is influenced by basal tissue metabolism, generation of electrical impulses, wall tension, and heart rate.

Oxygen consumption is directly related to heart rate, preload, and afterload. Increased heart rate also decreases diastolic filling time, decreasing oxygen supply.

Myocardial oxygen extraction is very high. Oxygen saturation in the coronary sinus blood is 30%, compared to 75% for the rest of the body. There is very little reserve to increase oxygen extraction in the myocardium; therefore increased oxygen demand must be met by increased delivery.

Table 69.1 Factors affecting myocardial contractility

Increase contractility	Decrease contractility
Sympathetic (innervate atria, ventricle, nodes)	Parasympathetic stimulation – minimal
Epinephrine and norepinephrine	Hypoxia, acidosis, hypercapnia
Hypercalcemia	Depletion of catecholamine stores in the heart (as seen in congestive heart failure, chronic hypertension, and elderly patients)
Digitalis	Loss of functioning muscle mass with ischemia/infarction
Glucagon	Anesthetics, especially potent inhalational agents, propofol, and thiopental
	Electrolytes: hyperkalemia, hypocalcemia
	Antiarrhythmic agents, including β-blockers and calcium blockers

Questions

1. Which of the following is TRUE regarding coronary circulation?
   a. Coronary dominance is defined by the origin of the LCX.
   b. The posteromedial papillary muscle is most susceptible to ischemic rupture.
   c. The arterial blood supply of the AV node is the LAD.
   d. Branches of the LCX are termed diagonal branches.

2. In Figure 69.6, point (c) corresponds to:
   a. aortic valve opening
   b. the end of isovolumetric contraction
   c. mitral valve closing
   d. end-systolic volume

3. In patients with aortic stenosis, left ventricular afterload is primarily determined by:
   a. systemic vascular resistance
   b. left ventricular wall thickness
   c. the resistance across the stenotic valve
   d. left ventricular diameter

Answers

1. b. The posteromedial papillary muscle is only supplied by the PDA, making it more susceptible to ischemic rupture. Coronary dominance is defined by the origin of the PDA. The blood supply of the AV node is the PDA. Branches of the LCX are termed obtuse marginal arteries.

2. d. (a) closure of the mitral valve, the beginning of isovolumetric contraction and systole, end-diastolic volume; (b) opening of the aortic valve; (c) closure of the aortic valve, end-systolic volume, beginning of isovolumetric relaxation and diastole; (d) opening of the mitral valve

3. c. In normal patients, left ventricular afterload is primarily determined by SVR. In patients with significant aortic stenosis, the primary determinant of afterload is the resistance to ventricular ejection by the stenotic valve. The diameter and wall thickness of the ventricle are determinants of the ventricular wall tension as determined by Laplace's law, but are not the primary determinants of ventricular afterload.

Further reading

Vacanti, C. A., Sikka, P. K., Urman, R. U., Dershwitz, M., and Segal, B. S. (2011). *Essential Clinical Anesthesia*, 1st edn. Cambridge University Press.

Sun, L. S. and Schwarzenberger, J. C. (2010). Chapter 16. Cardiac physiology. In *Miller's Anesthesia*, 7th edn. Philadelphia: Churchill-Livingstone Elsevier, pp. 393–410.

Chapter 70

Cardiovascular pharmacology

Erich N. Marks and Lauren J. Cornella

Keywords

Electrolytes (calcium, phosphorus); cardiovascular effects
Positive inotropes
Phosphodiesterase III inhibitors (inodilators); milrinone, others
Digitalis actions and toxicity
Vasoconstrictors
Non-adrenergic vasoconstrictors; vasopressin and congeners
Beta-blockers; anti-anginal drugs
Vasodilators – nitroprusside, nitroglycerin, hydralazine, calcium channel blockers, others
Angiotensin-converting enzyme inhibitors and angiotensin II receptor blockers

Cardiac performance and end-organ blood flow can be manipulated pharmacologically in order to maintain adequate tissue perfusion and oxygen delivery.

Oxygen delivery (DO_2) is determined by the following equation:

$$DO_2 = CO \times [1.39 \times Hgb \times SaO_2 + (0.003 \times PaO_2)]$$

Where CO = cardiac output

Hgb = hemoglobin concentation

SaO_2 = hemoglobin oxygen saturation

PaO_2 = partial pressure of oxygen in blood

With an adequate hemoglobin level and oxygen saturation, cardiac output becomes the main determinant of oxygen delivery.

The role of electrolytes in cardiovascular performance

Ca^{2+} is the dominant electrolyte involved in modulating myocardial contractility and vascular smooth muscle tone.

In the cardiac myocyte, intracellular calcium binds to *troponin C*, which allows actin to form cross-bridges with myosin and contraction occurs. For myocardial relaxation, calcium must be removed from troponin C. In normal hearts, only 25% of myofilaments are saturated with calcium, leaving a large reserve of potential contractility that can be activated by either increasing Ca^{2+} concentrations or sensitizing the myocytes to Ca^{2+} already present.

In myocytes, the messenger *cyclic adenosine monophosphate (cAMP)* controls Ca^{2+} concentrations. cAMP activates protein kinase A, which phosphorylates intracellular targets, increasing intracellular Ca^{2+} concentrations and enhancing Ca^{2+} reuptake. This results in both increased contraction during systole (inotropy) and enhanced relaxation during diastole (lusitropy).

In vascular smooth muscle, *calmodulin* regulates actin and myosin, leading to vasoconstriction in the presence of calcium. Here, cAMP has the opposite effect – it enhances reuptake of Ca^{2+} by the sarcoplasmic reticulum, decreasing its availability for contraction and promoting vasodilation.

All drugs used to manage myocardial contractility and vascular smooth muscle tone act by altering intracellular Ca^{2+} concentrations as shown in Figure 70.1.

Significant *hyperphosphatemia* can decrease intracellular Ca^{2+} levels by decreasing Ca^{2+} absorption in the gut and causing frank precipitation. The resulting hypocalcemia depresses myocardial contractility and decreases vascular tone.

Intravenous inotropic drugs

The most commonly used *inotropic drugs* all increase cardiac output by either increasing the amount of cAMP produced in the cardiac myocyte or inhibiting its breakdown. The major difference in these agents is their effect on the peripheral vasculature.

Inoconstrictors (calcium chloride) increase contractility and vasoconstriction.

Inodilators (dobutamine, milrinone, glucagon, levosimendan) increase contractility and promote vasodilation.

Essential Clinical Anesthesia Review: Keywords, Questions and Answers for the Boards, ed. Linda S. Aglio, Robert W. Lekowski, and Richard D. Urman. Published by Cambridge University Press. © Cambridge University Press 2015.

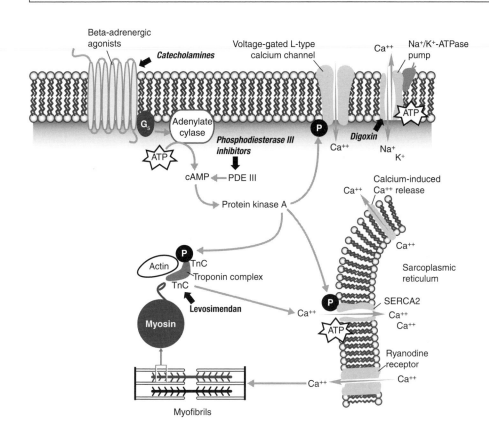

Figure 70.1 Effect of inotropic drugs on intracellular calcium. From: Vacanti et al., 2011. Cambridge University Press, p. 439.

Mixed inotropes (epinephrine, dopamine) increase contractility and have mixed effects on the peripheral vasculature depending on drug dosing. The most common inotropes are listed in Table 70.1.

Digitalis (digoxin)

Digitalis (digoxin) is an oral drug that acts as a modest positive inotrope and an antiarrhythmic. It increases intracellular Ca^{2+} through inhibition of the Na^+/K^+ ATPase, which normally exchanges intracellular Ca^{2+} for extracellular Na^+ and K^+ (see Figure 70.1). This also gives digoxin its antiarrhythmic property, as it slows electrical impulse propagation through the cardiac conduction system.

Digoxin has a narrow therapeutic window. The risk of toxicity increases with hypokalemia, hypercalcemia, hypomagnesemia, and renal impairment. Signs of toxicity include arrhythmias (atrial tachycardia with block, bradyarrhythmias, ventricular tachycardia), visual disturbances, and mental disturbances.

Vasoconstrictors

Vasoconstrictors induce contraction of vascular smooth muscle, resulting in increased systemic vascular resistance (SVR) and increased mean arterial pressure (MAP). Remember:

$$MAP = CO \times SVR$$

Where CO = cardiac output

End-organ perfusion must be monitored closely when these agents are used. Pharmacologic vasoconstriction may actually decrease end-organ perfusion despite increased MAP. For this reason, vasoconstrictors must not replace adequate volume resuscitation. See Table 70.2 for the commonly used vasoconstrictors.

Vasodilators

Vasodilators produce vascular smooth muscle relaxation and decrease SVR. They are primarily indicated for elevated SVR, myocardial ischemia, and heart failure. Some (nitroglycerin, nitroprusside) are converted to nitric oxide in the body, increasing the concentration of cGMP and producing venous and arterial vasodilation. Others (hydralazine, fenoldopam, nicardipine) act through different mechanisms described below.

Calcium channel blockers, nitrates, and beta-blockers have *anti-anginal effects* through either reduction of myocardial oxygen demand or increase in myocardial oxygen supply. Table 70.3 lists the most commonly used vasodilators in anesthesia and their mechanisms of action.

β-blocking drugs

β-blocking drugs bind to β-adrenergic receptors and antagonize their effects, resulting in decreased heart rate and contractility, decreased systemic blood pressure, decreased AV node conduction, and an increased refractory period of the pacemaker cells. Reduction of heart rate and slowing of conduction

Table 70.1 Inotropic drugs

Agent	Action	HR	Con	Preload	SVR/PVR	BP	CO	Indications	Use
Epinephrine	α_1, α_2, β_1, β_2-agonist							Reduced CO	2–10 μg IV bolus
	Dose-dependent action							Hypotension	Infusion 2–20 μg/min (central line)
	1–3 μg/min = β	↑	↑↑↑	↑	-/↓	↑	↑	Cardiac arrest / Anaphylaxis	Arrest: 0.5–1.0 mg IV bolus / Monitor end-organ perfusion closely
	3–10 μg/min = β > α	↑↑			-/↑	↑	-/↓		Short half-life (minutes)
	10+ μg/min = α > β	↑↑			↑↑		-/↓	Cardiogenic shock / Bronchospasm	
Dopamine	α_1, β_1, β_2, D_1-agonist							Low CO	Infusion 2–20 μg/kg/min (central line)
	Indirect NE release							Low SVR / Renal insufficiency (low dose)	Monitor end-organ perfusion (especially > 10 μg/kg/min)
	1–3 μg/kg/min = D_1	-			↓	Variable	↑		
	3–10 = $\beta_2 > D_1$	↑	↑↑	↑	-/↑	↑	↑/-↓		Short half-life (minutes)
	10+ = $\alpha_1 > \beta$, D_1	↑↑	↑↑	↑	↑↑	↑	↑/-↓		
Dobutamine	Strong $\beta_1 > \beta_2$	↑/	↑↑	-	-/↓	Variable	↑↑	Low CO (especially with ↑ SVR/PVR) / Right heart failure	Infusion: 2–30 μg/kg/min / Short half-life (minutes)
	Weak α_1	↑↑			↑ (in β-blocked patients)			Stress echocardiography	25–75 μg/kg load over 10 min
Milrinone	Inhibits phosphodiesterase III	-/↑	↑↑	↓	↓/↓↓	Variable	↑↑	Low CO (especially with ↑ SVR/PVR)	(beware ↓ BP, esp. with ↓ preload)
	Increases cAMP / Does not act at β receptors							Right heart failure / Synergistic with β-agonists	Infusion: 0.375–0.75 μg/kg/min / Longer half-life (2.4h)
Glucagon	Increases intracellular cAMP	↑	↑↑	-/↓	-/↓	↑	↑	Hypoglycemia / β-blocker toxicity / Low CO / Refractory CHF	Bolus: 1–5 mg IV slowly / Infusion: 25–75 μg/min / Rarely used because of multiple side effects (Nausea, emesis, tachycardia, hyperglycemia, hypokalemia, anaphylaxis)

Drug	Mechanism	HR	Con	SVR	PVR	BP	CO	Indications	Dose/Preparation	Side effects/Notes
Calcium chloride	Free Ca^{+2} ion	-/↓	↑	-		↑	↑/↓	Hypocalcemia	10% calcium chloride 100 mg/ml 200–1,000 mg slow IVP (prefer central line) Causes vein inflammation Do not use Immediately after reperfusion	Hyperkalemia Hypotension from hypocalcemia Calcium channel blockade Counteracts hypermagnesemia
Levosimendan*	Calcium-sensitizing agent cAMP-independent Vascular dilation via K^+-ATPase channels	-/↑	↑↑	↓	↓	Variable	↑↑	Low CO	Bolus: 6–24 µg/kg (10–20 min) Infusion: 0.05–0.4 µg/kg/min (up to 24 h) Active metabolite with 80 h half-life Effects last 24–48 h after infusion stopped	Right heart failure Supplement β-agonists Possible reduced proarrhythmic effect

IV, intravenous; HR, heart rate; Con, contractility; SVR, systemic vascular resistance; PVR, pulmonary vascular resistance; BP, blood pressure; CO, cardiac output; CHF, congestive heart failure; IVP, IV push; ATPase, adenosine triposphatase.

*Levosimendan (inodilator) (not available currently in the United States) – a calcium-sensitizing agent that acts as an inodilator. It exerts its inotropic effect by sensitizing calcium to troponin C, thereby enhancing the calcium sensitivity of the cardiac myofilaments. It does not increase intracellular calcium. It also causes vascular dilation by opening potassium-ATPase channels on vascular smooth muscle cell membranes. Levosimendan mildly inhibits phosphodiesterase III activity. Adapted from: Vacanti et al., 2011, *Essential Clinical Anesthesia*, Cambridge University Press, Chapter 71.

Table 70.2 Vasoconstrictors

Drug	Action	HR	Contractility	Preload	SVR/PVR	BP	CO	Indications	Use
Phenylephrine	α_1-agonist	-/↓ (reflex)	-	-	↑↑	↑	-/↓	Peripheral vasodilation Low SVR SVT (reflex vagal stimulation) TOF spell	40–80 µg IV bolus Infusion: 20–200 µg/min Short half-life (minutes)
Ephedrine	Indirect NE release Mild direct α, β_1, β_2 Acts like small-dose epinephrine	↑	↑	↑↑	↑	↑	↑	Low SVR (especially if HR low) Low CO (especially if HR low) Transient cardiac depression	5–10 mg IV bolus 25–50 mg IM Tachyphylaxis with repeat dosing Slightly longer duration of action
Norepinephrine	α_1; α_2; β_1-agonist Intense α_1 and α_2 constriction throughout dosing range	variable	↑	↑↑	↑↑↑	↑	-/↓	Peripheral vascular collapse Shock, vasoplegia,↓ SVR Need ↑ SVR with some ↑ Con Phenylephrine is not working	2–10 µg IV bolus (never more unless extremis) Infusion 2–20 µg/min (central line) Monitor end-organ perfusion closely Short half-life (minutes)
Vasopressin	Direct vasoconstriction via V_1 receptors No action at β or α receptors	-/↓	-	-	↑↑ (possible PVR sparing at lower doses)	↑	variable	Second-line agent: shock, vasoplegia, sepsis, ↓ SVR Pulmonary HTN with ↓ SVR Use with milrinone to counteract ↓ SVR ACEI/ARB-refractory hypotension	Infusion: 0.01–0.04 µg/min (pharm dose) Monitor end-organ perfusion closely Half-life 10–35 min
Methylene blue	Complex mechanism Inhibits NO/GMP Inhibits NO synthase	-	-	-	↑↑	↑	-	Not a first-line agent Limited clinical trials and case reports ↓ SVR, persistent vasoplegia	Bolus: 15–20 mg/kg over 15–30 min Effect of bolus lasts 2–3h Infusion: 0.25–1.0 mg/kg/h Monitor end-organ perfusion

NE, norepinephrine; NO, nitric oxide; HR, heart rate; SVR, systemic vascular resistance; PVR, pulmonary vascular resistance; BP, blood pressure; CO, cardiac output; CON, contraindications; SVT, supraventricular tachycardia; TOF, tetralogy of Fallot; HTN, hypertension; ACEI, angiotensin-converting enzyme inhibitor; ARB, angiotensin receptor blocker; IV, intravenous; IM, intramuscular.
From: Vacanti et al., 2011, Chapter 71.

Table 70.3 Vasodilators

Drug	Action	HR	Contractility	Preload	SVR/PVR	BP	CO	Indications	Use
Nitroglycerin	Direct vasodilator ↑ cGMP production Venous > arterial Excellent coronary effects	↑ (reflex)	-	↓↓	↓	↓	↑/↓	Myocardial ischemia Increased coronary spasm HTN Pulmonary HTN CHF	40–80 µg IV bolus Infusion: 10–200 µg/min At infusions higher than 200 µg/min, switch to SNP or another agent Tolerance if infused for long periods
Nitroprusside	Direct vasodilator ↑ cGMP production Arterial = venous	↑ (reflex)	-	↓	↓↓	↓	↑/↓	HTN, ↑ SVR Controlled hypotension	Infusion: 0.1–2.0 µg/kg/min Max infusion: 10 µg/kg/min (short periods only) Avoid prolonged doses >20 µg/kg/min (toxicity) Protect from light
Hydralazine	Direct vasodilator Arterial >> >> venous	↑ (reflex)	-	-	↓↓	↓	-/↑	HTN, ↑ SVR	Continuous BP monitoring (A-line) Use with caution in liver or kidney dysfunction
Fenoldopam	Synthetic dopamine receptor agonist Rapid-acting arterial dilator Maintains renal perfusion	↑ (reflex)	-	-	↓↓	↓	↑	Severe hypertension in patients with impaired renal function	IV infusion: 0.01–1.6 µg/kg/min Readjust dose every 15–20 min for effect
Nicardipine	Dihydropyridine calcium channel blocker Arterial >> >> venous	↑ (reflex)	-	-	↓↓	↓	-/↑	HTN To improve lusitropy in cardiac ischemia Coronary vasospasm	Infusion: 1–4 µg/kg/min Titrate to BP May cause phlebitis in peripheral IV (infused for >12 h)

HR, heart rate; SVR, systemic vascular resistance; PVR, pulmonary vascular resistance; BP, blood pressure; CO, cardiac output; HTN hypertension; CHF, congestive heart failure; IV, intravenous; SNP, sodium nitroprusside.
From: Vacanti et al., 2011, Chapter 71.

Table 70.4 β-blockers

Drug	Action	Onset	β half-life, h	Elimination	IV dose
Propranolol	β$_1$-, β$_2$-antagonist	2–5 min	3.5–4.0	Hepatic	0.5–1.0 mg prn
Labetalol	β$_1$-, β$_2$-, α$_1$-antagonist Ratio of α to β-blockade is 1:7	2–5 min	3–5	Hepatic	10–40 mg prn (max. 300 mg)
Metoprolol	Selective β$_1$-antagonist	5 min (peak 20 min)	3–4	Hepatic	1–5 mg prn (max, 15 mg)
Esmolol	Selective β$_1$-antagonist	Rapid	9 min	Red blood cell and plasma esterases	0.25–0.5 mg/kg prn Infusion: 50–300 µg/kg/min

prn, as needed.
From: Vacanti et al., 2011, Chapter 71.

Table 70.5 Calcium channel blockers

Drug	Action	Onset	β half-life	IV dose	Comments
Verapamil	Strong myocardial effects Arterial dilation	3–5 min	3–10 h Hepatic	1–2 mg prn (low dose, especially during anesthesia)	Myocardial depression > peripheral *arterial* vasodilation Use low doses in GA, unstable patients, or patients with reduced EF Rx: SVT, HTN, vasospasm, ischemia
Diltiazem	Weaker myocardial effects Arterial dilation	2–5 min	3–5 h Hepatic and renal	20 mg bolus, then 5–15 mg/h infusion Lower doses with hemodynamic instability	Less myocardial depression compared with verapamil Causes selective coronary artery vasodilation Rx: SVT, HTN, vasospasm, angina
Nicardipine (see vasodilators)	No myocardial effects Arterial dilation	Minutes	14 min Hepatic	1–4 µg/kg/min	Titrate to blood pressure May cause phlebitis in peripheral IV if infused for >12 h

prn, as needed
From: Vacanti et al., 2011, Chapter 71.

occurs by decreasing the availability of cAMP, which slows the inward current of Na$^+$ in the pacemaker cells, delaying spontaneous depolarization.

Each β-blocking drug is characterized by a different affinity for the β-adrenergic receptors (β$_1$ and β$_2$), metabolism, and half-life, as shown in Table 70.4.

Indications for β-blockade include: hypertension, tachyarrhythmias, myocardial ischemia and infarction (to decrease myocardial oxygen demand), and dynamic ventricular outflow obstruction. β-blockade may also decrease perioperative cardiac morbidity and mortality.

Toxicity may be treated with large doses of β-agonists, temporary pacing, or other inotropic drugs whose mechanism of action does not involve β-adrenergic receptors (calcium, milrinone, or glucagon).

Calcium channel blockers

Calcium channel blockers interact with L-type Ca^{2+} channels, blocking Ca^{2+} entry into the cell. Contractility, heart rate, and peripheral vascular tone (especially arterial) are decreased. The refractory period of pacemaker action potentials is increased.

Indications are hypertension, supraventricular arrhythmias, arterial and coronary vasospasm, and myocardial ischemia (to decrease myocardial oxygen consumption).

Angiotensin-converting enzyme (ACE) inhibitors and angiotensin II receptor blockers (ARBs)

ACE inhibitors block the conversion of angiotensin I to angiotensin II, causing vasodilation and reduction in salt and water reabsorption in the kidney. Indications include hypertension, CHF, and prevention of diabetic nephropathy. Side effects of these drugs include dry cough (from bradykinin increase), hyperkalemia, hypotension, and renal impairment. Common ACEIs are captopril, enalapril, lisinopril, and ramipril.

Patients who experience dry cough may be placed on an ARB. These drugs antagonize the effects of angiotensin II at binding sites. Common ARBs are losartan, irbesartan, and valsartan.

Caution for these drugs is advised in patients with renal dysfunction and volume depletion.

Proper drug selection

There is no gold standard for choosing an inotrope, vasoconstrictor, or vasodilator. The proper drug selection requires knowledge of Ca^{2+} modulation in the myocardium and vascular smooth muscle, understanding the mechanism of action of the chosen drug(s), and weighing the side effect profiles against the desired effect.

Questions

1. Oxygen delivery to tissues is least affected by which of the following?

   a. hemoglobin oxygen saturation
   b. cardiac output
   c. the partial pressure of oxygen in blood
   d. hemoglobin concentration

2. With high doses or prolonged infusions, methemoglobinemia is a possible side effect of which of the following medications?

   a. nitroglycerin
   b. nitroprusside
   c. milrinone
   d. methylene blue

3. All of the following drugs demonstrate preferential arterial dilation except for which?

   a. hydralazine
   b. nitroprusside
   c. nicardipine
   d. nitroglycerin

4. Which of the following is FALSE regarding the intracellular messenger cAMP?

   a. cAMP increases the release of Ca^{2+} by the sarcoplasmic reticulum within the myocardium.
   b. cAMP decreases myocardial lusitropy.
   c. cAMP promotes vasodilation in vascular smooth muscle.
   d. Concentrations of cAMP are increased by stimulation of β-adrenergic receptors.

Answers

1. c. Oxygen delivery to tissues is dependent on cardiac output and the oxygen content of the blood: $DO_2 = CO \times [1.39 \times Hgb \times SaO_2 + (0.003 \times PaO_2)]$. As can be seen from this equation, the PaO_2 contributes very little to the delivery of oxygen to tissues. In fact, it is often omitted from the equation in clinical decision making. The primary determinants of tissue oxygen delivery are cardiac output, hemoglobin concentration, and oxygen saturation.

2. a. Prolonged infusions and high doses of nitroglycerin can put a patient at risk for developing methemoglobinemia. Along with stopping the infusion, methylene blue is a potential therapy for methemoglobinemia. Nitroprusside can cause both cyanide and thiocyanate toxicity in patients with renal dysfunction and during prolonged infusions. Milrinone has no specific associated toxicities.

3. d. Hydralazine, nitroprusside, and nicardipine all preferentially dilate the arterial system, though all dilate the venous system at higher doses. Nitroglycerin preferentially dilates the venous system with minimal arterial dilation.

4. b. The intracellular messenger cAMP is linked to the action of many cardiovascular drugs by helping to control Ca^{2+} concentrations. In cardiac myocytes, cAMP increases intracellular Ca^{2+} concentrations and enhances Ca^{2+} reuptake, resulting in both increased contraction during systole (inotropy) and increased relaxation during diastole (lusitropy). In vascular smooth muscle, increased cAMP enhances reuptake of Ca^{2+} by the sarcoplasmic reticulum, decreasing its availability for contraction and promoting vasodilation.

Further reading

Vacanti, C. A., Sikka, P. K., Urman, R. U., Dershwitz, M., and Segal, B. S. (2011). *Essential Clinical Anesthesia*, 1st edn. Cambridge University Press.

Butterworth, J. F. (2103). Chapter 2. Cardiovascular drugs. In *A Practical Approach to Cardiac Anesthesia*, 5th edn. Philadelphia: Lippincott Williams & Wilkins, pp. 23–88.

Pagel, P. S. et al. (2010). Chapter 23. Cardiovascular pharmacology. In *Miller's Anesthesia*, 7th edn. Philadelphia: Churchill-Livingstone Elsevier, pp. 595–632.

Chapter 71

Adjunct cardiovascular drugs

Erich N. Marks and Lauren J. Cornella

Heparin

Anticoagulation is essential to the safe conduct of cardiopulmonary bypass (CPB) and the most common anticoagulant used is heparin. *Heparin* is a negatively charged mucopolysaccharide with a molecular weight that varies from 10 to 30 kDa. Heparin is derived from either bovine lung or porcine intestine.

Heparin binds to *antithrombin III* (AT III) via a specific pentasaccharide sequence on the heparin molecule, increasing the activity of AT III up to 4,000-fold. AT III primarily limits the action of thrombin, but also regulates several other factors in the coagulation cascade, including IXa, Xa, XIa, and XIIa, ultimately inhibiting clot formation.

Unfractionated heparin contains heparin molecules of many different sizes, with smaller heparin molecules having a greater anticoagulant effect. For this reason, the clinical effect of a dose of unfractionated heparin can be quite variable. The amount of circulating AT III, the underlying health of the patient, and preexisting liver disease can also affect the clinical response to a dose of heparin.

The anticoagulant effect of heparin is generally monitored by *activated partial thromboplastin time (aPTT) or activated clotting time (ACT)*. ACT is a point-of-care test that measures time to clot formation via the intrinsic coagulation pathway by the addition of Factor XII activators (kaolin, Celite, glass beads) and increases linearly with heparin concentration. Recommended ACT values for the commencement of CPB varies by institution but is usually >350 seconds.

Adverse effects of heparin include: allergic reactions (due to its porcine or bovine origin), bone demineralization (due to increased osteoclast activity), bleeding (due to a relatively narrow therapeutic window), and heparin-induced thrombocytopenia.

Protamine

Protamine is the only widely available agent for the reversal of heparin. Protamine is a polycationic compound derived from salmon sperm. It forms ionic bonds with circulating heparin, preventing its binding with AT III and reversing its clinical effect. The typical dosing is 1 mg/100 units of heparin to be reversed. Rapid administration of protamine (>50 mg/10 min) is ill advised.

Three types of *adverse reactions to protamine* have been described:

1. Hypotension related to histamine release from mast cells during rapid administration.
2. IgE-mediated allergic reactions in patients that have previously received protamine.
3. IgG-mediated anaphylactoid reactions leading to severe pulmonary vasoconstriction, pulmonary hypertension, and right heart failure.

Treatment of these reactions includes stopping the protamine infusion and instituting supportive therapy. If hypotension was due to histamine release, protamine can usually be restarted slowly once the patient is stable. If the adverse reaction was due to allergic or anaphylactoid means, protamine may be contraindicated.

Essential Clinical Anesthesia Review: Keywords, Questions and Answers for the Boards, ed. Linda S. Aglio, Robert W. Lekowski, and Richard D. Urman. Published by Cambridge University Press. © Cambridge University Press 2015.

Heparin-induced thrombocytopenia

The estimated incidence of heparin-induced thrombocytopenia (HIT) is between 10% and 20% of patients exposed to heparin. There are two distinct types of heparin-induced thrombocytopenia, HIT type 1 and HIT type 2. Studies have shown that the incidence of HIT is higher with heparin derived from bovine sources.

HIT type 1 is due to direct antiplatelet effects of heparin and produces a mild, transient, generally asymptomatic thrombocytopenia that rarely requires treatment. It generally appears two days after heparin exposure.

HIT type 2 is the result of plasma IgG antibody formation directed at heparin/platelet factor 4 (PF4) complexes, which causes a serious and potentially fatal clinical syndrome. It may occur in any patient exposed to heparin, but the use of unfractionated heparin, long-term exposure, large doses of heparin, the postsurgical setting, and a history of previous heparin exposure increase the risk.

The *diagnosis of HIT type 2* is suspected in the setting of an unexplained decrease in platelet count by at least 50% occurring four to ten days after heparin exposure. HIT causes thrombocytopenia and a prothrombotic state. Thrombosis may be seen in the venous and/or arterial circulation. Diagnostic tests for HIT include the commonly performed enzyme-linked immunosorbent assay (ELISA) for IgG antibodies to the heparin/PF4 complex, and the gold-standard serotonin release assay (SRA). The ELISA has a sensitivity of 97%, but a specificity of only 74% to 87%. If the ELISA is negative, the likelihood of HIT is very low. The SRA is both highly sensitive and specific, but is performed at very few laboratories and is thus often used as a confirmatory test in the setting of a positive ELISA and a high pretest probability.

Treatment of HIT consists of removing the patient from all heparin exposure, including heparin-coated vascular catheters and low molecular weight heparin, and initiating alternative anticoagulation. Platelet transfusions are contraindicated.

Heparin alternatives

Alternatives to heparin include the direct thrombin inhibitors lepirudin, bivalirudin, argatroban, and danaparoid, as well as the factor Xa inhibitor fondaparinux. Dosing recommendations for the direct thrombin inhibitors are given in Table 71.1. It should be noted that these doses are not absolute and actual doses will depend on types of monitoring devices available, need for CPB, and the patient's specific medical condition. The use of direct thrombin inhibitors for CPB is off label.

Danaparoid is not currently available in the United States. It has 17% cross-reactivity with heparin/PF4 antibodies and may cause or worsen HIT.

Bivalirudin is metabolized by plasma proteases and eliminated by the kidneys. Renal dysfunction may prolong its half-life.

Fondaparinux is a direct inhibitor of factor Xa, and thereby inhibits the conversion of prothrombin to thrombin. It has a long half-life (approximately 17 hours) and is cleared by the kidneys. Fondaparinux can form a complex with PF4; however, heparin/PF4 antibodies do not react with fondaparinux/PF4 complexes in such a way that causes platelet activation and HIT. Its use in patients with HIT for DVT prophylaxis is off label. Dosing is once daily, subcutaneously.

The direct thrombin inhibitors and fondaparinux have no antidote; the effects must be allowed to dissipate with time. The clinical effects may also be difficult to monitor, as the bleeding time, PTT, INR, and ACT are all increased by these drugs.

Antifibrinolytic drugs

Antifibrinolytic drugs are commonly used in trauma and surgery to decrease bleeding and the need for transfusion. These drugs include aminocaproic acid, tranexamic acid, and aprotinin.

Aminocaproic acid and *tranexamic acid* are lysine analogues that compete for the lysine binding sites on plasminogen and fibrinogen, thereby inhibiting plasmin formation and inhibiting fibrinolysis. Rapid administration may cause transient hypotension.

Aprotinin is a serine protease inhibitor that has intrinsic procoagulant effects as well as antifibrinolytic and anti-inflammatory effects. It is derived from bovine lung tissue and has been implicated in anaphylactic and anaphylactoid

Table 71.1 Dosing regimens of alternate drugs

Drug	Half-life	Elimination	Dose	Note
Argatroban	39–51 min	Hepatic	PCI 2–3 µg/kg/min CPB 5–10 µg/kg/min	
Danaparoid	~25 h	Renal	Not clearly defined	Unavailable in US Ab cross-reactivity
Lepirudin	~80 min	Renal	Bolus, 0.25 mg/kg Infusion, 0.5 mg/min	
Bivalirudin	25 min	Plasma proteases	Bolus, 1.5 mg/kg Infusion, 2.5 mg/kg/h	

Ab, antibody; CPB, cardiopulmonary bypass; PCI, percutaneous intervention.

reactions. Aprotinin has been linked to an increased risk of death and postoperative renal failure and is no longer available in the United States.

Questions

1. All of the following are true regarding heparin anticoagulation except which?
   a. The anticoagulant effect of heparin relies on proper levels and function of antithrombin III.
   b. Protamine reverses heparin anticoagulation by potentiating its enzymatic degradation.
   c. Heparin-induced thrombocytopenia (HIT) can be caused by exposure to heparin-coated catheters.
   d. Long-term heparin anticoagulation may cause bone demineralization.

2. If heparin-induced thrombocytopenia (HIT) is suspected in a patient:
   a. Low molecular weight heparin can be used as an alternative.
   b. All anticoagulation should be stopped in the patient.
   c. Platelet transfusion is indicated if the platelet count is low.
   d. All types of heparin should be stopped, heparin-coated catheters removed, and alternative anticoagulation started.

Answers

1. b. Protamine forms ionic bonds with circulating heparin, preventing its binding with AT III and reversing its clinical effect. The remaining statements regarding heparin anticoagulation are true.
2. d. If HIT is suspected in a patient, all heparin exposure must be discontinued. This includes low molecular weight heparin and exposure to heparin-coated catheters. The patient must be anticoagulated with an alternative agent because the patient is at high risk for thrombosis and thrombosis-related complications. Platelet transfusions are contraindicated in HIT.

Further reading

Mannucci, P. M. and Levi, M. (2007). Prevention and treatment of major blood loss. *New England Journal of Medicine* 356, 2301–2311.

Park, K. W. (2004). Protamine and protamine reactions. *International Anesthesiology Clinics* 42(3), 135–145.

Warkentin, T. E. and Greinacher, A. (2003) Heparin induced thrombocytopenia and cardiac surgery. *Annals of Thoracic Surgery* 76, 2121–2131.

Vacanti, C. A., Sikka, P. K., Urman, R. U., Dershwitz, M., and Segal, B. S. (2011). *Essential Clinical Anesthesia*, 1st edn. Cambridge University Press.

Chapter

72

Coronary artery bypass grafting utilizing cardiopulmonary bypass

Erich N. Marks and Lauren J. Cornella

Keywords

Indications for coronary artery bypass grafting

Myocardial oxygen supply and demand: determining factors

Monitoring considerations for coronary artery bypass grafting using cardiopulmonary bypass

Circulatory assist: cardiopulmonary bypass (CPB): components (pump, heat exchanger, oxygenator, filters)

CPB: cardiopulmonary bypass techniques

CPB: mechanisms of gas exchange

CPB: priming solutions, hemodilution

CPB: anesthetic considerations during bypass

CPB: cooling and warming

CPB: anticoagulation and antithrombin III deficiency

CPB: physiologic effects

Alpha-stat and pH-stat blood gas management

Indications for coronary artery bypass grafting

1. Left main coronary artery disease.
2. Left main equivalent disease, defined as 70% stenosis or greater in the proximal left anterior descending artery (LAD) and proximal left circumflex artery (LCX).
3. Multivessel coronary artery disease.
4. Stable angina and two-vessel disease with significant proximal LAD obstruction.
5. Stable angina and one- to two-vessel coronary artery disease without proximal LAD stenosis but with a significant amount of viable myocardium at risk.
6. Severe, incapacitating angina despite maximal medical therapy.

Myocardial oxygen supply and demand

Myocardial function depends on a balance of oxygen supply and demand. *Increased oxygen demand* results from increased contractility, increased heart rate, and increased wall tension.

Decreased myocardial oxygen supply results from decreased coronary artery blood flow, decreased arterial oxygen content, and increased oxygen extraction.

Monitoring for CABG using CPB

In addition to standard American Society of Anesthesiologists monitors, specialized monitors are used in CABG patients to guide management. A Foley catheter to monitor urine output, arterial catheter for blood pressure monitoring and frequent blood gas analysis, and central venous catheter for vasoactive infusions and central venous pressure monitoring are customary.

A pulmonary artery catheter may be considered in patients with cardiac failure or pulmonary hypertension. It also allows for transvenous pacing.

Transesophageal echocardiography (TEE) may be useful in select patients, particularly those with poor ventricular function or valvular disease.

Components of the CPB circuit

- A venous cannula drains blood from the right heart to the CPB circuit. It can be placed in the right atrium, superior vena cava and inferior vena cava, or femoral vein.
- A venous reservoir stores blood drained from the right heart.
- A pump head pumps blood through the circuit.
- A heat exchanger warms or cools the blood.
- The oxygenator receives blood from the heat exchanger and oxygenates it, adds anesthetic gas, and removes carbon dioxide. Two types of oxygenators are available – *bubble oxygenators* and *membrane oxygenators*. In a *bubble oxygenator*, small bubbles of oxygen make direct contact with the blood and passive diffusion of oxygen and carbon dioxide occurs. Oxygen diffusion is directly related to the surface area of the bubbles, while carbon dioxide removal is proportional to the total gas flow through the oxygenator. Trauma to the blood components is the major disadvantage of this oxygenator. *Membrane oxygenators*

Essential Clinical Anesthesia Review: Keywords, Questions and Answers for the Boards, ed. Linda S. Aglio, Robert W. Lekowski, and Richard D. Urman. Published by Cambridge University Press. © Cambridge University Press 2015.

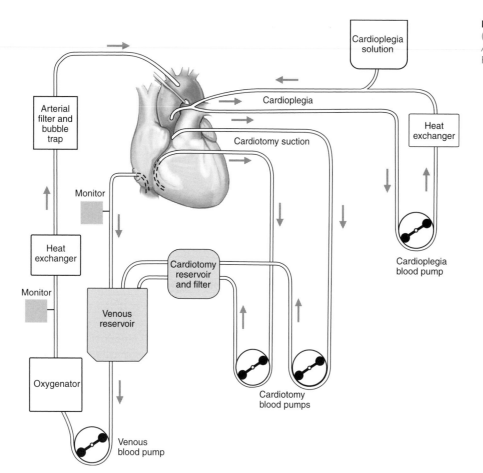

Figure 72.1 Components of the CPB circuit. (From Vacanti et al. 2011. *Essential Clinical Anesthesia*, Cambridge University Press, Figure 73.2.)

separate the blood and gas using a thin semipermeable membrane that allows for diffusion. The disadvantage is resistance to blood flow, which necessitates its position distal to the pump head.

- An arterial filter removes air and debris.
- An arterial cannula returns blood to the patient's systemic circulation. This cannula is usually placed in the ascending aorta, but can also be placed in the axillary or femoral arteries.

The **CPB circuit** also contains:

- a cardioplegia circuit on a separate pump head, which is used to deliver a high-potassium solution to arrest the heart
- cardiotomy suction(s) that return waste blood from the surgical field to the venous reservoir

Components of the CPB circuit are illustrated in Figure 72.1.

Physiologic effects of CPB

The physiologic effects of CPB are numerous. The nonpulsatile nature of CPB decreases lymphatic flow and increases the neuroendocrine response. The interaction between blood and nonphysiologic surfaces can cause coagulopathy, red cell hemolysis, thrombocytopenia, and a systemic inflammatory response (SIRS). Hyperglycemia from stress is common.

The CPB circuit is usually *primed* with lactated Ringer's solution with bicarbonate buffer. The priming volume of 800 to 1,500 cc causes a dilutional anemia.

Hypotension is frequently seen due to systemic vasodilation from SIRS, decreased blood viscosity, and low levels of calcium. Cardioplegia solution delivered in the aortic root (antegrade) or in the coronary sinus (retrograde) can cause systemic hyperkalemia.

Anesthetic considerations pre-CPB

During the anesthetic induction and in the pre-bypass period, myocardial oxygen supply must be matched to demand. *Anticoagulation* is established with heparin. Activated clotting time (ACT) is monitored throughout the bypass period. Recommended ACT is generally >350 seconds prior to CPB, but varies according to the institution. Heparin requires AT III to function as an anticoagulant (see Chapter 71). If the ACT fails to increase despite heparin dosing, *antithrombin (AT) III deficiency* should be suspected and may need treatment with fresh frozen plasma, AT III concentrate, or synthetic AT III.

Anesthetic management during CPB

Once on full-flow CPB (2 to 2.5 l/min/m^2), asystole is induced by placing a cross-clamp on the ascending aorta (proximal to the arterial cannula) and administering antegrade and/or retrograde cardioplegia.

In some institutions, the patient is *cooled* to decrease the body and heart's metabolic activity. Urine output and the patient's temperature should be monitored closely.

The patient must be *rewarmed* slowly to prevent the formation of gas bubbles within the blood and to prevent creating large temperature gradients between well-perfused organs and those that are vasoconstricted. As the patient is rewarmed, metabolic activity escalates and the patient is at risk for intra-operative awareness.

Arterial blood gas management

Acid–base management during hypothermic CPB is controversial. The two strategies currently employed are *alpha-stat* and *pH-stat management*. Alpha-stat management maintains the ionization state of histidine imidazole constant at low patient temperatures. The solubility of CO_2 increases with hypothermia, resulting in a lower partial pressure of CO_2. This suggests a "respiratory alkalosis," despite a constant total body CO_2. For example, if the $PaCO_2$ is 40 mm Hg at 37°C, it will decrease to 19 mm Hg at 20°C. Alpha-stat strategists maintain that this respiratory alkalosis is physiologically appropriate because the temperature-corrected $PaCO_2$ is normal.

pH-stat strategists maintain the $PaCO_2$ at 40 mm Hg, even when the patient is hypothermic. This is accomplished by adding CO_2 to the CPB circuit. This produces a total body hypercarbia and results in a temperature-corrected "respiratory acidosis."

Weaning from CPB

When the surgeon no longer needs asystole, the aortic cross-clamp is removed and the cardioplegia is washed out by the arterial perfusate. Cardiac activity will resume.

Before weaning from CPB, a checklist should be employed to ensure that:

- core temperature is at least 36°C
- lab values are within normal limits (especially pH, Hct, K, Ca)
- rate and rhythm are adequate to produce a cardiac output (pacing and/or defibrillation may be necessary)
- MAP and contractility are adequate (vasopressors and/or inotropes may be necessary)
- ventilation/oxygenation is resumed and is adequate

- the heart is de-aired and without new regional wall motion abnormalities or valvular disease (TEE is especially helpful here)

To wean from CPB, the venous cannula is clamped and all venous blood returns to the right heart. Residual blood in the circuit can be transfused into the patient via the arterial cannula.

Once safely weaned from CPB, protamine is given to reverse heparin anticoagulation according to the institution's protocol and the patient is decannulated. Communication between the anesthesia provider, perfusionist, and surgeon is essential during protamine administration.

Questions

1. All of the following are consequences of cardiopulmonary bypass except which?
   a. hyperglycemia
   b. coagulopathy
   c. increased pulse pressure
   d. anemia

2. A patient being managed with a pH-stat strategy is viewed by an alpha-stat strategist as having which of the following?
   a. metabolic acidosis
   b. metabolic alkalosis
   c. respiratory acidosis
   d. respiratory alkalosis

Answers

1. c. The cardiopulmonary bypass circuit uses a nonpulsatile pump. Only a mean arterial pressure can be displayed. Hyperglycemia is a result of the stress response generated by cardiopulmonary bypass. A dilutional anemia is common due to the CPB circuit priming solution. Coagulopathy can also be caused by activation and consumption of platelets and clotting factors by the circuit.

2. c. In the pH-stat approach to blood gas management, the patient's temperature-uncorrected $PaCO_2$ and pH are kept within the normal range by adding CO_2 to the CPB circuit (so that the patient's $PaCO_2$ is 40 even at low temperatures). When temperature-corrected (i.e., viewed by alpha-stat), this patient will appear to have a respiratory acidosis due to the high total body CO_2. In the alpha-stat approach, the temperature-corrected $PaCO_2$ is kept within the normal range, making the in vivo $PaCO_2$ appear low (i.e., respiratory alkalosis by a pH-stat strategist).

Further reading

Vacanti, C. A., Sikka, P. K., Urman, R. U., Dershwitz, M., and Segal, B. S. (2011). *Essential Clinical Anesthesia*, 1st edn. Cambridge University Press.

Green, M. S., Okum, G. S., and Horrow, J. C. (2013). Chapter 11. Anesthetic management of myocardial revascularization. In *A Practical Approach to Cardiac Anesthesia*, 5th edn. Philadelphia: Lippincott Williams & Wilkins, pp. 293–318.

Hessel, E. A. et al. (2013). Chapter 21. Cardiopulmonary bypass: equipment, circuits, and pathophysiology. In *A Practical Approach to Cardiac Anesthesia*, 5th edn. Philadelphia: Lippincott Williams & Wilkins, pp. 587–629.

Chapter

73

Off-pump coronary artery bypass

Zahra M. Malik and Martin Zammert

Advantages of off-pump coronary artery bypass (OPCAB) include avoiding the side effects and complications associated with cardiopulmonary bypass (CPB) such as the development of systemic inflammatory response and aortic manipulation with aortic cross-clamping (leading to atheroma embolization and thus stroke and neurocognitive impairment).

Absolute *contraindications to OPCAB* include hemodynamic instability and poor quality target vessels, which include intramyocardial vessels and diffusely diseased or calcified coronary vessels. Relative contraindications to OPCAB include cardiomegaly/congestive heart failure, critical left main disease, small distal targets, recent/concurrent myocardial infarction, cardiogenic shock, and left ventricular function <35%.

For optimal surgical exposure during OPCAB, the heart must be made immobile and be positioned appropriately, which may involve the use of apical or nonapical suction devices as well as deep pericardial retration sutures. Thus *surgical implications of OPCAB* include cardiac arrhythmias, hemodynamic changes from positioning the heart (especially for posterior RCA CABG), and temporary target vascular occlusion leading to local ischemia from mechanical manipulation. Intracoronary shunts may help to avoid transient ischemia during the suturing of anastomoses.

The implications for *anesthetic management of OPCAB* are similar to coronary bypass utilizing the heart–lung machine. Standard ASA monitors, large-bore IVs for rapid infusion, arterial line for beat-to-beat monitoring, and lab measurements. Central line for pressor and inotrope infusions and pulmonary artery catheter and transesophageal echocardiography are often used. Induction techniques are

similar to those undergoing myocardial revascularization with CPB. Preload should be increased to improve hemodynamic stability during positioning of the heart. *"Fast track" cardiac anesthesia* is administered using a limited dose of short-acting narcotics to facilitate in early postoperative extubation (one to four hours). Regional techniques utilizing thoracic epidurals may facilitate postoperative pain control, but the risk of epidural hematoma is unknown as OPCAB still requires some level of anticoagulation. Heparinization is used during OPCAB but to varying levels. Protamine reversal may or may not be given, and antifibrinolytic agents are generally not administered. Access to full cardiopulmonary bypass should be immediately available in case the patient does not tolerate OPCAB. This includes both medications (heparin and antifibrinolytics) and members of the perfusionist team.

Questions

1. Which one of the following is NOT an absolute patient contraindication to off-pump coronary artery bypass (OFCAB)?
   a. diffusely diseased target vessels
   b. calcified coronary vessels
   c. small distal targets
   d. intramyocardial vessels

2. Which one of the following is an advantage of OPCAB vs. traditional on-pump coronary artery bypass surgery?
   a. less technically demanding
   b. reduced risk of stroke
   c. reduced risk of cardiac arrhythmias
   d. reduced risk of epidural hematoma if utilizing regional anesthesia

Answers

1. c. Absolute contraindications to OPCAB include hemodynamic instability, poor quality target vessels, including intramyocardial vessels, diffusely diseased or

Essential Clinical Anesthesia Review: Keywords, Questions and Answers for the Boards, ed. Linda S. Aglio, Robert W. Lekowski, and Richard D. Urman. Published by Cambridge University Press. © Cambridge University Press 2015.

calcified coronary vessels. Repair of small distal targets is a relative contraindication to OPCAB.

2. b. Advantages of OPCAB include avoidance of the complications associated with cardiopulmonary bypass such as the development of systemic inflammatory response, aortic manipulation, embolization, and stroke.

Further reading

Chang, T. S. and Fox, J. A. (2011). Off-pump coronary artery bypass. In Vacanti, C. A., Sikka, P. K., Urman, R. U., Dershwitz, R., and Segal, B. S. (eds) *Essential Clinical Anesthesia*. New York, NY: Cambridge University Press, pp. 461–463.

Kim, J. Y., Ramsay, J. G., Licina, M. G., and Mehta, A. R. (2013). Alternative approaches to cardiac surgery with and without cardiopulmonary bypass. In Hensley, F. A., Martin, D. E., and Gravlee, G. P. (eds) *A Practical Approach to Cardiac Anesthesia*, 5th edn. Philadelphia, PA: Lippincott Williams & Wilkins, pp. 359–370.

Chapter

74

Transesophageal echocardiography

Zahra M. Malik and Martin Zammert

TEE indications

The 2010 revised practice guidelines for perioperative TEE by the American Society of Anesthesiologists and the Society of Cardiovascular Anesthesiologists state that "TEE should be used in all open heart (e.g., valvular procedures) and thoracic and thoracic aortic surgical procedures and should be considered in coronary artery bypass graft surgeries to: (1) confirm and refine the preoperative diagnosis, (2) detect new or unsuspected pathology, (3) adjust the anesthetic and surgical plan accordingly, and (4) assess the results of surgical intervention."

Technical aspects of TEE

The ultrasound transmitted to a patient interacts with tissue by reflection, refraction, scattering, and attenuation. Higher frequencies have better resolution but less penetration into tissue. The frequency of ultrasound used in TEE is approximately 3.5 to 7 MHz. Doppler echocardiography uses ultrasound reflected from red blood cells to measure the velocity and direction of blood flow. The Doppler effect increases the frequency of waves reflected from cells moving toward the transducer and decreases the frequency of waves from cells moving away from the transducer.

Modes of cardiac ultrasound imaging include:

- M-mode echocardiography – this was the primary imaging mode before 2D imaging. It uses a single linear beam of ultrasound directed into tissues. As M-mode has the highest temporal resolution it is useful in precisely timing events within the cardiac cycle such as allowing detection of high-frequency oscillating motion (e.g., aortic leaflet fluttering and premature systolic closure, pathognomonic for left ventricular outflow tract obstruction).
- Two-dimensional echocardiography utilizes a rapidly moving beam of ultrasound through a plane via phased array transducers to construct a 2D image.
- Pulsed-wave Doppler (PWD) measures the velocity and direction of blood flow in a specific location.
- Continuous-wave Doppler measures the velocity and direction of blood flow along the line of the ultrasound beam. It has no limit on the maximum velocity measured. It is used to measure maximum flow velocities in aortic and mitral stenosis.
- Color-flow Doppler is a form of PWD that superimposes velocity onto a simultaneous 2D image of the heart. Flow toward the transducer is usually mapped as red and away from the transducer as blue. Can be used to detect turbulence.
- Tissue Doppler is a form of PWD that measures the velocity of tissue motion at specific points in the heart. It is commonly used to measure the velocity of mitral or tricuspid annular motion to assess diastolic as well as systolic function of the left and right ventricle.

TEE views: perfusion distribution

The left ventricule is supplied with blood by three major coronary arteries: the left anterior descending artery, the left circumflex artery, and the right coronary artery. The transgastric short axis view of the ventricles at the level of the papillary muscle allows the assessment of the distribution areas of all three major coronary arteries.

TEE findings in pericardial effusion include fluid between the heart and the pericardium as well as chamber collapse when the pericardial pressure becomes greater than cardiac chamber pressure. Atrial collapse will be seen prior to ventricular collapse and will occur in diastole first and then progress into systole. The right side of the heart (lower pressure) is

Essential Clinical Anesthesia Review: Keywords, Questions and Answers for the Boards, ed. Linda S. Aglio, Robert W. Lekowski, and Richard D. Urman. Published by Cambridge University Press. © Cambridge University Press 2015.

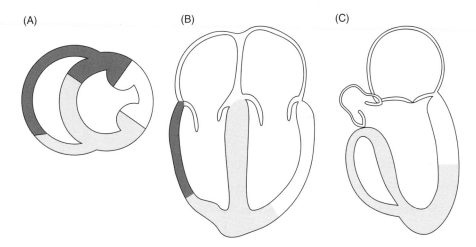

Figure 74.1 Coronary artery supply of the left and right ventricles in three views: the short-axis view (A), the four-chamber view (B), and the three-chamber view (C). Dark gray, RCA; light gray, LAD; white, CX.

affected before the left side. The most sensitive diagnostic indicator on TEE of *pericardial tamponade* is right ventricular collapse during systole in a patient with a pericardial effusion.

In comparison, the *TEE findings of hypovolemia* include uniform underfilling of all cardiac chambers' compression. Systolic papillary muscle contact ("kissing" papillary muscles) is classically seen on TEE. Additionally, a significant pericardial effusion is absent.

TEE findings in pulmonary embolism include increased size of pulmonary arteries, right ventricular dysfunction, severe tricuspid regurgitation, and a dilated right ventricle. Free RV wall akinesis with normal motion of the apex (also know as "McConnell's sign") has a high specificity for the detection of pulmonary embolism.

The rate of complications of TEE is 0.2%, but can increase in patients with esophageal or gastric disease. Absolute *contraindications of TEE* include a patient history of esophagectomy, severe esophageal obstruction, perforation or hemorrhage, and cervical trauma. *Complications of TEE* include oral, pharyngeal, or laryngeal trauma, esophageal injury, hoarseness, dislodgement of endotracheal tube, thermal injury, and arrhythmias.

Questions

1. Which of the following is the best mode of cardiac ultrasound imaging to assess severe aortic stenosis?
   a. pulsed-wave Doppler
   b. continuous-wave Doppler
   c. color-flow Doppler
   d. tissue Doppler

2. Which of the following is the best mode of cardiac ultrasound imaging to assess systolic function of the left ventricle?
   a. pulsed-wave Doppler
   b. continuous-wave Doppler
   c. color-flow Doppler
   d. tissue Doppler

3. Which of the following is an absolute patient contraindication to performing transesophageal echocardiography?
   a. history of esophageal varices
   b. history of esophageal radiation
   c. history of esophagectomy
   d. history of esophagitis

Answers

1. b. Continuous-wave Doppler measures the velocity and direction of blood flow along the line of the ultrasound beam, without a limit on the maximum velocity measured. It is used to measure maximum flow velocities in aortic and mitral stenosis.

2. d. Tissue Doppler is a form of pulsed-wave Doppler that measures the velocity of tissue motion at specific points in the heart. It is commonly used to measure the velocity of mitral annular motion to assess diastolic function of the left ventricle.

3. c. Absolute contraindications of TEE include a patient history of esophagectomy, severe esophageal obstruction, perforation or hemorrhage, and cervical trauma.

Further reading

Jervis, K. and Subramaniam, B. (2011). Transesophageal echocardiography. In Vacanti, C. A., Sikka, P. K., Urman, R. U., Dershwitz, R., and Segal, B. S. (eds) *Essential Clinical Anesthesia*. New York, NY: Cambridge University Press, pp. 464–472.

American Society of Anesthesiologists and Society of Cardiovascular Anesthesiologists (2010) Practice guidelines for perioperative transesophageal echocardiography. An updated report by the American Society of Anesthesiologists and the Society of Cardiovascular Anesthesiologists Task Force on Transesophageal Echocardiography. *Anesthesiology* 112(5), 1084–1096.

Beaulieu, Y. (2007). Bedside echocardiography in the assessment of the critically ill. *Critical Care Medicine* 35, S238–S240.

Wilson, W. C., Grande, C. M., and Hoyt, D. B. (eds) (2007). *Trauma: Critical Care*, Vol. 2, 1st edn. New York, NY: Informa HC, p. 401.

Morgan, G. E., Mikhail, M. S., and Murray, M. J. (eds) (2006). *Clinical Anesthesiology*, 4th edn. McGraw-Hill, p. 505.

Pacemakers and automated implantable cardioverter-defibrillators

Jessica Patterson and John A. Fox

Keywords

Pacemaker/AICD indications
Pacemaker/AICD codes
Pacemaker/AICD malfunction
Anesthetic device management

The use of artificial pacing is generally indicated for symptomatic bradycardia, the cause of which can be attributed to failure of impulse formation or failure of proper cardiac conduction. More *common indications for artificial pacing* include sick sinus syndrome, third-degree AV block, or advanced second-degree AV block.

Indications for AICD placement include (1) a history of life-threatening clinical event associated with a ventricular dysrhythmia or (2) cardiomyopathy with an ejection fraction of less than 35% for primary dysrhythmia prevention.

Temporary pacing is most commonly transvenous, but can also be endocardial, epicardial, transesophageal, or transcutaneous. Additionally, specialized pulmonary artery catheters now have temporary pacing ability.

The *pacemaker coding system* is derived from five letters to allow for a complete description of the pacemaker. See Table 75.1.

The *chamber paced* and *chamber sensed* are self-explanatory. The *response to the sensed event* can be for the pacemaker to trigger a stimulus (T) when it senses an absence of depolarization or the pacemaker can inhibit (I) itself from triggering a stimulus if it senses a native depolarization. The pacemaker can be programmed to do neither (O) or both (D) of these options.

Rate responsiveness refers to the ability of modern pacemakers to develop a higher or lower pacing speed depending on activity. This ability in modern pacemakers is referred to as *adaptive rate pacing* (ARP). Some devices can sense vibration, acceleration of the body, changes to the QT interval or minute ventilation to increase the pacing speed. Blood pH and oxygen saturation are some variables a few of the latest devices can detect to adjust pacing speed.

The fifth letter in the pacemaker/AICD code refers to *antitachycardia function*. Some of the available options are antitachycardia pacing (P), shock in the form of cardioversion or defibrillation (S), or no antitachycardia function (O).

AICDs function by sensing the R–R interval, and if the detected R–R interval is less than the programmed interval, the device readies itself for electrical therapy. Modern day AICDs also take into consideration the morphology and suddenness of onset in order to diagnose ventricular tachycardias.

Most AICDs are able to progress through different treatment options such as overdrive pacing, cardioversion, and defibrillation.

Table 75.1 Pacemaker/AICD codes

I	II	III	IV	V
Chamber paced	**Chamber sensed**	**Response to sensed event**	**Programmability/rate response**	**Antitachycardia function**
O = None	**O** = None	**O** = None	**O** = None	**O** = None
A = Atrium	**A** = Atrium	**I** = Inhibit	**R** = Adaptive rate	**P** = ATP
V = Ventricle	**V** = Ventricle	**T** = Triggered		**S** = Shock
D = Dual (A & V)	**D** = Dual (A & V)	**D** = Dual (I & T)		**D** = Dual (P & S)
S = Single	**S** = Single			

ATP, Antitachycardia pacing.
(From Atlee, J. L. and Bernstein, A. D. 2001. Cardiac rhythm management devices (part II): perioperative management. *Anesthesiology*, 95(5): 11265–11280.)

Essential Clinical Anesthesia Review: Keywords, Questions and Answers for the Boards, ed. Linda S. Aglio, Robert W. Lekowski, and Richard D. Urman. Published by Cambridge University Press. © Cambridge University Press 2015.

Overdrive pacing increases the heart rate in order to suppress certain arrhythmias. The ability to overdrive pace as a first option to treat tachyarrhythmias helps to conserve battery life and minimize damage to the myocardium, which occurs with shock therapy.

Cardioversion can be delivered in a synchronized fashion in order to avoid degeneration to fibrillation, and *defibrillation* can be delivered to treat ventricular tachycardia or fibrillation.

A number of malfunctions can occur with pacemakers/AICDs. Some of the more common include failure to capture or inappropriate shocks.

Failure to capture in pacemaker devices can be due to ischemia, fibrosis, severe acidosis, beta-blockers, hyperglycemia, and some antiarrhythmics.

AICDs may not deliver effective shocks that can be caused by altered morphologies of the rhythm caused by ischemia or acidosis. In contrast, AICDs may deliver *inappropriate shocks* to electrocautery artifacts, supraventricular tachycardia that is misdiagnosed at ventricular tachycardia, double counting of R and T waves during pacing, and lead artifacts.

In addition to determining the indication for the pacemaker/AICD, make and model, last interrogation, and status of battery, the *preanesthetic plan* for a patient with a device should include a 12-lead EKG and rhythm strip to determine if the patient is A, V, or AV paced or totally pacemaker dependent.

If the patient is pacemaker dependent, the device should be programmed to an asynchronous mode usually by placement of a magnet to avoid electrocautery interference. Additionally, AICDs should be deactivated with the use of a magnet to avoid delivery of an inappropriate shock in the setting of electrocautery interference. In this situation, the ability to defibrillate externally should be made readily available.

Use of bipolar cautery at the lowest current energy and placement of the grounding plate as far as possible from the device will reduce the risk of interference.

Following any surgery or anesthetic, the patient plans for proper follow-up by the electrophysiologist (cardiologist) should be in place to make sure that the device is properly functioning.

Questions

1. A 64-year-old man presents to the preoperative clinic for evaluation prior to his total reverse shoulder arthroplasty that is scheduled for one week later. His history is significant for sick sinus syndrome for which a DDD pacemaker programmed at a rate of 70 bpm was placed four years ago. Which of the following is FALSE?

   a. A preoperative EKG showing a paced rhythm at a rate of 58 bpm may indicate battery failure.

   b. Placement of a magnet should occur if the patient is pacemaker dependent and will adjust the mode to VVO.

   c. The asynchronous mode of the pacemaker can be activated by placing a magnet over the device and will usually be preprogrammed to 80 bpm.

   d. The asynchronous mode of pacemakers can lead to hemodynamic instability if the patient is reliant on their atrial kick.

   e. If the patient's heart rate exceeds that set in the asynchronous mode, there is a possibility of R on T phenomenon.

2. Immediately after induction, a patient's heart rate decreases to 44 bpm. The patient has a VVI pacemaker and he is pacemaker dependent at a programmed rate of 70 bpm. Additionally, pacemaker spikes are now no longer apparent on the intraoperative rhythm strip. Which of the following is a possible cause of this acute pacemaker malfunction?

   a. oversensing from electrocautery
   b. hypokalemia leading to failure to capture
   c. lead fracture or disruption
   d. battery failure
   e. succinylcholine-induced myopotential leading to inhibition of the VVI pacemaker

3. Which of the following is NOT a possible pacing option for a patient with a DDD pacemaker?

   a. atria sensed and ventricle paced
   b. atrial and ventricular pacing
   c. normal sinus rhythm
   d. atria paced and ventricle sensed
   e. none of the above, all of the choices are possible pacing options

Answers

1. b. All of the above choices are true of pacemakers, except for (b), because a magnet will typically switch to an asynchronous mode such as VOO where neither chamber will be sensed.

2. e. The scenario above describes a patient's heart rate dropping from the 70s to 40s with a pacemaker in place shortly after induction. Since it is unlikely that electrocautery is in use immediately after induction, this is incorrect. However, it is possible that electrocautery could be sensed by the pacemaker as intrinsic cardiac electroactivity and as a result the pacemaker will inhibit pacing. In this particular scenario, immediately after induction, the most likely cause is succinylcholine-induced myopotentials being sensed by the pacemaker and inhibiting pacing.

3. e. As stated above, the letters are in order of chambers paced, chambers sensed, and function. So a DDD pacemaker paces both the atrium and ventricle, senses both the atrium and ventricle, and has the ability to pace or inhibit pacing. All of the options listed are possible with this type of pacemaker depending on the patient's intrinsic cardiac electroactivity.

Further reading

Vacanti, C. A., Sikka, P. K., Urman, R. U., Dershwitz, M., and Segal, B. S. (2011). *Essential Clinical Anesthesia*, 1st edn. Cambridge University Press, pp. 473–478.

Kaplan, J. A. et al. (2011). *Kaplan's Cardiac Anesthesia: The Echo Era*. Saunders, Chapter 25.

Cheng, A. and Yao, F. (2012). Chapter 7. Pacemakers, implantable cardiactor-defibrillators, and cardiac asynchronization tropy clouces. In *Anesthesiology: Problem-Oriented Patient Management*. Lippincott Williams & Wilkins, pp. 217–239.

Chapter

76

Ventricular assist devices

Jessica Patterson and John A. Fox

Keywords

VAD definition
Benefits of VAD usage
Indications for VAD usage
VAD placement contraindications
VAD parameters
Anesthetic considerations for VAD placement
Complications of VADs

Ventricular assist devices (VADs) are mechanical devices that provide support to improve a patient's hemodynamics in the setting of a failing ventricle despite maximal inotropic and/or intra-aortic balloon pump support. Usual criteria are as follows:

- cardiac index <2 l/min/m^2
- systolic blood pressure <80 mm Hg
- UOP <20–30 ml/h

They can provide *left ventricular, right ventricular, or biventricular support*. In addition to providing left, right, or biventricular support, they can either be implanted inside or outside the body and either generate *pulsatile* or *continuous (axial) flow*. Patients with continuous flow VADs may not have a pulse (especially in the setting of a BiVAD) and blood pressure must be measured directly through an arterial catheter or with a sphygmomanometer.

Blood is removed from the respective side of the heart that is failing via an *inflow cannula* (named for inflow to the VAD, not the patient) to the pumping chamber of the VAD. The blood leaves the VAD via an *outflow cannula* and delivers the blood to the aorta or pulmonary arteries.

The VAD pumping chambers are dependent on an external power supply usually supplied by an electric or pneumatic console.

The *benefits of a VAD* include decompressing the failing ventricle and augmenting either systemic or pulmonary arterial perfusion, which can then result in an improvement of end-organ perfusion, a reduction of circulating catecholamines,

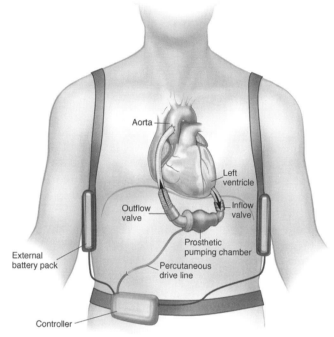

Figure 76.1 Basic components of a ventricular assist device. (Adapted from Vacanti et al. 2011. *Essential Clinical Anesthesia*, Cambridge University Press, Figure 77.1.)

renin-angiotensin and other cytokines, and ultimately recovery of the damaged myocytes.

Uses for VADs include: (1) short-term ventricular support for patients who have suffered an acute but potentially reversible myocardial insult, (2) bridge therapy to support heart transplant candidates until a donor heart becomes available, and (3) destination therapy for patients with refractory heart failure who are not transplant candidates.

Contraindications to VAD placement include renal failure, severe hepatic dysfunction, severe lung disease, or significant irreversible neurological deficits. Cancer and infection are also considered to be contraindications. Hepatic congestion leading

---

to hepatic failure can be a sign of right ventricular dysfunction, so if one finds elevated liver function tests in a patient being considered for an LVAD, it may be more appropriate to consider insertion of a BiVAD.

The *parameters* that are reported on a VAD are *flow estimate (l/min), pump speed (RPM)*, and *power (watts)*. For a given pump speed, the power values should run within an expected range.

If the power values are gradually increasing without changing the speed, one should consider an increase in volume status, decrease in afterload, or a thrombus on the rotor. Decreasing power at a constant speed may be attributed to occlusion of the flow.

VADs are very sensitive to volume and the first response to a low VAD output should be a volume challenge rather than increasing the VAD ejection rate for rotation speed. Because VADs are mechanical devices, there is no way to increase contractility to increase cardiac output and VAD flow is not particularly sensitive to increasing vascular resistance.

For *induction of anesthesia for VAD surgery*, it is important to be prepared to administer inotropes with induction, as these heart failure patients are dependent on the high amount of circulating catecholamines and the sympatholysis after induction of anesthesia needs to be minimized. Higher heart rates are generally desirable in these patients. Additionally, one must be aware that the low circulating time of these patients will result in a long induction time of intravenous anesthetics.

TEE evaluation is important in the precardiopulmonary bypass period to identify any of the following conditions that might need to be surgically addressed:

- Greater than *mild aortic insufficiency* (for LVADs) and *pulmonary insufficiency* (for RVADs) can cause retrograde flow back across the incompetent valve rather than through the VAD pump.
- *Ventricular or atrial septal defects* may lead to significant R to L shunt following initiation of VAD support.
- *Intracardiac thrombi* may lead to embolic events within the patient or within the VAD pump itself.

Major *complications of VAD therapy* include bleeding (due to anticoagulation), infection (requiring perioperative antibiotics), and thromboembolism (if postoperative anticoagulation is not monitored).

Questions

1. Which of the following is NOT true concerning VADs?
   a. The inflow cannula refers to the cannula coming from the VAD pump and into the ascending aorta.
   b. Increasing peripheral vascular resistance most likely does not decrease LVAD flow.
   c. Right ventricular dysfunction may impair flow to the left ventricle and the LVAD, so consideration for a BiVAD should be made if present.
   d. Perioperative prophylactic antibiotics are important to prevent infection.
   e. A contraindication to VAD placement is a creatinine >5 mg/dl.

2. A 54-year-old male with non-ischemic cardiomyopathy has undergone LVAD placement as bridge therapy for eventual heart transplant four days ago. His VAD has been functioning appropriately, but the nurse has just called to inform that he now has decreased VAD output. Which of the following should NOT be done?
   a. Increase the VAD rate or output.
   b. Attempt diuresis to mitigate volume overload.
   c. Initiate milrinone or another inotropic therapy.
   d. Obtain a TEE to assess for malposition of the inflow cannula.
   e. Initiate therapy with a pulmonary vasodilator such as nitric oxide or flolan.

Answers

1. a. The cannulas are named in reference to their flow toward the VAD, so the inflow cannula refers to the cannula that is carrying blood to the VAD from the left ventricle.
2. a. The cause of decreased VAD output may be because of cannula malposition, right ventricular overload, volume overload, or decrease in cardiac inotropy. The patient should be evaluated for possible causes and treated before just reflexively turning up the VAD rate or ouput.

Further reading

Vacanti, C. A., Sikka, P. K., Urman, R. U., Dershwitz, M., and Segal, B. S. (2011). *Essential Clinical Anesthesia*, 1st edn. Cambridge University Press, pp. 479–484.

Chapter

77

Anesthetic considerations for surgical repair of the thoracic aorta

Jessica Patterson and John A. Fox

Keywords

Anesthetic management of thoracic aortic surgeries
Cerebral protection during ascending aortic or aortic arch surgeries
Isoelectric EEG
Deep hypothermic circulatory arrest
Anterior spinal cord ishchemia
Great artery of Adamkiewicz
Spinal cord protection

Urgent or emergent thoracic aortic surgeries may include *thoracic aortic dissection, leaking aneurysm*, or a *contained traumatic transection*. Large-bore intravenous access and arterial blood pressure monitoring are important for volume resuscitation and continuous monitoring of hemodynamics.

Preoperatively, pain and anxiolytic premedications can help with patient comfort and can help to lower heart rate and blood pressure, which is desired to prevent extension of the dissection or aortic rupture.

Intraoperatively, tight control of hemodynamics is important to ensure adequate perfusion of vital organs and also to prevent further dissection or aortic rupture. Generally, to reach these two goals, systolic blood pressures should be between 100 and 120 mm Hg and diastolic blood pressures should be between 60 and 80 mm Hg. Additionally, a low heart rate (60 to 80 bpm) is desirable to reduce the number of blood flow pulsations to the intimal tear.

Vasodilators and *beta-blockers* are the usual medications to achieve the hemodynamics parameters described above.

In the setting of aortic surgery requiring cardiopulmonary bypass (CPB), systemic anticoagulation, stimulation of the inflammatory response, consumptive coagulopathy, and increased fibrinolysis can contribute to *massive bleeding*. If *deep hypothermic circulatory arrest* (DHCA) is needed, hypothermia may contribute to bleeding through platelet dysfunction.

Table 77.1 Common IV vasodilators used to control hypertension

Drug	Common dosages	Comments
Sodium nitroprusside	Start infusion at 0.5–1.0 μg/kg/min and titrate to effect. Cyanide toxicity has occurred with doses of 8–10 μg/kg/min	Rapid onset and offset. Vasodilates both arterial and venous smooth muscle. Central administration is ideal, but can be administered through a large peripheral IV line.
Nitroglycerin	Typical infusion range is 1.0–4.0 μg/kg/min	Rapid onset and offset. Less potent than sodium nitroprusside. May be particularly helpful in settings in which aortic dissection affects coronary arterial flow, as blood flow may be somewhat improved with coronary vasodilation.
Fenoldopam	Start infusion at 0.05–0.1 μg/kg/min and titrate to effect to a maximum dose of 0.8 μg/kg/min	Selective D1 dopamine receptor agonist with little affinity for D2 dopamine or other adrenoreceptors. Although fenoldopam results in dilation of many vascular beds, it may have some renal-protective benefits related to increasing renal blood flow.
Nicardipine	Typical infusion range is 5.0–15.0 mg/h and can be titrated to effect; also may be administered as an IV bolus (usually 05–2.0 mg)	A dihydropyridine calcium channel blocker that inhibits calcium influx into vascular smooth muscle, thereby causing vasorelaxation. It is marketed as having more selectivity for cerebral and coronary arteries than the other dihydropyridines.

(From Vacanti et al., *Essential Clinical Anesthesia*, Chapter 78.)

Essential Clinical Anesthesia Review: Keywords, Questions and Answers for the Boards, ed. Linda S. Aglio, Robert W. Lekowski, and Richard D. Urman. Published by Cambridge University Press. © Cambridge University Press 2015.

Table 77.2 Commonly used β-adrenergic receptor antagonists (β-blockers)

Drug	Common dosages	Comments
Propranolol	Start with IV bolus of 1 mg, but total doses as high as 8 mg may be required to achieve adequate heart rate control	Nonselective β-adrenergic receptor antagonist (β_1 and β_2) that has been used for many years in the setting of aortic dissection to slow heart rate. However, propranolol use is now often supplanted by β_1-selective adrenergic receptor antagonists (see below). The half-life of the main metabolite of propranolol is 5–7 h, so shorter-acting agents should be considered in patients who are hemodynamically labile.
Labetalol	Loading doses can be administered IV, with initial doses of 5–10 mg. Loading doses should subsequently be doubled approximately every 10 min (up to a maximum total dose of 300 mg) until target heart rate and blood pressure are achieved. Once target heart rate and blood pressure are achieved by IV loading doses, a continuous infusion may be initiated at 0.5–2 mg/min, or the patient may be redosed with small IV boluses approximately every 30 min	Provides a combination of α_1-, β_1-, and β_2-adrenergic receptor antagonism, and thus can be administered as an alternative to a combination of sodium nitroprusside and β-blocker. The disadvantage of the labetalol approach to blood pressure and heart rate control for aortic dissections is a longer time to onset of desired blood pressure effect and less ease of rapid titration than seen with strict vasodilators.
Esmolol	Bolus IV loading dose of 500 µg/µg over I min, then initiate IV infusion at 50 µg/kg/min titrated to effect, up to a maximum infusion of 300 µg/kg/min	β_1-selective adrenergic receptor blocker with rapid onset and short duration of action. Its β_1 selectivity makes it favorable for patients who are prone to bronchospasm. Its short half-life makes it easy to titrate and to terminate if a patient develops bronchospasm or becomes hemodynamically unstable.
Metoprolol	Typical initial IV bolus dose of 2.5–5.0 mg; may be repeated every 5–15 min up to a maximum total dose of 20 mg to achieve target heart rate	β_1-selective adrenergic receptor blocker with longer duration of action than esmolol, so it can be administered effectively without continuous infusion.

(From Vacanti et al., *Essential Clinical Anesthesia*, Chapter 78.)

The *three common steps to aortic surgery* include:
1. Occluding flow proximal and distal to the site of aortic injury to prevent further hemorrhage.
2. Restore blood flow to major organs that are perfused by arterial branches.
3. Repair or replace the portion of injured or diseased aorta.

Surgery of the ascending aorta or aortic arch is usually approached through a midline sternotomy and will require full CPB.

Cerebral protection strategies are employed when interruption of cerebral blood flow is expected. *Hypothermia*, reducing cerebral metabolic rate and cerebral oxygen consumption, can be mild to moderate (22–25°C) or profound (15–20°C).

In addition to hypothermia, achieving an *isoelectric EEG* by administering propofol or thiopental prior to initiation of DHCA may further reduce the cerebral metabolic rate and allow added cerebral protection. Although mannitol and systemic steroids are given for cerebral protection, the data for these medications is not strong.

Surgically selective anterograde cerebral perfusion through a right axillary (or carotid) cannula or retrograde cerebral perfusion through a superior vena caval cannula can be employed for cerebral protection during DHCA.

Descending thoracic aortic or thoracoabdominal aortic repairs may be done through a left thoracotomy incision and will typically need one-lung ventilation. These repairs frequently do not need CPB and thus do not require high doses of heparin for systemic heparinization.

The aorta is typically cross-clamped proximal and distal to the affected portion. The cross-clamp can cause a sudden increase in *left ventricular afterload* and can lead to significant hypertension and possibly left ventricular strain. To avoid left heart strain, the hypertension should be treated with short-acting antihypertensive agents such sodium nitroprusside or nitroglycerin.

Paraplegia from *anterior spinal cord ischemia* is the most serious complication from descending aortic and thoracoabdominal repairs. Compromised blood flow through the anterior spinal artery is more likely to occur in repairs that last longer than 30 minutes. Radicular branches of intercostal arteries collateralize with the anterior spinal artery. One of the radicular branches, *great artery of Adamkiewicz*, arises at the *T8–L4 level* and supplies a major portion of the anterior spinal cord.

Spinal cord protection can be employed with the use of a *CSF drain* placed at the L3–L4 or L4–L5 interspace.

Spinal cord perfusion pressure (SCPP) = Mean arterial pressure (MAP) – CSF pressure or CVP

The lumbar drain can be transduced during the surgery. CSF can be drained and MAP can be raised to help maintain an adequate SCPP. In general, it is not recommended to let CSF pressure go below 10 mm Hg because of complications such as intracranial hypotension and subdural hematoma.

Questions

1. A 72-year-old female with history significant for 60 pack 1 year tobacco abuse, hypertension, hyperlipidemia, and diabetes presents for thoracoabdominal aneurysm repair. Following aortic cross-clamp, which of the following physiologic changes would NOT be expected?
   a. increased mixed venous oxygen saturation
   b. increased segmental wall motion abnormalities
   c. increased coronary blood flow
   d. increased carbon dioxide production
   e. increased pulmonary capillary wedge pressure

2. In the case above, which of the following is NOT an appropriate measure to prepare for cross-clamping of the aorta?
   a. Prepare sodium nitroprusside infusion to treat possible hypertension.
   b. Administer lasix and/or mannitol.
   c. Consider bicarbonate infusion.
   d. Increase the depth of anesthesia.
   e. Increase minute ventilation.

Answers

1. d. All of the answer choices can be expected with cross-clamping of the aorta, except increased carbon dioxide production.
2. e. Because there is decreased carbon dioxide production with cross-clamping of the aorta, decreasing minute ventilation would be an appropriate measure.

Further reading

Vacanti, C. A., Sikka, P. K., Urman, R. U., Dershwitz, M., and Segal, B. S. (2011). *Essential Clinical Anesthesia*, 1st edn. Cambridge University Press, pp. 485–492.

Aortic cross clamp: CV complications (2013). http://openanesthesia. org/index.php?title=Aortic_crossclamp:_CV_complications

Chapter

78

Cardiac transplantation in the adult

Jessica Patterson and John A. Fox

Keywords

Hyperacute rejection
Acute RV failure following transplant
Post-bypass bradycardia
Cardiac denervation

Potential donors must be screened for *ABO blood type compatibility*, panel-reactive antibody screening, and heart size. Because of ABO and antibody screening, *hyperacute rejection* (resulting from preformed donor-specific antibodies in the recipient) is a rare occurrence. This complication occurs within minutes to hours.

During organ harvesting, hemodynamic goals include a MAP of 80 to 90 mm Hg, CVP of 5 to 12 mm Hg, urine output >100 ml/h, as well as normal electrolyte levels and ABG values. After explatation of the donor heart, the ex vivo ischemia time is approximately four to six hours.

Patients awaiting heart transplant frequently have an *AICD* in place and/or are taking *amiodarone* for risk of symptomatic *ventricular tachycardia or fibrillation*. These arrhythmias are the *most common cause of sudden death* in patients with severe heart failure awaiting transplantation.

Because some degree of pulmonary hypertension may exist prior to transplantation, weaning from CPB may prove to be difficult because of *acute RV failure*. Prostaglandin E_1 infusion, inhaled nitric oxide, or even placement of an RVAD may be necessary until the pulmonary vasculature changes normalize with time.

Frequently, *post-bypass bradycardia* is seen and may last for up to seven days. A heart rate of 90 to 100 bpm is desirable and can be achieved with isoproterenol, dopamine (or other catecholamine administration), or atrial pacing.

Signs of acute rejection include drop in voltage in leads I, II, III, V1, and V6, abnormal gallop rhythms, fever, and changes in urinary output or weight.

Anesthetic considerations for a heart transplant patient having noncardiac surgery.

- *Cardiac denervation* results in slower increases in heart rate and indirect sympathomimetic drugs such as ephedrine, atropine, and pancuronium will generally be ineffective.
- *Cardiac output* is mostly dependent on *increasing stroke volume* so it is important to maintain an adequate preload in these patients
- Both the donor and recipient sinus nodes may be present resulting in *P waves generated from both nodes.*
- Anticholinergics should be avoided as they may produce vasodilation without a compensatory tachycardic response, which can lead to hypotension.

Essential Clinical Anesthesia Review: Keywords, Questions and Answers for the Boards, ed. Linda S. Aglio, Robert W. Lekowski, and Richard D. Urman. Published by Cambridge University Press. © Cambridge University Press 2015.

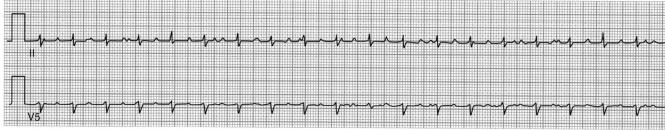

Figure 78.1 EKG for Quest 2.

Questions

1. A 32-year-old female presents with acute appendicitis for a laparascopic appendectomy. Her history is significant for heart transplant five years ago for non-ischemic cardiomyopathy following viral myocarditis. During insufflation of the abdomen, she develops bradycardia with a heart rate in the 30s. In addition to asking the surgeon to desufflate the abdomen, what is the appropriate pharmacologic measure?

   a. administer ephedrine
   b. administer glycopyrrolate
   c. administer epinephrine
   d. administer pancuronium
   e. administer atropine

2. The EKG in Figure 78.1 is obtained preoperatively from the patient described above. What is the diagnosis?

   a. wandering pacemaker
   b. second-degree AV block
   c. third-degree AV block
   d. normal finding in a post-heart transplant patient
   e. myocardial ischemia

Answers

1. c. Patients with cardiac transplants will not respond to drugs that block the parasympathetic system because this system was denervated during the transplant. So to raise the heart rate, drugs that act directly, such as epinephrine or isoproterenol, will need to be used.

2. d. Two distinct P waves is a common finding in patients with a history of cardiac transplant and it is due to the presence of the original SA node and the SA node of the transplanted heart.

Further reading

Vacanti, C. A., Sikka, P. K., Urman, R. U., Dershwitz, M., and Segal, B. S. (2011). *Essential Clinical Anesthesia*, 1st edn. Cambridge University Press, pp. 493–496.

Cohn, L. H. and Edmunds, L. H. (2003). *Cardiac Surgery in the Adult*, 2nd edn. New York: McGraw-Hill.

Chapter 79

Persistent postoperative bleeding in cardiac surgical patients

Rosemary Uzomba, Michael D'Ambra, and Robert W. Lekowski

Keywords

Surgical bleeding, medical bleeding, prolonged surgical bleeding, mild and excessive bleeding, primary hemostasis, platelet activation, platelet aggregation, platelet adhesion, marginalization of plts, vWF, secondary hemostasis, contact/surface activation, intrinsic coagulation pathway, extrinsic coagulation pathway, common (final) pathway, thrombin, fibrinolysis, plasmin, tissue plasminogen activator (tPA), lysine analog antifibrinolytics, protein C and S, antithrombin III (AT III), heparin, low molecular weight heparin (LMWH), direct thrombin inhibitors (DTI), warfarin, cyclo-oxygenase (COX) inhibitors, GP IIb/IIIa inhibitors, ADP receptor inhibitors, direct P2Y12 inhibitors, adenosine uptake inhibitor, cardiopulmonary bypass (CPB), liver disease, renal disease, cryoprecipitate, fresh frozen plasma (FFP), recombinant factor VIIa, profilinine®, DDAVP

During cardiac surgery there are many surgical and medical manipulations that can occur that adversely effect postoperative hemostasis:

- *Surgical bleeding*: inadequate surgical hemostasis or suture line leakage as a result of manipulation of the **vasculature** (aorta, pulmonary veins, coronary arteries, internal mammary artery), **the tissue** (atria and appendages), and **the planes of exposure** (mediastinal and pleural spaces).
- *Medical bleeding*, i.e., microvascular bleeding as a result of coagulopathy seen with the institution of CPB (which requires the administration of heparin and antifibrinolytics).
- *Prolonged surgical bleeding* postoperatively can lead to platelet and coagulation factor depletion thus leading to secondary (2°) coagulopathy.

Diagnostic modalities used postoperatively include *chest radiography* (which may demonstrate a widened mediastinum)

Table 79.1 Chest tube drainage indicative of excessive postoperative bleeding. Requires surgical re-exploration

>500 ml in first hour		
400 ml/h in first two hours	or	>20 ml/kg over first three hours
300 ml/h in first three hours		
200 ml/h in first four hours		

and *transesophageal echocardiography* (which may demonstrate classic tamponade or, more commonly, focal compression by hematoma).

Bleeding will occur after cardiac surgery and may be mild or excessive:

- *Mild bleeding*: for first six hours after surgery = 0.5–1.0 ml/kg/h; should respond to volume replacement.
- *Excessive bleeding*: >8–10 ml/kg/h *or* as a general guideline.

In order to understand the pathophysiology involved in persistent postoperative bleeding one must be intimately familiar with the normal processes involving primary hemostasis (platelet activation, adhesion, and aggregation) secondary hemostasis (the coagulation "cascade"), and the balancing anticoagulation system (fibrinolysis).

Primary hemostasis begins with formation of a platelet (plt) plug. Plt functionality requires a three-step process: **activation, aggregation, and adhesion**.

Platelet activation results from contact with collagen (in the subendothelial [SE] matrix) when a potent plt agonist binds to the plt membrane receptor.

- *Plt agonists* induce change in plt shape from disc to spherical shape revealing plt glycoproteins (GP).
- Potent agonists for plt activation include **thrombin** (clotting factor II_a, **most potent** plt agonist), adenosine diphosphate (**ADP, which binds to P2Y12 receptor**, a prominent participant in plt activation by collagen and thrombin), and thromboxane (**TXA_2**).
- As a result of plt activation plts release contents of dense granules and alpha granules.

Essential Clinical Anesthesia Review: Keywords, Questions and Answers for the Boards, ed. Linda S. Aglio, Robert W. Lekowski, and Richard D. Urman. Published by Cambridge University Press. © Cambridge University Press 2015.

Table 79.2 Clinical presentation

If you see…	Suggests
Bright red blood	Bleeding from left-sided cardiac structures (IMA, IC, aorta, LA, PV)
Dark blood	Bleeding from right-sided cardiac structures
Dilute serosanguinous fluid	3rd space fluid in thoracic cavity
Sudden increase in bleeding	Surgical etiology (esp. if normal PT/PTT)
Diffuse widespread oozing	Platelet abnormality, DIC or both

Abbreviations: IMA, internal mammary artery; IC, intercostal arteries; LA, left atrium; PV, pulmonary veins; DIC, disseminated intravascular coagulation. (Source: Vacanti et al. *Essential Clinical Anesthesia*, 2011.)

Table 79.3 Coagulation factors

Factor	Name	Plasma concentration, µg/ml	% of normal required for hemostasis
I	Fibrinogen	3,000	30
II	Prothrombin	100	40
III	Tissue factor	–	–
IV	Calcium	–	–
V	Proaccelerin	10	10–15
VII	Proconvertin	0.5	5–10
VIII	Antihemophilic	0.1	10–40
IX	Thromboplastin	5	10–40
X	Stuart	10	10–15
XI	Prethromboplastin	5	20–30
XII	Hageman	30	0
XIII	Fibrin stabilizing	30	1–5

(*Source*: Vacanti, C. (ed.) *Essential Clinical Anesthesia*, 2011.)

- *Dense granules* contain serotonin (**5-HT**, weak plt agonist), **Ca^{2+}** (needed for plt shape change, disc to sphere), and **ADP** (which recruits more plts to the site of injury as well as stimulates plt GP, which activates plt phospholipase leading to arachidonate formation and eventually TXA$_2$ formation via cyclooxygenase).
- *Alpha granules* contain von Willebrand factor (**vWF**), fibrinogen (**FG**), thrombospondin (**TSP**), and plt factor 4 (**PF4**) among others.
- When plts change shape (from disc to spherical), GP IIB/IIIA receptors are exposed.

Platelet aggregation occurs when **FG and TSP** form molecular bridges with **GP IIB/IIIA** receptors of nearby plts.

Platelet adhesion begins fast (within one minute) of vessel injury and is complete within 20 min.

- Plt adhesion requires *marginalization of plts* to allow for plt contact with endothelium.
- Since RBCs and WBCs travel in center of vessel, high hematocrits (Hct) aid in plt marginalization (whereas low Hct, as seen post CPB, leads to decreased marginalization and plt adhesion).
- GP IB and GP IX along with vWF mediate adhesion of plts to the vessel wall.
- *vWF* is a massive (multimer) protein that protects factor VIII in the plasma from proteolytic enzymes. In the presence of damaged endothelium, vWF **uncoils** to expose the section that has a high affinity for plt GP. The uncoiled vWF attaches to the GP slowing the plt down (against the shear force). This helps **activate** the plt and initiates membrane signaling and expression of GP IIB/IIIA (which leads to plt **aggregation**) and GP IB (which leads to plt **adhesion**).
- End-product is the bridging of normal plts to damaged endothelium.

Quantitative or qualitative plt abnormalities are the most common cause of postoperative bleeding after surgeries involving CPB. Often patients are receiving anti-plt and antithrombotic agents in the preoperative period. Table 79.3 illustrates some of these drugs that can lead to perioperative bleeding.

Secondary hemostasis involves the coagulation system (see Figure 79.1).

Contact/surface activation

- Contact coagulation factors are XII (12), XI (11– aka **pre-plasma thromboplastin**), and pre-kallikrein (PK).
- The cofactor high molecular weight kininogen (HMWK) binds factors 11 and PK to the damaged endothelial surface or to activated plts; whereupon, factor 12a cleaves factors 11 and PK to yield 11a and kallikrein (K). Factor 11a, with the help of calcium (Ca^{2+}) converts factor IX (9) to activated factor IXA (9a).

Intrinsic coagulation pathway

- Factor 9a, facilitated by factor VIII (8) converts factor X to activated factor XA (10a).
- Ca^{2+} (aka factor 4) binds factors 9a and 10 to the phospholipid membrane.
- The intrinsic pathway is monitored by partial thromboplastin time (**PTT**).

Extrinsic coagulation pathway

- Tissue factor III (TF) in the vascular SE activates factor VII (7) to Factor VIIA (7a).
- Factor 7a, along with Ca^{2+}, activates both factors 9 and 10. Additionally, Factor 7a can active factors 9 and 10 on the plt membrane in absence of TF (a lower affinity pathway).

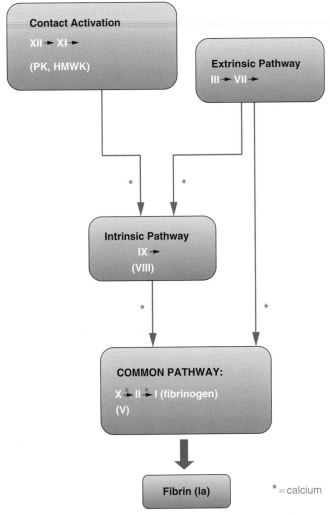

Figure 79.1 Simplified coagulation cascade. Abbreviations: PK, pre-kallikrien; HMWK, high molecular weight kininogen. (Source: Kaplan, J. (ed) *Cardiac Anesthesia: The Echo Era.* 6th edn, p.1111.)

- The extrinsic pathway is monitored by prothrombin time (**PT**).

Common (final) pathway

- The generation of 10a by the intrinsic and extrinsic pathways marks the beginning of the common pathway.
- Phospholipid-bound 10a binds to phospholipid-bound prothrombin (factor II, 2). The binding of 10a and thrombin is accelerated by activated factor VA (5a) (N.B. Factor 5 amplifies the clotting cascade 3,000×). The binding causes a fragment (F1.2) to be cleaved from prothrombin. Prothrombin (factor II) undergoes a conformational change thus becoming thrombin (activated factor II).
- The most important intermediary step in the common pathway is the generation of activated factor II (2a, i.e. **thrombin**).

- **Thrombin**
  - . activates:
    - – factors V (proaccelerin), VIII (anti-hemophilic), and XIII (fibrin stabilizing factor)
  - . cleaves:
    - – factor I (fibrinogen, FG)→ factor IA (1a, fibrin)
  - . stimulates:
    - – platelet recruitment
  - . releases:
    - – tissue plasminogen activator (tPA), therefore, aids fibrinolysis
    - – prostacyclin and nitric oxide from endothelial cells
  - . aids in anticoagulation by activation of:
    - – protein C (with the help of thrombomodulin)
    - – N.B. **protein C** (along with **protein S**, inactivates factor 5a and 8a).

Primary and secondary hemostasis is kept in balance by the anticoagulation systems: **fibrinolysis, protein C and S, and antithrombin III**.

Fibrinolysis remodels and removes clot when the endothelium has healed.

- *Plasmin* is the principle enzyme in fibrinolysis (just like thrombin is the principal enzyme in coagulation).
- Plasminogen, the inactivated precursor of plasmin, binds to fibrin at its lysine binding site. Fibrin also binds *tissue plasminogen activator (tPA)*, which cleaves plasminogen to yield plasmin. Plasmin, in turn, cleaves fibrin, fibrinogen, factors V and VIII. The action of tPA is magnified by its binding to fibrin.
- Agents that lead to the release of tPA from endothelial stores include: thrombin, factor XA, epinephrine, venous occlusion, and CPB.
- The end-products of fibrinolysis: fibrinopeptides, fibrin degradation products (FDPs), and D-dimers.
- The *lysine analog antifibrinolytics, episilon-aminocaproic acid (amicar®), and tranexamic acid,* bind to plasminogen at its lysine binding site, thus prohibiting fibrin from binding to plasminogen.

Protein C and S inactivate factors V and VIII (5 and 8). Coagulation is thus limited to the site of vascular injury.

- Thrombin, along with thrombomodulin, activates *protein C* ensuring that unbridled coagulation does not occur. (Thus thrombin both regulates and activates coagulation.)

Antithrombin III (AT III) slowly associates with thrombin (factor IIA) to inactivate factor IIA (thrombin) and XA.

- In the presence of heparin, the binding of AT III to factor IIA and XA is enhanced 2,000-fold and 1,200-fold, respectively.

There are many anticoagulant drugs used in the preoperative period that may contribute to postoperative bleeding. They include:

- Antithrombin III agonists:
  - *heparin*: a negatively charged acid. Derived from bovine lung or pig intestine. A specific pentasaccharide sequence in the heparin molecule binds to a lysine (positive charge) residue on AT III. This binding alters the configuration of AT III allowing it to bind at an accelerated rate to factors XA and IIA. Of note, heparin can only inhibit plasma-free thrombin (as opposed to clot bound thrombin)
  - *low molecular weight heparin (LMWH)*: possesses the pentasaccharide sequencing that allows it to bind to AT III and inhibit XA **only**. LMWH cannot inhibit thrombin. Examples of LMWH include: enoxaparin (**Lovenox**®), fondaparinux (**Arixtra**®).
- *Direct thrombin (IIA) inhibitors* (DTI) are drugs that directly inhibit the enzymatic site on thrombin and, in some instances, the fibrin binding site of thrombin as well. DTIs render thrombin inactive. Examples include: bivalrudin (**Angiomax**®), argatroban, dabigatran, (**Pradaxa**®). Dabigatran is the only FDA-approved oral DTI.
- *Direct XA inhibitors* inhibit factor XA from activating prothrombin to thrombin. Examples include: rovaroxiban (**Xarelto**®), apixaban (**Eliquist**®).
- *Warfarin* (**Coumadin**®) inhibits vitamin K synthesis and thus the synthesis of factors 2/7/9/10 and proteins C and S (which are all vitamin K dependent). Patients should have their warfarin held for at least five days prior to elective surgery. Treatment modalities to reverse warfarin include administration of fresh frozen plasma (FFP), prothrombin complex concentrate (PCC), recombinant activated factor VII (rVIIA) or vitamin k (takes at least eight hours to work).
- Antiplatelets:
  - *cyclooxygenase (COX) inhibitors*: prevent formation of TXA$_2$, a potent plt activator, e.g., **aspirin**.
  - *GP IIB/IIIA inhibitors*: prevent plt aggregation, e.g., abciximab (**Reopro**®), eptifibatide (**Integrelin**®), tirofiban (**Aggrastat**®). Because these agents work on the final common pathway of plt aggregation (along with fibrinogen) they are the most potent plt inhibitor (>90% inhibition)
  - *ADP receptor inhibitors*: prevent plt activation because ADP binds to P2Y12 receptor, which is a prominent participant in plt activation by collagen and thrombin, e.g., clopidogrel (**Plavix**®); prasugrel (**Effient**®); ticlodipine (**Ticlid**®). These have a slow onset of action because the pro-drug must be converted to the active form

Table 79.4 Half-life of vitamin K – dependent factors

Factor	Half-life
2	3 days
7	6 hours (second shortest half-life)
9	24 hours
10	2 days
Proteins C and S	shortest half-life

(*Source*: Kaplan J. (ed). *Cardiac Anesthesia: The Echo Era*. 6th edn, p. 1114.)

  - *direct P2Y12 inhibitors*: see above, e.g., ticagrelor (**Brilinta**®), cangrelor.
  - *adenosine uptake inhibitor*: prevents plt adhesion, e.g., dipyridamole (**Persantine**®).

Intraoperatively, the most profound insult to platelet function, the coagulation system, and fibrinolysis is the institution of *cardiopulmonary bypass* (CPB).

- On CPB, plt number decreases secondary to: hemodilution, heparin-induced thrombocytopenia, hypothermic-induced splenic sequestration, plt destruction from blood–gas and blood–tissue interfaces (e.g., cardiotomy suction, filters, oxygenators). However, plt count nadir rarely <50 k.
- CPB induces partial degranulation as well as depletion of GP IB and IIB/IIIA receptors. Therefore, plt activation, adhesion, and aggregation are impaired.
- Clotting factors are destroyed by use of cardiotomy suctions. Additionally, hemodilution of clotting factors occurs (however, not below that which is needed for adequate clot formation) see Table 79.3.
- CPB induces fibrinolysis, which leads to undesirable breakdown of clot after surgery. Additionally, the products of fibrinolysis prevents cross-linkage of fibrin strands and, therefore, clot formation.
- FDPs contribute to plt dysfunction post-CPB. Local plasmin formation affects plt membrane proteins. Thus **antifibrinolytics** help preserve platelet function.
- N.B. Unrestricted thrombin activity and fibrinolysis leads to consumption of both platelets and coagulation factors.
- Stimulation of inflammatory system by CPB → leucocyte activation → monocyte activation → TF expression → cascade of coagulation and fibrinolysis.
- Lastly, CPB requires heparinization, therefore adequate reversal of heparin's action must be ensured after the cessation of CPB.

In the immediate postoperative period, hypertension must be avoided as this may disrupt formed clot post CPB.

When a patient has persistent bleeding in the postcardiac surgical period, bleeding risk factors from the preoperative and intraoperative periods must be assessed.

Table 79.5 Risk factors associated with postoperative bleeding

Patient-specific	Surgery-specific
Female sex	Emergency surgery
Female insufficiency	"Redo" procedures
Increased age	Combined procedures
Poor nutrition	Long duration of cardiopulmonary bypass
History of excessive bleeding	Excessive operative bleeding
Smaller body mass index	
Preoperative cardiogenic shock	

(Data from Ferraris, V.A., Ferraris, S., Saha, S. P., Hessel, E. A. et al. 2007. Perioperative blood transfusion and blood conservation in cardiac surgery. The Society of Thoracic Surgeons and the Society of Cardiovascular Anesthsiologists Clinical Practice Guideline. *Annals of Thoracic Surgery*, 83527–86; From Vacanti et al. 2011. *Essential Clinical Anesthesia*, Cambridge University Press, p. 497.)

Preoperative bleeding risk factors include: a history of coagulopathy, plt dysfunction (quantitative or qualitative), organ dysfunction that predisposes to a bleeding diathesis (e.g., liver disease, kidney disease, or congestive heart failure with passive liver congestion as suggested by elevated PT and LFTs).

Liver disease can lead to a decrease in circulating levels of factors 2, 7, 10, AT III, and protein S, as well as a mild decreases in factors 13, 12, 11, HMWK, and PK. However, factor levels are not affected. Treatment would be the administration of FFP.

Renal disease: severe uremia (not mild to moderate renal disease) leads to impaired plt secretion and aggregation functions. The treatment is DDAVP, which stimulates release of factor VIII and large multimer vWF (needed for plt adhesion and aggregation).

Other patient- and surgery-specific risk factors for persistent bleeding after cardiac surgery (PBCS) are shown in Table 79.5.

Upon arrival to ICU the patient should be assessed for: amount of chest tube drainage, presence of generalized oozing, hypothermia, hypertension, signs of tamponade. Laboratory investigations include PT, PTT, CBC, and fibrinogen levels (to assess for coagulopathy, anemia, and thrombocytopenia).

Hypofibrinogenemia (fibrinogen <100 mg/dl; normal = 200–400 mg/dl), if due to disseminated intravascular coagulopathy (DIC) or massive transfusion, warrants treatment with *cryoprecipitate* (cryo) 0.25 µg/kg.

A unit (10 ml bag) of cryo contains: 250 mg of fibrinogen, 100 units of factor VIII, vWF, factor XIII, and fibronectin. It is often transfused as four to six pooled units. In general, cryo is reserved for treatment of specific deficiencies of the aforementioned factors.

A PT/PTT level 1.5 times control suggests a clotting factor deficiency (due to hemodilution, consumption, qualitative or quantitative reasons). Treatment includes FFP, replacement with specific factor therapy, recombinant factor replacement (e.g., NovoSeven®, Profilinine®) of prothrombin complex concentrates (PCC).

FFP contains *all* the clotting factors *and* AT III. The recommended dose is 10 to 15 ml/kg (therefore for 100 kg patient = 1,000–1,500 ml).

Recombinant factor VIIA (NovoSeven®) is activated clotting factor VII that is used "off label" to treat sustained severe bleeding post cardiac surgery. Must ensure that there is no obvious correctable surgical source of blood loss. Additionally, the thrombin-generation response to rVIIA depends on the availability of other coagulation factors and platelets and therefore these must be replaced. In the setting of uncontrolled post-cardiac surgical hemorrhage, the general recommended dose = 90 µg/kg (in hemophiliacs) or 30 µg/kg (in surgical patients), with second doses considered if no response is seen after 30 to 60 minutes. Risks include uncontrolled thrombosis. rVIIA is expensive (~US$4,500–8,500 depending on the dose used).

Profilinine® is a three-factor PCC that contains factors 2, 10, and nonactivated 9 (and very low levels of nonactivated factor 7). When used in a surgical patient with life-threatening bleeding, must provide source of fibrinogen (a unit of FFP) to encourage clot formation. Dosing is weight based and according to factor 9 activity (20–30 IU/kg). Often only one dose is needed. Currently it is the only three-factor PCC available in the United States. Risks include seroconversion of parvovirus, Creutzfeldt–Jakob disease (a small risk), PE, or thrombosis of renal vasculature requiring dialysis. Profilinine is expensive (~US$1,540 for a 25 IU/kg dose in a 70 kg patient).

Thrombocytopenia (plt count <100k/µl, normal 150–400k/µl) occurring during CPB is a result of hemodilution, heparin administration, hypothermia-induced plt splenic sequestration, destruction by cardiotomy suction/filters. Plt counts rarely decrease to <50k.

In general, plt transfusion is not required for plt counts >100k but is definitely required for plts <50k. Transfusion for counts between 50k and 100k requires insight into factors such as anticipation of continued bleeding, volume status, depletion/repletion of clotting factors and red blood cells, as well as the quality of plt function.

DDAVP improves plt function in severely uremic patients and cirrhotic patients by releasing factor VIII (2- to 20-fold increase) and large multimer vWF from the vascular endothelium. The optimal dose is 0.3 µg/kg (given intravenously, subcutaneously, or intranasally) with the optimal effect occurring 30 to 90 minutes after administration. Depletion of vWF stores account for the drug's tachyphylaxis.

Questions

1. Blockade of which factor would yield the greatest impact on the final common pathway?
   a. Factor II
   b. Factor VI
   c. Factor VII
   d. Factor IX
   e. Factor X

2. Cardiopulmonary bypass (CPB) affects:
   a. platelet function and number
   b. fibrinolysis
   c. clotting factors
   d. systemic inflammatory system
   e. all of the above

3. A 56-year-old female with a PMH of mild renal insufficiency, iron-deficient anemia, asthma, NIDDM, and three-vessel coronary artery disease is s/p a three-vessel CABG with left internal mammary and two saphenous vein grafts. In the postcardiac surgical ICU her BP is 180/90, temperature = 35.9°F, plt count is 85K, INR = 1.6, fibrinogen = 101k, and her chest tube output is 500 ml in the first hour and is bright red. What should you do next?
   a. administer rVIIA
   b. warm the patient and give DDAVP, her platelets are dysfunctional due to hypothermia and renal disease
   c. give prothrombin complex contrite (PCC)
   d. call the OR – take the patient back for surgical re-exploration
   e. do nothing

Answers

1. d. While all the factors mentioned would affect the common final pathway, factor IX is utilized by both the intrinsic (activation by factor XI) and the extrinsic (activation by factor VII) pathways.

2. e. CPB affects platelet function by inducing partial degranulation of the plt as well as depleting the glycoproteins IB, IIB/IIIA, thus impairing the platelets' ability to activate, adhere, and aggregate. CPB also induces fibrinolysis, which can lead to consumption of platelets and clotting factors. (N.B. clotting factors never fall below that which is needed for adequate coagulation.) Lastly, CPB stimulates the systemic inflammatory system, which can (via activation of leucocytes and monocytes) lead to tissue factor expression, and the initiation of the clotting cascade, as well as fibrinolysis.

3. d. >500 ml chest tube output in the first hour after surgery is excessive bleeding. Additionally the output is bright red, which hints to an arterial bleeding. The source of the bleed could be anything from bleeding from the internal mammary bed to disrupted sutures or disrupted clot (patient is relative hypotensive). rVIIA and PCC are not warranted (expensive, may cause thrombosis, and no transfusions had occurred yet). Mild renal deficiency does not cause plt dysfunction (severe uremia does). The best plan is to re-explore the chest to rule out surgical bleeding. Prolonged surgical bleeding can lead to depletion of plts and clotting factors and lead to a secondary coagulopathy.

Further reading

Spiess, B., Horrow, J., and Kaplan, J. (2011). Transfusion medicine and coagulation disorders. In Kaplan, J. (ed) *Cardiac Anesthesia: The Echo Era*, 6th edn. Philadelphia, PA: Elsevier Saunders, pp. 949–991.

Bethune, W. and Fitzsimons, A. E. (2011). Persistent postoperative bleeding in cardiac surgical patients. In Vacanti, C. A., Sikka, P. J., Urman, R. D., Dershwitz, M., and Segal, B. S. (eds) *Essential Clinical Anesthesia*. New York, NY: Cambridge University Press, pp. 497–502.

Deitcher, S. R. (2002). Interpretation of the international normalised ratio in patients with liver disease. *Lancet* 359, 47.

Richardson, A. et al. (2009) The role of recombinant activated factor VII in cardiac surgery. *HSR Procedures in Intensive Care Cardiovascular Anesthesia* 1(3), 9–12.

Chapter

80

Carotid endarterectomy

Agnieszka Trzcinka and Shaheen Shaikh

Keywords

Carotid sinus baroreceptor innervation
Carotid body chemoreceptors
Physiologic effects during carotid endarterectomy (CEA)
Carotid sinus reflex
CEA: blocking hemodynamic responses
Anesthetic techniques for CEA
Carotid endarterectomy: monitoring
Electroencephalogram (EEG): interpretation
EEG burst suppression
CEA complications
Carotid sinus baroreceptor denervation
Carotid body denervation
Ventilatory response following CEA
Neurologic deficits following CEA
Cerebral hyperperfusion syndrome

Carotid sinus baroreceptor innervation is via the glossopharyngeal nerve branch called the sinus nerve of Hering.

Carotid body chemoreceptors respond to partial pressure of oxygen changes.

Physiologic effects during carotid endarterectomy (CEA) include stimulation of carotid sinus baroreceptors, resulting in bradycardia and hypotension (*carotid sinus reflex*).

Blocking hemodynamic responses during CEA may be accomplished with use of local anesthetic injection in the area of carotid bifurcation and with preoperative administration of atropine or glycopyrrolate.

Anesthetic techniques for CEA include general anesthesia (ensuring availability of ephedrine, phenylephrine, and nitroglycerin) and regional anesthesia (blockade of C2–C4 dermatomes via superficial cervical plexus block or deep cervical plexus block).

Monitoring during CEA focuses on detection of myocardial ischemia (BP input via intra-arterial catheter, five-lead EKG with ST-segment monitoring) and cerebral ischemia (electroencephalogram, SSEP, transcranial Doppler, stump pressure, and cerebral oximetry).

Electroencephalogram (EEG) illustrates signals from the superficial cerebral cortex and may reveal ipsilateral decreased activity during carotid artery cross-clamping (possible if CBF is less than 15 ml/100g/min and dependent on inhaled anesthetic in use). EEG is sensitive to all anesthetic agents (inhaled anesthetic level may have to be maintained at ≤0.5 MAC to ensure reliable monitoring).

EEG interpretation is based on measured frequency and amplitude. Activity is divided into alpha, beta, delta, and theta wave patterns as outlined in Figure 80.1.

Increased depth of anesthesia above MAC of 1.5 results in longer periods of *EEG burst suppression* with no electrical signal activity.

Possible *CEA complications* include blood pressure instability (hypertension and hypotension), myocardial infarction, neck hematoma with airway obstruction, respiratory dysfunction, and neurologic deficit.

Postsurgical hypertension may be associated with *carotid sinus baroreceptor denervation*. It is most pronounced two to three hours after surgery and may last up to 24 hours.

Unilateral *carotid body denervation* may affect *ventilatory response* to decreased partial pressure of oxygen. This effect is especially pronounced after bilateral CEA, and such patients rely on central brainstem chemoreceptors for ventilatory response to changes in partial pressure of carbon dioxide and are prone to respiratory depression after opioid administration.

Neurologic deficits following CEA may range from focal injury stemming from particular nerve damage (recurrent laryngeal, hypoglossal, and superior laryngeal) to global cerebral injury resulting from thrombosis, embolic event, or occlusion of artery.

Cerebral hyperperfusion syndrome may manifest several days postoperatively in patients who develop severe hypertension. Symptoms include persistent ipsilateral headache, focal neurologic deficits, and possible progression to seizures. It is characterized by ipsilateral elevated CBF and occurs due to surgically restored normal cerebral perfusion pressure in previously ischemic areas with abnormal autoregulation.

Essential Clinical Anesthesia Review: Keywords, Questions and Answers for the Boards, ed. Linda S. Aglio, Robert W. Lekowski, and Richard D. Urman. Published by Cambridge University Press. © Cambridge University Press 2015.

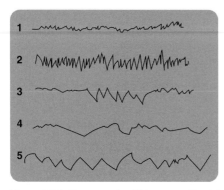

Figure 80.1 Representative EEG patterns. *Line 1*: Beta waves seen in the awake patient. *Line 2*: Alpha waves seen in a related patient. *Line 3*: Theta waves seen in the somnolent patient. *Line 4*: Sleep spindles seen in the sleeping patient. *Line 5*: Delta waives in the relatively deeply anesthetized patient. (Source: Gelfand, B. J. and Leeson, S. 2011. Carotid endarterectomy. From Vacanti et al. 2011. *Essential Clinical Anesthesia*, Cambridge University Press, p. 506.)

Questions

1. Select all TRUE statements. The carotid sinus:

   a. contains chemoreceptors that respond to changes in partial pressure of carbon dioxide

   b. is innervated by CN XI

   c. may be stimulated during carotid endarterectomy resulting in profound bradycardia

   d. may be denervated during carotid endarterectomy resulting in loss of ventilatory drive

2. Select all TRUE statements. Cerebral hyperperfusion syndrome:

   a. most often occurs immediately after CEA

   b. results from elevated CBF affecting vasculature with impaired autoregulation

   c. presents with symptoms of nausea, emesis, and photophobia

   d. is the most common cause of neurologic injury after CEA

3. All of the following statements are true EXCEPT which?

   a. Neurophysiologic monitoring during CEA decreases risk of stroke with improved prognosis.

   b. EEG monitoring does not register signals from brain areas deeper than superficial cerebral cortex.

   c. Delta waves on EEG strip indicate deep anesthetic level.

   d. Neurophysiologic monitoring during CEA may assist surgical team in appropriate use of shunting.

Answers

1. c. Carotid sinus is innervated by branch of CN IX (glossopharyngeal) and contains baroreceptors. Stimulation of this area may result in significant bradycardia and hypotension. Carotid body is composed of chemoreceptors that respond to changes in PO_2. Carotid body denervation may affect ventilatory response to decreased partial pressure of oxygen. Chemoreceptors in the brainstem respond to changes in partial pressure of carbon dioxide.

2. b. Cerebral hyperperfusion usually occurs three to eight days after surgical intervention with symptoms of persistent ipsilateral headache, focal neurologic deficits, and possible progression to seizure. It occurs due to surgically restored normal cerebral perfusion pressure in previously ischemic areas with abnormal autoregulation. It is not a common cause of neurologic morbidity after CEA.

3. a. The EEG illustrates signals from the superficial cerebral cortex and may reveal ipsilateral decreased activity during carotid artery cross-clamping. Neurophysiologic monitoring has not been shown to decrease risk of stroke, but may assist the surgical team in the appropriate use of shunting.

Further reading

Gelfand, B. J. and Leeson, S. (2011). Carotid endarterectomy. In Vacanti, C. A., Sikka, P. K., Urman, R. D., Dershwitz, M., and Segal, B. S. (eds) *Essential Clinical Anesthesia*. New York: Cambridge University Press, pp. 503–508.

Norris, E. J. (2009). Anesthesia for vascular surgery. In Miller, R. D., Eriksson, L. I., Fleisher, L. A., Wiener-Kronish, J. P., and Young, W. L. (eds) *Miller's Anesthesia*, 7th edn. New York: Churchill Livingstone, pp. 2026–2031.

Abdominal aortic aneurysm

Mohab Ibrahim and Linda S. Aglio

Keywords

Abdominal AO Xclamp
Heparin-induced thrombocytopenia
Hypotension
LMWH: cont vs. discount
LMWH and neuraxial anesthesia
LMWH: postoperative epidural
Low viscosity improves blood flow
Venous pressure: gravity effects

Abdominal AO Xclamp

A process in which a clamp is applied to the aorta by the surgeon for the surgical repair of aneurysms. The clamp site is proximal to the lesion of interest. The clamp prevents exsanguination and allows for dry conditions that are needed for surgical repair of the aorta. This maneuver usually constitutes the majority of hemodynamics seen with abdominal aortic aneurysm (AAA) repair.

Hemodynamics

Applying an aortic cross-clamp results in increase in blood pressure (BP) secondary to increased systemic vascular resistance (BP = systemic resistance × cardiac output). The increase in BP is a combination of the mechanical effects of the clamp, the release of vasoactive mediators (renin-angiotensin, catecholamines, etc.), and autotransfusion. Autotransfusion is the result of decreased venous capacity secondary to the vasoactive mediators. A supraceliac position of the aortic cross-clamp results in significant increase in preload. An infraceliac position attenuates the preload.

The application of an aortic cross-clamp may be associated with increased systolic wall tension (systolic wall tension = BP × radius/wall thickness). Increase in volatile anesthetics or using vasodilators may be needed.

Heparin-induced thrombocytopenia

Heparin-induced thrombocytopenia (HIT) is a clinical syndrome in which there are appreciable decreases in platelet count and thrombotic events associated with heparin administration. There are two types of HIT: type 1 is the result of direct effect of heparin on platelets; type 2 is IgG antibody mediated.

Management: once HIT is suspected, heparin, and all products containing heparin, must be stopped.

Treatment: if anticoagulation is desired in the setting of HIT, one must consider direct thrombin inhibitors as alternatives to heparin. Low molecular weight heparin (LMWH) has nearly 100% cross-reactivity and is better avoided in HIT. Currently available direct thrombin inhibitors include lepirudin, bivalirudin, and argatroban. Lepirudin is renally metabolized. Bivalirium is metabolized by plasma proteases and renally. Argatroban is hepatically metabolized.

Hypotension

A clinical situation in which the blood pressure drops below baseline. There are several reasons for the development of hypotension. Hypotension is observed secondary to either a decrease in systemic resistance, decrease in cardiac output, or a combination of both. Depending on the reason, a compensatory mechanism can be better appreciated or designed. Induction of anesthesia can be associated with hypotension secondary to decrease in both systemic vascular resistance and cardiac output. The patient may benefit from small doses of both direct alpha-1 agonist such as phenylephrine and a sympathomimetic such as ephedrine. In case of preexisting hypovolemia, an IV fluid bolus may improve hypotension. Surgical causes include significant bleeding or compression of major vessels. Replacing the lost volume with either crystalloids, colloids, or blood products and addressing the vascular compression may be sufficient to treat the hypotension.

Neuraxial anesthesia may result in hypotension because of blocking the sympathetic outflow. In this case, small doses of

Essential Clinical Anesthesia Review: Keywords, Questions and Answers for the Boards, ed. Linda S. Aglio, Robert W. Lekowski, and Richard D. Urman. Published by Cambridge University Press. © Cambridge University Press 2015.

phenylephrine, ephedrine, and IV fluids may attenuate the hypotension. Sepsis may also result in hypotension. Fluids and pressors may be needed until the source of sepsis is identified and treated.

Intrinsic mechanisms to address hypotension include activation of the renin-angiotensin system, fluid shift from intracellular compartment into the vascular compartment, decrease urine output, and increasing the thirst drive.

LMWH: cont vs. discount

In certain clinical situations, the risks of employing neuraxial anesthesia may outweigh the benefits. Probably the greatest risk associated with neuraxial anesthesia is epidural/spinal hematoma. One of the factors, which may increase the risk of hematoma formation, is anticoagulants such as LMWH. LMWH may be prescribed as a prophylactic therapy for conditions such as factor V Leiden mutation, protein C deficiency, pulmonary embolism, DVT, and other medical conditions that may predispose to increased blood clot formation. In such a scenario, the anesthesiologist must engage both the surgical team and the patient to decide the risk and benefit of neuraxial anesthesia for pain control. Surgical patients are already at increased risk of forming blood clots secondary to surgical trauma, decreased physical activity, and possible damage to blood vessels. For a patient with a condition predisposing them to develop blood clots, the cessation of LMWH needed for initiating or discontinuing neuraxial anesthesia may have severe consequences. Therefore a careful review of risks and benefits, may need to be undertaken.

LMWH and neuraxial anesthesia

Neuraxial anesthesia is used either as a primary mode of anesthesia or as a secondary mode for better pain control. However, there are some risks associated with neuraxial anesthesia. Probably one of the most significant risks is spinal or epidural hematoma, which may require neurosurgical intervention for immediate decompression and evacuation of the hematoma. The risk of spinal or epidural hematoma are increased when LMWH are used.

There are several medications that are considered LMWH, such as ardeparin, delteparin, danaparoid, enoxaparin, and tinzaparin.

For preoperative LMWH consideration, the American Society of Regional Anesthesia (ASRA) recommends waiting 12 hours for prophylactic dosing and 24 hours for therapeutic dosing, after the last dose before starting neuraxial anesthesia.

LMWH: postoperative epidural

For twice/day dosing, the first dose of LMWH should not be administered until 24 hours postoperatively. If a continuous technique is used, then the catheter should be removed on postoperative day one and the first dose of LMWH should be held for at least two hours after the catheter is removed.

For once/day dosing, the first dose of LMWH may be given six to eight hours postoperatively. The second dose should be started at least 24 hours after the first dose of LMWH. Indwelling catheters may be removed 10 to 12 hours after the last dose of LMWH. Additional doses of LMWH must be held for an additional two hours after catheter removal.

Low viscosity improves blood flow

Blood flow in small vessels and capillaries is a function of many factors including viscosity. As viscosity decreases, less driving force becomes necessary to move red blood cells in vessels. When the driving force is kept the same, blood with lower viscosity will be better and will perfuse tissue more efficiently.

Blood viscosity varies inversely with temperature and directly with hematocrit concentration. Decreasing blood viscosity may be achieved by hemodilution. Decreasing blood viscosity allows for increased venous return, and increasing cardiac output through the increase in stroke volume and contractility. Though the oxygen-carrying capacity of hemodiluted blood is reduced, the better perfusion of tissue coupled with increased cardiac output compensate for the decreased oxygen-carrying capacity.

Venous pressure: gravity effects

Gravity plays a crucial role in hemodynamics. When a person stands up, venous blood is pooled to the lower extremities. If no compensatory mechanism existed, such phenomena would result in decreased preload, leading to decreased cardiac output. When a person moves from a standing position to a laying down position, less venous blood is pooled in the lower extremities, resulting in increased preload and increased cardiac output. A similar argument can be made regarding the Trendelenburg position, in which the lower extremities are at higher elevation than the heart at a supine position. Such position encourages better return of venous blood to the heart, increasing the preload and resulting in increased cardiac output.

In the event of blood pooled by gravity to the lower extremities, certain mechanisms are initiated to compensate for the decreased preload. These mechanisms include increased heart rate and increased sympathetic output to facilitate vasoconstriction. The baroreceptors located in the carotid sinus plays a significant role in initiating the compensatory mechanisms. This is known as the baroreceptor reflex. The carotid sinus sends signals through the glossopharyngeal nerve to the nucleus of the solitary tract (NTS) in the brainstem, which ultimately effects the sympathetic outflow. Decreased blood pressure, such as seen when a person stands up from a sitting position, initiates the baroreceptor reflex causing disinhibition, resulting in increased sympathetic tone.

Questions

1. A postoperative patient receiving heparin for anticoagulation prophylaxis suddenly develops thrombocytopenia – what is the next course of action?

a. Continue heparin therapy until a serotonin release assay has been conducted. If positive, switch to a direct thrombin inhibitor.
b. Continue heparin therapy until enzyme-linked immunosorbent assay I is performed to identify heparin-dependent IgG antibodies. If positive, switch to a direct thrombin inhibitor.
c. Look for other causes of thrombocytopenia. If no other causes can be identified, continue with heparin.
d. Stop heparin. Switch to a direct thrombin inhibitor. Run enzyme-linked immunosorbent assay to identify heparin-dependent IgG antibodies.

2. A 75-year-old male with a history of congestive heart failure is undergoing AAA open repair. After placement of a supraceliac clamp, his blood pressure drops. Which is the best course of action?
    a. administer fluid bolus
    b. decrease the volatile anesthetics
    c. administer phenylephrine
    d. carefully titrate nitroglycerin

3. All the following factors contribute to blood viscosity except which?
    a. temperature
    b. hematocrit
    c. amount of IV fluid given
    d. blood pressure

Answers

1. d. HIT is a clinical diagnosis when no other reason for thrombocytopenia can be identified. Once suspected, heparin should be stopped and a direct thrombin inhibitor should be used. Serotonin release assay is expensive and time consuming. Enzyme-linked immunosorbent assay I performed to identify heparin-dependent IgG antibodies may require time to be performed, which may place the patient at increased risk.

2. d. The hemodynamic response of the aortic cross-clamp depends not only on the position of the clamp, but also on the heart condition. If the cross-clamp is placed in a supraceliac position, a significant splanchnic venous constriction takes place, resulting in increased preload. In congestive heart failure, the heart may not be able to accommodate both the increase in preload and afterload. A fluid bolus may exacerbate the CHF. Decreasing volatile anesthetics may increase the afterload and preload, which could lead to further deterioration of the hemodynamics. Administering phenylephrine will increase the afterload, placing more stress on an already stressed heart. Careful titration of nitroglycerin may cause vasodilation and may reduce the preload, allowing the heart to have better contractility and output.

3. d. Blood viscosity is inversely proportional to temperature and directly proportional to hematocrit. If enough IV fluid is given, this may decrease the hematocrit, resulting in decreased viscosity (mass of hematocrit remains the same, while IV fluids increase the total volume, resulting in relative decrease in hematocrit concentration). Blood pressure does not play a role in determining blood viscosity.

Further reading

Vacanti, C. A., Sikka, P. K., Urman, R. U., Dershwitz, M., and Segal, B. S. (2011). *Essential Clinical Anesthesia*, 1st edn. Cambridge University Press, Chapters 72, 82, and 83.

Yao, F. (2012). *Anesthesiology: Problem-Oriented Patient Management*, 7th edn, Chapters 6 and 9.

www.openanesthesia.org

Chapter 82

Endovascular abdominal aortic aneurysm repair

Andrea Girnius and Annette Mizuguchi

Keywords

Abdominal aortic aneurysm (AAA)
Abdominal aortic cross-clamp: hemodynamics
Abdominal aneurysm resection: anesthetic management
Surgical considerations
Endoleak

An *abdominal aortic aneurysm* is present when the diameter of the aorta is >3 cm (>50% of expected size). It can be detected clinically by a pulsatile abdominal mass or can be found incidentally on imaging studies. Aneurysms enlarge by about 0.5 cm/year, and once they reach 5 to 6 cm in diameter, *surgical repair is indicated*.

The *endovascular* approach to AAA repair was introduced in 1991. Its advantages include a less invasive nature, reduced blood loss, and no need for aortic cross-clamping leading to relative hemodynamic stability.

Anesthetic considerations: patients with abdominal aortic aneurysms have a high likelihood of coexisting coronary artery disease as well as other significant comorbidities. AAA repair is a high-risk surgery, and all endovascular repairs have the potential to be converted to open repairs. Therefore, thorough preoperative evaluation and optimization with an emphasis on the cardiovascular system is warranted before this surgery.

Monitoring for this procedure typically includes standard ASA monitors, large-bore intravenous access, and invasive arterial blood pressure monitoring. Decisions about central venous monitoring should be made on a case-by-case basis and should take into account the likelihood of conversion to open repair.

Anesthetic management can include both regional and general anesthesia. The choice depends on the preferences of the anesthesiologist, surgeon, and patient. Patient cooperation is required for regional techniques. The various techniques have not been shown to affect mortality or postoperative complication rates.

In the event of conversion to an *open procedure*, an *aortic cross-clamp* will be needed to complete the repair. This

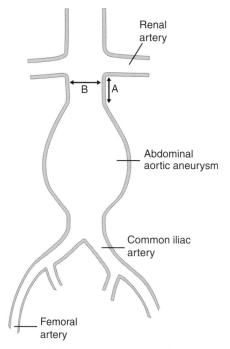

Figure 82.1 Anatomic requirements for infrared EVAR are listed as follows: the aneurismal aortic neck ("landing zone") should be at least 15 mm (A); the infrarenal aortic neck diameter range should be 19 to 36 mm (B); one femoral artery must be free from significant occlusive disease and have a diameter of >7.7 mm; if the larger iliac is being used, it must be free from toruosity or excessive calcification; the distal attachment site must be nonaneurysmal and of sufficient length to accommodate the graft; and there should be at least one straight iliac artery that can be used as a conduit for the delivery system. (From Vacanti et al. 2011. *Essential Clinical Anesthesia*, Cambridge University Press, Figure 83.1.)

has important *hemodynamic* implications. An aortic cross-clamp increases afterload, which increases left ventricular systolic wall tension and predisposes the patient to myocardial ischemia. Vasodilators are typically used to offset this effect. The more proximal on the aorta the cross-clamp is placed, the more afterload increases. Most consistently, hypertension is seen above the clamp and hypotension is seen below the clamp.

Essential Clinical Anesthesia Review: Keywords, Questions and Answers for the Boards, ed. Linda S. Aglio, Robert W. Lekowski, and Richard D. Urman. Published by Cambridge University Press. © Cambridge University Press 2015.

Surgical considerations: there are certain anatomic requirements that must be met in order for an infrarenal stent to be deployed successfully (see Figure 82.1). The endograft is placed via iliofemoral arterial access under fluoroscopic guidance. Systemic anticoagulation with heparin is achieved before stent deployment.

Complications of endovascular AAA repair include endoleak, migration of stent graft, conversion to open procedure, acute rupture (most likely during stent deployment), embolic events, paralysis, infection, and problems with wound healing.

Endoleak describes continued blood flow into the aneurysmal sac after deployment of the stent. It can occur at any time after the deployment of the stent. There are four types of endoleak:

(I)   Leakage at the proximal or distal graft attachment sites
(II)   Retrograde flow from collateral branches
(III) Leak from overlapping parts of the stent
(IV)   Leakage through the graft wall

Type IV endoleaks usually resolve with time. Type I and III endoleaks should be repaired urgently. Management of type II endoleaks is controversial, as some will resolve with time and others lead to aneurysm enlargement. They are usually followed by serial CT scan.

Renal dysfunction is commonly seen after endovascular AAA repair (EVAR). The etiology is likely multifactorial but includes the use of contrast dye during the procedure and the position of the graft. Renal-protective strategies for the prevention of contrast-induced nephropathy include hydration, bicarbonate infusion, and N-acetylcysteine pretreatment.

Questions

1. Which of the following surgical considerations for endovascular AAA repair is NOT true?
    a. Length of the aneurysmal aortic neck does not matter.
    b. The infrarenal neck diameter should be 19 to 36 mm.
    c. One femoral artery must be free from occlusive disease.
    d. The femoral artery being used must have a diameter >7.7 mm.

    e. The iliac artery being used should be free of tortuosity or excessive calcifications.

2. Which of the following endoleaks does NOT require repair?
    a. Type I endoleak
    b. Type III endoleak
    c. Type II endoleak with evidence of aneurysm enlargement on repeat CT scan
    d. Type IV endoleak
    e. none of the above

3. Which of the following statements regarding the anesthetic management for endovascular AAA repair is TRUE?
    a. The likelihood of conversion to an open repair is low.
    b. Patients undergoing this procedure usually have minimal comorbidities.
    c. Regional anesthesia can be an option for this procedure given a cooperative patient and a willing surgeon.
    d. In an open procedure, aortic cross-clamp placement causes systemic hypotension.
    e. Expected blood loss for both the open and endovascular repair is similar.

Answers

1. a. Certain anatomical conditions must be met for the endovascular technique to be used successfully. One of these conditions is an adequate aortic neck length in order for the stent to have a place to land. All other choices are true.
2. d. Type IV endoleak, or leakage through the graft wall, usually resolves over time and does not necessitate surgical management. Type II endoleak can be followed with CT scan, but if there is evidence of enlargement, then it should be managed surgically.
3. c. Anesthetic management can include both regional or general anesthesia. The endovascular procedure can be done under regional anesthesia given a cooperative patient and surgeon.

Further reading

Mizuguchi, K. A. (2011). Endovascular abdominal aortic aneurysm repair. In Vacanti, C. A., Sikka, P. K., Urman, R. U., Dershwitz, M., and Segal, B. S. (eds)

Essential Clinical Anesthesia. New York, NY: Cambridge University Press, pp. 516–518.

Norris, E. J. (2009). Anesthesia for vascular surgery. In Miller, R. D., Eriksson, L. I.,

Fleisher, L. A., Wiener-Kronish, J. P., and Young, W. L. (eds) *Miller's Anesthesia,* 7th edn. New York: Churchill-Livingstone, pp. 1985–2044.

Chapter

83

Peripheral vascular disease

Andrea Girnius and Annette Mizuguchi

Keywords

Peripheral arteriosclerotic disease
Peripheral vascular disease (PVD)
Atherosclerosis
Claudication
Ankle–brachial index (ABI)
Surgical indications for peripheral vascular disease
Evaluation of peripheral vascular disease
Preoperative assessment for peripheral vascular
    surgery
Anesthetic techniques

The major cause of *peripheral vascular disease* (PVD) is *atherosclerosis*. The major *risk factors for PVD* correspond to those for atherosclerosis. They include smoking, diabetes, obesity, hyperlipidemia, hypertension, and homocysteine elevation.

Claudication is reproducible ischemic pain induced by activity and relieved by rest. It is due to insufficient blood flow to muscles during exercise. Pain that is present without exercise is called *rest pain* and indicates critical ischemia.

Medical management of PVD includes risk factor modification and exercise.

The severity of PVD can be assessed using an *Ankle–Brachial Index (ABI)*, which compares the blood pressures in the upper and lower extremities.

$$ABI = P_{leg}/P_{arm}$$

Where P_{leg} = systolic blood pressure of the dorsalis pedis or posterior tibial arteries, and P_{arm} = highest of left vs. right arm brachial systolic blood pressure.

Table 83.1 ABI index

ABI value	Interpretation
>1.2	Abnormal vessel hardening from PVD
0.9–1.2	Normal range
0.5–0.9	Mild-moderate PVD
<0.5	Severe PVD

An ABI above 1.2 indicates abnormal vessel hardening from PVD, which makes the ABI inaccurate.

Indications for surgery to correct PVD include: (1) intermittent activity limiting claudication nonresponsive to medical management; (2) ischemic rest pain; (3) ischemic ulcer; (4) gangrene.

Preoperative considerations: peripheral revascularization is classified as a high-risk surgery (>5% risk of perioperative cardiac event). These patients often have significant comorbidities, including coronary artery disease (CAD), diabetes mellitus (DM), and renal dysfunction.

Preoperative evaluation should focus on evaluating comorbidities with a focus on the cardiovascular system. A preoperative EKG should be obtained as a baseline. Renal function should be evaluated as contrast dye is often used in vascular surgeries. If the patient is on anticoagulation, coagulation studies (PT/INR and PTT) should be obtained.

Perioperative beta-blocker management is critical in this patient population. Patients already on beta-blocker treatment should continue taking them through the perioperative period. Patients who are not already on a beta-blocker but are at high cardiac risk (coronary artery disease, positive stress test, significant cardiac risk factors) may benefit from perioperative initiation of beta-blocker therapy.

The decision to hold or continue other medications such as statins, angiotensin-converting enzyme (ACE) inhibitors, or aspirin should be made on a case-by-case basis. Decisions about *aspirin* should be made in conjunction with the surgical team as it can increase surgical bleeding. However, it has not been shown to increase morbidity and mortality. In addition, discontinuing aspirin may increase the risk of cardiovascular events.

For patients with coronary artery disease (CAD), studies have not shown a difference in outcome between medical management and interventional revascularization (including percutaneous and surgical treatment). Medical management includes beta-blockade, statins, aspirin therapy, and management of hypertension and any existing heart failure.

Essential Clinical Anesthesia Review: Keywords, Questions and Answers for the Boards, ed. Linda S. Aglio, Robert W. Lekowski, and Richard D. Urman. Published by Cambridge University Press. © Cambridge University Press 2015.

Anesthetic techniques include regional and general anesthesia. The decision about anesthetic technique should be made on a case-by-case basis.

Patients with peripheral vascular disease are at high risk for intraoperative *blood pressure lability*, likely due to underlying comorbidities such as hypertension and atherosclerosis.

Most peripheral vascular surgery requires *arterial cross-clamping* for vascular repair. Release of the cross-clamp and reperfusion of the affected area causes vasodilatory metabolites, carbon dioxide, and oxygen free radicals to enter circulation. Thus vasoactive agents should be available at the time of cross-clamp release, as *hypotension* is expected.

Monitoring should include standard ASA monitors, including monitoring of a precordial EKG lead (V4 or V5), as this is very sensitive for detecting coronary ischemia. In selected patients, *invasive arterial pressure monitoring* is indicated. Central venous and pulmonary artery pressure monitoring is not routinely used.

Contrast dye may be used in peripheral revascularization. As many of these patients may have underlying renal dysfunction, there is concern for contrast-induced nephropathy. *Renal-protective strategies* that can be used include hydration, sodium bicarbonate infusion, and N-acetylcysteine pretreatment.

Questions

1. Which of the following is an indication for surgical treatment of peripheral vascular disease?
   a. ischemic rest pain
   b. ischemic ulcer
   c. gangrene
   d. activity limiting claudication
   e. all of the above

2. Which of the following statements about renal function during surgery for peripheral vascular disease is NOT true?
   a. Hydration is not effective as a strategy for renal protection.
   b. Contrast-induced nephropathy is unlikely to occur.
   c. Patients undergoing peripheral vascular surgery are unlikely to have underlying renal disease.
   d. Sodium bicarbonate infusions are never used for renal protection.
   e. All of the above.

3. A 68-year-old male scheduled to undergo right-sided femoral to popliteal bypass for symptomatic claudication has a medical history of CAD, chronic renal insufficiency, and diabetes mellitus type 2. His CAD is medically managed with a beta-blocker, statin, and aspirin. He is able to climb two flights of stairs without shortness of breath or chest pain, but his activity is limited by his claudication. Which of the following statements about perioperative management of his CAD is true?
   a. He should stop his aspirin seven days before surgery.
   b. Continuing his beta-blocker perioperatively is likely to reduce his risk of perioperative cardiac events.
   c. He should undergo cardiac catheterization before surgery, as interventional revascularization will improve his outcome.
   d. A baseline EKG will not be helpful in this case as it is likely to be abnormal.
   e. Statins should never be continued perioperatively.

Answers

1. e. All of the above are indications for surgery for PVD.
2. e. Kidney function is an important consideration in patients with peripheral vascular disease. These patients are likely to have underlying kidney disease and are at risk for kidney injury from contrast dye. Hydration and sodium bicarbonate infusions are two strategies to help prevent renal injury.
3. b. Beta-blocker therapy has been proven to reduce perioperative cardiac events in patients with CAD, which is a common comorbidity in patients with peripheral vascular disease. Aspirin use should be discussed with the surgeon but can be continued perioperatively.

Further reading

Leduc, L. H. and Helstrom, J. L. (2011). Peripheral vascular disease. In Vacanti, C. A., Sikka, P. K., Urman, R. U., Dershwitz, M., and Segal, B. S. (eds) *Essential Clinical Anesthesia*. New York, NY: Cambridge University Press, pp. 519–522.

Norris, E. J. (2009). Anesthesia for vascular surgery. In Miller, R. D., Eriksson, L. I., Fleisher, L. A., Wiener-Kronish, J. P., and Young, W. L. (eds) *Miller's Anesthesia*, 7th edn. New York: Churchill-Livingstone, pp. 1985–2044.

POISE Study Group (2008). Effects of extended-release metoprolol succinate in patients undergoing non-cardiac surgery (POISE trial): a randomised controlled trial. *Lancet* 371(9627), 1839–1847.

Chapter

84

Respiratory physiology

Hanjo Ko and George P. Topulos

Keywords

Pulmonary circulation
Work of breathing: resistance and compliance
Dead space: anatomical and physiological
Shunt
Ventilation and perfusion mismatch
Hypoxic pulmonary vasoconstriction
West zones
Pulmonary function testing

Dual pulmonary circulations

The pulmonary artery carries mixed venous blood from the right ventricle to the pulmonary capillaries, where gas exchange takes place. The arterialized blood is then carried to the left atrium via the pulmonary vein. Compared to the systemic circulation, the blood flow is the same (cardiac output), but at much lower pressures due to lower resistance.

The separate bronchial arteries, with flows that are a small fraction of the cardiac output, are branches of the aorta. They are the nutrient vessels for the conducting airways and associated blood vessels. Part of the bronchial circulation empties into the pulmonary vein forming part of the normal anatomic shunt.

Compliance is the ratio of change in volume to change in transmural pressure ($\Delta V/\Delta P_{tm}$). Unless the chest is open due to trauma or surgery, the lung and chest wall change volume by the same amount. Therefore the compliance of the respiratory system is less than the compliance of the either the lung or chest wall alone.

Airway *resistance* is predominantly determined by total airway cross-sectional area, which in turn is influenced by lung volume and elastic recoil. Resistance is increased by decreased elastic recoil (emphysema), and increased airway smooth muscle tone and airway inflammation and secretions (chronic bronchitis and asthma), as well as foreign bodies and increased lung water. In healthy subjects, intermediate-sized bronchi contribute most of the resistance to flow, and distal small

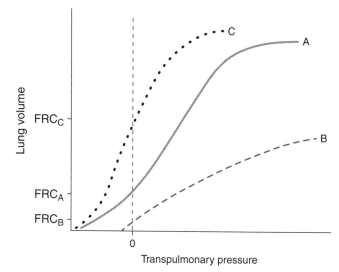

Figure 84.1 Pulmonary pressure–volume relationships in (A) normal lung, (B) severe restrictive disease, and (C) obstructive disease. Note that total lung capacity (indicated by the highest volume achieved), FRC, and complaince *(curves)* all change with disease.

airways contribute the least, because of their large number and total cross-sectional area.

In a given airway (or blood vessel) flow may be laminar, turbulent, or intermediate.

Patients with decreased compliance and stiff lungs (e.g., pulmonary fibrosis) or chest walls tend to favor a rapid, shallow breathing pattern, to decrease elastic work. Patients with increased airway resistance (e.g., tracheomalacia, tracheal stenosis, severe asthma, or COPD) tend to breathe with larger tidal volumes, slower rates, and lower gas flows, to decrease resistive work.

Dead space is an area that is ventilated but not perfused, $\frac{V_A}{Q} = \infty$. *Anatomical dead space* = 2 cc/kg = 150 cc in an average adult = upper airway, trachea, and other conducting airways. Total dead space = anatomic + alveolar. Under normal circumstance in young healthy adults, there is no alveolar dead space and the dead space to tidal volume ratio, $V_D/V_T = 20–30\%$. Dead space is slightly increased with mask

Essential Clinical Anesthesia Review: Keywords, Questions and Answers for the Boards, ed. Linda S. Aglio, Robert W. Lekowski, and Richard D. Urman. Published by Cambridge University Press. © Cambridge University Press 2015.

Table 84.1 Laminar or turbulent flow

	Necessary driving pressure proportional to	Flow characteristics
Laminar	1/**4th** power radius Tube length Flow rate Gas **viscosity**	**More** efficient **Parabolic** flow profile, streamlines with highest velocity in the center of the airway **Low** Reynolds number
Turbulent	1/**5th** power radius Tube length Flow rate **squared** Gas **density**	**Less** efficient **Blunt** flow profile, uniform velocities across airway **High** Reynolds number

ventilation, and decreased by an ETT. In disease, alveolar (not anatomic) dead space often increases. In special cases (e.g., failure of circuit one-way valve), equipment dead space may increase enormously. The ratio of *physiological dead space* to tidal volume, V_D/V_T is found using the Bohr equation (below), and includes anatomic and alveolar dead space, where $PaCO_2$ is arterial PCO_2 and $PECO_2$ is *mixed exhaled* (not end-tidal) PCO_2. Because some dead space is always present, $PETCO_2$ is usually slightly lower than arterial. A large increase in the difference between $PaCO_2$ and $PETCO_2$ is very suggestive of an increased dead space, for example by a pulmonary embolism. Because of alveolar dead space, the $PETCO_2$ may not always be high even though $PaCO_2$ is high. However, if the $PETCO_2$ is high, the $PaCO_2$ will always be high:

$$\frac{V_D}{V_T} = \frac{PaCO_2 - P\bar{E}CO_2}{PaCO_2}$$

Shunts occur in areas that are perfused but not ventilated, $\frac{V_A}{Q} = 0$. Two normal anatomic shunts, <1% of cardiac output flow from the aorta to the left atrium, bypassing the pulmonary circulation altogether: (1) part of the bronchial circulation, and (2) part of the coronary circulation that drains into Thebesian veins. Pathology can also cause R → L intracardiac shunts. Pulmonary shunts may be due to (1) atelectasis, (2) disease of the parenchyma, or (3) airway obstruction by a foreign body. All shunts cause hypoxemia. Because, by definition, flow through pure shunt does not come in contact with alveolar gas, 100% FiO_2 does not fully correct the hypoxemia. This distinguishes pure shunt from less extreme V/Q mismatch. The ratio of *physiological shunt* to total blood flow, $\frac{\dot{Q}_S}{\dot{Q}_T}$ is found using the shunt equation (below), and includes anatomic and alveolar shunt, where $Cc'O_2$ is pulmonary end capillary O_2 content, CaO_2 is arterial O_2 content, and $C\bar{V}O_2$ is *mixed* venous O_2 content. Typically, shunt is not associated with hypercarbia because a small increase in $PaCO_2$ results in compensatory increased ventilation:

$$\frac{\dot{Q}_S}{\dot{Q}_T} = \frac{Cc'O_2 - CaO_2}{Cc'O_2 - C\bar{V}O_2}$$

V/Q mismatch

Normally, at rest the average V/Q ratio is close to 1.0, with V/Q highest at the apex and lowest at the base (range 0.3–2). Pulmonary diseases broaden the distribution of V/Q ratios (i.e., more alveolar units with high and/or low V/Q). More alveolar units with low V/Q ratios (i.e., more shunt-like) leads to hypoxemia, and should result in hypercarbia, but usually does not due to the resulting increased minute ventilation. Increased minute ventilation can correct the hypercarbia caused by blood flow to low V/Q regions. However, because the oxyhemoglobin dissociation curve plateaus, lung units with high V/Q ratios cannot correct the hypoxemia caused by blood flow to low V/Q regions. Pulmonary embolism is a special case that should result only in an increase in dead space ventilation. However, the release of unknown injurious factors results in increased blood flow to low V/Q regions and hypoxemia, which along with tachypnea are the primary signs of a PE.

Hypoxic pulmonary vasoconstriction is one of the primary mechanisms that preserve matching of ventilation and perfusion. Low alveolar oxygen tension leads to vasoconstriction of the small arterioles supplying that region of the lung. Local blood flow is profoundly reduced. As a result, blood flow is diverted to areas of higher ventilation and higher alveolar PO_2.

West zones

Zone 1 – Can be seen in low arterial pressure (shock) and high alveolar pressure (PEEP ventilation) = areas that are ventilated but not perfused = increasing the physiological dead space.

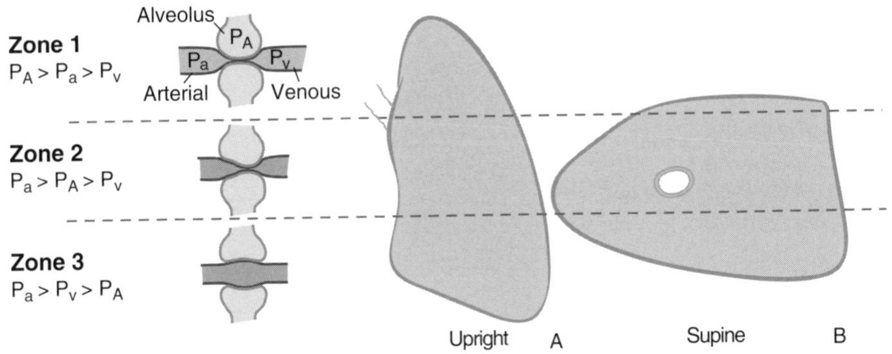

Figure 84.2 West zones. From: Vacanti et al., 2011, p. 256.

Zone 1
$P_A > P_a > P_v$

Alveolus
P_A
P_a P_v
Arterial   Venous

Zone 2
$P_a > P_A > P_v$

Zone 3
$P_a > P_v > P_A$

Upright   A

Supine   B

Table 84.2 Causes of decreased PaO_2

Normal A–a O_2 gradient	Increased A–a O_2 gradient
Low FiO_2 Low alveolar ventilation	Increased shunt Increased V/Q mismatch Diffusion abnormality

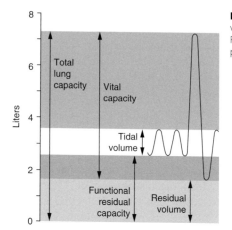

Figure 84.3 Lung volumes and capacities. From: Vacanti et al., 2011, pp. 528–529.

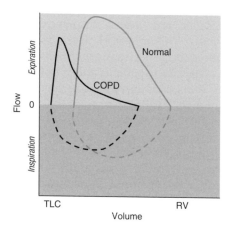

Figure 84.4 Flow volume loops normal COPD. From: Vacanti et al., 2011, pp. 528–529.

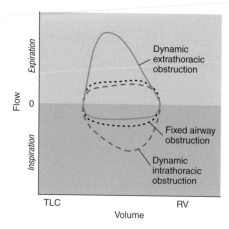

Figure 84.5 Flow volume loops airway obstruction. From: Vacanti et al., 2011, pp. 528–529.

Pulmonary function test

FRC = volume of gas in the lungs after normal expiration = residual volume + expiratory reserve volume.

Normal FEV1 = 80% of VC (effort dependent).

Restrictive lung disease = ↓ FEV1, ↓ FVC, normal FEV1/FVC.

Obstructive lung disease = ↓ FEV1, normal or somewhat ↓ FVC, ↓ FEV1/FVC.

↓ DLCO = seen in pulmonary fibrosis and sarcoidosis.

Extrathoracic obstructions have a greater effect on inspiratory flow, while intrathoracic obstructions have a greater effect on expiratory flow, as shown in the idealized figure. However, unlike what is shown in Figure 84.5, almost all obstructions affect both inspiration and expiration.

Questions

1. Which of the following results is least likely in a patient with massive ascites?
   a. normal FRC
   b. low FEV1
   c. low FVC
   d. normal FEV1/FVC

2. Which of the following is associated with an increase in FRC?
   a. COPD
   b. exercise
   c. older age
   d. PEEP or CPAP
   e. all of the above

Answers

1. a. Recall that the "chest wall" = thorax + diaphragm + abdomen. Massive ascites increases the volume of and pressure within the abdomen, this results in increased elastic recoil of the chest wall, a caudad shift in the position of the diaphragm, and so decreased resting lung volume.

2. e. Exercise leads to increased tidal volume as well as higher respiratory rate, which may not allow for sufficient lung emptying, leading to hyperinflation.

Further reading

Vacanti, C. A., Sikka, P. K., Urman, R. U., Dershwitz, M., and Segal, B. S. (2011). *Essential Clinical Anesthesia*, 1st edn. Cambridge University Press, Chapter 85.

Kodali, B. S. (2013) Capnography: an educational website dedicated to patient safety, 7th edn. www.capnography.com.

Nurok, M. and Topulos, G. P. (2012). Chapter 2. Respiratory physiology. In Hartigan, P. M. (ed) *Practical Handbook of Thoracic Anesthesia*. New York: Springer, pp. 17–39.

Chapter

85

Oxygen and carbon dioxide transport

Hanjo Ko and George P. Topulos

Keywords

Oxygen–hemoglobin dissociation curve
Bohr effect
Haldane effect
Mixed venous saturation
Oxygen toxicity
Hamburger shift

Oxygen–hemoglobin dissociation curve

Cooperative binding refers to the fact that with the binding of each successive oxygen molecule, hemoglobin's affinity for oxygen increases. The P50, the partial pressure at which hemoglobin is 50% saturated, is 26.5 mm Hg for adult Hb and 19 mm Hg for fetal Hb. At high atitudes, more 2,3-DPG is produced over hours to days, to increase Hb affinity for O_2, and compensate for lower PiO_2.

Bohr effect: ↑ $[H^+]$ or ↑ $PaCO_2$ decreases Hb affinity for O_2, shifts the dissociation curve to the R, thus facilitating delivery of oxygen to peripheral tissues.

Haldane effect: binding of oxygen to Hb decreases its affinity for CO_2.

Both the Bohr and Haldane effects work by changing the conformation of hemoglobin molecules. The effects work in opposite directions in the lungs and peripheral tissues, enhancing transport of both O_2 and CO_2.

Blood O_2 content, cc O_2, ml O_2/100 ml blood =

cc O_2 = (1.39 × hemoglobin × O_2 saturation) + (0.03 × PO_2).

At rest, normal oxygen extraction ratio = 25%. When arterial oxygen content decreases, or metabolic demand increases (e.g., exercise), oxygen extraction ratio and cardiac output (CO) initially increase to make up the difference.

O_2 consumption = CO × (arterial O_2 content – mixed venous O_2 content)

or,

Mixed venous O_2 content = arterial O_2 content – (O_2 consumption/CO)

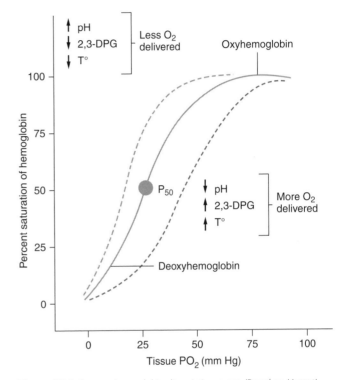

Figure 85.1 Oxygen–hemoglobin dissociation curve. (Based on Vacanti et al. 2011. *Essential Clinical Anesthesia*, Cambridge University Press, Figure 86.1.)

Despite how the Fick equation is normally written (upper), under normal circumstances, O_2 consumption is an independent variable set by the metabolic rate, and mixed venous O_2 content is the dependent variable (result). However, when oxygen supply (CO × arterial O_2 content) decreases below a critical threshold, it becomes impossible to compensate with higher extraction, and anaerobic metabolism begins. This leads to lactate accumulation and an O_2 debt. In critically ill patients, but not in normal, an increase in oxygen supply may lead to an increase in oxygen consumption; this response to supranormal oxygen supply, reflects the oxygen debt.

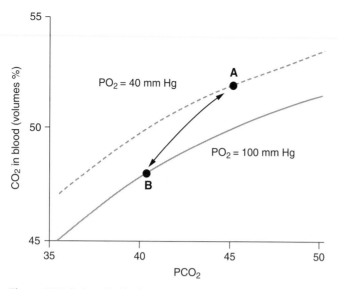

Figure 85.2 Carbon dioxide dissociation curve and the Haldane effect (shift from A to B). (Based on Vacanti et al. 2011. *Essential Clinical Anesthesia*, Cambridge University Press, p. 534.)

Mixed venous saturation = oxygen saturation measured in the pulmonary artery where all three sources of venous return (superior vena cava, inferior vena cava, coronary sinus) are completely mixed. Since it is a whole body average, normal mixed venous O_2 does not assure all tissues are well oxygenated. As can be seen from the equations just above, four factors determine mixed venous content, and so saturation:

- cardiac output
- hemoglobin concentration
- arterial O_2 content
- O_2 consumption

Oxygen toxicity

1. Pulmonary: airway inflammation and reduced vital capacity are seen after high PiO_2 for 24 hours. PaO_2 of 255 mm Hg has been established as safe. On the other hand, there is evidence of improved outcomes regarding wound infection with higher inspired oxygen.
2. Retrolental fibroplasia in newborns.
3. CNS: very high PiO_2 (>2 ATA), seen only under hyperbaric conditions, may cause seizures.

While not a toxic effect, absorption atelectasis increases as the FiO_2 increases.

Hamburger shift or chloride shift: as bicarbonate generated within red blood cells leaves the cells, chloride ions from the extracellular space are pumped in to prevent intracellular alkalosis and maintain electrical neutrality.

Questions

1. Which of the following statements regarding carbon monoxide poisoning is FALSE?
   a. Treatments for carbon monoxide poisoning include 100% oxygen and hyperbaric oxygen until patient is asymptomatic (usually with COHb <10%).
   b. Clinical features of CO poisoning include headache, myocardial ischemia, nausea/vomiting, and fetal distress in pregnant patients.
   c. COHb levels are commonly used to determine the need for treatment.
   d. CO binds to hemoglobin at same site as oxygen with 200 times greater affinity.
   e. CO shifts the oxygen–hemoglobin dissociation curve to the left.

2. Which of the following statements regarding methemoglobinemia is FALSE?
   a. Methemoglobinemia happens when the iron moiety in the hemoglobin molecule is converted from its reduced state (Fe^{2+}) to its oxidized state (Fe^{3+}).
   b. Methemoglobinemia can be due to administration of nitrates, nitrites, prilocaine, benzocaine, or sulfonamides.
   c. Treatment consists mainly of administration of methylene blue, but hyperbaric oxygen and exchange transfusion can also be utilized.
   d. Methemoglobinemia shifts the oxygen-hemoglobin dissociation curve to the right.

3. Which of the following conditions leads to an increased amount of 2,3-DPG?
   a. high altitude
   b. chronic lung disease
   c. congestive heart failure
   d. sickle cell disease
   e. all of the above

Answers

1. c. Unfortunately COHb concentrations correlate poorly with clinical status. Normal individuals have up to 3% COHb, and smokers up to 9%.
2. d. The oxidized hemes of methemoglobinemia are unable to bind to oxygen so the oxygen-hemoglobin dissociation curve is shifted to the left.
3. e. The production of 2,3-DPG is increased in hypoxemia, chronic lung disease, anemia, sickle cell disease, and high altitude as an adaptive mechanism to compensate for diminished peripheral tissue oxygen availability.

Further reading

Vacanti, C. A., Sikka, P. K., Urman, R. U., Dershwitz, M., and Segal, B. S. (2011). *Essential Clinical Anesthesia*, 1st edn. Cambridge University Press, Chapter 86.

Kodali, B. S. (2013). Capnography: an educational website dedicated to patient safety, 7th edn. www.capnography.com.

Hsia, C. C. (1998). Respiratory function of hemoglobin. *New England Journal of Medicine* 338, 239–247.

86

Lung isolation techniques

Yuka Kiyota, Philip M. Hartigan, and George P. Topulos

Keywords

Indications for lung isolation
Tracheobronchial anatomy
Double-lumen tubes (DLT)
Bronchial blockers
One-lung physiology
Hypoxic pulmonary vasoconstriction (HPV)

The *indications for lung isolation* are divided into absolute and relative indications. There is no absolute contraindication.

A basic understanding of the normal *tracheobronchial anatomy* is essential for successful lung isolation.

- The average distance from the teeth to the carina: 20–25 cm.
- The left mainstem bronchus branches from the carina at a 45° angle.
- The left mainstem bronchus is 5.4 cm long in men and 5 cm in women.
- The right mainstem bronchus branches from the carina at a 10° angle.
- The right mainstem bronchus is 1.9 cm in men and 1.6 cm in women.

The right upper lobe bronchus usually trifurcates almost immediately, creating what is often referred to as the "Mercedes-Benz" sign.

Double-lumen tube (DLT)

The *DLT* is the most common tool for lung isolation. It has tracheal and bronchial lumens, each with inflatable cuffs to provide a seal. Typical DLT sizes for pediatric patients are 26F and 28F, and for adult patients are 35F, 37F, 39F, and 41F.

Proper size selection of the DLT is important to provide good lung isolation while causing minimal trauma to the airway. Below is a rough guide for initial size selection based on patient sex and height.

Because of the short right mainstem bronchus, it is easy to unintentionally obstruct the opening of the right upper lobe, thus the left-sided DLT is easier to place than the right-sided

Table 86.1 Indications for OLV

Absolute:
Isolation of lungs to prevent spillage from hemorrhage or infection
Therapeutic need to ventilate only one lung
    Bronchopleural fistula
    Unilateral cysts or bullae
    Unilateral bronchial disruption or trauma
Unilateral lung lavage
Video-assisted thoracoscopic surgery (VATS)

Relative:
Surgical exposure: high priority
    Thoracic aortic aneurysm
    Pneumonectomy
    Upper lobectomy
Surgical exposure: lower priority
Esophageal surgery
Middle or lower lobectomies
Thoracoscopy under general anesthesia

Table 86.2 Rough DLT sizing guide based on patient height

DLT size	35F	37F	39F	41F
Female	≤5 ft 1 inch	5 ft 2 inches–5 ft 11 inches	≥6 ft	–
Male	–	≤5 ft 5 inches	5 ft 6 inches–5 ft 11 inches	≥6 ft

DLT. The indications for the right-sided DLT are operations that involve left main bronchus (e.g., left single lung transplant, left pneumonectomy, left main bronchus sleevectomy), or when pathology of the left mainstem precludes a left DLT. Advantages of *DLT* compared to *bronchial blockers*:

- large internal diameter, lower resistance, and possibly faster deflation of the lung
- easier passage of suction catheter
- ability to pass a pediatric fiberoptic bronchoscope

Essential Clinical Anesthesia Review: Keywords, Questions and Answers for the Boards, ed. Linda S. Aglio, Robert W. Lekowski, and Richard D. Urman. Published by Cambridge University Press. © Cambridge University Press 2015.

Disadvantages of *DLT*:

- need for the tube exchange
- potential for airway trauma due to its large diameter and stiffness
- more difficult to intubate patients with difficult airways due to DLT size and stiffness

Bronchial blockers

- A small diameter catheter with an inflatable occlusive balloon at its distal end.
- Advantages:
  - tube exchange is not needed
  - comes in a variety of sizes, allowing it to be used for size 4.5 ETT
  - can be used for patients with difficult airway or for pediatric patients
  - can be used for primary lung isolation or rescue device for inadequately functioning DLT
  - can be used to isolate individual lobes.
- Disadvantages:
  - possibly slower lung collapse
  - lumen inadequate for suctioning (but can be used for CPAP)
  - potential displacement into trachea, particularly when used on right.
- Stand-alone bronchial blockers (*BB*):
  - Arndt Wire Guided BB (Cook Inc.), Cohen BB (Cook Inc.) has tip control, EZ Blocker (Teleflex) Y-Tipped double BB:
    - all are analogous, but with different steering mechanisms; all require bronchoscopy for placement
    - all come with a multiport connector to fit onto the 15 mm connector of the ETT
    - Arndt BB comes in 5F, 7F, and 9F, for use with minimum ETT size of 4.5
    - the Arndt wire is removable, which leaves 1.4 mm lumen that can be used for CPAP or limited suctioning
  - Fogarty catheter:
    - made from latex
    - no central lumen to provide CPAP or suctioning
    - easy to place. Central wire stylet can be bent 45 degrees at tip, and directed, under fiberoptic observation, to target bronchus by rotating and advancing
    - spherical cuff, not low pressure/high volume.
- *Bronchial blocker* bound to an SLT:
  - univent:
    - an SLT with a separate channel fused along the anterior concave surface that houses a sliding bronchial blocker

- the blocker can be guided into the right, left, or secondary bronchi with the aid of a fiberoptic bronchoscope
- outer diameter is markedly larger than standard ETT with same internal diameter.

One-lung physiology

Lateral decubitus position is the standard position for pulmonary resection.

Perfusion is directly influenced by gravity but it is not altered by the induction of anesthesia or paralysis.

Ventilation depends on whether the patient is awake, anesthetized, paralyzed, or has an open chest.

The $\dot{V}_A/\dot{Q}$ ratio is preserved close to baseline in an awake spontaneously breathing subject in the lateral position, as gravity increases both ventilation and perfusion to the dependent lung.

$\dot{V}_A/\dot{Q}$ mismatch is increased in a spontaneously breathing, laterally positioned, anesthetized patient due to the decreased functional residual capacity (FRC), making the dependent lung less compliant, and the nondependent lung more compliant. Gas exchange is further worsened because gravity increases perfusion to the dependent lung.

$\dot{V}_A/\dot{Q}$ mismatch is further increased in a paralyzed (mechanically ventilated), laterally positioned, anesthetized patient because the weight of the abdominal contents, mediastinum, and chest wall further restricts the dependent lung, functionally decreasing its compliance and shifting ventilation to the nondependent lung.

The situation is further worsened when the chest is opened by additional compression of the dependent lung, and elimination of confinement of the nondependent lung.

Isolation of the operative lung, so it is not ventilated, causes a large right-to-left intrapulmonary shunt in the unventilated lung, resulting in a widening of alveolar–arterial oxygen gradient. Normally this would result in hypoxemia. However, the use of an FiO_2 of 1.0 prevents the hypoxemia in about 90% of patients. In addition, both gravity and *HPV* decrease the shunt by redirecting more of the pulmonary blood flow to the dependent ventilated lung. However, the restrictive physiology of the dependent lung makes that lung prone to atelectasis (and shunt).

Hypoxic pulmonary vasoconstriction (HPV) diminishes blood flow to areas of the lung where the alveolar PO_2 is low:

- accomplished via pulmonary arteriolar vasoconstriction
- decreases the shunt fraction by as much as 50%
- primary trigger is low alveolar PO_2
- secondary trigger is low mixed venous PO_2
- mechanism incompletely understood
- a rapid, exquisitely local phenomenon
- an intrinsic property of pulmonary arterial vascular smooth muscle
- independent of autonomic nervous system, endothelium, or known secondary messengers

Factors that directly affect HPV

Alkalosis globally inhibits HPV, and acidosis (hypercarbia) globally accentuates it.

Vasodilating agents such as nitroglycerin, nitroprusside, dobutamine, calcium channel blockers, and hydralazine can inhibit HPV.

Factors that indirectly affect HPV

Elevated pulmonary artery pressure or flow in the non-ventilated lung from any cause may diminish the effectiveness of HPV, such as: increased airway pressures in the dependent lung, hypoxia in the ventilated (dependent) lung, or preexisting pulmonary hypertension.

Inhalational anesthetics inhibit HPV directly in a dose-dependent manner, but within clinically relevant dosages (<1.5 MAC), their indirect effects through cardiac output and mixed venous oxygen tension result in no significant net effect on one-lung oxygenation.

Questions

1. All are FALSE statements except for which?
   a. A Fogarty catheter, used as a bronchial blocker, can provide CPAP to the distal airway.
   b. A Mac blade is preferred for the placement of DLT.
   c. DLT allows the use of an adult bronchoscope.
   d. A univent tube and a standard ETT with equal internal diameters will also have comparable external diameters.

2. Which is the correct statement?
   a. In a patient who is spontaneously breathing, laterally positioned, with a closed chest, $\dot{V}_A/\dot{Q}$ mismatch is largely increased.
   b. Vasodilating agents such as nitroglycerin can increase HPV.
   c. Patients with chronic pulmonary hypertension have more effective HPV.
   d. Hypoxia in the ventilated (dependent) lung may diminish the effects of HPV in the nondependent lung.

Answers

1. b. A Fogarty catheter lacks a central lumen, therefore is unable to provide CPAP or suction. The DLT does not accommodate an adult bronchoscopy. The univent has a larger external diameter than a standard ETT with the same internal diameter.

2. d The $\dot{V}_A/\dot{Q}$ ratio is preserved relatively close to one in a spontaneously breathing, laterally positioned patient with a closed chest.

Further reading

Vacanti, C. A., Sikka, P. K., Urman, R. U., Dershwitz, M., and Segal, B. S. (2011). *Essential Clinical Anesthesia*, 1st edn. Cambridge University Press.

Chapter 87. Lung isolation techniques.

Hartigan, P. M. (ed.) (2011). *Practical Handbook of Thoracic Anesthesia*. Springer, Chapter 5.

Kodali, B. S. (2013). Capnography, an educational website dedicated to patient safety, 7th edn. www.capnography.com.

Chapter

87

Anesthetic management for pulmonary resection

Yuka Kiyota, George P. Topulos, and Philip M. Hartigan

Keywords

ppoFEV$_1$ (predicted postoperative forced expiratory
volume in 1 second)
Postoperative pulmonary complications
Thoracic epidural anesthesia (TEA)
Bronchospasm
Air trapping (auto-PEEP)
One-lung ventilation (OLV)
Hypoxic pulmonary vasoconstriction
Ventilator-induced lung injury (VILI)
Post-pneumonectomy pulmonary edema (PPPE)
High-risk criteria for pneumonectomy
Cardiac herniation
Right-to-left intracardiac shunt

Preoperative evaluation for pulmonary resection needs to
clarify the surgical plan (extent of incision), the maximum
tolerable extent of resection (based on respiratory mechanics,
cardiopulmonary reserve, and lung parenchymal function),
and the plan for lung isolation and postoperative pain
control.

Predicted postoperative forced expiratory volume in 1 second
(ppoFEV$_1$) is used to estimate the impact of resection on
pulmonary mechanics.

ppoFEV$_1$ = preoperative FEV$_1$ [1 − (% functional lung
tissue to be removed)/100]

This can be roughly estimated by proportionally adjusting
FEV$_1$ based on the number of subsegments to be removed,
or more accurately calculated by the formula above using
information obtained from ventilation–perfusion scans. The
lower limit of acceptable ppoFEV$_1$ is controversial. ppoFEV$_1$
<0.8 l or <40% predicted are widely quoted as thresholds for
increased risk for postoperative respiratory failure.

Lung parenchymal function is grossly assessed by diffusing
capacity of lung for carbon monoxide (DLCO) or arterial
blood gas values. Cardiopulmonary reserve is estimated from
tests for maximum oxygen consumption (MVO$_2$), exercise
tolerance, or exercise desaturation tests.

Postoperative pulmonary complications include respiratory
failure, pulmonary edema, acute lung injury, atelectasis,
infection, aspiration, bronchospasm, mucous plugging, upper
airway obstruction, air leak, pneumothorax, bronchopleural
fistula, etc. Preoperative pain control strategies may help prevent many postoperative pulmonary complications by facilitating early extubation and deep breathing, effective coughing,
and early ambulation, while limiting respiratory depression,
sedation, and delirium. Narcotic-sparing pain control strategies such as thoracic epidural analgesia are particularly
important to this.

Thoracic epidural anesthesia (TEA) is the most widely used
means of controlling postthoracotomy pain. Compared with
parenteral opiates, TEA is superior for control of the dynamic
pain associated with deep breathing and coughing, and for the
preservation of lung function as measured by incentive spirometry. TEA reduces perioperative pulmonary complications
following thoracotomy compared to parenteral opiates.

Induction considerations: four issues related to induction
of thoracic patients deserve special considerations.
Bronchospasm:

- Bronchospasm is narrowing of small airways due to
  constriction of bronchiolar smooth muscle, resulting in
  airway obstruction, air trapping, increased work of
  breathing and expiratory wheezing.
- Airway hyperreactivity is common among pulmonary
  resection patients due to the high prevalence of smoking,
  COPD, and infection/inflammation.
- Preoperative bronchodilator treatment may be of benefit.
- Adequate depth of anesthesia at the time of airway
  instrumentation is the best preventive measure.
- Recent URI and COPD exacerbations should ideally be
  under control two weeks prior to the surgery.

Air trapping (auto-PEEP):

- Defined as incomplete expiration to relaxation volume
  before beginning of next inspiration.
- Synonymous with "auto-PEEP" and "intrinsic PEEP," and
  results in dynamic hyperinflation over time.

Essential Clinical Anesthesia Review: Keywords, Questions and Answers for the Boards, ed. Linda S. Aglio, Robert W. Lekowski, and Richard
D. Urman. Published by Cambridge University Press. © Cambridge University Press 2015.

- In extreme cases, may cause volutrauma, tension pneumothorax, and cardiac arrest.
- Patients with severe COPD (FEV_1 <40%) are particularly prone.
- Best minimized by setting long expiratory times (low I:E ratio and avoiding fast respiratory rates).

Mass-effect on cardiac output (see keyword *anterior mediastinal mass*):

- Thoracic tumors or effusions reduce cardiac output by decreasing the gradient for venous return to the thorax and heart, or by direct compression.
- Reclining to the supine position, induction of general anesthesia, and initiation of positive pressure ventilation may exacerbate these effects.
- Postural symptoms, echocardiographic data, and CT evidence of a mass effect on heart or great vessels are the principal tools for identification of high-risk patients.
- Compression of SVC mandates IV placement in the lower extremity.

Mass effect on airway patency (see keyword *anterior mediastinal mass*):

- The FRC reduction imposed by the supine position and induction of anesthesia leads to a reduction in the caliber of major airways.
- In addition, the supine position exacerbates airway compression directly as the vector of gravitational force becomes more perpendicular to the airway.
- Physiology is that of variable central airway obstruction.
- Management principles for high-risk patients include awake fiberoptic assessment, possibly stenting the stenotic portion with a tube prior to induction, and positive pressure ventilation.

Intraoperative considerations include lung isolation decisions, *one-lung ventilation* (OLV), positioning, choice of anesthetics, and recruitment of the operative lung prior to chest closure. Only OLV will be discussed here. The reader is referred to the references for the other topics.

One-lung ventilation requires lung isolation by use of a double-lumen tube (left or right), bronchial blocker, or by endobronchial intubation.

One-lung ventilator settings should be tailored to the individual's physiology. Typical recommendations are:

- tidal volumes of 5 to 6 ml/kg ideal body weight to avoid ventilator-induced lung injury
- PEEP (5 cm H_2O +/−) to discourage dependent lung atelectasis and atelectrauma
- respiratory rate and I:E adjusted to roughly target normocapnea (or mild permissive hypercapnia)
- FiO_2 initially at 1.0 – then weaned to target SpO_2 >90%
- recruitment maneuvers intermittently to the dependent lung

Table 87.1 Treatment of hypoxemia during OLV

Confirm $FiO_2 = 1.0$
Bronchoscopy to rule out obstruction/malposition
Temporary reinflation of operative lung
Recruitment maneuver to nonoperative lung
CPAP to operative lung
PEEP to nonoperative lung
Cross-clamp of pulmonary artery, or branch thereof

(From Vacanti et al., Table 88.4.)

Patients with obstructive pulmonary disease will likely have auto-PEEP, making extrinsic (machine) PEEP unnecessary. Patients with pulmonary hypertension or right heart dysfunction should receive higher FiO_2 and more aggressive ventilation to prevent hypercapnia. Those with restrictive physiology may require higher ventilatory pressures and PEEP levels, and higher I:E ratios.

Hypoxemia (SpO_2 <90%) is unusual during OLV, barring a misplaced double-lumen tube or blocker, excessive secretions, or severe pathophysiology. Assuming none of the above and delivery of 100% oxygen to the dependent lung, hypoxemia during OLV is due to excessive shunt in the dependent and/or the nondependent lung. Therapy for the latter is CPAP, if tolerated by the surgeons. Therapy for dependent lung shunt consists of recruitment maneuvers, PEEP, and bronchoscopy to rule out obstruction. Excessive PEEP will redirect blood to the nondependent lung and increase total shunt. In severe abrupt desaturation, the patient should be stabilized by recruiting the operative lung prior to further diagnostics. If cross-clamp of the pulmonary artery by surgeons is imminent, this will reliably reduce nondependent lung shunt.

Hypoxic pulmonary vasoconstriction (HPV)

- Constriction of small (<200 micron) pulmonary arterioles in response to low alveolar oxygen tension, or (secondarily) low mixed venous oxygen tension.
- Physiologic mechanism to reduce intrapulmonary shunting and improve V/Q matching.
- Exquisitely local and rapid response of pulmonary vascular smooth muscle.
- Independent of autonomic innervation or endothelial messengers.
- Mechanism incompletely understood.
- During OLV, gravity plus HPV reduce the nondependent lung blood flow from 45–55% to approximately 22% of cardiac output (on average).
- HPV is inhibited by most vasodilators.
- Inhaled anesthetics inhibit HPV dose dependently in vitro, but do not cause hypoxemia during OLV in clinically relevant doses.
- TIVA agents (propofol, remifentanil, dexmedetomidine) do not inhibit HPV.

Ventilator-induced lung injury (VILI)

- Results from excessive overdistention (volutrauma) and/or from the shear stresses of repeated collapse and reexpansion of lung units (atelectotrauma).
- During OLV, VILI to the dependent lung may result in acute lung injury.
- The dependent lung is especially vulnerable to VILI because of the contralateral open pneumothorax, resulting in propensity for overinflation due to air trapping during surgery.
- Protective ventilatory strategies (5–6 ml/kg plus PEEP) have been adopted for OLV in effort to minimize this risk.

Post-pneumonectomy pulmonary edema (PPPE)

- Historical term for idiopathic pulmonary edema/acute lung injury following lung resection.
- Occurs in 2% to 4% of pneumonectomies; less common following lesser resections.
- Diagnosis of exclusion.
- High mortality following pneumonectomy (50%).
- More common following right pneumonectomy.
- Impaired lymphatic drainage and inflammatory response are contributing causes.
- Associated with more positive fluid balance.
- May be associated with higher ventilatory pressures/volumes during OLV.

High-risk criteria for pneumonectomy

- $PaCO_2$ >45 mm Hg (room air)
- PaO_2 <50 mm Hg (room air)
- FEV_1 <2 l
- $ppoFEV_1$ <0.8 l (or <40% predicted)
- FEV_1/FVC <50% predicted
- max. breathing capacity <50% predicted
- max. O_2 consumption <10 ml/kg/min
- exercise desaturation >4%
- stair climb < two flights with dyspnea
- ppoDLCO <40% predicted
- pulmonary hypertension or decreased right heart function

Cardiac herniation

- Displacement of heart into empty hemithorax following pneumonectomy.
- Can cause abrupt cardiovascular collapse from torsion of great vessels.
- More likely following right pneumonectomy with a pericardial defect that was inadequately reconstructed.
- Most often happens at resumption of the supine position.

- Returning the patient to the lateral position usually restores the circulation. If not, drugs and CPR are ineffective with the heart displaced into the empty hemithorax. Must emergently reopen thoracotomy and perform open-chest cardiac massage.

Right-to-left intracardiac shunt

- Normal = 0.3% of cardiac output from Thebesian veins.
- Pathologic shunts may occur from septal or congenital structural defects.
- Rarely, following pneumonectomy, mediastinal shift with cardiac rotation directs inferior vena caval flow toward the foramen ovale resulting in right-to-left intracardiac shunt. The resulting desaturation is termed platypnea orthodeoxia.

Questions

1. Which statement is INCORRECT?
   a. In clinically relevant dosages, volatile agents have minimal effect on oxygenation during OLV.
   b. If $ppoFEV_1$ <40%, patients are at high risk for postoperative respiratory failure.
   c. Treatment of hypoxia during OLV includes applying PEEP to the operative lung and CPAP to the nonoperative lung.
   d. Platypnea orthodeoxia is a relatively uncommon syndrome and defined as dyspnea and deoxygenation accompanying a change from a recumbent to an upright position.

2. A patient with severe COPD is scheduled for left upper lobectomy. One-lung ventilation was just establibed and the patient's oxygen saturation suddenly drops to 75% from 98% with FiO_2 of 100%. What is the appropriate next step?
   a. apply CPAP of 5 cm H_2O to the nondependent (operative) lung
   b. increase the tidal volume to 15 cc/kg
   c. resume two-lung ventilation
   d. ask the surgeon to ligate the left pulmonary artery

Answers

1. c. In the event of hypoxia during OLV, applying CPAP to the operative lung (nondependent lung) attempts to direct the blood flow away from the operative lung to the nonoperative lung (dependent lung), and applying PEEP to the nonoperative lung (dependent lung) would recruit collapsed alveoli.
2. c. Severe hypoxia during one-lung ventilation mandates resuming two-lung ventilation as an appropriate next step. PEEP is unlikely to help because auto-PEEP is likely present in excess of ideal (due to COPD).

Further reading

Wiser, S. H. and Hartigan, P. M. (2011). Chapter 88. Anesthetic management for pulmonary resection. In Vacanti, C. A., Sikka, P. J., Urman, R. D., Dershwitz, M., and Segal, B. S. (eds) *Essential Clinical Anesthesia*. New York: Cambridge University Press.

Hartigan, P. M. (2012). Chapter 16. Principles of anesthetic management for pulmonary resection. In Hartigan, P. M. (ed) *Practical Handbook of Thoracic Anesthesia*. New York: Springer.

Slinger, P. and Darling, G. (2011). Chapter 2. Preanesthetic assessment for thoracic surgery. In Slinger, P. (ed) *Principles and Practice of Anesthesia for Thoracic Surgery*. New York: Springer.

88 Lung transplantation for end-stage lung disease

Stephanie Yacoubian and Ju-Mei Ng

Keywords

Lung transplantation: types performed in the United States
Lung allocation score system
Pulmonary fibrosis: indications to qualify for a transplant
Chronic obstructive pulmonary disease (COPD): indications to qualify for a transplant
Cystic fibrosis: indications to qualify for a transplant
Bronchiectasis: indications to qualify for a transplant
Pulmonary hypertension (primary or secondary): indications to qualify for a transplant
Connective tissue disorders: indications to qualify for a transplant
Lung transplantation: contraindications
Single lung transplantation (SLT): common indications
Bilateral sequential lung transplantation (BSLT): common indications
Heart–lung transplantation: common indications
Pediatric transplantation: major indications
Living donor lung transplantation: indications
Donor lung: procurement
Lung preservation
Ischemic time
Ex vivo lung preservation
Anesthesia monitors for lung transplantation: essential and additional
Test clamp: PA
Lung-protective ventilator settings
Sequence of anastomosis
Pulmonary edema: transplanted lungs
Indications for CPB
Pulmonary hypertension: treatment (systemic, inhaled)
Inhaled prostaglandin: PGI_2 (iloprost)
Inhaled NO
Transesophageal echocardiography: lung transplantation
Pulmonary venous obstruction
Primary graft dysfunction (PGD)

Lung transplantation: types performed in the United States

Patients with end-stage lung disease, who are failing optimal and maximal medical therapy, get referred for transplant evaluation when:

1. The predicted two- to three-year survival is less than 50%.
2. The New York Heart Association (NYHA) level of function reaches class III or IV.

Lungs are allocated through government-sponsored organizations. All candidates are listed and assigned a *lung allocation score* from 0 to 100, relating to the extent and progress of disease and likelihood of survival after a transplant. The score is updated every six months and reflects the patient's cardiopulmonary disease progress, functional status, laboratory values, oxygen dependence, and comorbidities.

The specific type of operation is performed based on institutional preferences and recipient factors:

- single lung transplantation (SLT)
- bilateral sequential lung transplantation (BSLT): with or without cardiopulmonary bypass (CPB)
- heart–lung transplantation
- living donor transplantation (one lobe from each donor, ×2)
- pediatric lung transplantation

Pretransplant work-up

Evaluate underlying lung pathology, comorbidities, ability to tolerate and to comply with long-term immunosuppressive therapy.

Patients with stable coronary artery disease with or without stents or angioplasty may still qualify. A proposed plan for antiplatelet therapy is essential in patients presenting with stents deployed within the last year.

- Work-up includes:
- chest radiographs
- chest CT scans

Essential Clinical Anesthesia Review: Keywords, Questions and Answers for the Boards, ed. Linda S. Aglio, Robert W. Lekowski, and Richard D. Urman. Published by Cambridge University Press. © Cambridge University Press 2015.

- spirometry
- V/Q scans
- serologic tests (ABG, electrolyte panels, liver function tests, CBC, coagulation profile, ABO blood type, viral serology (CMV, HIV))
- cardiovascular evaluation (EKG, echocardiography, cardiac catheterization)

Pulmonary disease related specific indications

Pulmonary fibrosis: indications to qualify for a transplant

- diffusing capacity of lung for carbon monoxide (DLCO) <39%
- decrease in pulse oximeter saturation to <88% (6-min walk test)
- honeycombing (high resolution CT)

Chronic obstructive pulmonary disease (COPD): indications to qualify for a transplant

- recurrent acute exacerbations with hypercapnia, PCO_2 >50 mm Hg
- pulmonary hypertension
- cor pulmonale
- forced expiratory volume in the first second of expiration (FEV_1) <20% predicted

Cystic fibrosis: indications to qualify for a transplant

- frequent exacerbations requiring antibiotic therapy
- exacerbations with hospital and intensive care unit admissions
- FEV_1 <30%, or a rapid decline
- recurrent hemoptysis

Bronchiectasis: indications to qualify for a transplant

- pulmonary hypertension
- recurrent infections
- recurrent hemoptysis

Pulmonary hypertension (primary or secondary): indications to qualify for a transplant

- New York Heart Association class III or IV despite maximal medical therapy
- cardiac index (CI) <2
- no improvement with intravenous pulmonary vasodilators

Connective tissue disorders (sarcoidosis, eosinophilic granuloma, lymphangioleiomyomatosis): indications to qualify for a transplant

- hypoxia
- poor functional status
- severe impairment of lung function

Lung transplantation: contraindications

Major contraindications

- malignancy
- advanced dysfunction of other organ systems
- incurable chronic systemic infection (e.g., HIV, HCV)
- psychiatric conditions that would hinder the patient's compliance with posttransplant medical therapy

Relative contraindications

- age >65 years (no hard upper limit set)
- critical unstable conditions
- colonization with highly virulent organism
- mechanical ventilation or ECMO (extracorporeal membrane oxygenation)
- severe chest wall deformity or pleural disease

SLT: common indications (%)

- chronic obstructive pulmonary disease (COPD) (50)
- idiopathic pulmonary fibrosis (28)
- alpha 1-Antitrypsin deficiency (7)
- cystic fibrosis (2)
- retransplant (2)
- primary pulmonary hypertension (1)
- other indications (10)
- SLT is performed with one-lung ventilation with CPB on standby.
- CPB used in case of hemodynamic instability, hypoxia, or hypercarbia.

BSLT: common indications (%)

- cystic fibrosis (28)
- COPD (24)
- idiopathic pulmonary fibrosis (14)
- alpha 1-antitrypsin deficiency (8)
- primary pulmonary hypertension (6)
- retransplant (2)
- other indications (18)
- mostly used for any infectious pathology (cystic fibrosis, bronchiectasis) that would result in contamination of the transplanted lung, e.g., when SLT performed
- Performed with or without CPB.
- BSLT offers higher long-term mortality and graft function compared to SLT.

Heart–lung transplantation: common indications

- pulmonary hypertension
- Eisenmenger's syndrome
- primary pulmonary hypertension with right ventricular (RV) dysfunction

- Operation performed under CPB.
- Single donor organs are transplanted en bloc.

Pediatric transplantation: major indications

- cystic fibrosis
- primary pulmonary hypertension
- bronchopulmonary dysplasia
- arteriovenous malformation
- hypoplastic lungs (congenital diaphragmatic hernia)
- Extracorporeal circulation used in this process.

Living donor lung transplantation: indications

Cystic fibrosis is the most common indication.

Requires two living donors: one lobe from each donor transplanted into recipient.

Donor lung: procurement

ABO compatibility and appropriate donor–recipient size match.

Donor lungs are procured from cadaveric brain-dead donors with preserved pulmonary function who have had:

1. Strict fluid management.
2. Normal bronchoscopy (no evidence of infection, pathology, or aspiration).
3. Normal chest X-ray.
4. Normal arterial blood gases.

Lung preservation

Allograft is cooled, flushed with pulmoplegic solution (+/– high-dose steroids, pulmonary vasodilators) and kept partially inflated with continuous positive airway pressure (CPAP).

Ischemic time

From time of organ harvest to reperfusion in the recipient. Recommended time is less than six hours.

As the ischemic time is shortened, the damage from reperfusion injury is likely to decrease.

Ex vivo lung preservation

Involves applying therapy to pretransplanted donor lungs (ex vivo) in order to optimize the organ's quality.

It is currently in active phase of research.

Anesthesia monitors for lung transplantation: essential and additional

Essential monitors:

- standard ASA monitors
- invasive arterial pressure (radial/femoral)
- central venous pressure (CVP)/pulmonary artery (PA) catheter

- Serial arterial blood gases (ABGs)

Additional monitors:

- transesophageal echocardiography (TEE)
- depth of anesthesia
- cerebral oximetry

Anesthetic considerations: pre induction

- Update history and note any recent antibiotics or culture results.
- Assess NPO status.
- Assess airway.
- Determine oxygen and steroid dependance.
- Be vigilant with sedation, light sedation with monitoring.
- Consider antacid prophylaxis.
- Consider bronchodilator therapy.
- Have a plan for turning off the IV prostaglandin.
- Large-bore IV.
- Arterial line.
- Consider thoracic epidural if CPB is very unlikely.

Anesthetic considerations: induction

- Communicate with procurement team to assess timing and confirm incision time.
- Careful induction.
- Intubate with single-lumen endotracheal tube.
- Bronchoscopy and pulmonary toilet.
- Double-lumen tube, usually a left double-lumen tube except during left single lung transplant.
- Double stick internal jugular vein with central venous and pulmonary artery catheter placed.
- Femoral lines (artery and vein in case of SLT, artery only in case of BSLT).
- Prophylactic antibiotics.
- Immunosuppression (high-dose steroid and antithyomocyte globulin).

Anesthetic considerations: pre-pneumonectomy

- Establish single-lung ventilation in setting of SLT.
- Anticipate hypoxia and hypercarbia, and manage accordingly.

Test clamp

This is done during single lung transplants and involves placement of a clamp on the PA by the surgeon prior to explantation. Hemodynamic profile pre- and post-test clamp needs to be monitored.

Indications for CPB:

- SaO_2 90% on FiO_2 of 1.0
- baseline PAP >40 mm Hg
- MPAP >50 mm Hg during test clamp
- CI < 2 l/min/m^2 or severe systemic hypotension

Anesthetic considerations: pneumonectomy

- Withdraw the PA catheter prior to stapling of the PA.
- Reposition the double-lumen tube if necessary.

Anesthetic considerations: anastomosis

- Close attention to EKG and ST changes.
- Consider using clean bronchoscopes.
- New lung ventilated gently with low FiO_2 (as tolerated) with peak pressures <25 cm H_2O and PEEP.

Reperfusion

Expect systemic hypotension secondary to:

- ischemia reperfusion and metabolic byproducts now circulating
- delayed filling of the LV
- humoral factors
- pulmoplegia washout

Lung-protective ventilator settings

Once implanted and the anastomoses are complete, the new lung is slowly reperfused and gently ventilated. Lung-protective strategies are used:

- tidal volume 4–6 ml/kg
- peak pressures <25 cm H_2O
- 5–15 cm H_2O PEEP
- suctioning of the transplanted lung

Sequence of anastomosis during lung transplantation

pneumonectomy of recipient lung
implantation of donor lung
anastomosis performed posterior to anterior

Bronchial anastomosis followed by pulmonary artery (PA) anastomosis, and anastomosis of a cuff of the left atrium, which contains the donor pulmonary veins (PV), to the recipient's left atrium.

Most tenuous is the bronchial anastomosis, as the central airway is supplied by a watershed blood supply. Proximal bronchial anastomoses tend to do better than more distal ones.

The circumflex coronary artery may be obstructed by clamps or retractors while the atrial (pulmonary veins) anastomosis is being performed. Rotational deformities may obstruct the pulmonary veins.

Pulmonary artery (PA) anastomosis may kink as the chest is closed, if the segment is too long.

Stenosis of the PA anastomosis is usually a delayed complication.

It is key to remember that the bronchial circulation, lymphatics, and nerves are not restored. Which makes the *post-transplant patient* more vulnerable to pulmonary edema.

Pulmonary edema: transplanted lungs

Early pulmonary edema

Obstructive atrial anastomosis presents with pulmonary edema similar to an early graft failure.

More delayed pulmonary edema

- >4 h after unclamping
- pulmonary edema secondary to cytokine-related endothelial injury
- lack of lymphatic drainage exacerbates this condition

Transplanted lungs are very prone to pulmonary edema due to the capillary leak that results from reperfusion injury to the microvasculature, and because of an impaired lymphatic drainage as the transplanted lungs do not have a lymphatic drainage system.

Indications for CPB

- high PA pressures
- RV dysfunction
- severely dilated PAs
- severe hypoxia, hypercarbia, and acidosis during one-lung ventilation (OLV)

Some centers use CPB for all BSLTs.
Advantages of CPB:

- hemodynamic stability
- less likelihood of hypoxia and hypercarbia
- less stress on RV
- better vascular control

Potential disadvantages of CPB:

- heparin-induced thrombocytopenia
- greater blood loss/more transfusions
- greater inflammatory response

Initiation CPB:

- ACTs >350 s
- cannulation sites (aorta or femoral artery, RA or femoral vein)
- warm CPB with a beating heart
- consider antifibrinolytics

An emerging alternative to CPB = ECMO.

Pulmonary hypertension and RV dysfunction: treatment

Pulmonary hypertension and RV dysfunction is exacerbated by: hypoxia, acidosis, hypercarbia, light anesthesia, hypothermia, and vasoconstricting drugs.
Systemic pulmonary vasodilators:

- nitroglycerin
- alprostadil
- sodium nitroprusside

Disadvantages:

- reversal of hypoxic pulmonary vasoconstriction
- hypotension

Supplement with inotropic therapy:

- dobutamine
- milrinone (also reduces PA pressures)
- epinephrine

Inhaled prostaglandin: PGI₂ (iloprost)

- reduces pulmonary pressures
- does not have systemic effects
- increases right ventricle (RV) performance

Inhaled nitric oxide (NO)

- NO (10–20 ppm)
- selective pulmonary vasodilator
- reduces pulmonary vascular resistance
- improves unloading of the right ventricle
- evidence of anti-inflammatory properties

Transesophageal echocardiography: lung transplantation

- Presently not considered an essential monitor.
- Excellent for assessing biventricular function and volume status.
- Can assess flow across the pulmonary venous anastomosis.

Pulmonary venous obstruction

Rare but fatal complication and cause of posttransplant graft failure

Primary graft dysfunction

- serious complication
- multifactorial
- alloantigen dependent: immune response to allograft
- alloantigen independent: non-immune mediated (e.g., mechanical trauma during surgery)
- ischemia reperfusion injury = pulmonary edema, hypoxia, alveolar damage

Treatment is supportive with mechanical ventilation, diuresis, inhaled NO.
ECMO may be life saving if all other modalities fail.

Questions

1. You are performing a BSLT for COPD using one-lung ventilation (OLV) and no CPB. Half an hour into starting OLV, blood gas analysis shows: pH = 7.10, PaO_2 = 47, $PaCO_2$ = 93, base excess = –6. Vent settings: pressure control ventilation with PIP = 45 mm Hg, PEEP = 10, RR = 25, TV = 300, FiO_2 = 100%. Patient is on 160 µg/h of phenylephrine with mean arterial pressures less than 50 mm Hg for the past 15 minutes. What is your next step?

   a. Increase PEEP to 15 mm Hg.
   b. Increase pressure to 60 mm Hg and change higher alarm limit. Recheck blood gas ten minutes after change.
   c. Inform surgeon to initiate CPB.
   d. Start epinephrine and bicarbonate infusion. Titrate to MAP of greater than 60 mm Hg. Repeat ABG in 15 minutes.

2. Inhaled nitric oxide is characterized by all except which of the following?

   a. it is cheap and cost-effective in most centers
   b. does not cause systemic vasodilation
   c. inhibits platelet aggregation
   d. reduces neutrophil adherence to the endothelium

Answers

1. c. Severe hypoxia, hypercarbia, and acidosis are major indications for initiating CPB while performing BSLT with OLV. Cannulation may occur either through the femoral vessels or the chest. Increasing PEEP or PC settings will not be effective in this setting and may exacerbate the situation by increasing shunt. Epinephrine infusion may be used as a bridge until CPB is initiated, and bicarbonate infusion will only exacerbate the acidosis and hypercarbia in a situation where increasing minute ventilation is not a viable option.

2. a. Inhaled NO is usually expensive and therefore most centers use inhaled prostaglandins as a first measure. Inhaled NO has the extra benefit of having anti-inflammatory properties as it reduces neutrophil adherence to the endothelium and inhibits platelet aggregation.

Further reading

Vacanti, C. A., Sikka, P. K., Urman, R. U., Dershwitz, M., and Segal, B. S. (2011). *Essential Clinical Anesthesia*, 1st edn. Cambridge University Press.

Hartigan, P. M. (2012). *Practical Handbook of Thoracic Anesthesia*, 1st edn. New York, NY: Springer.

Chapter

89

Bronchoscopy and mediastinoscopy: anesthetic implications

Stephanie Yacoubian and Ju-Mei Ng

Keywords

Flexible fiberoptic bronchoscope: definition and anesthetic requirements
Rigid bronchoscope: definition and anesthetic requirements
Rigid bronchoscopy: contraindications
Ventilation options through rigid bronchoscope
Apneic oxygenation
Jet ventilation
Foreign body aspiration
Mediastinum: anatomy
Cervical mediastinoscopy
Anterior mediastinoscopy
Mediastinoscopy: innominate artery compression
Mediastinoscopy: complications
Endobronchial ultrasound: transbronchial biopsy

Flexible fiberoptic bronchoscope: definition and anesthetic requirements

It is a flexible long scope that uses a fiberoptic system to transmit an image from the tip of the instrument to an eyepiece or video camera at the proximal end. There is usually a working channel through which instruments, e.g., wires or suction, can be applied.

Common indications for flexible bronchoscopy

- staging of lung cancer
- tracheobronchial tree assessment (stenoses, hemoptysis, internal or external obstruction)
- unexplained chronic cough
- localized wheeze
- bronchoalveolar lavage, brushings, biopsies
- stent deployment, adjustment, or evaluation
- transbronchial biopsy
- foreign body retrieval

- balloon dilation (airway)
- delivery of laser or photodynamic therapy
- placement of brachytherapy cannulae
- evaluation of aspiration, burn, or chemical injury
- evaluation or treatment of bronchopleural fistulae
- evaluation of tracheo esophageal fistulae
- evaluation of rejection after lung transplant
- delivery of devices for bronchoscopic lung volume reduction surgery
- anesthetic applications: difficult intubation, confirmation of endotracheal tube position, lung isolation

Anesthetic requirements

The anesthetic plan has to be tailored to the patient's comorbidities and the specifics imposed by the target lesion (e.g., airway compression, obstruction, bleeding).

Flexible bronchoscopy can be performed either under general anesthesia or in an awake patient with good topicalization of the airway.

The airway mucous membranes have a high vascular surface area, and vigilance in calculating the maximum tolerable dose of local anesthetic is important.

During bronchoscopy under sedation, dexmedetomidine should be considered as it does not blunt the respiratory drive. An antisialologue (e.g., glycopyrrolate) may be helpful in decreasing secretions. Prophylactic bronchodilator therapy can be used in a patient with reactive airways.

Any of the following may be utilized as a conduit for bronchoscopy, whether in the awake patient or under general anesthesia:

- bite block
- laryngeal mask airway (LMA)
- nasotracheal route
- endotracheal tube (ETT)

Under general anesthesia, a larger ETT with a minimum of 7.5 mm outer diameter is needed in order to allow the passage of an adult flexible bronchoscope.

Essential Clinical Anesthesia Review: Keywords, Questions and Answers for the Boards, ed. Linda S. Aglio, Robert W. Lekowski, and Richard D. Urman. Published by Cambridge University Press. © Cambridge University Press 2015.

Suctioning through the bronchoscope will hinder the delivery of inhaled anesthetics, and may not allow delivery of adequate tidal volume. Frequent suctioning will also inhibit the ability to measure end-tidal CO_2. Therefore, total intravenous anesthesia (TIVA) should be considered if the case is prolonged.

Rigid bronchoscope: definition and anesthetic requirements

These bronchoscopes are rigid, metal tubular instruments with attached lighting devices. They come in various diameters but in general are larger than flexible bronchoscopes. They are designed to pass from the oral cavity through the glottis and into the trachea or a major bronchus.

Common indications for rigid bronchoscopy

- mechanical core-out of obstructive lesions of the airway
- retrieval of foreign bodies in the airway
- delivery of laser therapy
- deployment, adjustment, removal of airway stents
- evaluation and treatment of hemoptysis
- rescue ventilation of patients with tracheal collapse
- back-up when flexible bronchoscopy is inadequate

Anesthetic requirements

- Requires general anesthesia preferably with muscle relaxation.
- Positioning: full neck extension.
- Dental guards to protect the upper teeth.
- Specific anesthetic tailored toward the patient's coexisting conditions and lesion-specific considerations.
- Consider steroids before the end of the case, in order to decrease trauma-related airway edema.
- In cases of more extensive airway trauma, racemic epinephrine nebulizer may be helpful.

Complications of rigid bronchoscopy

- neck injury
- dental trauma
- vocal cord injury
- tracheobronchial tree trauma
- pneumomediastinum/pneumothorax
- hemorrhage/hemoptysis
- loss of airway
- sympathetic surge (myocardial ischemia, arrhythmias)
- hypoxemia
- hypercarbia
- postoperative upper airway obstruction
- fire (if a laser is used)
- total airway obstruction (when stents are utilized)

Rigid bronchoscopy: contraindications

- carotid artery pathology
- instability of cervical spine

Ventilation options through rigid bronchoscope

- spontaneous ventilation
- positive pressure ventilation (PPV) (side port of ventilating rigid bronchoscope)
- jet ventilation, high-frequency jet ventilation, or oscillatory ventilation

Apneic oxygenation

During PPV through a side port, the proximal viewing port needs to be occluded, and the posterior pharynx packed in order to decrease air leak at the glottis.

With prolonged apneic oxygenation, patient may be able to preserve adequate oxygen saturation, but CO_2 exchange will not be possible. This needs to be timed and communication with the surgeon is important.

In the first minute of apnea, $PaCO_2$ increases by approximately 6 mm Hg/min. For every other minute of apnea, $PaCO_2$ increases by approximately 3 mm Hg/min.

TIVA is an optimal anesthetic for rigid bronchoscopy.

Jet ventilation

- Cannot assess fraction of inspired oxygen (FiO_2).
- Tidal volume is unknown.
- End-tidal CO_2 is unknown.
- Since exhalation is passive, this mode of ventilation carries a high risk of barotrauma, specially in inexperienced users.
- Hypoventilation is difficult to assess.
- Monitor ventilation by observing bilateral adequate chest rise, frequent arterial blood gas measurements, or transcutaneous CO_2 monitoring.

Foreign body aspiration (FBA)

The foreign body may be of unknown size, shape, or nature, and there may not be a clear picture of the extent of the obstruction or the edema caused by the object.

- If the patient is stable, consider a chest radiograph and/or a CT scan.
- Flow-volume loops are rarely used, but may provide information on the location of the object.
- Intrathoracic obstruction = truncated expiratory limb.
- Extrathoracic obstruction = truncated inspiratory limb.

On physical exam:
- Inspiratory stridor = extrathoracic obstruction.
- Expiratory stridor = intrathoracic obstruction.

- General anesthesia and rigid bronchoscopy should be immediately available even in the setting of examination under local anesthesia.
- Coughing or manipulation of the foreign body should be avoided to prevent potential complete airway obstruction.
- Extraction can be performed by the surgeon through retrieval instruments like baskets, snares, or balloon-tipped catheters.
- Aspiration of organic matter (e.g., nuts) may cause a reactive mucosal edema. This makes retrieval more challenging.
- Friable foreign bodies may break apart into pieces.
- In case of tracheal obstruction, foreign body can be pushed into a mainstem bronchus as a last resort. Ventilation can then be achieved through the contralateral lung.
- Anesthetic options range from spontaneous ventilation to paralysis with PPV.
- Pediatric anesthesiologists tend to prefer inhalation induction despite a full stomach, especially in a crying child.
- There is no evidence that general anesthesia with an inhalation induction with spontaneous ventilation as opposed to PPV will prevent airway obstruction.

Mediastinum: anatomy

From thoracic inlet to diaphragm.

- anterior border = sternum, chest wall
- posterior border = spine
- lateral borders = right and left lungs

Divided into two parts:

1. Upper portion (superior mediastinum):
   superior limit = superior thoracic aperture
   inferior limit = plane of sternal angle to T4-T5
2. Lower portion divided into three parts:
   a. anterior mediastinum, in front of the pericardium. Contains: loose areolar tissue, lymphatic vessels, lymph nodes, small branches of the internal thoracic artery, thymus
   b. middle mediastinum, includes pericardium and its contents. Contains: heart, pericardium, ascending aorta, superior vena cava, azygos vein, carina, mainstem bronchi, pulmonary artery and its branches, right and left pulmonary veins, phrenic nerves, lymphatic glands, pericardiophrenic vessels
   c. posterior pericardium, behind the pericardium. Contains: thoracic descending aorta, azygos vein, hemiazygos vein, vagus nerve, splanchnic nerves, esophagus, thoracic duct, lymph glands.

Cervical mediastinoscopy (C-med)

- The incision is made above the manubrium and the mediastinoscope slides in a plane created by dissecting between the pretracheal fascia and trachea.

- C-med can access the majority of mediastinal lymph nodes.
- Vulnerable adjacent structures: innominate artery, innominate vein, pulmonary artery, azygos vein.

Anterior mediastinoscopy (A-med)

- This is a left parasternal incision made between the second and third rib.
- Ideal for accessing anterior mediastinal and aortopulmonary window lymph nodes.
- Vulnerable adjacent structures: internal mammary vessels, aorta, pulmonary artery.

Mediastinoscopy: innominate artery compression

- General anesthetic tailored toward patient's coexisting diseases.
- Mediastinoscope may transiently compress the innominate artery. This can compromise perfusion through the right carotid.
- Consider EEG monitoring in patients with L-carotid stenosis or history of cerebrovascular accidents.
- Placement of pulse oximeter and/or arterial line (if indicated) on the right upper extremity is encouraged, as it may signal innominate artery compression.

Mediastinoscopy: complications

- Major complications: hemorrhage (azygos vein, pulmonary artery, rarely aorta), tracheobronchial laceration, esophageal perforation, recurrent laryngeal nerve paralysis, phrenic nerve paralysis, thoracic duct injury, cerebrovascular accident, air embolism.
- Minor complications: pneumothorax, recurrent nerve paresis, minor bleeding, autonomic reflex bradycardia.
- When significant hemorrhage occurs, call for blood and extra help, obtain more IV access, and secure invasive pressure monitor. Have heparin available as there may be the rare need to go on CPB.
- The surgical management may range from packing to emergent sternotomy or thoracotomy with possible CPB.

Endobronchial ultrasound (EBUS): transbronchial biopsy

EBUS bronchoscope has a curvilinear ultrasound probe at its distal end with color Doppler capability to aid identification of vascular structures. Proximal to that is a biopsy channel.

Used for evaluating and obtaining biopsies of mediastinal structures.

Complications:

- hemoptysis
- tracheal obstruction (as saline-filled balloon tip is inflated)

Questions

1. A 76-year-old lady is scheduled for a C-med. All of the following are considered relative contraindications for this procedure, except for which?
   a. coagulopathy
   b. SVC syndrome
   c. prior C-med
   d. prior thoracotomy

2. A 45-year-old male is undergoing A-med for a hilar lymph node biopsy. To improve visualization, the L-lung is isolated using a bronchial blocker. Why is one-lung oxygenation harder to maintain when the patient is in the supine position, compared to the lateral decubitus position?
   a. Bronchial blockers are not effective in these situations.
   b. There is decreased blood flow to the deflated lung.
   c. There is greater blood flow to the deflated lung.
   d. The less effective one-lung ventilation is not likely related to the patient's position.

Answers

1. d. All of the other answers are considered relative contraindications. A few additional relative contraindications are: SVC syndrome, ascending thoracic aneurysm, severe kyphosis, prior radiation to the region. The risk/benefit ratio should be assessed and evaluated with the surgical team.

2. c. Due to the effect of gravity, there is increased shunting to the deflated lung and therefore a greater blood flow.

Further reading

Vacanti, C. A., Sikka, P. K., Urman, R. U., Dershwitz, M., and Segal, B. S. (2011). *Essential Clinical Anesthesia*, 1st edn. Cambridge University Press.

Hartigan, P. M. (2012). *Practical Handbook of Thoracic Anesthesia*, 1st edn. New York, NY: Springer.

Chapter

90

Management of mediastinal mass

Stephanie Yacoubian and Ju-Mei Ng

Keywords

Mediastinum: anatomy
Common mediastinal pathologies: adults
Common mediastinal pathologies: young children
Mediastinal mass: symptoms and signs
Tracheobronchial tree compression or infiltration
Pulmonary artery compression
Heart/right ventricular outflow tract
    obstruction (RVOT)
Superior vena cava (SVC) syndrome
Positive pressure ventilation and dynamic
    hyperinflation
Anterior mediastinal mass (AMM): algorithm
Tracheal cross-sectional area
Postural spirometry
Peak expiratory flow rate
Heliox
Local anesthesia for biopsy of AMM

Mediastinum: anatomy

From thoracic inlet to diaphragm.

- anterior border = sternum
- posterior border = vertebral column
- lateral borders = right and left parietal pleura

Divided into compartments:

- anterosuperior
- middle
- posterior

Common mediastinal pathologies: adults

- Most likely located in anterosuperior mediastinal
  compartment.
- Most common lesions: lymphoma, thymoma, germ cell
  tumors.

Common mediastinal pathologies: young children

- Most likely located in posterior mediastinal compartment.
- Most common masses are of neurogenic origin.

Mediastinal mass: symptoms and signs

- Most adults with mediastinal lesions are asymptomatic.
- 70% of children with mediastinal masses present with
  symptoms and signs.

Signs and symptoms of compression or infiltration

1. Tracheobronchial tree:

   - cough
   - stridor
   - wheeze
   - dyspnea
   - recurrent pulmonary infections
   - hemoptysis

2. Esophagus:

   - dysphagia

3. RVOT:

   - dyspnea
   - syncope

4. Recurrent laryngeal nerve:

   - hoarseness
   - vocal cord paralysis

5. Sympathetic chain:

   - Horner's syndrome

6. Phrenic nerve:

   - elevated hemidiaphragm

7. Superior vena cava:

   - dyspnea
   - cough

Essential Clinical Anesthesia Review: Keywords, Questions and Answers for the Boards, ed. Linda S. Aglio, Robert W. Lekowski, and Richard
D. Urman. Published by Cambridge University Press. © Cambridge University Press 2015.

- upper body edema
- plethora
- cyanosis
- venous engorgement
- syncope
- orthopnea
- stridor
- headache
- decreased mentation

Tracheobronchial tree obstruction

- History of orthopnea with AMM is an indication of high risk of obstruction with general anesthesia.
- Airway obstruction is the most common complication seen with anterior mediastinal masses.
- Caution needs to be exerted with supine positioning, induction of general anesthesia, positive pressure ventilation, and paralysis.
- Supine positioning reduces functional residual capacity (FRC) and thoracic volumes.
- General anesthesia leads to additional loss of FRC and thoracic volumes.
- Positive pressure ventilation increases airflow velocities across a stenosis, by changing from a laminar flow to a turbulent flow.
- Paralysis likely associated with exacerbation of a mass effect caused by an AMM.
- Single-lumen or double-lumen endobronchial tubes can be used to stent open the airway.
- Rigid bronchoscopy has also been used to relieve obstruction.
- Consider low-frequency or high-frequency jet ventilation.

Compression of pulmonary artery (PA), RVOT, and heart

Supine or altered posture, induction of anesthesia, mechanical ventilation, hypovolemia, and decreased cardiac contractility may contribute to cardiovascular collapse.

Positive pressure ventilation is associated with *dynamic hyperinflation*, as it forces air during inspiration, which later becomes trapped as expiratory gas flow is obstructed. This will cause an increase in intrathoracic pressure. The high intrathoracic pressure will lead to a drop in venous return and a rise in right ventricular pressure, and hence worsen the gravity of any vascular obstruction.

Superior vena cava syndrome (SVC syndrome)

- SVC syndrome may lead to airway edema.
- It is essential to obtain lower extremity venous access.

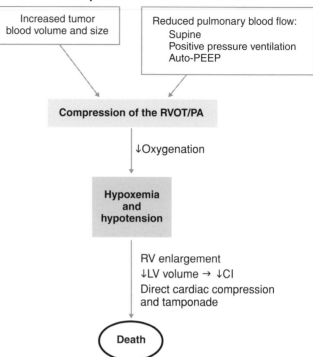

Compression of the PA and Heart

Figure 90.1 Effects of anesthesia on compression of the pulmonary artery. (From Vacanti et al. 2011. *Essential Clinical Anesthesia*, Cambridge University Press, Figure 91.3, p. 569.)

- Large-bore IVs need to be in place, given the potential for massive hemorrhage.
- With induction of anesthesia, the decreased venous return from the SVC coupled with pharmacologic vasodilation may lead to a severe hypotension.
- SVC syndrome is exacerbated by: straining, coughing, Trendelenburg positioning.
- Maintenance of sitting position is crucial during induction of anesthesia.

Anterior mediastinal mass (AMM): algorithm

Radiologic evaluation: tracheal cross-sectional area

- Chest CT scan or MRI is indicated for evaluating the location of the mass, and determining the extent of compression and involvement of crucial structures.
- Cross-sectional area of the trachea is correlated with degree of perioperative respiratory problems.
- Tracheal cross-sectional area <50% predicted was associated with total airway obstruction with general anesthesia in children.
- More than 50% tracheal compression is also associated with postoperative respiratory complications.

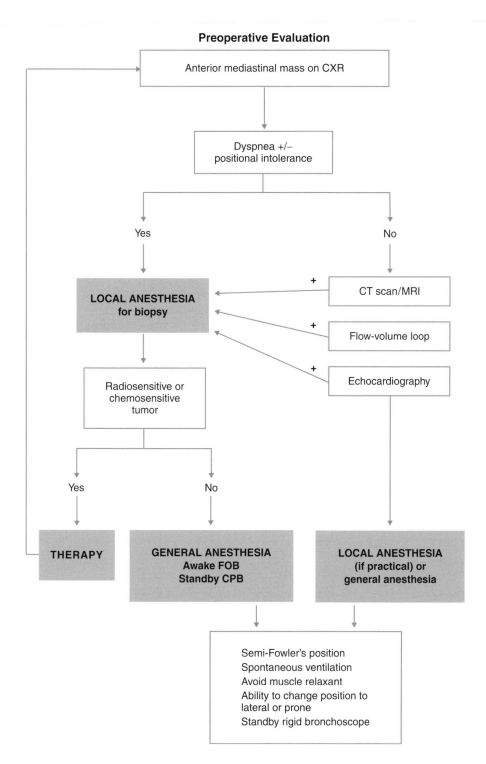

Figure 90.2 Preop evaluation. (From Vacanti et al. 2011. *Essential Clinical Anesthesia*, Cambridge University Press, Figure 91.4, p. 570.)

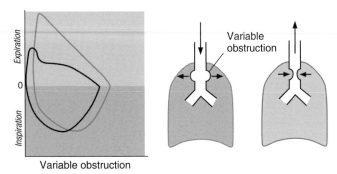

Figure 90.3 Variable obstruction. (From Vacanti et al. 2011. *Essential Clinical Anesthesia*, Cambridge University Press, Figure 91.5, p. 571.)

Postural spirometry

- Postural change from upright to supine = increased midexpiratory plateau on spirometry.
- Pathognomonic sign for variable intrathoracic airway obstruction (e.g., anterior mediastinal mass).
- Increased risk of airway obstruction with initiation of general anesthesia.

However, flow-volume loop studies are not very sensitive predictors of perioperative airway obstruction and do not add further information than what is already obtained from chest imaging and clinical signs and symptoms.

Peak expiratory flow rate (PEFR)

PEFR of 40% or less of predicted is associated with a ten-fold increased risk of perioperative complications.

Heliox

- Heliox = 20% oxygen and 80% helium.
- Decreases the density of the inspiratory gas, as a result it decreases airway resistance through turbulent flows seen in the setting of airway compression.
- Heliox, along with corticosteroids and racemic epinephrine, can also be used during postoperative periods.

Local anesthesia for biopsy of AMM

Prevent situations (e.g., anxiety, pain) that increase minute ventilation that may exacerbate airflow dynamics by inducing turbulence.

Anesthetic management of an anterior mediastinal mass

Management of Mediastinal Masses

Anesthetic Goals

- Avoid complete airway obstruction
- Avoid loss of cardiac output from increased compression of the heart and great vessels
- Avoid complications in cases with SVC obstruction
- Avoid general anesthesia for high-risk patients when feasible

Preoperative Interventions

- Identify the high-risk patient
- XRT for high-risk patients with radiosensitive tumors
- Chemotherapy for high-risk patient
- Assess for ability to perform procedure under local anesthesia

Specific Interventions

Airway Obstruction
- Awake fiber optic intubation
- Spontaneous ventilation
- Position change if obstruction increases
- Intubate distal to mass with armored tube
- Endobronchial intubation
- Rigid bronchoscopy
- Cardiopulmonary bypass

Loss of Cardiac Output
- Rotate patient (mass into dependent position)
- Maintain preload
- Avoid vasodilators
- Avoid negative inotropes
- Cardiopulmonary bypass

SVC Obstruction
- IVC distribution access
- Keep head of bed elevated
- Steroids
- Diuretics (if tolerated)
- Be prepared for significant blood loss

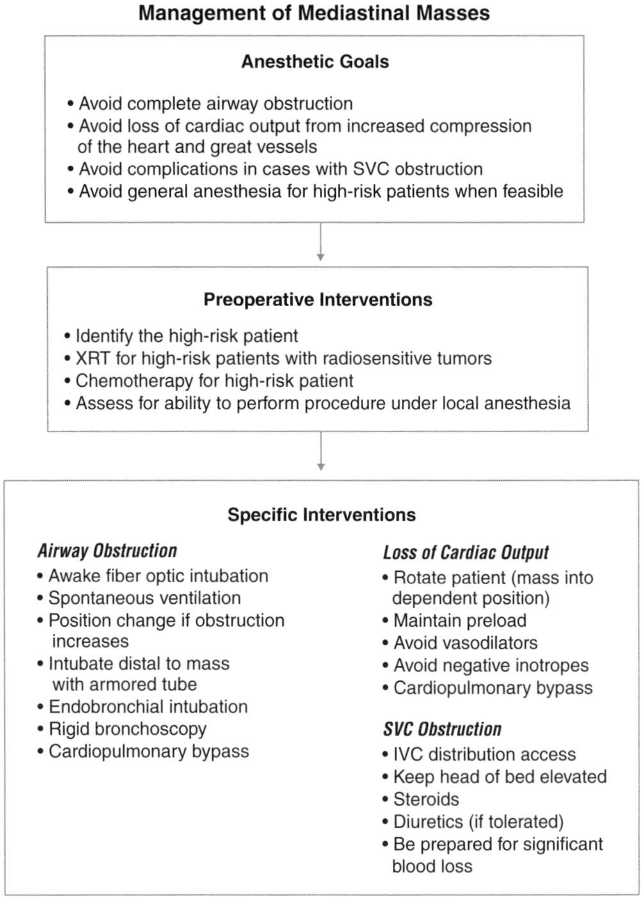

Figure 90.4 Mediastinal mass. (From Vacanti et al. 2011. *Essential Clinical Anesthesia*, Cambridge University Press, Figure 91.6.)

Questions

1. Which of the listed preoperative evaluations for anterior mediastinal mass is most likely to predict a high-risk patient with an increased likelihood of airway collapse with induction of general anesthesia?

   a. Peak expiratory flow rate (PEFR) 35% predicted with a chest CT showing a cross-sectional area of less than 50% predicted.

   b. PEFR 45% predicted with a chest CT showing 50% tracheal compression.

   c. PEFR not obtained. CT chest showing 30% tracheal compression. Patient reports no orthopnea and is able to sleep using one pillow.

d. PEFR is normal. CT chest unavailable. Patient is asymptomatic.

2. You are evaluating a patient with an anterior mediastinal mass. The patient is not cooperating and is unable to tell whether or not he is having cardiovascular symptoms secondary to a possible compression. What is the next appropriate step?
   a. Cancel the case as the patient is not providing an adequate history.
   b. Refer the patient to a cardiologist.
   c. Proceed with the case and have CPB on standby.
   d. Perform echocardiography.

3. A 20-year-old male has an anterior mediastinal mass with more than 50% decrease in tracheal cross-sectional area. He is scheduled fo a supraclavicular lymph node biopsy under local anesthesia. What would be your drug of choice (safety and comfort) as the surgeon is infiltrating the surgical site with local anesthetic?
   a. 10 mg IV ketamine, then titrate to comfort.
   b. 100 µg IV remifentanil.
   c. 100 mg IV propofol.

d. Do not medicate even if patient is anxious and has pain.

Answers

1. a. Shamberger et al. reported that patients who have a PEFR and tracheal cross-sectional area more than 50% did well under general anesthesia.

2. d. Echocardiography can provide information regarding the extent of cardiac, systemic, or pulmonary vascular compression. Echocardiography is recommended in patients presenting with cardiovascular symptoms, or patients with inadequate history.

3. a. Crucial to provide comfort in these situations, as explained in this chapter. Ketamine is the drug of choice as it preserves chest wall tone and functional residual capacity.

Further reading

Vacanti, C. A., Sikka, P. K., Urman, R. U., Dershwitz, M., and Segal, B. S. (2011). *Essential Clinical Anesthesia*, 1st edn. Cambridge University Press.

Hartigan, P. M. (2012). *Practical Handbook of Thoracic Anesthesia*, 1st edn. New York, NY: Springer.

91 Principles of neurophysiology

Whitney de Luna and Linda S. Aglio

Keywords

Autonomic nervous system: anatomy
CBF autoregulation: physiologic inferences
CBF: autoregulation
Cerebral perfusion pressure: determinants
$CMRO_2$ and hypothermia
Anesthetics and $CMRO_2$
CBF: perioperative regulation

The autonomic nervous system (ANS) controls the visceral, involuntary functions of the body. Two main divisions:

1. Central ANS (hypothalamus, medulla oblongata, and pons).
2. Peripheral ANS (sympathetic nervous system (SNS) and parasympathetic nervous system (PNS)).

Preganglionic and postganglionic neuron synapse are in the autonomic ganglia (exception: adrenal medulla – directly connected to preganglionic neuron). Pre/postganglionic neurons connect the PNS/SNS system with the effector organ.

Sympathetic nervous system:

- Originates from cell bodies in intermediolateral columns (T1-L2).
- Preganglionic fibers exit with anterior nerve roots and synapse with paravertebral (stellate ganglion), prevertebral (celiac/superior mesenteric/inferior mesenteric ganglion), or terminal sympathetic ganglion (rectal, bladder, cervical ganglion).
- Postganglionic fibers travel longer distances with somatic nerves to target organs.
- Preganglionic neurons are cholinergic – release acetylcholine.
- Postganglionic neurons are adrenergic – release norepinephrine/epinephrine; or dopaminergic – release dopamine (exception: sweat glands – cholinergic).

Parasympathetic nervous system: originates from cell bodies in midbrain, medulla, and sacral spinal cord (CN III,

VII, IX, X, and S2–S4). Preganglionic/postganglionic neurons are cholinergic.

Cerebral perfusion pressure (CPP) is the difference between mean arterial pressure and intracranial pressure (ICP) or central venous pressure, whichever is greater. CPP is primarily dependent on MAP.

Normal *cerebral blood flow (CBF)* is 50 cc/100 g/min.

The normal *cerebral metabolic rate for the oxygen* is 6 cc/100 g/min for gray matter and 2 cc/100 g/min for white matter.

Jugular oxygen saturation is about 65 to 70%.

CBF rates between 15 and 20 cc/100 g/min typically produce a flat (isoelectric) EEG. Values below 10 cc/100 g/min are associated with irreversible brain damage.

Brain energy is derived from oxidative glucose metabolism with small amounts of lactic metabolism. During starvation hyperglycemic ketones are metabolized. The brain has no energy stores. Seven minutes of total ischemia results in ATP levels falling to zero.

CBF is influenced by: (1) blood pressure, (2) metabolism, (3) certain dioxides, (4) oxygen, (5) viscosity.

CBF remains constant over a wide range of mean arterial blood pressure. The limits of *autoregulation* are 60 to 160 mm Hg. Chronic hypertension causes a right shift of the autoregulatory curve. Autoregulation is impared by hypoxia and hypercapnia, volatile anesthetic agents, and clinical states such as head injury, subarachnoid hemorrhage, and cerebrovascular disease.

Volatile anesthetics result in a dose-dependent depression of cerebral autoregulation.

CBF is closely linked to cerebral metabolism (flow-metabolism coupling).

Activation of the cortex results in an immediate focal increase in flow.

CBF changes 5% to 7% per 1°C change in *temperature*. Hypothermia decreases both CMR and CBF. Pyrexia has the opposite effect.

The most important extrinsic influence on CBF are the respiratory gas tensions, particularly $PaCO_2$.

CBF increases energy between 20 to 80 mm Hg of *arterial* PCO_2.

Essential Clinical Anesthesia Review: Keywords, Questions and Answers for the Boards, ed. Linda S. Aglio, Robert W. Lekowski, and Richard D. Urman. Published by Cambridge University Press. © Cambridge University Press 2015.

Parasympathetic (craniosacral) nerve distribution

Sympathetic (thoracolumbar) nerve distribution

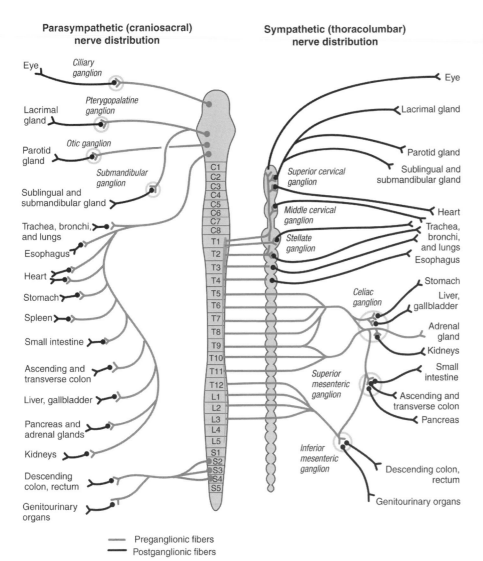

Figure 91.1 Parasympathetic/sympathetic nerve distributions. (From Vacanti et al. 2011. *Essential Clinical Anesthesia*, Cambridge University Press, Figure 92.3.)

Blood flow changes 1 to 2 cc/100 g/min per mm Hg change in PCO_2.

The change in CBF is complete within two minutes of the change in PCO_2. CBF reverts to normal within a few hours; reactivity to carbon dioxide is attenuated in patients with carotid stenosis, cardiac failure, severe hypotension, and after brain injury. If carbon dioxide recovery is reduced, a "steal" may occur in diseased areas. Here, blood is diverted into normally sensitive areas when PCO_2 rises.

Effects of inhalation agents on cerebral metabolic rate

Halothane, desflurane, sevoflurane, and isoflurane produce dose-dependent decreases in $CMRO_2$. Isoflurance produces the greatest depression; there can be up to 50% reduction. Desflurane and sevoflurane seem to be similar. Halothane produces the least effect, usually about <25% reduction.

Unlike hypothermia, no further reduction in $CMRO_2$ occurs once the EEG is isoelectric. The reduction is not uniform throughout the brain, for example isoflurane reduces $CMRO_2$ mainly in the neocortex.

Effect of intravenous agents on cerebral metabolic rate

All intravenous agents have no effect or reduce $CMRO_2$ and CBF. Changes in the metabolic rate generally parallel the changes in metabolic rate. Ketamine is the only exception.

Cerebral autoregulation and CO_2 responsiveness are presented with all agents.

Isoflurane is the only inhalation agent that increases CSF absorption. It is similar to the intravenous agents in this regard, except for ketamine.

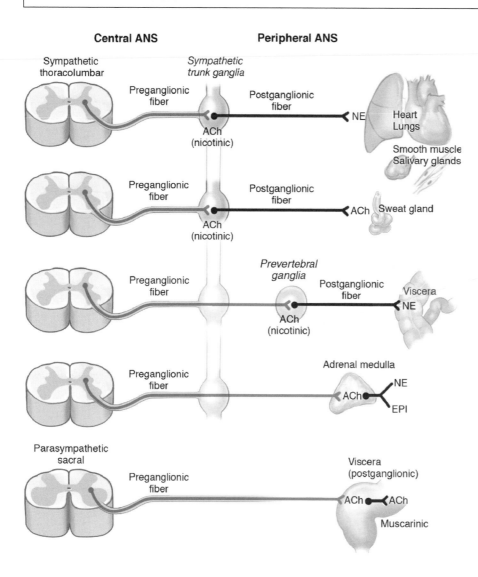

Figure 91.2 Automonic nervous system organization. (From Vacanti et al. 2011. *Essential Clinical Anesthesia*, Cambridge University Press, Figure 92.1.)

Questions

1. Carbon dioxide:

   a. adjusted to low arterial partial pressure reduces CBF as long as CO_2 level is reduced
   b. causes constriction and increased cerebral blood flow
   c. is not linearly related to cerebral blood flow
   d. the BBB is highly permeable to CO_2 but impermeable to hydrogen ions; respiratory acidosis renders rapid changes in CSF pH, while metabolic acidosis has a minimal effect

2. Which of the following anesthetics decreases cerebral blood flow?

   a. nitrous oxide 70% and oxygen 30%
   b. air, oxygen, remifentanil 0.125 µg/kg/min
   c. nitrous oxide 70%, oxygen 29%, isoflurane 1%
   d. air, isoflurane, propofol, fentanyl, 1.0 µg/kg/min

3. Which of the following agents increases cerebrospinal fluid absorption?

   a. desflurane
   b. sevoflurane
   c. ketamine
   d. isoflurane

Answers

1. d. Carbon dioxide is a cerebral vasodilator, thereby increasing cerebral blood flow, and is not linearly associated with cerebral blood flow at every level.
2. b. The inhalation agents are cerebral vasodilators, which increase cerebral blood flow, while the IV agents are cerebral vasoconstrictors, which decrease cerebral blood flow.
3. d. All the other agents listed increase CSF absorption.

Further reading

Miller, R. D. (2010). *Miller's Anesthesia*. Philadelphia, PA: Churchill-Livingstone/Elsevier.

Vacanti, C. A., Sikka, P. K., Urman, R. U., Dershwitz, M., and Segal, B. S. (2011). *Essential Clinical Anesthesia*, 1st edn. Cambridge University Press.

Chapter 92

Cerebral protection

Whitney de Luna and Linda S. Aglio

Keywords

Cerebral blood flow and metabolism
Cerebral blood flow: temperature effect
Cerebral blood flow: interventions
Hypocarbia and cerebral perfusion
Hypothermia: systemic effects
Mild hypothermia complications
Cerebral ischemia: deep hypothermia
Barbiturates: cerebral protection, CNS effects,
   mechanism of action

Cerebral blood flow

Global CBF is maintained at 50 ml/100 g/min.

- At CBF of 20 ml/100 g/min, EEG shows evidence of ischemia.
- At CBF of 15 ml/100 g/min, EEG is isoelectric
- At CBF <10 ml/100 g/min, there is potentially irreversible membrane failure evident if flow is not restored within three to eight minutes.

Cerebral metabolism is spent on electrical activity (55%) and basal cellular homeostasis (45%). The brain is dependent on continuous production of ATP and has little high-energy phosphate compound reserve. Stored phosphocreatinine is used during ischemia to preserve ATP levels.

Cerebral blood flow: temperature effect. Cerebral metabolic rate decreases 4% for each decreased degree Celsius, CBF decreases proportionally. The maximum decrease in $CMRO_2$ occurs between 27 and 14°C, or once the EEG is isoelectric.

Hyperthermia increases CMR and thus CBF until 42°C, where $CMRO_2$ declines due to toxic threshold from protein denaturation.

Cerebral blood flow: interventions

1. Induced hypertension: vessels during ischemia are maximally dilated and pressure dependent. Pressure and

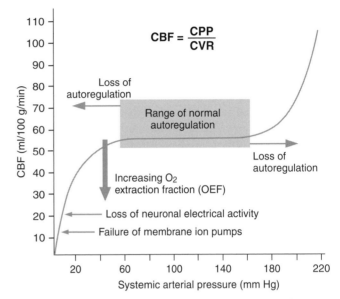

Figure 92.1 Cerebral blood flow during ischemia. (From Zabramski, J. M. and Albuquerque, F. C. 2004. Cerebral protection. In Le Roux, P. D., Winn, H. R. and Newell, D. W. eds. *Management of Cerebral Aneurysms*. Philadelphia: Saunders, p. 548.)

blood viscosity are the only parameters used to increase blood flow (Hagen–Poiseuille equation).

2. Hypothermia: *systemic effects of hypothermia* include decreases in brain metabolism, cerebral blood flow, cerebral blood volume, and CSF production. Hypothermia also inhibits excitatory neurotransmitters, lipid perioxidation, and free radical formation.

Clinical advantage of mild hypothermia is inconclusive (i.e., for aneurysm surgery, TBI patients). Mild hypothermia is only shown effective in comatose survivors of cardiac arrest. Hyperthermia, however, is associated with adverse effects.

Deep hypothermic circulatory arrest (DHCA)

DHCA to 15°C is used during cardiopulmonary bypass and can be used safely for up to 60 minutes. $CMRO_2$ during DHCA decreases to 10% of normal.

Essential Clinical Anesthesia Review: Keywords, Questions and Answers for the Boards, ed. Linda S. Aglio, Robert W. Lekowski, and Richard D. Urman. Published by Cambridge University Press. © Cambridge University Press 2015.

Table 92.1 Cerebral protection strategy

Physiologic	Pharmacologic
Induced hypertension	Barbiturate
Avoid hyperthermia	Nimodipine
Mild hypothermia	Prostaglandin synthesis inhibitor
Normoglycemia	$Mg^{3}+$
Normocapnia	Vitamins C and E
Normal pH	Lidocalne
Avoidance of seizure	Erythropoietin
ICP control	

(From Vacanti, C. A., Sikka, P., Segal, S., and Urman, R. eds. 2011. *Essential Clinical Anesthesia*. New York: Cambridge University Press, p. 589.)

The major risk of hypothermia is coagulopathy. Patients also need to be monitored for rebound intracranial pressure during rewarming. Note that mild hypothermia (33–34°C) is not associated with morbidity.

3. Normocapnia is the goal. Hypocapnia will reduce CBF and increase the risk of cerebral ischemia. Hypercapnia will increase CBF, but will also increase ICP and compromise CPP.

4. Normoglycemia: both hyper-and hypoglycemia are associated with cerebral injury.

5. *Barbiturates* are the gold standard for *cerebral protection* in focal ischemia, but not beneficial in global ischemia when neuronal/metabolic activities are already shut down. *Mechanism* is through potentiation of GABA receptors/inhibition of synaptic transmission. Barbiturates also block Na^+ channels, reduce Ca^{2+} influx, block excitatory neurotransmitter release, and inverse vascular steal. Barbiturates decrease CBF and reduce $CMRO_2$. Associated with a 30% reduction for general anesthesia and 50% reduction during EEG suppression with no further decrease in $CMRO_2$ once EEG is isolectric.

6. Other pharmacologic agents (etomidate, propofol, volatile anesthestics) have been shown to reduce injury through $CMRO_2$ reduction experimentally, but none superior. Calcium channel blockers can cause vasodilation and improve CBF, used for subarachnoid hemorrhage.

Questions

1. Which of the following is true about induced hypertension to increase CBF?
   a. It is effective for global ischemia.
   b. It is without substantial risk in the context of cerebral ischemia.
   c. It works primarily through shunting flow away from collateral circulation.
   d. It is most effective in the setting of impaired autoregulation.

Table 92.2 Complications of deep hypothermia (18 to 22°C)

Cardiovascular	Myocardial depression, arrhythmia, hypotension, ↓ tissue perfusion, ↓ ADH, ↑ viscoslty, vasoconstriction
Coagulation	Thrombocytopenia, platelet dysfunction, fibrinolysis, sludging
Metabolism	Slow metabolism of anesthetic agents, prolonged neuromuscular blockade
Shivering	Increased O_2 consumption
Surgical	Increased wound infection

(From Vacanti, C. A., Sikka, P., Segal, S., and Urman, R. eds. 2011. *Essential Clinical Anesthesia*. New York: Cambridge University Press, p. 588.)

2. At what temperature is the EEG isoeletric?
   a. 15°C
   b. 20°C
   c. 25°C
   d. 30°C

3. Which intervention decreases both basal CMR in addition to electrophysiologic CMR?
   a. hypothermia
   b. barbiturates
   c. calcium channel blockers
   d. xenon

Answers

1. d. Induced hypertension is most effective with impaired autoregulation. It is mainly used to increase collateral circulation when CBF drops below the ischemic threshold. There is no circulation in global ischemia so induced hypertension will have no effect. Serious complications include edema leading to more ischemia or conversion of an infarct to a hemorrhagic stroke.

2. b. EEG is isoeletric at 20°C.

3. a. Hypothermia causes a reduction in both electrophysiologic energy consumption and basal CMR (related to maintenance of cellular integrity) and preferentially basal CMR. Pharmacologic drugs reduce the component of CMR associated with electrophysiologic activity, which is 60% of $CMRO_2$ in the awake state. Xenon works through noncompetitive blockade of NMDA receptors.

Further reading

Hypothermia after Cardiac Arrest Study Group (2002). Mild therapeutic hypothermia to improve the neurologic outcome after cardiac arrest. *New England Journal of Medicine* 346(8), 549–556.

Miller, R. D. (2010). *Miller's Anesthesia*. Philadelphia, PA: Churchill-Livingstone/Elsevier, pp. 327–331.

Vacanti, C. A., Sikka, P. K., Urman, R. U., Dershwitz, M., and Segal, B. S. (2011). *Essential Clinical Anesthesia*, 1st edn. Cambridge University Press, pp. 585–590.

Craniotomy

93

Whitney de Luna and Linda S. Aglio

Keywords

- Intraoperative awareness: risk factors
- Intraoperative fluid management
- Bradycardia during neurosurgery: causes
- Hypotensive drugs and intracranial pressure (ICP)
- Lumbar cerebral spinal fluid (CSF) drainage
- Positioning
- Venous air embolism: detection
- Somatosensory evoked potentials (SSEPs): pathways and spinal column function
- SSEPs: interpretation, anesthetic effects, moderating factors
- Motor evoked potentials: spinal cord
- Brainstem auditory evoked responses: anesthetic implications

General approach to maintenance of general anesthesia for craniotomies

1. Induction with minimal coughing/straining.
2. Full stomach precautions.
3. Achieving hypocapnia quickly.
4. Avoiding hypoxia/hypercarbia.
5. Emergence with minimal coughing.
6. Rapid emergence for postoperative neurological examination.

Intraoperative awareness occurs from an imbalance between anesthetic requirement and delivery. A patient may have:

1. normal requirement with low anesthetic delivery – from error in expertise or vaporizer/circuit/end-tidal gas monitor malfunctions
2. lower requirement because of hypovolemia/cardiac failure, but amount of anesthetic required is too high to be tolerated by cardiovascular system
3. higher requirement if the patient is tolerant to sedatives/analgesics

Less anesthetics are required when the dura is opened as the brain parenchyma is devoid of sensation. Use of EEG-based BIS monitoring may reduce but not eliminate awareness.

Management of intracranial pressure (ICP) during neurosurgery

Intraoperative fluid management during neurosurgery is governed by osmolar gradient, as blood–brain barrier endothelial junctions prevent the passage of ions. Normal saline (NS) and lactated Ringer's are used most often.

NS is slightly hyperosmolar causing hyperchloremic metabolic acidosis. LR are hypo-osmolar – can increase ICP with large-volume administration. Free water solutions lower plasma osmolality and increase edema and ICP. Dextrose-based fluids worsen neurologic outcomes (metabolism of glucose to lactic acid lowers cerebral tissue pH).

Causes of bradycardia

Increased intracranial pressure (ICP) resulting in pressure/stretching of brainstem (Cushing reflex). This leads to reflexive hypertension, bradycardia, and apnea. The Cushing reflex pathway preserves adequate cerebral perfusion pressure despite increased ICP.

Other causes of bradycardia: lesion compressing the brain parenchyma during neurosurgical procedures, i.e., placement of extradural drains, seizures, trigemino-cardiac reflex, cerebellar lesions, spinal lesions.

Hypotensive drugs and ICP: β-adrenergic blockers (i.e., propranolol and esmolol) and combined α- and β-adrenergic blocker (i.e., labetalol) can reduce systemic blood pressure in patients with raised ICP with minimal or no effect on CBF or ICP.

Lumbar CSF drainage can be used when dura is open and patient is mildly hyperventilating (to prevent brain herniation). Drainage of 10 to 20 ml of CSF can reduce tension.

Essential Clinical Anesthesia Review: Keywords, Questions and Answers for the Boards, ed. Linda S. Aglio, Robert W. Lekowski, and Richard D. Urman. Published by Cambridge University Press. © Cambridge University Press 2015.

Positioning

Prone – used for midline lesions, posterior fossa. Disadvantages: difficult ventilation, limited access to ET tube, airway pressure necrosis, ocular edema and blindness from retinal artery thrombosis, venous air embolism (less common than with sitting position).

Sitting – posterior surgeries. Improved CSF and venous drainage, less bleeding.

However, the highest risk of VAE is, risk of quadriplegia in elderly with spinal stenosis, supratentorial hemorrhage. Contraindications: intracardiac defects, pulmonary AV malformations, carotid stenosis.

Other:

Supine – head laterally rotated and flexed, not for patients with severe joint disease. Risk of impaired jugular venous drainage/brain edema.

Lateral – used for lateral/cerebellopontine angle lesions. Low risk for VAE but high risk of rapid sinus bleeding. Possible postoperative brachial plexus and popliteal nerve damage.

Venous air embolism (VAE) is caused by large volumes of air entering the sinuses when sinuses are tented open by attachments to the dura. Precordial Doppler ultrasound is the most sensitive noninvasive monitor for *detection*. "Mill-wheel" murmur characteristic.

Evoked potentials

Somatosensory evoked potentials (SSEPs) are used to assess intraoperative spinal cord, brainstem, and cortical pathways during surgical manipulation. Pathway injury results in increased latency or decreased amplitude of evoked waveform.

SSEP pathway: applied sensory stimulus leads to afferent nerve impulse detected by surface electrodes. SSEPs are elicited by stimulation of peripheral nerve at distal sites (upper extremities – median/ulnar nerves at wrist; lower extremities – posterior tibial/peroneal nerves). SSEP enter dorsal nerve roots and ascend the spinal cord.

SSEP interpretation: 50% decrease in latency or 10% decrease in amplitude indicates significant compromise.

Motor evoked potentials (MEP) descend the dorsolateral and ventral spinal cord.

Anesthetics prolong latency and amplitudes in a dose-dependent fashion. MEPs are more sensitive to inhalational anesthetics and deliver anesthetics at constant levels. Avoid boluses and changes to inhalation agents. Volatile administration typically limited to 0.50 to 1 MAC.

Levels of 60% or less nitrous oxygen decrease SSEP amplitude but does not affect latency. Additive use with inhaled agent decreases SSEP amplitude but does not increase latency more than with inhaled agent alone.

IV anesthetics affect SSEP and MEP only in high concentrations. Induction doses of thiopental, ketamine, etomidate, and fentanyl preserve SSEP.

- Etomidate: increases amplitude and latency of SSEP in elderly patents.
- Benzodiazepines: have minimal effects on SSEP and no effect on auditory evoked responses.
- Opioids: minimal changes even at relatively high doses.
- Propofol: increases latency and decreases amplitude in cortical SSEPs.

Physiologic factors such as *temperature (hypo-/hyperthermia), systemic blood pressure, PaO_2, and $PaCO_2$ moderate SSEPs*. This reflects changes in blood flow/oxygen to neuronal structures. Irrigation of surgical field with unwarmed fluids also affects recordings despite normal core temperature.

For *brainstem auditory evoked responses (BAER)*, significant response is correlated with latency >1 millisecond. BAERs are less affected by anesthetics than SSEP/visual evoked potentials such that most anesthetic regimens are tolerated.

Questions

1. What is the most common cause of postoperative visual loss from prone positioning?
   a. occlusion of central retinal artery
   b. occlusion of central retinal vein
   c. ischemic optic neuropathy
   d. cerebral embolism causing cortical blindness
   e. corneal abrasion

2. Which statements are true regarding fluid administration?
   a. Lactated Ringer's may increase ICP at large volumes.
   b. Mannitol never causes an increase in ICP.
   c. Hetastarch, not dextran solutions, interfere with platelet function.
   d. Dextrose-containing solutions have no effect on neurological outcome.

3. All of the following are part of the management for a venous air embolism EXCEPT for which?
   a. increase oxygen flow
   b. attempt to aspirate entrained air
   c. keep patient's head stable
   d. occlude air entry sites

Answers

1. c. Ischemic optic neuropathy (ION) is a more frequent cause of postoperative visual loss than loss due to occlusion of central retinal vessels. ION is likely a result of multiple factors, including low arterial pressure, low hematocrit, and lengthy procedures. In addition, risk factors for vascular diseases such as hypertension, diabetes, smoking, and hyperlipidemia may put patients at higher risk, as well as anatomic variation of the optic nerve head.

2. b. Mannitol can transiently increase ICP with prolonged use by disrupting the blood–brain barrier and diffusing into the brain parenchyma. LR is mildly hyponatremic and can

increase ICP with large volumes. Both hetastarch and dextran solutions interfere with platelet function. Hetastarch also interferes with factor VIII complex. Dextrose are known to worsen neurologic outcome during focal ischemia.

3. c. If a VAE is detected, surgeons should be notified and asked to flood the field and cover sites of possible air entry. O_2 flow should be increased while N_2O should be discontinued. Air can be aspirated via an arterial catheter. However, the patient should be placed head down. Other management techniques may include cardiovascular support or jugular compression to increase cranial venous pressure.

Further reading

Barash, P., Cullen, B., and Stoelting, R. (2006). *Clinical Anesthesia*. New York: Lippincott Williams & Wilkins, pp. 767–775.

Miller, R. D. (2010). *Miller's Anesthesia*. Philadelphia, PA: Churchill-Livingstone/Elsevier, pp. 2045–2062.

Vacanti, C. A., Sikka, P. K., Urman, R. U., Dershwitz, M., and Segal, B. S. (2011). *Essential Clinical Anesthesia*, 1st edn. Cambridge University Press, pp. 591–596.

Chapter

94

Cerebrovascular diseases

Agnieszka Trzcinka and Shaheen Shaikh

Keywords

Subarachnoid hemorrhage (SAH)
Cerebral circulation: circle of Willis, anterior circulation, posterior circulation
Ruptured cerebral aneurysm: signs and symptoms
Cerebral aneurysm: determination of rupture
Ruptured cerebral aneurysm: treatment options
Cerebral aneurysm: endovascular coiling
Cerebral aneurysm clipping: neurophysiologic monitoring
Cerebral aneurysm: rupture at induction
Cerebral aneurysm clipping: anesthetic management
Cerebral aneurysm clipping: intravenous fluid
Cerebral aneurysm clipping: intraoperative osmotherapy, brain volume
Ruptured cerebral aneurysm: intraoperative rebleeding risk, transmural pressure
Cerebral aneurysm clipping: temporary clips, cerebral ischemia protection
Cerebral aneurysm clipping: circulatory arrest, deep hypothermia
Elevated intracranial pressure after SAH
SAH: neurogenic pulmonary edema
SAH: cardiac dysfunction, EKG findings
SAH: electrolyte abnormalities
SAH: hyponatremia
Ruptured cerebral aneurysm: prognosis
Cerebral vasospasm: characteristics
Cerebral vasospasm: treatment
Cerebral vasospasm: triple H therapy
Cerebral vasospasm: nimodipine
Postoperative diabetes insipidus: treatment
Arteriovenous malformation
AVM: normal perfusion pressure breakthrough
AVM: treatment

Subarachnoid hemorrhage (SAH) results from rupture of cerebral vessels (i.e., due to cerebral aneurysm or arteriovenous

malformation). Most cerebral aneurysms arise in anterior circulation and have better outcomes compared to aneurysms within posterior circulation.

Cerebral circulation: anterior circulation is derived from internal carotid arteries and provides blood supply to the majority of the cerebrum. *Posterior circulation* is derived from vertebral arteries and provides blood supply to the brainstem, cerebellum, and visual cortex. These two systems are connected to form the *circle of Willis*.

Signs and symptoms of ruptured cerebral aneurysm include headache, range of focal neurologic deficits, mental status change, neck stiffness, sensitivity to light, nausea, and vomiting.

Determination of cerebral aneurysm rupture is via noncontrast CT or lumbar puncture (obtained for evidence of xanthochromia if imaging is negative). Cerebral angiogram is performed to further elucidate the aneurysm's characteristics.

Ruptured cerebral aneurysm treatment options are surgical clipping (definitive treatment) and endovascular coiling based on aneurysm characteristics and patient's medical condition.

Endovascular aneurysm coiling is recommended for cerebral aneurysm involving the basilar artery and cases with high Hunt–Hess grade or major comorbidities. Compared to aneurysm clipping, this therapy may not offer definitive treatment and carries a risk of rupture (ranging from 1.4% to 2.7%), with mortality greater than 30%.

Monitoring during *cerebral aneurysm clipping* includes standard ASA monitors, intra-arterial catheter, and *neurophysiologic monitoring* chosen based on aneurysm characteristics (EEG, SSEP, BAEP). Occasionally, CBF analysis via jugular bulb catheter and transcranial Doppler is implemented.

Steps must be taken to prevent *cerebral aneurysm rupture at induction*. Risk of rupture increases with increase in transmural gradient (MAP minus intracranial pressure). Slow controlled induction is recommended with adequate depth of anesthesia and muscle paralysis. Pressor response to intubation can be blunted by use of IV lidocaine, fentanyl, esmolol, or additional propofol.

Essential Clinical Anesthesia Review: Keywords, Questions and Answers for the Boards, ed. Linda S. Aglio, Robert W. Lekowski, and Richard D. Urman. Published by Cambridge University Press. © Cambridge University Press 2015.

The goal of *anesthetic management for cerebral aneurysm clipping* cases includes ensuring stable intraoperative ICP level until dura is surgically opened. Intravenous anesthetic agents are useful in such circumstances because they decrease cerebral blood flow (CBF) coupled with reduction in cerebral metabolic rate of oxygen consumption ($CMRO_2$). A regimen of propofol and remifentanil can be implemented in cases of markedly elevated ICP. Otherwise, inhalational anesthetic below 1 MAC and opioid infusion may be used. Nitrous oxide should be used with caution as it elevates CBF and ICP.

Recommended *intravenous fluid for intracranial aneurysm clipping* is isotonic crystalloid without dextrose. Ringer's lactate is considered hypotonic.

Intraoperative osmotherapy decreases interstitial fluid content and *brain volume* via administration of mannitol at 0.25 to 1.0 g/kg (effective with intact blood–brain barrier) and furosemide.

Intraoperative rebleeding risk is proportional to aneurysmal vessel *transmural pressure*, which is equal to the difference between mean arterial pressure and intracranial pressure (MAP – ICP). In a setting of rebleeding, MAP can be temporarily decreased to 50 mm Hg until bleeding is controlled and temporary clips are placed. Giant aneurysms (size greater than 25 mm) increase risk of rupture and rebleeding.

At the time of placement of *temporary clips, cerebral protection* maneuvers are used to minimize ischemic injury. Such strategies include EEG burst suppression and mild hypertension (20–30% BP increase above baseline), to increase collateral flow, avoiding hyperthermia, and maintaining low normal PCO_2 level.

Surgical clipping of giant aneurysms (>25 mm in size) may require use of cardiopulmonary bypass or *circulatory arrest* with *deep hypothermia* for *cerebral protection*.

Elevated intracranial pressure is often seen *after SAH* and may be due to obstructed CSF outflow, hematoma displacing surrounding tissue, and cerebral vasospasm contributing to ischemia and edema. ICP in such cases may be temporarily lowered via hyperventilation until definitive treatment.

Neurogenic pulmonary edema is thought to be related to large catecholamine release from intracranial hypertension, but the exact pathophysiology is not known. Presenting hypoxemia must be quickly addressed to prevent increased CBF.

SAH is associated with *cardiac dysfunction* in the setting of elevated catecholamine levels. Echocardiography may reveal temporary wall motion abnormality and significantly decreased ejection fracture (stunned myocardium). Electrocardiogram (EKG) may reveal ST/T wave abnormalities, QT prolongation, and arrhythmias (premature ventricular contractions, atrial flutter, atrial fibrillation, ventricular arrhythmias). There is no indication for work-up in a setting of these abnormal *EKG findings* except in cases of compromised hemodynamic status or presence of many known cardiac risk factors.

Electrolyte abnormalities associated with SAH: hyponatremia, hypokalemia, hypomagnesemia, hypocalcemia.

Hyponatremia in the setting of SAH is most likely due to cerebral salt wasting (CSW) syndrome with decreased volume status, but may also be due to inappropriate secretion of antidiuretic hormone (SIADH).

The prognosis for ruptured cerebral aneurysm is based on several factors: Hunt–Hess grade on admission, patient's age, occurrence of cerebral vasospasm, and the aneurysm's anatomical characteristics.

Cerebral vasospasm after SAH presents most often three to four days after rupture and peaks six to seven days after the initial event with new mental status changes. It is characterized by vasoconstriction of cerebral vasculature mediated by multiple substances including oxyhemoglobin. Transcranial Doppler (TCD) is a good bedside diagnostic tool.

Proposed *cerebral vasospasm treatment* includes craniotomy and evacuation of the remaining clotted blood, triple H therapy, and neuroradiological intervention including intracerebral nicardipine, verapamil, angioplasty, and stenting.

Triple H therapy for cerebral vasospasm includes the use of hypertension, hypervolemia, and hemodilution to increase cerebral blood flow to the affected ischemic brain tissue. BP goal is based on whether aneurysm has been clipped (systolic BP of 160 to 200 mm Hg without surgical treatment versus 120 to 150 mm Hg in clipped aneurysm cases). Hypervolemia is titrated to central venous pressure of 10 to 12 mm Hg or pulmonary capillary wedge pressure of 12 to 18 mm Hg. The goal of hemodilution is to decrease blood viscosity without compromising oxygen delivery and increase CBF (goal hematocrit of 30% to 35%).

Cerebral vasospasm treatment with nimodipine improves prognosis by dilating collateral vasculature and regulating intracellular calcium movement.

Postoperative central diabetes insipidus may occur if hematoma is present near sella turcica with signs of hypernatremia, decreased volume status, and low urine concentration. Administration of hypotonic saline is initiated and refractory cases are treated with desmopressin.

Arteriovenous malformation stems from congenital abnormality of vasculature involving cerebral arteries and veins, creating a low-resistance arrangement leading to cerebral steal.

Patients may present with seizures, syncope, or intracranial hemorrhage. Bleeding risk varies depending on AVM size.

Vasculature in brain tissue surrounding AVM is chronically dilated and lacks autoregulation. These areas are vulnerable to *normal perfusion pressure breakthrough* (NPPB) after AVM resection (increased blood flow toward vessels that lack the ability to vasoconstrict) and bleeding in such a setting has a poor outcome. BP is often kept below normal postoperatively to prevent NPPB and intracranial hemorrhage.

Quite often patients present for resection following glue embolization of a large AVM in the neuroradiology suite to prevent NPPB.

AVMs are stratified via the Spetzler–Martin system according to size, characteristics of brain tissue surrounding the AVM, and venous outflow. Its grade is used to decide on best *treatment* option, including embolization, surgical resection, or a combination of these two modalities.

Questions

1. Triple H therapy for cerebral vasospasm includes:
   a. hemodilution to hematocrit level of 25%
   b. increasing intravascular volume to CVP of 10 to 12 mm Hg
   c. maintaining relative hypotension with systolic BP below 120 mm Hg
   d. use of isoproterenol to increase heart rate 20% above patient's baseline

2. Subarachnoid hemorrhage may be associated with all of the following abnormalities EXCEPT which?
   a. hyponatremia
   b. EKG evidence of QT prolongation
   c. hyperkalemia
   d. CXR evidence of bilateral infiltrates

3. Which of the following statements about cerebral aneurysms is TRUE?
   a. The majority of cerebral aneurysms are located in posterior cerebral circulation.
   b. Risk of rebleeding is proportional to aneurysmal transmural pressure.
   c. The Hunt–Hess classification estimates mortality risk based on cerebral aneurysm size.
   d. Vasospasm is a rare cause of morbidity after cerebral aneurysm rupture.

Answers

1. b. Triple H therapy for cerebral vasospasm includes the use of hypertension, hypervolemia, and hemodilution. BP goal is based on whether the aneurysm has been clipped: 160–200 mm Hg without surgical treatment versus 120–150 mm Hg in clipped aneurysm cases. Hypervolemia is titrated to CVP of 10–12 mm Hg. The goal of hemodilution is to decrease blood viscosity without compromising oxygen delivery. Therefore the goal hematocrit is between 30% and 35%.

2. c. SAH is associated with cardiac dysfunction in the setting of elevated catecholamine levels and EKG may reveal QT prolongation. Electrolyte abnormalities associated with SAH include hyponatremia and hypokalemia. Patients with SAH may also present with CXR infiltrates, indicating presence of neurogenic pulmonary edema.

3. b. Most cerebral aneurysms arise in the anterior circulation and have better outcomes compared to aneurysms within the posterior circulation. Intraoperative rebleeding risk is proportional to aneurysmal vessel transmural pressure. The Hun–Hess classification is based on a patient's symptoms and physical examination findings. Vasospasm is a major cause of morbidity after cerebral aneurysm rupture.

Further reading

Kim, G. Y. (2011). Cerebrovascular diseases. In Vacanti, C. A., Sikka, P. J., Urman, R. D., Dershwitz, M., and Segal, B. S. (eds) *Essential Clinical Anesthesia*. New York: Cambridge University Press, pp. 597–610.

Chapter
95
Anesthesia for electroconvulsive therapy

Agnieszka Trzcinka and Shaheen Shaikh

Keywords

Electroconvulsive therapy
ECT: seizure threshold
ECT: physiologic effects
ECT: anesthetic considerations
ECT: anesthetic agents and seizure duration
ECT: side effects
ECT: contraindications, relative contraindications
ECT and heart disease: anesthetic considerations

Table 95.1 Standard anesthesia protocol. From: Vacanti et al., 2011, p. 613.

Premedication	No atropine No benzodiazepines
Monitors	Noninvasive blood pressure EKG Pulse oximetry
IV access	20–22-gauge IV catheter
Induction	Methohexital 0.75 mg/kg
Muscle relaxation	Succinylcholine 0.75 mg/kg
Mask	Ventilation oxygen
Muscle relaxation confirmed	Foot sole reflex
Bite block	Between molars bilaterally
Terminate seizure (if >2 min)	Propofol, midazolam, lorazepam

Electroconvulsive therapy (ECT) may be used to treat cases of depression, schizophrenia, and mania that are either not responsive to medication treatment or associated with unacceptable medication side effects. It is proposed that ECT provides effective treatment by causing a grand mal seizure after application of electrical stimulation to the patient's scalp.

ECT seizure threshold is the minimum energy stimulation needed to produce a seizure. It can vary depending on the patient's age or ECT treatment repetition. It can be increased by benzodiazepines, propofol, or hypoxia and lowered by theophylline, caffeine, or low PCO_2 levels.

ECT therapy has certain *physiologic effects*. The immediate response is mediated via the parasympathetic system and results in bradycardia. Subsequent delayed response is mediated via the sympathetic system with tachycardia and hypertension. Premature ventricular contractions and flattened T waves may be observed during and after treatment. CBF and cerebral metabolic rate of oxygen consumption are both increased. Hormonal secretion is increased including release of ACTH, vasopressin, prolactin, and cortisol. Gastric and intraocular pressures are both increased during ECT treatment.

Anesthetic considerations for ECT treatment include: (1) avoidance of benzodiazepines and barbiturates, (2) neuromuscular blockade with succinylcholine or nondepolarizing muscle relaxant depending on patient factors. Premedication with glycopyrrolate may help prevent bradycardia. Ventilation is accomplished via mask, LMA, or ETT (patients with high risk of aspiration including pregnant patients and those with

symptomatic GERD). Tachycardia and HTN after ECT may be treated with beta-blockers.

Anesthetic agents have different effects on *ECT seizure threshold and duration* as outlined in Table 95.2.

Possible *ECT side effects* include short-term memory deficit and agitation.

ECT complications stem from the physiologic effects of ECT therapy, which may result in marked HTN, myocardial infarction, and congestive heart failure.

ECT contraindication is issued for patients with pheochromocytoma. *Relative ECT contraindication* is listed for patients with recent myocardial ischemia, cardiac arrhythmias, aortic aneurysms, recent stroke, elevated intracranial pressure, cerebral aneurysms, and high-risk pregnancy. In these cases, risks and benefits of ECT are considered against risk of patient's mental illness treated with medications.

Anesthetic considerations for ECT in patients with *heart disease* are multifold. Patients with recent myocardial infarction are observed for three to six months before ECT is administered. Beta-blockade may be considered for suspected demand ischemia prior to ECT therapy on a case-by-case basis, and additional testing may be required in pacemaker-dependent patients (potassium level, EKG, CXR). External

Essential Clinical Anesthesia Review: Keywords, Questions and Answers for the Boards, ed. Linda S. Aglio, Robert W. Lekowski, and Richard D. Urman. Published by Cambridge University Press. © Cambridge University Press 2015.

Table 95.2 Anesthetic agents suitable for ECT

Drug	Dose	Seizure threshold	Seizure duration	Comments
Methohexital	0.5–1 mg/kg IV	Minimal anticonvulsant effects	↔	Induction agent of choice by APA Short duration of action Pain upon injection
Thiopental	2–4 mg/kg IV	↑	↔ ↓	Longer duration of action
Ketamine	0.5–2 mg/kg IV	↓	↓	Slower onset Delayed recovery Hypersalivation Ataxia Increased hemodynamic variability
Propofol	1–2.0 mg/kg IV	↑ ↑	↓	Rapid onset Short duration of action Use in patients with excessive seizure duration after standard dose of methohexital or with severe PONV
Etomidate	0.15–0.3 mg/kg IV	↓ ↔	↑	Delayed recovery Emetogenic Accentuated hemodynamic response
Opioids	The short-acting opioids remifentanil and alfentanil allow for a reduced dose of barbiturates or propofol and thus prolong seizure duration.			

APA, American Psychiatric Association; PONV, postoperative nausea and vomiting.
From: Vacanti et al., 2011, p. 614.

magnet, atropine, and isoproterenol should be readily available. Patients with critical aortic stenosis are considered high risk for ECT therapy and should be carefully monitored with postprocedure hospital or ICU admission. Patients with aortic aneurysm may be treated with beta-blocker two to three days prior to ECT and nitroprusside infusion during the procedure. Arterial line monitoring would be implemented during such cases with postprocedure hospital admission.

Questions

1. Which of the following agents prolongs seizure duration?
   a. propofol
   b. ketamine
   c. etomidate
   d. methohexital
   e. thiopental

2. All of the factors below lower seizure threshold EXCEPT for which?
   a. high PaO2 level
   b. serial ECT treatments
   c. caffeine
   d. low $PaCO_2$ level

3. All of the following statements are true regarding antidepressant treatment during ECT therapy EXCEPT for which?
   a. Lithium can be safely used during ECT treatment sessions.

   b. Use of meperidine should be avoided in patients treated with MAOIs.
   c. Neuroleptic medications should be discontinued prior to ECT treatment.
   d. Inability to tolerate antidepressant side effects is one of the indications for ECT treatment.

4. ECT treatment typically results in which of the following physiologic responses?
   a. decreased cortisol release
   b. self-limited hypotension
   c. troponin enzyme elevation
   d. immediate short period of bradycardia

Answers

1. c. Among listed agents, only etomidate prolongs seizure duration. Please refer to Table 95.2 for additional details.
2. b. High PaO_2 level, caffeine, and hypocapnia lower seizure threshold. Serial ECT treatments result in progressively higher seizure threshold.
3. a. Lithium therapy must be stopped before ECT due to concern for severe confusion when these treatments are concurrently used.
4. d. Hypotension is very rarely seen after ECT. This treatment is usually immediately followed by a short period of bradycardia and subsequent tachycardia and hypertension. ECT treatment is associated with increased cortisol release and troponin enzyme elevation is not usually seen.

Further reading

Drop, L. (2011). Anesthesia for electroconvulsive therapy. In Vacanti, C. A., Sikka, P. J., Urman, R. D., Dershwitz, M., and Segal, B. S. (eds) *Essential Clinical Anesthesia*. New York: Cambridge University Press, pp. 611–616.

Stensrud, P. E. (2009). Anesthesia at remote locations. In Miller, R. D., Eriksson, L. I., Fleisher, L. A., Wiener-Kronish, J.P., and Young, W.L. (eds.) *Miller's Anesthesia*, 7th edn. New York: Churchill-Livingstone, pp. 2477–2479.

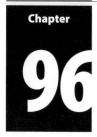

Chapter

96

Renal physiology

Michael Vaninetti and Assia Valovska

Keywords

Renal blood flow: physiology
Glomerular filtration rate
Renal blood flow autoregulation
Tubuloglomerular feedback
Renal medulla
Renin
Renal plasma flow

Combined *renal blood flow* is approximately 1.25 l/min, which is 25% of cardiac output. Most of this flow (90%) supplies the renal cortex. 1 l/min goes to the glomeruli, resulting in the production of 125 ml/min of filtrate (*glomerular filtration rate*, or GFR).

The afferent and efferent arterioles, which flow to and from the glomerulus, respectively, contain granular cell, which produce varying amounts of *renin*. Renin secretion is stimulated by afferent arteriolar hypotension, increased sympathetic stimulation, and decreased NaCl delivery to the macula densa.

Renin catalyzes the conversion of angiotensinogen to angiotensin I, which is then converted to angiotensin II. Angiotensin II stimulates the release of aldosterone from the adrenal cortex, which enhances sodium reabsorption, and ADH from the posterior pituitary, which enhances water reabsorption.

Renal blood flow autoregulation occurs largely due to the action of afferent arterioles. An increase in afferent vascular resistance decreases GFR, whereas a decrease in afferent vascular resistance increases GFR. In contrast, an increase in efferent vascular resistance increases GFR, whereas a decrease in efferent vascular resistance decreases GFR.

Autoregulation allows RBF and GFR to remain relatively constant as mean arterial pressure (MAP) varies between 80 and 180 mm Hg.

GFR is also regulated in part by *tubuloglomerular feedback* (TGF), in which the filtrate flowing within the thick ascending limb produces signals that are picked up by the granular cells of the afferent and efferent arterioles. Increased filtrate flow

results in afferent constriction and therefore reduced GFR, whereas decreased filtrate flow results in increased renal blood flow as well as GFR.

Nonpulsatile flow, such as that on cardiopulmonary bypass or on ECMO, tends to decrease RBF and GFR and increase renin production via TGF.

Following the production of ultrafiltrate at the glomerulus, a series of reabsorption and concentration steps occur along the nephron to reclaim water and electrolytes.

The *renal medulla* is highly metabolically active yet receives relatively little blood flow. Because of this, it has a high oxygen extraction and is particularly vulnerable to ischemia due to hypoperfusion.

Directly measured *plasma creatinine concentration* is the most common method of evaluating renal function, and depends on creatinine production as well as clearance by the kidneys. Creatinine production is dependent on lean body mass. Creatinine clearance is dependent on GFR.

Effective *renal plasma flow* (RPF) is calculated by measuring para aminohippurate (PAH) clearance, which is essentially fully cleared (by filtration and secretion) in one passage through the tubules (receiving the plasma flow). RBF is calculated as RPF/1 – hematocrit.

Questions

1. Renin secretion is stimulated by which of the following?
   a. afferent arteriolar hypertension
   b. decreased sympathetic stimulation
   c. decreased NaCl delivery to the macula densa
   d. hypernatremia

2. Glomerular filtration rate would be increased by which of the following?
   a. afferent arteriolar vasoconstriction
   b. efferent arteriolar vasoconstriction
   c. increased filtrate flow within the thick ascending limb
   d. efferent arteriolar vasodilation

Essential Clinical Anesthesia Review: Keywords, Questions and Answers for the Boards, ed. Linda S. Aglio, Robert W. Lekowski, and Richard D. Urman. Published by Cambridge University Press. © Cambridge University Press 2015.

3. In response to which of the following changes in mean arterial pressure (MAP) would renal blood flow (RBF) and glomerular filtration rate (GFR) remain relatively constant?
   a. 40 to 60
   b. 70 to 120
   c. 130 to 160
   d. 170 to 200

Answers

1. c. Renin is an enzyme produced by granular cells in the afferent and efferent arterioles of the glomerulus. Its function is regulation of the body's mean arterial blood pressure. Renin secretion is stimulated by afferent arteriolar hypotension, increased sympathetic stimulation, and decreased NaCl delivery to the macula densa.

2. b. GFR is largely regulated by vascular resistance in the afferent and efferent arterioles. An increase in efferent vascular resistance increases GFR, whereas a decrease in efferent vascular resistance decreases GFR.

3. c. Renal blood flow autoregulation occurs largely due to the action of afferent arterioles. Autoregulation allows RBF and GFR to remain relatively constant as mean arterial pressure (MAP) varies between 80 and 180 mm Hg.

Further reading

Garcia, E. R. (2011). Renal physiology. In Vacanti, C. A., Sikka, P. J., Urman, R. D., Dershwitz, M., and Segal, B. S. (eds) *Essential Clinical Anesthesia*. New York: Cambridge University Press, pp. 617–620.

Koeppen, B. M. and Stanton, B. A. (2013). *Renal Physiology*, 5th edn. Mosby Physiology Monograph Series. Mosby.

Chapter

Urology

97

Michael Vaninetti and Assia Valovska

Keywords

Cystourethroscopy
Ureteroscopy
Lithotomy position
Common peroneal nerve injury
Autonomic hyperreflexia
Transurethral resection of the prostate (TURP)
TURP syndrome (OA)
Extracorporeal shock wave lithotripsy (ESWL)
Prostatectomy
Nephrectomy
Lateral flexed position

Table 97.1 Factors influencing the amount of irrigation fluid absorbed during TURP

Duration of resection (20 ml of fluid are absorbed per minute of resection time on average)
Number and size of venous sinuses breached
Prostatic venous pressure
Hydrostatic pressure (height of irrigation fluid relative to patient)

(From Vacanti, C. A., Sikka, P. K., Urman, R. D., Dershwitz, M. and Segal, B. S. eds. 2011. *Essential Clinical Anesthesia*. Cambridge University Press, p. 620, Table 98.2.)

Diagnostic *cystourethroscopy* and *ureteroscopy* are among the most common urologic procedures and involve minimal surgical stimulation. Because of this, they are amenable to conscious sedation and local anesthetic techniques.

When cystoscopy or ureteroscopy are performed in conjunction with one or more of a variety of therapeutic interventions, such as lithotripsy, stenting, or tumor resection, more stimulation is encountered, often necessitating general or regional anesthesia.

In the absence of a contraindication, LMA is often an effective means of airway management for general anesthesia during urologic procedures. For axial anesthetic techniques, a T6 level is required for upper urologic procedures, and a T10 level is required for lower urologic procedures.

Lithotomy position involves elevation and abduction of the lower extremities, and results in decreased FRC, acutely increased venous return, and increased MAP with relatively stable cardiac output. It is also associated with *common peroneal nerve injury*, which results in foot drop and sensory defects of the dorsum of the foot.

Urologic procedures are common in patients with spinal cord injuries. *Autonomic hyperreflexia* is a phenomenon most common in patients with spinal cord damage above the T6 level, and is associated with severe bradycardia, hypertension,

and arrhythmias. Prevention involves adequate general or regional anesthesia, and treatment is with intravenous antihypertensive medications.

Transurethral resection of the prostate (TURP) is a common treatment for benign prostatic hyperplasia. Large amounts of urethroscopic irrigation are typically used to allow for visualization and clearing of the surgical field. Depending on the number of venous sinuses breached during the procedure, the duration of the procedure, and the type of irrigation solution used, excessive absorption of the irrigation solution can cause complications such as circulatory overload, hyponatremia, glycine or ammonia toxicity, hyperglycemia, and hypothermia.

The term *TURP syndrome* refers to the collective symptoms of volume overload, hyponatremia, and cerebral edema associated with excessive absorption of irrigation fluid used during TURP. The syndrome is associated with mental status changes and/or seizure, and is treated with:

1. fluid restriction
2. loop diuretics
3. hypertonic saline no faster than 100 cc/h for symptomatic hyponatremia
4. midazolam or phenytoin for seizure activity
5. intubation for airway protection

Essential Clinical Anesthesia Review: Keywords, Questions and Answers for the Boards, ed. Linda S. Aglio, Robert W. Lekowski, and Richard D. Urman. Published by Cambridge University Press. © Cambridge University Press 2015.

Table 97.2 Irrigation fluids used for TURP

Solution	Osmolality, mOsm/l	Precautions
Glycine 1.5%	220	Glycine toxicity, hyperammonemia, transient visual loss
Sorbitol 3.5%	165	Hyperglycemia, infection
Mannitol 5%	275	Acute circulatory volume expansion, osmotic diuresis
Cytal (sorbitol/ mannitol mixture)	178	Same as for sorbitol and mannitol

Table 97.3 Physiologic changes associated with lateral flexed position

Decreased FRC in the dependent lung
V/Q mismatching as a result of increased blood flow to the dependent lung with greater ventilation to the nondependent lung
Increased dead space ventilation proportional to the duration of procedure
Elevation of kidney rest may decrease venous return by compressing IVC
Inadvertent entry into the pleural space, a potential for a pneumothorax
Venous air embolism may occur through venous structures located above the level of the heart

(From Vacanti, C. A., Sikka, P. K., Urman, R. D., Dershwitz, M., and Segal, B. S. eds. 2011. *Essential Clinical Anesthesia*. Cambridge University Press, p. 626, Table 98.7.)

Extracorporeal shock wave lithotripsy (ESWL) is a procedure commonly used to treat nephrolithiasis in which an acoustic pulse is directed at the calculi causing stone fragmentation. These acoustic pulses may cause tissue damage if they encounter air–tissue interfaces, such as found in the lung or GI tract. Careful positioning must be used to ensure these structures are not in the path of the acoustic pulse.

Synchronization of shock waves during ESWL to approximately 20 ms after the R wave from the EKG, corresponding to the ventricular refractory period, decreases the incidence of arrhythmias during ESWL.

Prostatectomy is a common procedure and can be performed as an open operation, laparoscopically, or robotically. Open prostatectomy is amenable to primary neuraxial anesthesia, which offers potential benefits, including reduced blood loss, reduced postoperative pain, lower rates of DVT, and potentially lower rates of tumor recurrence. Robotic and laparoscopic prostatectomies are best managed with general anesthesia and endotracheal intubation due to the often high ventilatory pressures associated with steep Trendelenburg positioning and the need for precise CO_2 management.

Open *nephrectomy* is accomplished in the "kidney rest" or *lateral flexed position* via a lumbar flank, transabdominal midline, or thoracoabdominal incision. Such positioning has numerous effects on patient physiology.

Questions

1. Which of the following neuraxial techniques would be most appropriate as the primary anesthetic for ureteroscopic renal stone extraction?
   a. single shot spinal anesthesia covering to T8 level
   b. continuous epidural anesthesia covering to T10 level
   c. single shot spinal anesthesia covering to T6 level
   d. continuous epidural anesthesia covering to T4 level

2. Autonomic hyperreflexia is often characterized by all of the following EXCEPT which?
   a. bradycardia
   b. arrhythmia
   c. hypertension
   d. hyperthermia

3. Treatments for TURP syndrome typically include all of the following EXCEPT which?
   a. IV antihypertensives
   b. hypertonic saline infusion
   c. fluid restriction
   d. loop diuretics

Answers

1. c. When performing upper urologic procedures, such as a ureteroscopic renal stone extraction, a spinal anesthetic at the T6 level is required. If the procedure to be performed were in the lower urinary tract, e.g., below the ureters, then T10 level spinal anesthesia would be sufficient.

2. d. Autonomic hyperreflexia is an exaggerated reaction of the autonomic nervous system. It is primarily characterized by paroxysmal hypertension, bradycardia, and hypertension. Although patients with autonomic hyperreflexia may exhibit sweating, hyperthermia is not typically an associated symptom.

3. a. TURP syndrome refers to volume overload, hyponatremia, and cerebral edema associated with excessive absorption of irrigation fluid used during TURP. It is treated with a combination of fluid restriction, loop diuretics, hypertonic saline, midazolam or phenytoin for seizure activity, and intubation for airway protection. Antihypertensives are not routinely used and, in fact, could be harmful to the patient, as they could impair cerebral perfusion.

Further reading

Nathan, N. and Bhalla, T. (2011). Urology. In Vacanti, C. A., Sikka, P. J., Urman, R. D., Dershwitz, M., and Segal, B. S. (eds) *Essential Clinical Anesthesia*. New York: Cambridge University Press, pp. 621–627.

Payal Kohli, M. D. (2010). Anesthesia for urological surgery. In Ehrenfeld, J. Urman, R. D., and Segal, B. S. (eds) *Anesthesia Student Survival Guide*. New York: Springer, pp. 341–352.

Lebowitz, P., Richards, M., and Bryan-Brown, C. (2010). Anesthesia and management of anesthetic complications of laparoscopic urological surgery. In Ghavamian, R. (ed) *Complications of Laparoscopic and Robotic Urologic Surgery*. New York: Springer, pp. 7–17.

Chapter

98

Kidney and pancreas transplantation

Michael Vaninetti and Assia Valovska

Keywords

End-stage renal disease (ESRD)
Preoperative immunosuppression for renal
  transplantation
Intraoperative immunosuppression for renal
  transplantation
Anesthesia induction for renal transplantation
Pre-reperfusion optimization during renal
  transplantation
Postoperative care for renal transplantation
Mannitol in renal transplantation
Transplanted pancreas endocrine function

End-stage renal disease (ESRD) requiring hemodialysis (HD) is caused most frequently by diabetes mellitus, glomerulonephritis, polycystic kidney disease, and arterial hypertension.

Preoperative immunosuppression is often initiated with mycophenolatemofetil the day prior to kidney and pancreas transplantation.

Renal transplantation: anesthesia induction

Induction medications should not depend on renal function for their clearance.

- Safe medications include thiopental, propofol, fentanyl, and hydromorphone. Succinylcholine can be used if the serum potassium level is not elevated and if there are no contraindications, such as concurrent neuromuscular disorders, history of burns, or malignant hyperthermia. Rocuronium can be an alternative to succinylcholine if RSI is required.
- Unsafe medications include morphine (active metabolites morphine 3- and 6-glucuronide are renally excreted and can cause overdose) and meperidine (normeperidine is dependent on renal excretion, and build up can cause seizures).

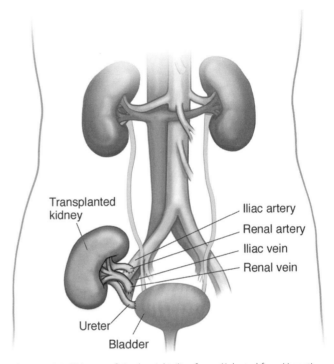

Figure 98.1 Kidney graft in the right iliac fossa. (Adapted from Vacanti et al. 2011. *Essential Clinical Anesthesia*, Cambridge University Press, Figure 99.1.)

Intraoperative immunosuppression is administered following induction and prior to transplanted kidney reperfusion. Commonly used immunosuppressants include methylprednisolone, sodium succinate, basiliximab, and thymoglobulin. Premedication with diphenhydramine and acetaminophen is used prior to thymogobulin administration.

The transplanted kidney is most often placed in the right iliac fossa (unless a combined kidney–pancreas transplant is being performed, in which case the pancreas is placed in the right iliac fossa and the kidney in the left).

Essential Clinical Anesthesia Review: Keywords, Questions and Answers for the Boards, ed. Linda S. Aglio, Robert W. Lekowski, and Richard D. Urman. Published by Cambridge University Press. © Cambridge University Press 2015.

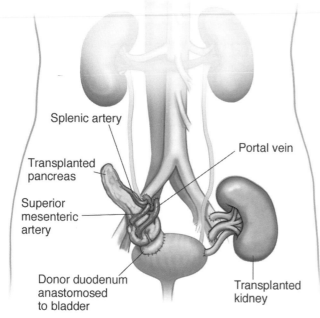

Figure 98.2 Combined kidney and pancreas transplantation. Pancreatic secretions are drained from a short segment of donor duodenum into the jejunum. (Adapted from Vacanti et al. 2011. *Essential Clinical Anesthesia*, Cambridge University Press, Figure 99.2.)

Pre-reperfusion optimization of intravascular filling and cardiac output should be attained prior to cross-clamp release by administering crystalloid to reach a CVP of 15 mm Hg and SBP >140 mm Hg or MAP >70 mm Hg. Vasopressors should be avoided but, if necessary, low-dose dopamine is preferred as it improves renal perfusion while minimizing vasoconstriction and graft ischemia.

Renal transplantation: mannitol

Use of mannitol during renal transplantation has been shown to decrease postoperative acute tubular necrosis. The mechanism of action is thought to be due to increased renal blood flow due to release of intrarenal vasodilating prostaglandins and atrial natriuretic peptide (ANP), as well as mannitol's role as an oxygen free-radical scavenger.

Renal transplant: postoperative care

Monitor urine output and CVP closely to assess graft function and intravascular volume. Avoid medications altering prostaglandin-mediated vasoregulation in the new kidney (e.g., ketorolac, celecoxib, and other nonsteroidal anti-inflammatory drugs). Also avoid epidural anesthesia to minimize risk of hypotension.

Pancreas transplantation considerations

- The dextrose-free form of medications should be administered to avoid hyperglycemia.

- Baseline lipase and amylase levels should be recorded as a reference for later rejection monitoring.
- Reperfusion of the new pancreas can cause hypotension from diffuse bleeding from the graft as well as from vasodilation from mediators in the pancreas.
- Low-dose dopamine (<5 μg/kg/min) should be administered if a CVP of 10 to 14 mm Hg does not suffice to maintain a MAP of at least 70 mm Hg.
- *Transplanted pancreas endocrine function* typically begins soon after reperfusion, thus glucose levels are monitored every 30 minutes.
- Any glucose or insulin administration should be communicated to the surgical team because it will alter the assessment of the graft.

Questions

1. Use of which of the following intraoperative medications can help prevent ATN after renal transplant?
   a. furosemide
   b. insulin
   c. dobutamine
   d. mannitol

2. Use of which medication should be limited during renal transplant?
   a. hydromorphone
   b. morphine
   c. fentanyl
   d. thiopental

3. What are the hemodynamic parameter goals when assessing reperfusion optimization of intravascular filling and cardiac output during renal transplantation?
   a. CVP of 15 and SBP >140 mm Hg or MAP >70 mm Hg
   b. CVP of 15 and SBP >120 mm Hg or MAP >60 mm Hg
   c. CVP of 10 and SBP >120 mm Hg or MAP >60 mm Hg
   d. CVP of 10 and SBP >110 mm Hg or MAP >50 mm Hg

Answers

1. d. Mannitol helps to prevent ATN following renal transplantation by increasing renal blood flow and by acting as an oxygen free-radical scavenger.
2. b. Morphine should be avoided in patients with renal failure as its active metabolites, morphine 3- and 6-glucuronide, are renally excreted. Failure to properly excrete these metabolites can lead to overdose.
3. a. When assessing reperfusion optimization of intravascular filling and cardiac output during renal transplantation, goal parameters include CVP of 15 mm Hg and SBP >140 mm Hg or MAP >70 mm Hg.

Further reading

Edrich, T. and Malek, S. (2011). Kidney and pancreas transplantation. In Vacanti, C. A., Sikka, P. J., Urman, R. D., Dershwitz, M., and Segal, B. S. (eds) *Essential Clinical Anesthesia.*

New York: Cambridge University Press, pp. 628–630.

ABA Key Words (2013). *Open Anesthesia.* Media Wiki. www.openanesthesia.org

Hilmi, I. A., Abdullah, A. R., and Planinsic, R. M. (2013). Chapter 20. Anesthetic management of pancreatic transplant recipients. In Al-Khafaji, A. (ed) *ICU Care of Abdominal Organ Transplant Patients.* Oxford University Press, pp. 195–197.

Anesthesia for intra-abdominal surgery

Kelly G. Elterman and Suzanne Klainer

Keywords

Aspiration of gastric contents: risk factors
Carcinoid crisis: prevention
Carcinoid-induced bronchospasm
FRC and general anesthesia
FRC: factors reducing
Intra-abdominal procedures: fluid management
Intra-abdominal procedures: postoperative
   considerations

Intra-abdominal surgery encompasses procedures involving the GI system, as well as genitourinary, gynecologic, and endocrine organs. Principles specific to gastrointestinal surgery can be applied to procedures involving other intra-abdominal organs.

Risk of aspiration

While rare, the *risk for aspiration* (approximately <5/10,000 general anesthetics) should always be considered for patients undergoing intra-abdominal surgery.

The risk of aspiration increases with abnormalities of the gastro esophageal sphincter (GES) tone, which plays a significant role in aspiration prevention. *Obesity, hiatal hernia, and anesthetic agents may decrease GES tone. Impaired gastric emptying,* such as may occur with diabetic gastroparesis or bowel obstruction, further increases the risk. Emergency surgeries and trauma patients should be considered to have a full stomach.

Fluid management

Intra-abdominal surgery is often associated with *significant fluid loss* and/or *fluid shifts*. Preoperatively, patients may be hypovolemic due to bowel preparation, vomiting, diarrhea, gastric decompression, fluid sequestration, or bleeding. Intra-operatively, fluid loss may be due to bleeding, drainage of ascites, and insensible losses. Blood loss should be replaced 3:1 with crystalloid and 1:1 with colloid. Insensible losses can

be estimated by type of surgery and amount of exposure, and ranges from minimal to 10 ml/kg/h.

Due to the potential for significant fluid shifts, *large-bore IV access is frequently considered.* Arterial lines and central venous lines may also be required, if close hemodynamic monitoring or frequent blood sampling is necessary.

Patients with bowel perforation and/or sepsis may be hemodynamically unstable preoperatively, or immediately after induction. Invasive monitors should be strongly considered and all fluid and electrolyte abnormalities should be corrected as much as possible preoperatively. Patients with a history of inflammatory bowel disease may be severely volume depleted, and may require stress–dose steroids if they receive chronic steroid therapy.

An assessment of the patient's volume status, based on physical exam as well as laboratory studies, is crucial to guide resuscitation management. The choice of crystalloid or colloid is frequently left to the individual anesthesiologist.

Anesthetic considerations for intra-abdominal surgery

General endotracheal anesthesia with regional anesthesia as an adjunct for postoperative pain control is the mainstay of management for intra-abdominal surgical procedures. Epidural anesthesia, usually placed in the low thoracic region for these procedures, has been shown to improve pain control while simultaneously decreasing *respiratory complications* and *postoperative ileus* due to decreasing postoperative opioid requirements. However, epidural anesthesia has no effect on mortality. Standard considerations with respect to risks of neuraxial anesthesia apply to placement of epidurals for elective intra-abdominal procedures.

Maintenance of anesthesia can be accomplished with inhalational agents, a balanced technique, or intravenous anesthesia. Some anesthesiologists avoid nitrous oxide due to the theoretical possibility that with diffusion into air-filled cavities it can distend the bowel and make surgical exposure difficult.

Muscle relaxation is necessary, as it improves surgical exposure and allows for ease of closure.

In the absence of large fluid shifts or administration of large amounts of blood products, patients can be extubated in the operating room postoperatively. *Those deemed at risk for facial or airway edema, or hemodynamic instability, should remain intubated and be ventilated in the ICU until edema resolves or hemodynamic stability returns.*

Intraoperative considerations

Abdominal surgery is associated with *significant heat loss*. For this reason, temperature monitoring and measures to avoid hypothermia, such as warmed air blankets or fluid warmers, are imperative. Raising the ambient OR temperature may also be necessary.

Hypoxia and hypoventilation as a result of Trendelenburg positioning, retraction, carbon dioxide insufflation, and decrease in FRC associated with general anesthesia are important considerations in intra-abdominal surgery, particularly laparoscopy. *The use of PEEP and PCV rather than VCV may be able to increase FRC and improve tidal volumes, which may improve oxygenation and ventilation.*

Mesenteric traction during surgical manipulation may lead to bradycardia and hypotension. Given the possibility of prostacyclin and antihistamine release as the causative mechanism, use of COX inhibitors and antihistamines may prevent symptoms.

Postoperative ileus is a major concern in abdominal surgery. Use of epidural analgesia with resultant minimization of opioids, as well as decreased sympathetic activity, may prevent or shorten the duration of ileus. Additional supportive measures, such as instituting early feeding and mobility, may also help bowel function return sooner. Choice of anesthetic does not influence the development of ileus.

Intra-abdominal surgery is an *independent risk factor for surgical site infections. Hypoxia, hypothermia, hyperglycemia, and blood transfusion increase this risk.* Timely and appropriate administration of antibiotics is crucial.

Intra-abdominal surgery – procedure-specific considerations

Splenectomy: patients with hematologic disorders may present for splenectomy. It is important to investigate the nature of the patient's hematologic disorder, as these patients may present with anemia, thrombocytopenia, or coagulopathy. They may also be on chronic steroids or have systemic manifestations of prior chemotherapy.

Trauma patients may present with a ruptured spleen. These patients may present with a difficult airway, multiple injuries, hemodynamic instability, and a full stomach. As previously mentioned, large-bore IVs and invasive monitors are necessary.

Of note, platelet transfusion for splenectomy patients, if necessary, should occur once the splenic vessels are ligated. Otherwise, the newly transfused platelets will be sequestered in the spleen.

Pancreatic surgery is often performed for pancreatitis or pancreatic cancer. Pancreatitis is associated with *fluid shifts and electrolyte abnormalities*, thus investigation and correction of volume and/or electrolyte abnormalities preoperatively is extremely important. Large-bore IVs and invasive monitoring is frequently necessary. Epidural analgesia may be a useful adjunct.

Carcinoid syndrome is a rare syndrome caused by carcinoid masses. *Key symptoms include flushing, tachycardia, hypo- or hypertension, bronchospasm, and diarrhea.* Cardiomyopathy, specifically right-sided valvular lesions, may result from long-standing disease. Presence of left-sided lesions should alert the anesthesiologist to the possibility of liver or lung metastases, or a patent foramen ovale.

The syndrome occurs as a result of *increased serotonin secretion*, frequently in the setting of anxiety, stress, or surgical manipulation. Intraoperative use of *octreotide may prevent or blunt symptoms.* Intraoperative considerations are the same as for intra-abdominal surgery, with the addition of avoidance of histamine-releasing medications (morphine, succinylcholine, mivacurium, atracurium).

Questions

1. Intra-abdominal surgery is often associated with which of the following?
   a. hyperthermia
   b. increased urine output
   c. minimal blood loss
   d. significant fluid shifts

2. Which of the following is most likely to occur in a patient undergoing laparoscopy upon being placed in the Trendelenburg position?
   a. tachycardia
   b. hypoventilation
   c. decreased peak airway pressures
   d. increased oxygen saturation

3. Carcinoid syndrome is associated with which of the following?
   a. bronchodilation
   b. left-sided valvular lesions
   c. hypertension
   d. pallor

4. Management of carcinoid crisis involves which of the following?
   a. fluid administration
   b. octreotide
   c. avoidance of histamine-releasing agents
   d. all of the above

Answers

1. d. Significant fluid shifts occur during intra-abdominal surgery due to preoperative and intraoperative factors. Preoperative factors include bowel preparation, vomiting, and/or diarrhea, or NG suctioning. Intraoperative factors include blood loss, as well as insensible losses.

2. b. Hypoventilation is common during laparoscopy in the Trendelenburg position due to decreased FRC and elevation of the diaphragm as a result of pneumoperitoneum. Additionally, intra-abdominal pathology, such as a large mass or abdominal compartment syndrome, may in and of itself limit diaphragm movement and result in hypoventilation.

3. c. Carcinoid syndrome may present with hypo- or hypertension. Additional symptoms include bronchoconstriction and flushing. Left-sided lesions are not typically seen.

4. d. Fluids, octreotide, and avoidance of histamine-releasing agents are very important in the management of all patients with carcinoid syndrome, as this may prevent the occurrence of a carcinoid crisis.

Further reading

Faris, K. and Syed, F. (2011). Anesthesia for intra-abdominal surgery. In Vacanti, C. A., Sikka, P. J., Urman, R. D., Dershwitz, M., and Segal, B. S. (eds) *Essential Clinical Anesthesia*. New York: Cambridge University Press, p. 1061.

Kinney, M. A. O., Warner, M. R., Nagorny, D. M. et al. (2001). Perianesthetic risks and outcomes of abdominal surgery for metastatic carcinoid tumours. *British Journal of Anaesthesia* 87, 442–452.

Finfer, S., Bellomo, R., Boyce, N. et al. (2004). A comparison of albumin and saline for fluid resuscitation in the intensive care unit. *New England Journal of Medicine* 350, 2247–2256.

Ebert, T., Shankar, H., and Haake, R. (2006). Perioperative considerations for patients with morbid obesity. *Anesthesiology Clinics* 24, 621–636.

Chapter

100

Principles of laparoscopic surgery

Olutoyin Okanlawon and Richard D. Urman

Keywords

Physiologic effects of laparoscopic procedures
Capnography during laparoscopic surgery
Complications of laparoscopic procedures
Anesthetic considerations

Physiologic effects of laparoscopic procedures

The physiologic effects of laparoscopy are related to the combination of three main factors: (1) creation of pneumoperitoneum by CO_2 insufflation, (2) alteration of patient position, (3) effects of systemic absorption of CO_2.

The hemodynamic effects on the cardiopulmonary system are shown in Figure 100.1.

Capnography during laparoscopic surgery

Three important applications of capnography during laparoscopy include: (1) noninvasive monitoring of $PaCO_2$ during CO_2 insufflation and can be used to adjust ventilation, (2) helping detect accidental intravascular CO_2 insufflation, (3) helping detect other complications of CO_2 insufflation such as pneumothorax or pneumomediastinum.

Periods of prolonged intra-abdominal CO_2 insufflation does not affect the reliability of partial end-tidal CO_2 ($PETCO_2$) in healthy ASA I and II subjects. However, in ASA III and IV patients who tend to have more significant cardiopulmonary diseases and increased alveolar dead space secondary to reduced cardiac output or V/Q mismatch, $PETCO_2$ may not reflect changes in $PaCO_2$. Therefore, direct arterial $PaCO_2$ monitoring is recommended via an arterial line.

Anesthetic considerations

Choice of anesthetic technique: general anesthesia endotracheal tube (GETA) with controlled mechanical ventilation is preferred due to requirement of pneumoperitoneum (and corresponding respiratory implications) and change in patient position (e.g., side effects of Trendelenburg position). The choice to use LMAs during laparoscopic procedures remains controversial despite recent studies pointing to the safety and feasibility of LMAs for such operations. LMAs have demonstrated decreased postoperative analgesic requirements, lower incidence of postoperative nausea and vomiting, and successful use of positive pressure ventilation, in spite of predisposing the patient to regurgitation and aspiration of gastric contents.

Monitoring

As previously noted, invasive monitoring (e.g., arterial line) may be indicated for ASA III and IV patients to evaluate the cardiovascular response to pneumoperitoneum and during position changes. Intermittent ABGs are recommended for patients with severe pulmonary disease. Placing the monitor

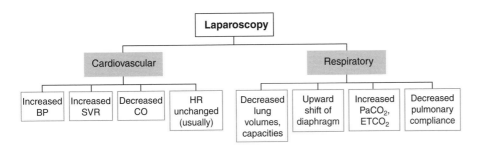

Figure 100.1 Physiologic effects of laparoscopy. (From Vacanti et al. 2011. *Essential Clinical Anesthesia*, Cambridge University Press, p. 637.)

settings on pressure–volume loop curves may identify airway complications by the variable compliance throughout an operation.

Maintenance: balanced anesthetic technique consisting of opiates, muscle relaxants, and volatile agents is used. Even though the pneumoperitoneum is a CO_2-filled space that has no relevant diffusion, nitrous oxide use should be avoided.

An orogastric tube is inserted to decompress the stomach. A urinary catheter may be inserted to decompress the bladder. Upon induction and prior to insulation, the patient is hyperventilated to approximately 30 mm Hg. Trocar insertion may cause a vagal response and inadvertent movement, so muscles should be adequately relaxed beforehand.

Treatment of intraoperative hypertension consists of adequate pain control, deepening of anesthetic, and administration of antihypertensive agents, if indicated. Multimodal analgesia is the best approach, with ketorolac (30 mg) being increasingly administered near the end of procedures.

Patients typically have an increased risk of postoperative nausea and vomiting (PONV). Although serotonin receptor antagonists (e.g., ondansetron) alone are proven to be highly efficacious, combining antiemetics with different mechanisms of action and sites may be even better, especially in high-risk PONV patients (i.e., adding dexamethasone, scopolamine patch to ondansetron, etc.).

Special populations and considerations
Pregnant patients

Evidence suggests that laparoscopic surgery is safer than laparotomy and does not have significant impact on the pregnancy or fetus. Since cardiac output decreases from baseline values during insufflation, it is important to maintain blood pressure within 20% of baseline with boluses of ephedrine. Use of a wedge under the right side is important to ensure left uterine displacement, maximize venous return, and maintain near-normal uterine perfusion. Opioids should be administered with caution, especially since they can depress ventilator drive and contribute to further increase in $PaCO_2$.

Infants and children

Capnogaphy has been proven to be an excellent guide in adjusting ventilation during CO_2 insufflation. Monitoring $PETCO_2$ in children often overestimates $PaCO_2$. Long procedures may necessitate the use of intermittent ABGs to avoid hyperventilation.

Obese patients

Laparoscopic procedures usually take longer in obese patients, with prolonged exposure to general anesthetic. An increased A–a gradient is often found due to impaired arterial oxygenation secondary to the pneumoperitoneum and the Trendelenburg position.

Cephalad displacement of the diaphragm, especially due to increased weight of the abdominal wall, may cause increased airway pressure due to decreased lung compliance.

Ventilation difficulties may lead to hypercarbia and hypoxemia when patients undergo laparoscopic procedures. Incidence of pulmonary atelectasis is higher in morbidly obese patients.

Complications of laparoscopic procedures

Table 100.1 Intraoperative complications during laparoscopy

Traumatic injuries associated with blind trocar or Veress needle insertion	• Injury of vascular structures aorta, inferior vena cava, iliac vessels, retroperitoneal hematoma • Injury of gastrointestinal structures: small and large bowel, liver, spleen, and mesentery • Minimization of the risk of accidental organ by mini-laparotomy insertion of Veress needle
Venous CO_2 embolism	• Inadvertent intravenous placement of the Veress needle • Passage of CO_2 into the abdominal wall or peritoneal vessels during insufflations • Passage of CO_2 into open vessels of the liver surface during laparoscopic cholecystectomy • Symptoms include hypotension with cardiovascular collapse, hypoxema, mill–wheel murmur, decrease in $ETCO_2$ because of a reduction of pulmonary blood flow • The incidence of undetected CO_2 embolism may be as high as 79% of patients during laparoscopic cholecystectomy
Pneumothorax, pneumomediastinum, pneumopericardium	• Tracking of insufflated CO_2 around aortic or esophageal hiatus of the diaphragm into the mediastinum with subsequent rupture into the pleural space • Passage of gas through embryogenic defects of the diaphragm • Pleural tears • Rupture of emphysematous bullae • Inadvertent placement of needle in extraperitoneal spaces

Table 100.1 (cont.)

Surgical emphysema	• Intentional extraperitoneal insufflation of CO_2 during inguinal hernia repair • Accidental extraperitoneal insufflations of CO_2; subcutaneous emphysema of abdomen, chest, neck, and groin
Vascular injury	Instrument insertion may cause concealed bleeding, particularly in the retroperitoneal space, may result in delayed diagnosis of vascular injury
Cardiac arrhythmias	Due to hypercarbia or increased vagal tone, due to peritoneal stretch (bradycardia, asystole)

(From Vacanti et al. 2011. *Essential Clinical Anesthesia*, Cambridge University Press, p. 639.)

Postoperative considerations

Laparoscopic procedures have been suggested to reduce the incidence of postoperative pulmonary complications. Increased intra-abdominal pressure → venous stasis, increased risk of DVT, and PE. For laparoscopic cholecystectomy, in particular, diaphragmatic dysfunction may last for up to 24 hours. Bile duct injuries are more common. Adequate PONV treatment is necessary prior to discharge.

Questions

1. The hemodynamic effects of laparascopy on the cardiopulmonary system include the following EXCEPT for which?

    a. increased blood pressure
    b. increased pulmonary compliance
    c. decreased cardiac output
    d. increased $PaCO_2$

2. A 48-year-old female with Parkinson's disease is scheduled for a laparoscopic cholecystectomy. She has had no previous problems with general anesthesia except for significant postoperative nausea and vomiting. Which will be the preferred antiemetic for this patient?

    a. metoclopramide
    b. promethazine
    c. ondansertron
    d. domperidone

Answers

1. b. Insufflation of the abdomen with CO_2 will further elevate the diaphragm and compress the lung volumes, thereby affecting the pulmonary filling pressures and decreasing compliance.

2. c. In this particular patient, the choice of antiemetic is based on the pathology behind the disease. Parkinson's disease results from the depletion of dopaminergic neurons, and therefore any pharmacological agent that is a dopamine antagonist will worsen symptoms. Ondansetron, a serotonin receptor antagonist, is considered safe in this population.

Further reading

Miller, R. D. et al. (2011). *Miller's Basics of Anesthesia*, 6th edn. Saunders, Chapter 33, p. 538.

Joshi, G. (2001). Complications of laparoscopy. *Anesthesiology Clinics of North America* 19, 89–105.

Chapter

101

Principles of anesthesia for esophageal and gastric surgery

Olutoyin Okanlawon and Richard D. Urman

Keywords

Esophageal surgery: preoperative assessment,
  intraoperative management
Postoperative management, respiratory complications
Bariatric surgery: preoperative assessment,
  intraoperative management
Postoperative management

Esophageal surgery

Patients have numerous presentations for esophageal surgery including gastro esophageal reflux disease, esophageal cancer, motility disorders, strictures, and perforation.

Esophagogastrectomy

The surgical technique for treating esophageal carcinoma depends on the location of the tumor itself. For lesions in the bottom third of the esophagus, a left thoracobdominal incision is made, followed by esophagogastrectomy, and the anastomosis of the jejunum to the proximal esophagus. In the middle third of the esophagus, an Ivor Lewis approach is used, which involves the mobilization of the stomach via an abdominal incision. The upper third of the esophagus may be managed by combined laparotomy with cervical incision.

Preoperative assessment

Comprehensive preoperative evaluation of patients with esophageal disease is a multisystem approach with emphasis on the nutritional, hematologic, and cardiopulmonary systems. While these patients usually have poor nutritional status and dehydration due to dysphagia, an improvement in nutritional status preoperatively has decreased the incidence of wound infections, sepsis, and perioperative morbidity and mortality. After reviewing the patient's history and physical examination, further tests may be necessary to evaluate cardiopulmonary status. Pulmonary function tests and ABGs can predict complications intraoperatively and the need for

postoperative mechanical ventilation. EKG, echocardiogram, or a cardiac stress test can aid in overall cardiac function evaluation and may be important given possible intraoperative hemodynamic instability. Laboratory tests are indicated based on initial examination. Of note, many of these patients have anemia and therefore a complete blood count (CBC) is recommended with blood bank sample (for possible perioperative blood transfusion). If chemoradiation was used in patients, this may impact intraoperative patient management. Pancytopenia is a main side effect of commonly used chemotherapy agents to treat esophageal cancer, such as doxurubicin and bleomycin. The former drug, doxorubicin, may lead to dose-related cardiomyopathy that can either be acute or slowly progressive. Bleomycin has a high incidence of pulmonary toxicity.

Intraoperative management

Initial set up includes standard ASA monitoring with the addition of an arterial line if tight blood pressure control and frequent laboratory sampling. The need for more invasive equipment, such as a central line and pulmonary artery catheter, depends on the patient's cardiopulmonary status. A preoperative placement of a thoracic epidural may be helpful for postoperative pain management and to facilitate early extubation, which is thought to be from the blunting of stress response to pain. Furthermore, postoperative morbidity and mortality from cardiopulmonary complications are reduced when adequate analgesia is provided. Due to the location of surgery, general endotracheal tube is the obligate anesthetic technique. Patients with esophageal disease typically are in a high-risk category for pulmonary aspiration and therefore induction should be either rapid sequence IV with cricoid or awake. Maintenance of anesthesia generally uses combination of volatile anesthetic and supplementation through the epidural with opioids and/or local anesthetics. Nitrous oxide is contraindicated due to bowel distension. Nondepolarizing muscle relaxants are suitable to use. The combination of general and regional anesthesia may necessitate a decrease in inhalational anesthetic and relaxant. Intraoperative complication

Essential Clinical Anesthesia Review: Keywords, Questions and Answers for the Boards, ed. Linda S. Aglio, Robert W. Lekowski, and Richard D. Urman. Published by Cambridge University Press. © Cambridge University Press 2015.

of esophageal surgery can include hypotension, bradycardia, dysrhythmias, tracheal damage, hypoxia, and hemorrhage. The decision to extubate in the operating room is multifactorial and largely dependent upon the extent of the surgery and the patient's condition. Alternatively, a patient can be mechanically weaned off the ventilator and extubated in the PACU. Often the ultra short-acting opioid, remifentanil, is used to assist in a smooth wake up with the hope of minimizing increases in intrathoracic pressure.

Postoperative management

Adequate pain control is essential to facilitate deep breathing, cough, chest physiotherapy, and early ambulation. Postoperative complications from esophageal surgery include aspiration, acute lung injury, atelectasis, pneumothorax, hemothorax, and esophageal anastomotic leak.

Respiratory complications, such as acute lung injury and acute respiratory distress syndrome, are common after an esophagectomy and lead to significant respiratory morbidity and mortality. In particular, the longer the one-lung ventilation time and operative time, the greater the incidence of acute lung injury. During the thoracic phase of the procedure, the collapsed lung incurs ischemia-reperfusion injury, whereas the dependent lung is exposed to microbarotrauma. Leakage of the anastomosis is another serious complication. Thoracic epidural analgesia is associated with a decrease in its incidence by improving intensive chest physiotherapy that preserves postoperative pulmonary function and prevents hypoxemia. Overall oxygenation is improved as well.

Nissen fundoplication

Patients who have esophageal stricture, ulcerations, Barrett's esophagus, or related respiratory problems, may benefit from an esophageal fundoplication. By wrapping the fundus of the stomach around a 3 to 4 cm segment of the lower esophagus, this operation increases lower esophageal sphincter pressure to prevent esophageal reflux. Anesthetic management for open Nissen fundoplication is similar to that for esophageal surgery, whereas laproscopic Nissen fundoplication is managed like an intra-abdominal laparoscopic case. Due to the anatomic reconfiguration of the stomach, it is possible that carbon dioxide insufflations above the diaphragm are high and can complicate ventilation management. Aggressive nausea and vomiting prophylaxis should be administered to prevent postoperative retching, which impacts the viability of the fundoplication.

Bariatric surgery

The most recent classification of obesity based on BMI (kilograms divided by meters squared) defines BMI >28 to be obese. BMI >35 is considered morbidly obese. Procedures to treat morbid obesity are divided into malabsorptive versus restrictive procedures. Within the bowel, manipulation of and/or bypassing the small bowel (the main portion of the GI tract responsible for absorption in the GI tract) render a state of chronic malabsorption. These procedures include jejunoileal bypass and biliopancreatic bypass.

Restrictive procedures include vertical banded gastroplasty and adjustable gastric banding. Effectively, the operation decreases the size of the gastric pouch, therefore limiting the amount of food that can be consumed at once. Gastroplasty creates a small upper pouch while an adjustable inflatable band limits stomach capacity.

Roux-en Y gastric bypass (RYGB) combines gastric restriction with minimal malabsorption. It involves anastomosis of the proximal gastric pouch to a segment of the proximal jejunum, bypassing most of the stomach and duodenum. Patients lose an average of 50% to 60% of excess bodyweight, with a corresponding BMI decrease of 10 kg/m^2 within 24 postoperative months. Laparoscopic bariatric surgery is minimally invasive and associated with less postoperative pain, lower morbidity, and faster recovery than an open procedure. Unlike open RYGB, the laparoscopic approach has a reduced incidence of wound infection and fewer overall complications. Rhabdomyolysis is more common in patients undergoing a laparoscopic procedure.

Preoperative assessment

Like any surgery involving morbidly obese patients, a thorough multisystem approach with emphasis on cardiopulmonary status and airway is needed. Obese patients have an increased incidence of difficult mask ventilation and intubation. Patients tend to have a larger tongue, redundant palate, and pharyngeal tissue causing a narrowing of the airway. Neck circumference is identified as the single best predictor of problematic intubation in morbidly obese patients.

Obese patient should be evaluated for obstructive sleep apnea with coexisting pulmonary hypertension, signs of right and/or left ventricular failure, ischemia disease, and system hypertension. As such, appropriate preoperative tests include echocardiogram, EKG, chest radiotherapy, and baseline ABG. Obese patients tend to increase intra-abdominal pressure and gastric volume, which increase the risk of pulmonary aspiration of gastric contents. In addition to routine laboratory tests, it maybe useful to get a few tests that reflect the history and physical examination of an obese patient. Patients may have chronic hypoxemia reflected in a CBC. Since obese patients may also have Type II DM, preoperative glucose and intraoperative monitoring is ideal. In terms of medications, patients should be instructed to continue until the time of surgery.

Intraoperative management

Routine preoperative medications including premedication with IV or oral benzodiazepines causes few side effects; however, they should be used with caution in patients with a history of obstructive sleep apnea. Other considerations include DVT prophylaxis given for increased risk for sudden death and acute postoperative pulmonary embolism, large-bore IV access when fluid shifts are anticipated, and adequate preparation for difficult mask ventilation and/or intubation. It is important to create the optimal patient position prior to induction as this will facilitate airway access. Adequate preoxygenation is vital because obese patients tend to have rapid desaturation, attributed to increased tissue oxygen consumption, and decreased baseline functional residual capacity (FRC). Given the high risk for aspiration and location of surgery, patients should be intubated either awake or after rapid sequence induction with cricoid pressure. A nasogastric tube should be inserted to properly suction stomach contents and can be used to check the anastomic integrity of the surgery. However, it should be removed before gastric division to avoid unplanned stapling or transaction. Maintenance of anesthesia is commonly with inhalational anesthetics. Some providers and studies point to the use of desflurane due to its rapid recovery profile. An epidural catheter, if present, can be used in combination with an inhalational anesthetic. Dexmedetomidine infusions can be used to decrease anesthetic and opioid requirements.

Proper positioning is important in this patient population. Obese patients tend to have multiple pressure areas, often not seen, which need to be protected and supported. The Trendelenburg position is not well tolerated by obese patients. Even when extubation criteria are met (including full reversal of muscle relaxants in a hemodynamically stable and cooperative patient) the decision to extubate depends on the patient's underlying cardiopulmonary status and the extent of the procedure.

Postoperative management

There is an increased incidence of atelectasis in morbidly obese patients after general anesthesia that may ultimately require continuous positive airway pressure (CPAP) or bilevel positive airway pressure (BiPAP) to combat obstruction. Pain causes patients to avoid taking deep breaths and ambulate. Adequate pain control is crucial to aid in breathing and improving pulmonary toilet. Epidural analgesia with local anesthetics, opioids, or both is an effective form of analgesia and can also aid in DVT prevention and earlier recovery of bowel motility. PCA pumps are equivalent to low thoracic/high lumbar epidural analgesia with continuous infusions. Surgical

complications for the anesthesiologist to be aware of include gastric pouch outlet obstruction, jejunostomy obstruction, DVT, PE, respiratory failure, GI bleeding, and wound infection. RYGB may also cause a "dumping syndrome," resulting in diarrhea and abdominal cramps secondary to a high-sugar liquid diet.

Questions

1. Bleomycin, a common chemoradiation agent for esophageal cancer, is known to have the following side effects EXCEPT for which?
   a. pancytopenia
   b. pulmonary toxicity
   c. cardiomyopathy
   d. hyperpigmentation

2. Anesthetic considerations for patients planning to undergo esophageal surgery include the following EXCEPT for which?
   a. rapid sequence intubation with cricoid is preferred for induction
   b. use of sevoflurane for maintenance
   c. propofol and opioids are safe
   d. nitrous oxide with any volatile agent for maintenance

Answers

1. c. The most serious side effect of bleomycin is pulmonary fibrosis and impaired lung function. Doxorubicin, another chemothereupetic agent used, is known for its cardiotoxic side effect.
2. d. The use of nitrous oxide is contraindicated in this type of surgery. It may diffuse into preformed gaseous bubbles, for example in the GI tract, thus leading to bowel distension.

Further reading
Dupont, F. W. (2000). Anesthesia for esophageal surgery. *Seminars in Cardiothoracic and Vascular Anesthesia* 4, 2–17.

Longnecker, D. E. et al. (eds) (2012). Chapter 53. Thoracic anesthesia. In *Anesthesiology*. New York: McGraw-Hill.

Principles of anesthesia for breast and gynecologic surgery

Olutoyin Okanlawon and Richard D. Urman

Breast surgery

Breast tumor surgery

Breast surgery is relatively low risk and perioperative risk is mainly dependent on the presence and severity of comorbidities and age of the patient. Common breast surgeries include lumpectomy, enlarged excisional biopsy, and modified radical mastectomy for breast cancer, and can be done through different anesthetic plans.

For example, breast biopsy and lumpectomy can be done with local anesthesia and sedation, whereas major breast cancer surgery is usually done under general anesthesia. Severe postoperative pain seems to be prevalent in nearly 60% of women. Risk factors include non-white race, obesity, and high post anesthesia care unit opioid use.

Regional vs. general anesthesia

For procedures such as mastectomy, lumpectomy, and reconstructive surgery, many suggest that a regional technique rather than general anesthesia may contribute to fewer side effects (e.g., lower PONV) and better pain control. Some retrospective data show that the use of regional analgesia and avoidance of systemic opioids may result in lower cancer recurrence rates, possibly due to inhibition of cellular and humoral immune function in humans. Thoracic epidural anesthesia initiated at the T3–T4 level has been

described for modified radical mastectomy, breast augmentation, and mastectomy with transverse rectus abdominus myocutaneous (TRAM) flap reconstruction. Thoracic paravertebral nerve block can be used to augment, or as an alternative to, general anesthesia in a high-risk patient undergoing breast surgery. Procedures involving the anterior chest wall may require blockage up to C5 to include pectoral nerves.

Augmentation mammoplasty

Often performed for cosmetic reasons or in patients who have undergone breast cancer surgery, augmentation mammoplasty involves prosthesis insertion either under or above the pectoralis muscle. While this is more commonly done under general anesthesia, local anesthetic with IV sedation can be used. Regional anesthesia can also be employed with various local anesthetic techniques including intercostal nerve blocks and pump infusion.

Of note, many of these patients who have undergone breast surgery with chemoradiation may have significant effects on cardiac, pulmonary, and other systems, including difficult IV access.

Gynecological surgery

Since the 1970s an increasing number of procedures have been done in the ambulatory setting. Improved surgical techniques and instrumentation, such as minimally invasive surgery and new smaller flexible scopes, respectively, have become commonplace.

Anesthetic options for common gynecologic procedures are shown in Table 102.1.

With a distended medium such as saline, dextran, or CO_2, *hysteroscopy* involves direct visual examination of the uterine cavity through a flexible hysteroscope. IV sedation or paracervical block is adequate if prolonged manipulation is not required. Resections of submucosal leiomyomas and endometrial ablation may require regional or GA. In conjunction with hysteroscopy, curettage and laparoscopy can be performed.

Essential Clinical Anesthesia Review: Keywords, Questions and Answers for the Boards, ed. Linda S. Aglio, Robert W. Lekowski, and Richard D. Urman. Published by Cambridge University Press. © Cambridge University Press 2015.

Table 102.1 Anesthetic options for common gynecologic procedures

Gynecologic procedure	Common anesthetic options
Transabdominal or transvaginal hysterectomy	GA or regional
Diagnostic laparoscopy	GA
LEEP, cervical biopsy	MAC or GA
Dilation & curettage	MAC or GA
Tubal ligation	GA or regional

GA, general anesthesia; MAC, monitored anesthesia care.
(Source: Goulson, D. T. 2007. *Current Opinion in Anesthesiology* 2013, 195–200.)

Table 102.2 Major approaches to gynecologic surgeries

Laparoscopy	Hysteroscopy
Endometriosis	Myamectomy
Ectopic pregnancy	Septum resection
Hysteroscopy	Endometrial ablation
Myomectomy	Polypectomy
Tubal sterilization	Adhersions/Asherman's
Ocpherectomy	Proximal tubal cannulation
Ovarian cystectomy	Hysterosalpingogram
Adnexal mass removal	
Salpingostomy/salpingectomy	
Bladder neck suspension	
Infertility	
Sling/Burch procedures	

Vaginal	Abdominal
Hysterectomy	Hysterectomy
Myomectomy (rare)	Myomectomy (low transverse incision)
Dilation & curettage	Tumor debulking
Dilation & evacuation	Urinary stress incontinence surgery
Laser therapy	

(Source: Vacanti et al. 2011. *Essential Clinical Anesthesia*, 2011)

Most common complications include uterine perforation, bleeding, and infection.

Loop electrosurgical excision procedure (LEEP) is a therapy for vulvar and cervical lesions. Low-voltage, high-frequency alternating current is used to limit thermal damage and permit adequate hemostasis. This can be done under local with IV sedation or GA.

Tubal ligation is most commonly performed via laparoscopy under GA but can be done via a regional technique. Worldwide, more than 75% of tubal ligation procedures are performed under local anesthesia.

Gynecological laparoscopy

Compared to laparotomy, laparoscopy offers shorter hospitalization, less postoperative pain, less morbidity, and a shorter recovery period. Laparoscopy can either be diagnostic or operative.

Anesthetic techniques for laparoscopy

Possible anesthetic techniques for laparoscopic surgery include general anesthesia with an endotracheal tube or a laryngeal mask airway or spontaneous ventilation. Regional anesthesia alone or a combined technique with regional/general anesthesia can be done. Local anesthesia with intravenous sedation is also an option. As more laparoscopic procedures are performed on an outpatient basis, there is a greater emphasis on using short-duration drugs to promote rapid recovery and fast tracking while minimizing and effectively treating postoperative complications (e.g., pain and PONV). Maintenance may include shorter acting volatile agents such as sevoflurane or desflurane, and continue IV infusions of propofol. Remifentanil is often used to promote such fast tracking. Regional anesthesia provides some advantages such as decreased PONV, reduced postoperative pain, and shorter stay; however, it can be controversial during laparoscopy.

Robotic-assisted gynecologic surgery: a relatively new, but increasingly popular technique. Anesthetic considerations include positioning the patient in a modified dorsal lithotomy with a steep Trendelenburg position after induction and insufflating the abdomen with CO_2. Due to stereotactic positioning of robotic arms, muscle paralysis is highly recommended. Limited volume of IV fluids is advisable when a patient is in the Trendelenburg position.

Commonly, for most gynecological laparoscopic procedures, induction is achieved with an IV agent such as propofol, although volatile agents can also be used. LMAs in lieu of tracheal intubation can theoretically be used, especially in nonobese ASA I to II patients with no airway issues, as studies have shown that they can permit higher airway pressures without leaking. Decision to use an endotracheal tube can be dictated by duration of surgery and positioning (i.e., a steep Trendelenburg position).

Some surgeons are performing laparoscopic surgery under local anesthesia. The inherent simplicity of this technique is increasing, especially in office-based settings. In the postoperative setting, anesthesiologists can use a transverse abdominis plane (TAP) block, which can be done using the "double-pop" technique or US guidance.

Postoperative analgesia: Table 102.3 reviews the various analgesic modalities for laparoscopic surgery. This multimodal

Table 102.3 Analgesic modalities for laparoscopic surgery

Modality	Clinical
Nonselective COX or selective COX-2 inhibitors	Multimodal approach to pain management, unless contraindicated
Intraperitoneal local anesthesia	More effective for pelvic procedures
Wound infiltration with local anesthesia	Better in combination with above
Removal of gas (and gasless surgery)	Possible decrease in shoulder pain
Intraperitoneal NS irrigation	Need large volumes (25–30 ml/kg) +/– local
Low intra-abdominal pressure	Decrease in analgesic requirements up to a week postoperatively
N_2O pneumoperitoneum	Pain reduction up to 24 h
Heated, humidified CO_2	Less pain and earlier return to activities
Phrenic nerve block	Decrease in the incidence of shoulder pain, but not analgesic requirements
Mesosalpinx/tubal block	Significant decrease in pain post tubal ligation
Rectus sheath block	Earlier discharge and decreased analgesic requirements
Pouch of Douglas block	+/– catheter, especially helpful post bilateral tubal ligation

(From Vacanti et al. 2011. *Essential Clinical Anesthesia*, Cambridge University Press, p. 650.)

approach is widely accepted and proven to provide optimal care for patients.

Prolapse repair

Genital prolapse includes cystocele, rectocele, and uterine prolapse. While the laparotomy approach has a fairly high risk of operative hemorrhage (from laceration of sacral veins), this can be minimized by the gynecologist's use of local anesthesia with epinephrine to obtain hydrodissection.

Obliterative vaginal operations such as LeFort's procedure and colpocleisis can be performed under local or regional anesthesia. Surgical operations for female urinary stress incontinence include the midurethral sling procedure, either retropubic or transobturator, with tension-free vaginal tape (TVT). These procedures have been successfully performed under local anesthesia, sedation, or general anesthesia.

Laparoscopic hysterectomy and myomectomy

Ellstrom et al. performed a prospective randomized study to evaluate pain with respect to pulmonary function in the first 48 hours after abdominal versus laparoscopic surgery. Pain scores were lower after laparoscopic hysterectomy on both the first and second postoperative days. For laparoscopic myomectomy, the potential of blood loss due to myometrial vasulatory exists and therefore needs to be monitored. Surgical techniques to minimize blood loss and subsequent need for blood transfusion include applying a tourniquet in the lower uterine segment, injecting vasopressin intramyometrially, using intraoperative blood-scavenging devices, and even rarely requiring simultaneous hysterectomy.

Questions

1. All of the following considerations should be given for a patient undergoing a robotic-assisted laparoscopic surgery EXCEPT for which?
    a. Minimizing fluids while in a Trendelenburg position.
    b. Optimal muscle relaxant when robotic arms are in the trocar position.
    c. Use of an LMA instead of an endotracheal tube when the patient is placed in variable positions.
    d. Operation with a surgeon-administered local anesthetic can be done under conscious sedation.

2. Known risk factors for significant postoperative pain include the following EXCEPT for which?
    a. non-white race
    b. obesity
    c. high post-anesthesia care unit opioid use
    d. young age

Answers

1. c. While there is increasing use of LMA in laparascopic procedures, it is relatively contraindicated in situations when a patient is placed in certain positions that will ultimately compromise an airway if such a device is no longer secure (i.e., steep Trendelenberg). When in doubt, an endotracheal tube is the safest way.
2. d. Randomized control trials have identified risk factors for postoperative pain. Older age seems to be associated with more postoperative pain issues.

Further reading

Longnecker, D. E. et al. (eds) (2012). Chapter 61. Anesthesia for obstetric care and gynecologic surgery. In *Anesthesiology*. New York: McGraw-Hill.

Westbrook, A. J. and Buggy, D. J. (2003). Anesthesia for breast surgery. *British Journal of Anesthesia: Continuing Education in Anesthesia, Critical Care & Pain Reviews* 3(5), 151–154.

Chapter

103

Anesthesia for liver transplantation

Julia Serber and Evan Blaney

Keywords

Orthotopic liver transplant
Ascites
Venovenous bypass
Preanhepatic phase
Anhepatic phase
Neohepatic phase

Orthotopic liver transplant: the first successful orthotopic liver transplant was performed in 1967. Orthotopic indicates that the transplanted liver is placed into the normal liver position once the diseased liver has been resected. There are numerous indications for liver transplantation. The most common is hepatocellular disease caused by alcohol and/or hepatitis.

Preanesthetic evaluation

In addition to the standard history and physical examination, an assessment of *ascites* is a key component. The presence of ascites increases the risk of gastric regurgitation and aspiration.

Numerous preoperative laboratory tests and diagnostic studies are required for liver transplant patients. These tests focus on cardiac performance, pulmonary function, hepatic synthetic and excretory function, coagulation status, hemoglobin level, and renal function. Significant coronary disease that is left untreated greatly increases the risk of mortality in the perioperative period. Patients with moderate to severe portopulmonary hypertension are typically not approved for liver transplantation.

Perioperative management

Typically, ASA standard monitors as well as several invasive monitors are employed. Arterial lines are placed to direct blood pressure management. Central venous pressure measurement is a useful tool to help guide intravascular volume replacement and assess right heart. A pulmonary artery catheter is sometimes placed. Transesophageal echocardiography can also be utilized to provide information about cardiac function and intravascular volume status. The risks and benefits of TEE must be weighed carefully in the setting of esophageal varices.

Multiple large-bore IV catheters placed above the diaphragm are usually sufficient for access.

Venovenous bypass (VVB) decompresses the inferior venous systemic and/or portal circulations while maintaining venous return to the heart by bypassing the portal circulation after the hepatic vessels have been cross-clamped.

Induction and maintenance of anesthesia

Induction is usually accomplished with standard methods. Patients with ascites should be considered to have a full stomach. Therefore a rapid sequence induction with cricoid pressure should be performed if there are no contraindications to this method. Patients with ascites have significantly reduced FRC. Adequate denitrogenation is very important.

Once induction is complete, any commonly used halogenated inhalational agent (i.e., isoflurane, sevoflurane) may be used for maintenance. Intermediate-acting opioids are titrated and paralysis is maintained.

There are three phases of the surgery: (1) *preanhepatic phase* (the time during which the total hepatectomy is being performed), (2) *anhepatic phase* (occurs from the time of hepatic artery clamping of the native liver until the new liver is reperfused), (3) *neohepatic phase* (this phase starts at the time of reperfusion of the liver).

Anesthetic concerns

Clamping of the portal triad and clamping of the IVC are two key moments of the surgery. Clamping of the portal triad results in decreased venous return, and variable effects on cardiac output and blood pressure. In contrast, cross-clamping of the IVC decreases systemic blood pressure as well as causing a decrease in cardiac output due to the reduction in venous return. Maintaining a CVP between 7 and 10 mm Hg has been shown to reduce the 30-day mortality as well as the incidence of postoperative renal failure.

Essential Clinical Anesthesia Review: Keywords, Questions and Answers for the Boards, ed. Linda S. Aglio, Robert W. Lekowski, and Richard D. Urman. Published by Cambridge University Press. © Cambridge University Press 2015.

Anhepatic phase

Metabolic acidosis may develop during this phase. Hyperkalemia must be treated to avoid cardiac arrhythmias.

Neohepatic phase

Graft reperfusion

The start of the neohepatic phase is marked by the initial reperfusion of the transplanted liver. Before this occurs, volume status and hemodynamics must be optimized. The event of graft reperfusion can greatly affect cardiovascular performance due to the release of residual preservative solution, air, clot, debris, and acidic blood. In preparation, the patient is often hyperventilated to a lower end-tidal CO_2 and blood pH. Vasopressors will likely be required at this time.

Postgraft reperfusion

There are often derangements in clotting activity during the initial reperfusion time period. There is an increase in fibrinolysis due to reduced clearance of tissue plasminogen activator. A goal at this point in the case should be to stop clot lysis and provide adequate levels of platelets and clotting factors.

Questions

1. During which phase of liver transplantation is citrate intoxication from rapid transfusion most likely to occur?
   a. preanhepatic phase
   b. anhepatic phase
   c. neohepatic phase

2. All coagulation factors are made by the liver EXCEPT for which?
   a. VII
   b. VIII, II
   c. VIII and von Willebrand factor

3. During which phase of a liver transplant would you expect to see the greatest degree of hemodynamic instability?
   a. preanhepatic
   b. anhepatic
   c. neohepatic

Answers

1. b. During the anhepatic phase, citrate intoxication from rapid transfusion is more likely because of the lack of liver metabolic function. Calcium should be administered to prevent hypocalcemia.
2. c. All coagulation factors except for factor VIII and von Willebrand factor are made by the liver.
3. c. Although hemodynamic instability can be seen at any point during a liver transplant, it is during the first part of reperfusion, when the vascular clamps are removed from the liver graft, that there is likely to be significant hemodynamic instability. Profound hypotension, decreased cardiac contractility, cardiac arrhythmias, or hyperkalemic arrest can all occur.

Further reading

Modak, R. (2008). Liver transhepatic phase: transfusion. In *Anesthesiology Keywords Review*. Philadelphia: Lippincott Williams & Wilkins, pp. 254–255.

Morgan et al. (1996). Chapter 3. Anesthesia for patients with liver disease. In *Lange Clinical Anesthesiology*, 4th edn. New York; McGraw-Hill.

Vacanti, C., Sikka, P., Urman, R., Dershwitz, M., and Segal, B. (eds) (2011). Chapter 8.

Liver disease. In *Essential Clinical Anesthesia*. Cambridge: Cambridge University Press.

Thyroid disorders

104

Hyung Sun Choi and Vesela Kovacheva

Keywords

Hyperthyroidism: metabolic and circulatory effects
Hyperthyroidism: preoperative management
Hyperthyroidism: intraoperative management
(thyroid storm)
Hyperthyroidism: postoperative complications
Hyperthyroidism: medications
Hypothyroidism: metabolic and circulatory effects
Hypothyroidism: myxedema coma
Hypothyroidism: substitute therapy
Hypothyroidism: anesthetic implications

Table 104.1 Thyroid diseases and the laboratory tests

	TSH	T4	T3	T3RU
Hyperthyroidism	↓	↑	↑	↑
1° Hypothyroidism	↑	↓	↓	↓
2° Hypothyroidism	↓	↓	↓	↓
Pregnancy	Normal	↑	Normal	↓

(Modified from Barash, P. G. *Clinical Anesthesia*, 6th edn. Table 41.1.)

Hyperthyroidism: metabolic and circulatory effects

Thyroid gland secretes T3 and T4 hormones. The secretion of thyroid hormones is regulated by the anterior pituitary and hypothalamus.

- **Thyroxine (T4)** is a prohormone product of thyroid gland:

  o Half-life of T4 in circulation is six to seven days, therefore missing the morning dose on the day of surgery has little impact.

  o T4 is metabolized to T3 or rT3; T3 is biologically active, while rT3 is not a biologically active form.

- **Tri-iodothyronine (T3):**

  o T3 is more potent and less protein-bound than T4.

  o T3 mediates most effects of the thyroid hormones.

- **T3RU (T3 Resin Uptake):**

  o T3RU is inversely proportional to TBG free binding sites.

  o T3RU is increased if T3 and T4 are high (hyperthyroidism) or TBG levels are low.

  o Increased T3RU means more sites are occupied.

- **Thyroid binding globulin (TBG):**

  o Increased with pregnancy, liver disease, OCP, opioids.

  o Decreased with nephrotic syndrome, cirrhosis.

Hyperthyroidism is associated with various signs and symptoms (i.e., tachycardia, anxiety, tremor, heat intolerance, fatigue, goiter, weight loss, cardiac dysrhythmia, and CHF).

Hyperthyroidism: preoperative management

- Defer elective surgery until euthyroid status is achieved.
- Expect potential difficult airway due to goiter (consider the need for awake fiberoptic intubation).
- Patients could be chronically hypovolemic → hydrate preoperatively to avoid exaggerated hypotensive episode.
- Rule out MEN prior to surgery (medullary thyroid carcinoma associated with pheochromocytoma).
- Extra caution is required for protecting the eyes since ophthalmopathy is common with Grave's disease.

Hyperthyroidism: intraoperative management

- MAC is not increased with hyperthyroidism, but ↑ cardiac output → ↑ anesthetic uptake.
- β-blocker to achieve HR <100 beats/min.

Essential Clinical Anesthesia Review: Keywords, Questions and Answers for the Boards, ed. Linda S. Aglio, Robert W. Lekowski, and Richard D. Urman. Published by Cambridge University Press. © Cambridge University Press 2015.

Thyroid crisis/thyroid storm

- Life-threatening exacerbation of hyperthyroidism.
- Precipitated by surgery, infection, trauma and stress.
- Most likely occurs postoperatively but can occur intraoperatively, mimicking malignant hyperthermia.

Treatment:

- volume resuscitation
- beta-blockers (esmolol or labetalol)
- sodium iodide 250 mg IV q 6 h
- propyl thiouracil
- hydrocortisone 50 to 100 mg IV q 6 h
- cooling blankets, acetaminophen, meperidine if shivering
- treatment of arrhythmias

Hyperthyroidism: postoperative complications

- Laryngeal nerve injury:
  - Superior laryngeal nerve injury → damage to motor input to cricothyroid muscle → vocal cord remains abducted → ↑ aspiration risk.
  - Recurrent laryngeal nerve injury → damage to motor input to larynx except for cricothyroid muscle:
    - unilateral damage can cause hoarseness and stridor
    - acute bilateral damage can cause total airway obstruction.
- Inadvertent removal of parathyroid glands → hypoparathyroidism → hypocalcemia → laryngospasm.
- Tracheal compression by hematoma or tracheomalacia:
  - hematoma causing compression → all the sutures should be cut open at the bedside and the patient taken emergently to the OR
  - tracheomalacia could develop after prolonged compression by large goiter, consider cuff leak test prior to extubation.

Hypothyroidism: metabolic and circulatory effects

- Hypothyroidism symptoms: fatigue, lethargy, weakness, cold intolerance, constipation, dry skin, bradycardia, delayed relaxation of deep tendon reflexes.
- Complications of hypothyroidism: CAD, CHF, adrenal crisis (unmasked by treatment), psychosis with delusions, increased sensitivity to opioids.

Hypothyroidism: myxedema coma

- rare, severe form of hypothyroidism
- precipitated by surgery, infection, trauma, and stress
- more common in elderly women
- signs and symptoms: severe hypothermia, hypoventilation, hyponatremia, hypoglycemia, hypotension, seizures, and mental status changes
- mortality rate: 25 to 50%
- only lifesaving surgery should proceed

Table 104.2 Hyperthyroidism: medications

Drug	Mechanism of Action
Thiourea derivatives: Propylthiouracil Methimazole	• Inhibit thyroid hormone synthesis • Prevent secretion of T3 and T4 • Prevent peripheral conversion of T4 to T3
β-Blockers	• Ameliorate β-adrenergic activity • Propranolol decreases conversion of T4 to T3 • Acute treatment
Iodine-containing compounds	• Inhibit T3 and T4 release
Glucocorticoids	• Inhibit T4 to T3 conversion • Immunosuppressive actions

(Adapted from Goldman, L. and Schafer, A. I. *Goldman's Cecil Medicine*, 24th edn. Chapter 233, e71–e72.)

Treatment:

- intubation and mechanical ventilation
- levothyroxine 200 to 300 μg IV over 5 to 10 minutes, then 100 μg IV q 24
- hydrocortisone 100 mg IV, then 25 mg IV q 6
- fluid and electrolyte therapy as indicated
- conserve body heat; careful rewarming

Hypothyroidism: substitute therapy

T4 (levothyroxine):

- Intravenous form 100% bioavailable, but only 50% for oral doses → IV dose should be half the oral dose.
- Caution in patients with coronary artery disease.

Hypothyroidism: anesthetic implications

- Elective surgery should be delayed in symptomatic patients.
- More susceptible to hypotension:
  - ↓ CO, blunted baroreceptor reflexes, ↓ intravascular volume
  - ↓ sensitivity to myocardial depressant drugs → volatile anesthetics NOT recommended.
- Ketamine can be used for induction.
- MAC is NOT decreased, although slow drug metabolism.
- Impaired ventilatory response to hypoxemia and hypercarbia.

Questions

1. Which of the following does NOT result in upper airway obstruction after thyroid surgery?
   a. tracheomalacia
   b. bilateral recurrent laryngeal nerve injury
   c. bilateral superior laryngeal nerve injury

d. tetany

e. cervical hematoma

2. Which of the following drugs used for patients with hyperthyroidism does NOT affect the synthesis and secretion of thyroid hormone?

   a. iodine-containing compounds

   b. propranolol

   c. sodium iodide

   d. propylthiouracil

   e. ^{131}I

3. Which of the following statements regarding myxedema coma is CORRECT?

   a. Intravenous T3 is the only treatment indicated.

   b. Hyperventilation is a prominent feature.

   c. All surgery is contraindicated.

   d. The condition is especially common in young women.

e. Mortality rate is between 25% and 50%.

4. What is the glucocorticoid's mechanism of action in the treatment of hyperthyroidism?

   a. prevents thyroid gland secretion of T3 and T4

   b. decreases thyroid gland production of T3 and T4

   c. suppresses peripheral conversion of T4 → T3

   d. adrenal suppression

Answers

1. c. Superior laryngeal nerve injury does not innervate the motor component of the upper airway.

2. b. Propranolol decreases the conversion of T4 to T3 and also ameliorates the beta-adrenergic activity.

3. e. Myxedema coma is a rare, severe form of hypothyroidism, for which mortality rate is as high as 25% to 50%.

4. c. Glucocorticoid suppresses the conversion of T4 to T3.

Further reading

Roizen, F. (2009). Chapter 35. Anesthetic implications of concurrent diseases. In Miller, E. (ed) *Miller's Anesthesia*, 7th edn. Elsevier, pp. 1086–1089.

Schwartz, J. J., Akhtar, S., and Rosenbaum, R. H. (2009). Chapter 49. Endocrine function. In Barash, P., Cullen, B., and Stoelting, R. (eds) *Clinical Anesthesia*, 6th edn. Lippincott Williams & Wilkins pp. 1279–1305.

Ladenson, K. (2012). Chapter 233. Thyroid. In Goldman, L. and Schafer, A. I. (eds) *Goldman's Cecil Medicine*, 24th edn. Elsevier. pp. 1450–1463.

Chapter

105

Parathyroid disorders

Hyung Sun Choi and Vesela Kovacheva

PTH effects: calcium and phosphate

Calcium metabolism

Plasma calcium exists in three forms:

- 50% protein, mostly albumin bound
- 45% free, ionized
- 5% phosphate, citrate bound

Normal total serum calcium is 8.8 to 10.4 mg/dl:

- Corrected serum calcium = Serum calcium + $(0.8 \times [4 - Albumin])$

Ionized calcium is involved in skeletal muscle contraction, coagulation, and neurotransmission. Its levels are affected by temperature and blood pH. For example, alkalosis increases negative charges on serum proteins and thus leads to a decrease in free calcium.

Parathyroid hormone (PTH)

- Maintains extracellular fluid calcium concentration via:
  - increased bone osteoclast activity
  - increased renal distal tubular reabsorption of calcium
  - increased synthesis of 1,25 dihydroxycholecalciferol
- Decreases renal absorption of phosphate and bicarbonate.

PTH secretion:

- regulated primarily by serum calcium
- influenced by phosphate, magnesium, and catecholamine levels

Hyperparathyroidism: physiological effects

Hyperparathyroidism: etiology:

- Primary – due to excess PTH secretion by parathyroid adenoma, and hyperplasia.
- Secondary – due to compensatory increase in PTH due to hypocalcemia (chronic renal disease).
- Ectopic – associated with lung cancer.

Hyperparathyroidism: signs and symptoms:

Hypercalcemia mnemonic – "**stones**, **bones**, abdominal **groans** and psychiatric **overtones**" (i.e., kidney **stones**, **bone** diseases, **pancreatitis**, and **psychosis**).

Hyperparathyroidism: anesthetic implications

- Preoperative:
  - treat hypercalcemia before surgery (especially if serum calcium >15 mg/dl)
  - hydrate with normal saline then furosemide to decrease calcium levels
  - bisphosphonates, mithramycin, and calcitonin can be used.
- Intraoperative:
  - avoid hypoventilation (acidosis increases calcium levels)
  - altered response to NMB agents (preexisting weakness)
  - osteopenic patients require careful positioning.
- Postoperative (similar to thyroid surgery postop):
  - laryngeal nerve injury can be associated with aspiration or hoarseness
  - hypocalcemia can lead to laryngospasm.

Hypoparathyroidism: postoperative manifestations and treatment

Hypoparathyroidism: etiology:

- Following thyroidectomy:
  - usually transient, but may be permanent.

Essential Clinical Anesthesia Review: Keywords, Questions and Answers for the Boards, ed. Linda S. Aglio, Robert W. Lekowski, and Richard D. Urman. Published by Cambridge University Press. © Cambridge University Press 2015.

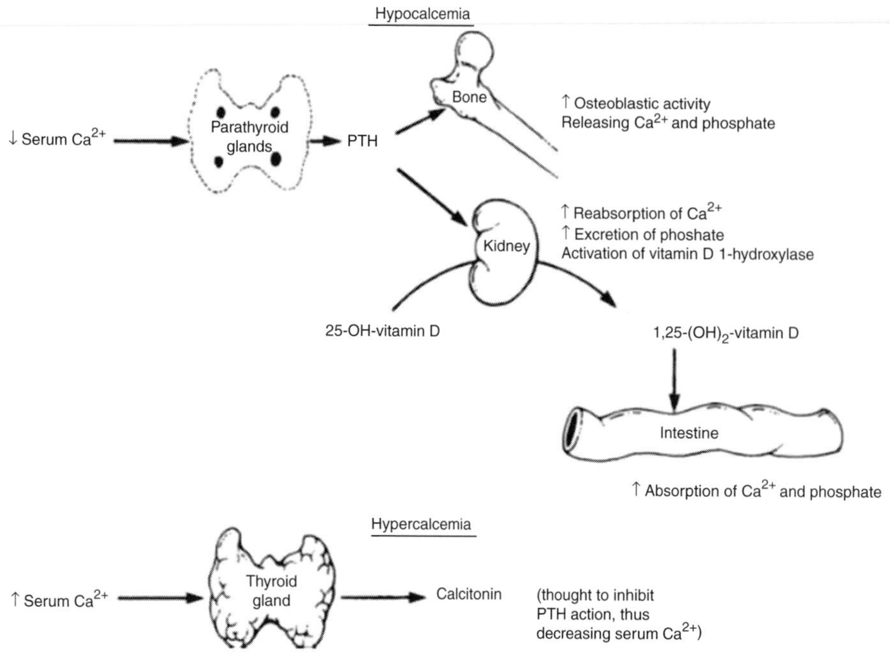

Figure 105.1 Hypocalcemia and hypercalcemia. (From Barash, P. G. *Clinical Anesthesia*, 5th edn., Figure 41.2.)

- After removal of parathyroid adenoma:
  - suppression of remaining parathyroid glands and accelerated remineralization of skeleton ("hungry bone syndrome").
- Other causes – neck trauma, severe hypomagnesemia, granulomatous disease, pseudohypoparathyroidism:
  - hypocalcemia due to renal resistance to PTH (genetic disease).

Hypoparathyroidism: manifested as hypocalcemia (serum calcium less than 4.5 meq/l):

- **Neurologic**: paresthesias (Chvostek, Trousseau signs), tetany, hyperactive reflexes, muscle.
- Cramps/weakness, seizures:
  - Chovstek's sign – Facial twitching after tapping on facial nerve
  - Trousseau's sign – Carpopedal spasm with tourniquet inflation above SBP for 3 min.
- **Respiratory**: laryngospasm, bronchospasm.
- **Cardiac**: arrhythmias, hypotension, bradycardia, QT prolongation.

Hypoparathyroidism: treatment:

- Airway – if vocal cord palsy, consider CPAP or intubation.
- IV calcium gluconate administration to maintain normal serum calcium.
- Myocardial depressants should be avoided.
- Alkalosis (hyperventilation, sodium bicarbonate) should be avoided.

Questions

1. A 67-year-old patient with multiple myeloma and hypercalcemia is scheduled for laparotomy. Which of the following is the primary risk associated with anesthetizing a patient with hypercalcemia?
   a. laryngospasm
   b. fluid imbalance
   c. coagulopathy
   d. hypotension

2. Hypercalcemia may be treated by each of the following EXCEPT for which?
   a. administration of mithramycin
   b. intravenous hydration
   c. correction of hypophosphatemia
   d. administration of calcitonin
   e. furosemide diuresis

3. A 38-year-old woman underwent subtotal thyroidectomy for Graves' disease. Twelve hours after the operation, the patent becomes irritable, complains of circumolar tingling, and develops stridor. Which of the following therapeutic interventions is most appropriate at this time?
   a. opening the surgical wound at the bedside
   b. administration of oral vitamin D
   c. start intravenous infusion of insulin and glucose
   d. administration of intravenous calcium gluconate

Answers

1. b. Hypercalcemia patients are often dehydrated. Therefore preoperative hydration is required.

2. c. Hyperparathyrodism is related to hypophosphatemia. Hypercalcemia is not related to hypophosphatemia.

3. d. Patient is showing signs/symptoms of hypocalcemia probably due to inadvertent removal of parathyroid gland. Calcium repletion is required at this point.

Further reading

Roizen, F. (2009). Chapter 35. Anesthetic implications of concurrent diseases. In Miller, E. (ed) *Miller's Anesthesia*, 7th edn. Elsevier, pp. 1089–1092.

Schwartz, J. J., Akhtar, S., and Rosenbaum, R. H. (2009). Chapter 49. Endocrine function. In Barash, P., Cullen, B., and Stoelting, R. (eds) *Clinical Anesthesia*, 6th edn. Lippincott Williams & Wilkins. pp. 1279–1305.

Wysolmerski, J. J. and Insogna, K. L. (2012). Chapter 253. The parathyroid glands, hypercalcemia and hypocalcemia. In Goldman, L. and Schafer, A. I. *Goldman's Cecil Medicine*, 24th edn. Elsevier, pp. 1591–1601.

Chapter

106

Pheochromocytoma and carcinoid tumors

Hyung Sun Choi and Vesela Kovacheva

Pheochromocytoma: manifestation and diagnosis

Pheochromocytoma is a heterogeneous group of neuroendocrine-secreting tumors that arise from chromaffin cells.

The manifestation of pheochromocytoma is the result of elevated levels of plasma catecholamines combined with an upregulated sympathetic nervous system.

Catecholamines are stress hormones, and thus stimulate lipolysis and glycogenolysis and lead to hyperglycemia.
Presentation:

- hypertension
- headache
- excessive sweating
- palpitations

Diagnosis:

- Traditionally, urinary metanephrines and VMA has been used.
- The plasma-free metanephrines test has proven superior (sensitivity >95%, specificity >80%).

Pheochromocytoma: preoperative management

Preoperative management:

- Hydration – pheochromocytoma patients are usually chronically hypovolemic.

- Hypertension management – α blockade (phenoxybenzamine) before β-blockade.

Medical management:

- Alpha blockers – give before beta-blockers to avoid unopposed alpha vasoconstriction:
  - phenoxybenzamine, prazosin
  - phentolamine (the only IV alpha blocker).
- Beta-blockers:
  - atenolol, propanolol
  - labetalol (also has alpha-blocking activity).
- Calcium channel blockers:
  - nicardipine.
- Alpha-methyl tyrosine
  - combined with alpha blockers
  - inhibits catecholamine synthesis by inhibition of tyrosine hydroxylase.

Roizen criteria:

- No BP reading >160/90 mm Hg for 24 h before surgery.
- Orthostatic hypotension with BP >80/45 should not be present.
- EKG should be free of ST/T changes for at least one week.
- No more than 1 PVC every 5 minutes.

Pheochromocytoma: intraoperative management

- Preoperative anxiolysis.
- Aggressive treatment of hemodynamic fluctuations, arterial catheter and central venous catheter indicated preinduction.
- Avoid sympathetic stimulants (i.e., ephedrine, ketamine)
- Avoid histamine-release drugs and halothane.
- Tumor isolation:
  - *hypertension* before isolation and *hypotension* after isolation → antihypertensives and vasoactive drugs

Essential Clinical Anesthesia Review: Keywords, Questions and Answers for the Boards, ed. Linda S. Aglio, Robert W. Lekowski, and Richard D. Urman. Published by Cambridge University Press. © Cambridge University Press 2015.

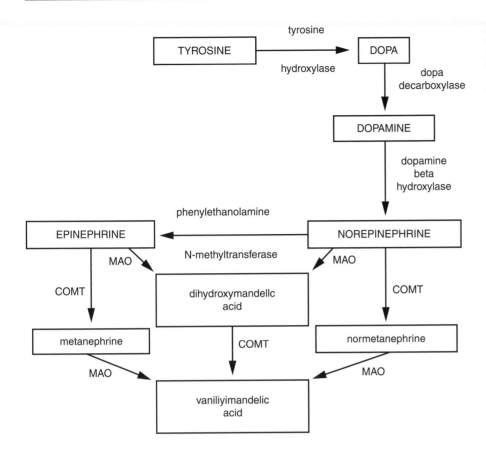

Figure 106.1 The synthesis and metabolism of endogenous catecholamines. COMT, catochol-O-methyltransferase; MAO, monoamine oxidase. (Reprinted with permission from Stoelting, R. K. and Dierdorf, S. F. eds. *Anesthesia and Co-existing Disease*. New York: Churchill-Livingstone.)

should be prepared (hypotension should be managed primarily by fluid replacement with adjunct vasoactive medecines)

- *hyperglycemia* before isolation and *hypoglycemia* after isolation warrants frequent glucose checks and tight control.
- Perioperative steroids should be considered if bilateral resection.

Pheochromocytoma: postoperative management

- Postoperative hemodynamic instability warrants close monitoring of patient's hemodynamics.
- Blood pressure and glucose should be closely monitored postoperatively.
- Some patients might still be hypertensive after the surgery due to elevated catecholamine stores in adrenergic nerve endings.

Carcinoid syndrome: manifestations

- Carcinoid syndrome – caused by secretion of vasoactive substances from carcinoid tumors:
    - serotonin
    - bradykinin
    - histamine

- Carcinoid is a rare tumor that arises from enterochromaffin cells mainly in the GI tract or bronchi.
- Since liver metabolizes all vasoactive substances, carcinoid syndrome implies pulmonary carcinoid or hepatic metastases.
- Symptoms: flushing, bronchoconstriction, diarrhea, right-sided heart disease.

Carcinoid syndrome: anesthetic implications

- Preoperative electrolyte and volume correction (diarrhea and high gastric output).
- *Octreotide* for morning of surgery and for intraoperative crises (i.e., hypotension, bronchospasm):
    - Octreotide – mimics somatostatin → reduces release of vasoactive agents.
- Consider ondansetron (serotonin 5-HT3 receptor antagonist) for antiemesis.
- Intraoperative measurement of electrolytes and glucose.
- Avoid drugs that induce histamine release.
- Consider invasive monitoring.
- Possible delayed awakening due to elevated serotonin.
- Multiple endocrine neoplasia (MEN).
- **MEN I:**
    - pancreatic islet cell tumors
    - pituitary adenoma

- parathyroid hyperplasia or neoplasm
- **MEN IIa:**
  - medullary thyroid CA
  - pheochromocytoma
  - parathyroid hyperplasia
- **MEN IIb:**
  - medullary thyroid CA
  - pheochromocytoma
  - multiple mucosal neuromas (IIb or III)

Questions

1. Each of the following drugs is useful for the preoperative preparation of patients with pheochromocytoma prior to surgical resection EXCEPT for which?
   a. phenoxybenzamine
   b. α-methyl-para-tyrosine
   c. octreotide
   d. prazosin

2. Which of the following is most likely to coexist with pheochromocytoma?
   a. pituitary adenoma
   b. medullary carcinoma of the thyroid
   c. insulinoma
   d. carcinoid tumor
   e. Conn syndrome

3. Which of the following statements concerning carcinoid tumors is TRUE?
   a. Carcinoid heart disease most commonly presents with mitral regurgitation.
   b. Carcinoid syndrome occurs in more than 50% of patients with carcinoid tumors.
   c. Carcinoid syndrome cannot occur unless liver metastases are present.
   d. Rectal tumors are most likely to metastasize to the liver.
   e. Treatment for symptomatic carcinoids is usually surgical.

4. Which of the following intraoperative complications would be most likely to occur during a resection of an isolated appendiceal carcinoid tumor?
   a. flushing
   b. hypotension
   c. bronchospasm
   d. hypertension
   e. none of the above

Answers

1. c. Both alpha blockers and alpha-methyl tyrosine can be used preoperatively to block the circulating catecholamine effect. Octreotide is used for carcinoid syndrome.
2. b. Both MEN IIa and IIb have the component of medullary thyroid cancer and pheochromocytoma.
3. e. Carcinoid heart disease presents with right heart valve disease. Liver metabolizes all the vasoactive substances, therefore carcinoid syndrome is rare. Carcinoid syndrome implies either pulmonary or hepatic metastases that bypass the liver.
4. e. Appendiceal tumor will not cause carcinoid syndrome unless it is metastasized to liver or lung, which bypasses the liver.

Further reading

Roizen, F. (2009). Chapter 35. Anesthetic implications of concurrent diseases. In Miller, E. (ed) *Miller's Anesthesia*, 7th edn. Elsevier, pp. 1084–1085.

Kinney, M. A., Narr, B. J., and Warner, M. A. (2002). Perioperative management of pheochromocytoma. *Journal of Cardiothoracic and Vascular Anesthesia* 16(3), 359–369.

Young, W. F. (2012). Chapter 235. Adrenal medulla, catecholamines, and pheochromocytoma. In Goldman, L. and Schafer, A. I. (eds) *Goldman's Cecil Medicine*, 24th edn. Elsevier, pp. 1470–1475.

Hande, K. (2012). Chapter 240. Carcinoid syndrome. In Goldman, L. and Schafer, A. I. (eds) *Goldman's Cecil Medicine*, 24th edn. Elsevier, pp. 1509–1511.

Chapter

107

Syndrome of inappropriate antidiuretic hormone, diabetes insipidus, and transsphenoidal pituitary surgery

Syed Irfan Qasim Ali and Vesela Kovacheva

Keywords

Syndrome of inappropriate antidiuretic
  hormone (SIADH)
Diabetes insipidus (DI)
Antidiuretic hormone (ADH)

Pituitary gland

The hypophysis is an organ that lies immediately beneath the hypothalamus, resting in a depression at the base of the skull called the sella turcica ("Turkish saddle"). It is comprised of two parts: anterior pituitary (adenohypophysis) secreting protein hormones and posterior pituitary (neuro hypophysis), which is an extension of the hypothalamus. Hypothalamic hormones control anterior pituitary hormonal secretion. Pituitary tumors are often hypersecretory, and therefore require surgical treatment. Depending on the size, they can be classified as macroadenomas larger than 10 mm in size, or microadenomas, smaller than 10 mm. They can be also functioning tumors causing hyperprolactinemia (prolactin), acromegaly (growth hormone), Cushing's disease (ACTH), or nonfunctioning tumors like craniophyrangiomas. Here we will discuss the physiology of *ADH* and anesthetic implications for transsphenoidal surgery for pituitary tumor resection.

Antidiuretic hormone

ADH or vasopressin is secreted by the posterior pituitary and synthesized in the hypothalamus as a response to elevated serum osmolarity (detected by osmoreceptors in the hypothalamus) and decreased extracellular volume (detected by stretch receptors in the left atrium). Arteriolar constriction of coronary, renal, and splanchnic vessels is seen with high *ADH* levels. By increasing the levels of factor VIII and von Willebrand factor, *ADH* helps with coagulation.

SIADH

Caused by excessive *ADH* production and manifested by oliguria, concentrated urine, and signs of hyponatremia.

Signs and symptoms of SIADH

Early presentation at serum sodium less than 125 mEq/l includes nausea, anorexia, and oliguria due to hyponatremic-related fluid shift.

Later on, as serum sodium further deceases, the symptoms progress to confusion, weakness, agitation, muscle cramps, obtundation, seizures, and, ultimately, coma.

Rate of sodium correction should not be faster than 12 mEq/l in first 24 hours due to risk of cerebral pontine myelinosis.

Hyponatremia and polyuria may indicate cerebral salt wasting syndrome.

Pseudohyponatremia occurs with severe hyperlipidemia and hyperproteinemia (as in multiple myeloma).

Table 107.1 Diagnosis and treatment of SIADH

Diagnosis	Treatment
Both hypothyroidism and glucocorticoid deficiency must be ruled out	Fluid restriction if serum sodium less than 120
Serum hyponatremia	Consider 3% hypertonic saline
Urine osmolarity >200 mOsm/l	Diuretics if fluid restriction not possible
FeNa >1% and urine sodium more than 30 mEq/l	Lithium/demeclocycline
Plasma osmolarity <270 mOsm/kg water	Euvolemic volume status

(Source: *Essential Clinical Anesthesia*, p. 673.)

Essential Clinical Anesthesia Review: Keywords, Questions and Answers for the Boards, ed. Linda S. Aglio, Robert W. Lekowski, and Richard D. Urman. Published by Cambridge University Press. © Cambridge University Press 2015.

Table 107.2 Causes of SIADH

Causes of SIADH	
Paraneoplastic syndromes	Small cell lung cancer
CNS processes	Multiple sclerosis, tumors, head trauma, delirium tremens, Guillain–Barré syndrome, infection
Pulmonary processes	Pneumonia, tuberculosis, positive pressure ventilation
Drugs	TCAs, chlorpropamide, clofibrate, NSAIDs, nicotine
Endocrine	hypothyroidism
Sympathetic activation	postoperative pain

CNS, central nervous system; TCAs, tricyclic antidepressants; NSAIDs, nonsteroidal anti-inflammatory drugs.
(Source: *Essential Clinical Anesthesia*, p. 673.)

Table 107.3 Correction of serum sodium level

Sodium deficit:

Na deficit = (Desired Na – Measured Na) × 0.6 × (Weight in kg)

Volume of hypertonic saline needed for correction:

Volume of 3% saline = (Na deficit)/513 mEq Na/l

Time needed for correction = (Desired Na – Measured Na)/0.5 mEq/l per hour

Rate of infusion = (Volume of 3% saline)/(Time needed for correction).

Elective surgeries should be postponed until serum sodium level is corrected to above 130 mEq/l.
(Source: *Essential Clinical Anesthesia*, p. 674.)

Diabetes insipidus

Water wasting is a result of *ADH* insufficiency. Central *diabetes insipidus* is due to decreased production or secretion of *ADH,* while nephrogenic *diabetes insipidus* is a result of kidney resistance to the effects of ADH.

Diagnosis of DI

DI is manifested by polyuria, polydipsia, hypovolemia, and hypernatremia. The diagnosis is based on serum hypernatremia, urine specific gravity 1.005 or less, urine osmolality <200 mOsm, and plasma osmolality of >287 mOsm.

Treatment

Central *DI* can be treated with aqueous *ADH* (100–20 mU/h), IM vasopressin, or intranasal desmopressin.

Nephrogenic *DI* is treated by resolving the underlying cause.

Table 107.4 Causes of diabetes insipidus

Central idiopathic (up to 50% of cases) autoimmune process with destruction of cells of the hypothalamus
Surgery: transsphenoidal resection of an adenoma may result in *DI* in up to 60% of patients with large tumors
Trauma: severe head injury, basal skull fracture, subarachnoid hemorrhage
Tumors: craniopharyngioma, pineal tumors
Other: hypoxic encephalopathy, anorexia nervosa, sarcoidosis, arteriovenous malformations
Nephrogenic drugs: lithium, demeclocycline, foscarnet, glyburide, methoxyflurane, amphotericin B
Familial: (rare) autosomal dominant
Collecting system insults: medullary cystic disease, ureteral obstruction

(Source: *Essential Clinical Anesthesia*, p. 674, Table 108.3.)

Table 107.5 Syndrome of inappropriate antidiuretic hormone (SIADH) versus diabetes insipidus (DI)

	SIADH	DI
Presentation	Hyponatremia	Polyuria
Plasma volume (awake patients)	Euvolemic (or slightly hypervolemic)	Euvolemic
Serum	Hypotonic (<275 mOsm/l)	Hypertonic (>310 mOsm/l)
Serum sodium	Decreasing (<135 mEq/l)	Increasing (>145 mEq/l)
Urine volume	Low (but not normally absent)	Voluminous (4 to 18 l/d)
Urine osmolarity	Relatively high (>100 mOsm/l)	Relatively low (<200 mOsm/l)
Urinary sodium	>20 mEq/l	>20 mEq/l
Treatment	Fluid restriction. If Na <120 mEq/l, hypertonic saline to correct sodium (but no faster than 1 mEq/l/h). Intravenous urea. Demeclocycline. Lithium (rarely used)	Consider supportive DDAVP (Desmopressin)

(Source: Nemergut et al. 2005. *Anesthesia and Analgesia* 101, 1170–1181, Table 2.)

Anesthetic considerations for pituitary surgery

1. Endocrine side effects from functional tumors.
2. Macroadenomas could cause increased intracranial pressure, visual disturbances, glucose intolerance leading to diabetes, and also airway obstruction.
3. Incidence of DI is less with an endonasal approach.

Preoperative management

1. Consider checking the CBC and electrolytes.
2. Particular attention to specific endocrine disorder like prolactinoma, acromegaly, or hyperthyroidism.
3. Careful assessment of airway.

Intraoperative management

1. Performed with mild head-up position to improve venous drainage, has slightly increased risk of venous air embolism.
2. Infiltration of nasal mucosa with lidocaine and epinephrine to reduce bleeding could lead to arrhythmia or hypertension.
3. Hypertensive episodes are common with this type of surgery, the goal is to keep the blood pressure close to baseline.
4. Potential risk for massive hemorrhage due to close proximity to major vessels.
5. Potential for CSF leak, perform Valsalva.

Postoperative complications

Common postoperative complications include pan-hypopituitarism, SIADH, DI, pain, CSF leak, or cranial nerve injury.

Questions

1. A 57-year-old 70 kg male after transsphenoidal resection of pituitary tumor was admitted in ICU, on postop day 1, his urine output is 150 ml/h, serum sodium is 124 mEq/l, CVP is 4, and the best course of action for this diagnosis should be:
   a. DDAVP
   b. fluid restriction
   c. 3% hypertonic saline
   d. careful monitoring

2. A 54-year-old woman has undergone transsphenoidal resection of a pituitary tumor, on her transfer to the ICU she is noticed to have a urine output of 150 ml/h and serum sodium of 151 mEq/l, the most likely diagnosis is:
   a. cerebral salt wasting syndrome
   b. SIADH
   c. diabetes insipidus
   d. normal response to surgery

3. Which of the following hormones are released by the posterior pituitary gland?
   a. TSH
   b. ACTH
   c. prolactin
   d. ADH

Answers

1. c. This is a case of cerebral salt wasting syndrome, which often occurs after intracranial surgery. Urine is relatively dilute and the flow rate is often high in cerebral salt wasting syndrome; urine is usually very concentrated and the flow rate is low in SIADH. So that is why dehydration and low CVP are noticed.
2. c. Diabetes insipidus is characterized by polyuria, hypernatremia, and hypertonic serum with hypotonic urine.
3. d. ADH is produced by the hypothalamus and secreted by the posterior pituitary.

Further reading

Summers, J. and Balachundhar, S. (2011). SIADH, diabetes insipidus and transsphenoidal pituitary surgery. In Vacanti, C. A., Sikka, P. J., Urman, R. D., Dershwitz, M., and Segal, B. S. (eds) *Essential Clinical Anesthesia.* Cambridge: Cambridge University Press, pp. 673–675.

Nemergut, E. C., Dumont, A. S., Barry, U. T., and Laws, E. R. (2005). Perioperative management of patients undergoing transsphenoidal pituitary surgery. *Anesthesia and Analgesia* 101, 1170–1181.

Chapter 108

Disorders of the adrenal cortex

Syed Irfan Qasim Ali and Vesela Kovacheva

Keywords

Cortisol
Aldosterone
Renin angiotensin
Cushing's syndrome
Conn syndrome
Addison's disease

The adrenal cortex is responsible for the synthesis of gluco-corticoid, mineralocorticoid, and androgen hormones.

Glucocorticoids

Most important glucocorticoid in the body is *cortisol,* which performs the following functions:

1. Mobilizes amino acids from extrahepatic tissues.
2. Stimulates gluconeogenesis (converting amino acids and fatty acids into glucose).
3. Stimulates glycogenesis in the liver (glycogen is the stored form of glucose).
4. Suppresses the inflammatory and immune responses.
5. Inhibits glucose uptake in muscle and adipose tissues.
6. Helps in mood and emotional stability.
7. In plasma, *cortisol* is free (10%), active form, and bound (90%), inactive form. The latter is bound to corticosterone binding protein, which prolongs the half-life and acts as a buffer.

Physical or physiological stress stimulates the release of ACTH and CRH, while *cortisol* inhibits it. Under normal conditions ACTH levels are highest after waking up followed by another lesser surge later in the day.

Cushing's syndrome

Cushing's syndrome is the result of an overproduction of glucocorticoids. *Cushing's* disease is caused by ACTH-producing pituitary adenoma, and ectopic ACTH-secreting bronchial or pancreatic carcinoid tumors, small cell lung cancer, and others.

ACTH-independent *Cushing's syndrome* is caused by adrenocortical adenoma, carcinoma, and other rare causes.

Signs and symptoms of Cushing's syndrome

They include weight gain, central obesity, brittle skin, easy bruising, osteoporosis and osteopenia, muscle weakness, hypertension, hypokalemia, glucose intolerance, diabetes, decreased libido, depression, irritability, increased risk of infections, deep venous thrombosis, and pulmonary embolism.

In addition, there may be hypervolemia and a hypokalemic metabolic alkalosis due to some mild mineralocorticoid effect.

Anesthetic considerations

1. Electrolyte corrections like hypokalemia.
2. Volume overload can be responsive to spironolactone.
3. Evaluate for difficult airway and difficult mask ventilation due to moon facies.
4. Fragile veins could make IV placement challenging.
5. Careful positioning since patients are prone to easy bruising.
6. Stress-dose steroids should be considered in patients with exogenous steroid use.

Mineralocorticoids

Aldosterone, the primary mineralocorticoid, works by increasing potassium and hydrogen excretion and sodium reabsorption. The *renin-angiotensin* system is the primary regulator of aldosterone.

Addison's disease

Adrenal insufficiency results from underproduction of steroid hormones. Destruction of adrenal cortex leads to primary adrenal insufficiency and is associated with both glucocorticoid and mineralocorticoid depletion. Tuberculosis is the most common cause in third world countries and autoimmune destruction is the most common in the Western world.

Essential Clinical Anesthesia Review: Keywords, Questions and Answers for the Boards, ed. Linda S. Aglio, Robert W. Lekowski, and Richard D. Urman. Published by Cambridge University Press. © Cambridge University Press 2015.

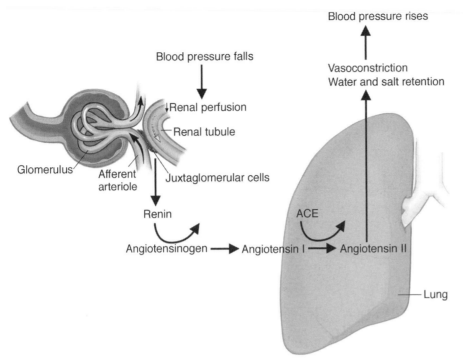

Blood pressure rises

Vasoconstriction
Water and salt retention

Blood pressure falls

↓Renal perfusion

Renal tubule

Glomerulus

Afferent
arteriole

Juxtaglomerular cells

Renin

ACE

Angiotensinogen → Angiotensin I → Angiotensin II

Lung

Figure 108.1
(From Vacanti et al. 2011. *Essential Clinical Anesthesia*, Cambridge University Press, Figure 109.2.)

Decreased ACTH → interruption of feedback inhibition HPA axis → elevated levels of corticotropin and melanocytes stimulating hormone (MSH) → bronze appearance of skin.

Signs and symptoms of adrenal insufficiency

A wide range of symptoms are due to glucocorticoid insufficiency, including fatigue, lack of energy, weight loss, joint pain, myalgia, fever, anemia, elevated TSH, hypoglycemia, and postural hypotension. Mineralocorticoid insufficiency causes abdominal pain, nausea, vomiting, hypotension, hyponatremia, and hyperkalemia. Mineralocorticoid deficiency or cutaneous hyperpigmentation are not seen in secondary adrenal insufficiency, which is caused due to insufficient ACTH production by the pituitary. Diarrhea, vomiting, abdominal pain, hypotension, or shock could be manifestations of *Addisonian crisis*, it may be difficult to distinguish from sepsis in critically ill patients.

Anesthetic considerations

Addisonian crisis is a life-threatening emergency. Therapeutic goals are as follows:

1. 100 mg IV hydrocortisone bolus with an additional 100 mg every 6 h for 24 h.
2. Hyperkalemia, hyponatremia, and other electrolytes need to be corrected.
3. Isotonic fluids.

4. Intraoperative glucocorticoid administration may lead to glucose intolerance and poor wound healing.

Primary hyperaldosteronism

Primary hyperaldosteronism is caused by a hyperactive adrenal cortex due to adenoma or hyperplasia (*Conn syndrome*), associated with increased secretion of *aldosterone*, which can cause hypokalemic metabolic alkalosis, hypervolemia without edema, hypertension, and depressed *renin* activity.

Anesthetic considerations

1. Address fluid overload and electrolyte abnormalities with potassium supplements and a potassium-sparing diuretic such as spironolactone.
2. Patients could also present with glucose intolerance and low ionized calcium.

Hypoaldosteronism

Hypoaldosteronism can be congenital or associated with certain medical conditions such as diabetes and renal failure. Metabolic abnormalities include hyponatremia and hyperkalemic metabolic acidosis. The patients are usually treated with 0.05–0.1 mg of fludrocortisones preoperatively and monitored closely perioperatively.

Etomidate can cause adrenal suppression for 24 hours, especially in critically ill patients.

Table 108.1 Glucocorticoid treatment regimens

Patients currently taking glucocorticoids	Prednisone 5 mg/day or dexamethasone 1 mg/day or equivalent	Minor surgery (e.g., herniorraphy) Moderate surgery (e.g., TAH) Major surgery (e.g., CABG)	Hydrocortisone 25 mg at induction Usual daily glucocorticoid dose + hydrocortisone 25 mg at induction + 100 mg/d for 24 h Usual daily glucocorticoid dose + hydrocortisone 25 mg at induction + 100 mg/d for 48–72 h
	High-dose immunosuppression	Any surgery	Give usual immunosuppressive doses during perioperative period
Patients who have taken glucocorticoids within the last year	Prednisone 5 mg/d or dexamethasone 1 mg/day or equivalent	Minor surgery (e.g., herniorraphy) Moderate surgery (e.g., TAH) Major surgery (e.g., CABG)	Hydrocortisone 25 mg at induction Hydrocortisone 25 mg at induction + 100 mg/d for 24 h Hydrocortisone 25 mg at induction +100 mg/d for 48–72 h

TAH, total abdominal hysterectomy; CABG, coronary artery bypass graft.
(Source: *Essential Clinical Anesthesia*, p.678, Table 109.1.)

Questions

1. A 55-year-old patient presents with hypotension, hypoglycemia, hyponatremia, hyperkalemia, metabolic acidosis, and bronze skin appearance; you suspect which of the following?
   a. primary adrenal insufficiency
   b. secondary adrenal insufficiency
   c. Conn syndrome
   d. Cushing's syndrome

2. A 79-year-old patient presents with hypertension, hypervolemia, hyperkalemia, and metabolic alkalosis. Which of the following adrenal disorders may you consider in this patient?
   a. primary adrenal insufficiency
   b. secondary adrenal insufficiency
   c. Conn syndrome
   d. Cushing's syndrome

3. Etomidate causes adrenal suppression by inhibiting which of the following enzymes?
   a. 3β-hydroxysteroid dehydrogenase
   b. 21-hydroxylase
   c. 11β-hydroxylase
   d. 3β-hydroxysteroid dehydrogenase

Answers

1. a. In primary adrenal insuffiency hyperkalemia, hypovolemia, hyponatremia, and metabolic acidosis are present, and elevated levels of corticotropin and melanocytes stimulating hormone (MSH) cause a bronze appearance of the skin.
2. c. Increased secretion of aldosterone (Conn syndrome) causes hypertension, hypervolemia (without edema), suppressed renin activity, and hypokalemic metabolic alkalosis.
3. c. Etomidate causes adrenal suppression by inhibiting 11β-hydroxylase.

Further reading

Summers, J. and Balachundhar, S. (2011). Disorders of the adrenal cortex. In Vacanti, C. A., Sikka, P. J., Urman, R. D., Dershwitz, M., and Segal, B. S. (eds) *Essential Clinical Anesthesia*. Cambridge: Cambridge University Press, pp. 676–680.

Arlt, W. (2012). Chapter 342. Disorders of the adrenal cortex. In Longo, D. L., Fauci, A.S., Kasper, D.L., Hauser, S.L., Jameson, J.L., and Loscalzo J. (eds), *Harrison's Principles of Internal Medicine*, 18th edn. www.accessmedicine.com/content.aspx?aID=9140931.

Chapter

109

Malignant hyperthermia

Zinaida Chepurny and Alvaro A. Macias

Keywords

Malignant hyperthermia (MH): pathophysiology
MH triggering agents
Masseter muscle rigidity (MMR)
Signs of MH
Differential diagnosis of MH
Neuroleptic malignant syndrome (NMS)
MH treatment
Caffeine halothane contracture test (CHCT)
Management of MH-susceptible patient
Diseases associated with MH

Table 109.1 Drugs that can trigger MH

Halogenated general anesthetics
Cyclopropane
Desflurane
Enflurane
Ether
Halothane
Isoflurane
Methoxyflurane
Sevoflurane
Depolarizing muscle relaxants (e.g., succinycholine)

(*Source*: Vacanti, C.A., Sikka, P.K., Urman, R.D., et al. 2011. *Essential Clinical Anesthesia*. New York: Cambridge University Press, p. 681.)

Malignant hyperthermia is a disease that can either be a result of an autosomal dominant inheritance pattern, or a de novo mutation with mutations of either RyR gene (ryanodine receptor, which is a calcium-release channel found on sarcoplasmic reticulum SR) on chromosome 19 and accounts for 50% to 80% of cases, or DHPR gene (dihydropyridine receptor, a voltage-gated Ca^{2+} channel). Mutations in these genes lead to altered function of the calcium-release channels, causing increased calcium release from SR and intracellular build up of Ca^{2+}.

MH triggering agents: all depolarizing muscle relaxants and all volatile general anesthetics. Upon exposure, rapid release of Ca^{2+} from SR occurs, increase in muscle metabolism ensues, activation of contractile elements causes contracture of skeletal muscle, and consumption of ATP increases aerobic and anaerobic metabolism. Hypermetabolic state of O_2, glucose consumption, and CO_2 production lead to acidemia, hyperkalemia, rhabdomyolysis, and cardiac dysrhythmia.

Contracture of skeletal muscle seen in MH is not responsive to relaxation with nondepolarizing neuromuscular relaxants.

Diseases associated with MH: *central core disease, multiminicore disease and King–Denborough syndrome*.

Masseter muscle rigidity (MMR) is a contraction of the jaw, which prevents full mouth opening following administration of succinylcholine, with flaccid paralysis elsewhere. Incidence of MH following MMR depends on the degree of muscle tone

increase. In patients who experience extreme jaw muscle tension, 50% of them may be susceptible to MH. Patient should be closely monitored for early signs of MH and elective surgery postponed based on clinical assessment. In case of emergency, procedure may continue with nontriggering anesthetic. If there are clinical signs of MH postoperatively, individuals should be treated and have serum CK measured at 6-hour intervals over the next 24 hours or until it plateaus, urine should be analyzed for myoglobinuria, and monitor for temperature changes. If there is no clinical evidence of MH, patients may be discharged that day.

Signs of MH: following exposure to a triggering agent, tachycardia and tachypnea can be seen. In cases of mechanical ventilation, the first signs are hypercarbia or increase in end-tidal CO_2 unresponsive to increase in minute ventilation. Late signs of MH include hyperthermia, whole body rigidity, cyanosis, mottling, and sweating. It is important to remember that many individuals have had prior exposures to triggering agents that did not initially result in an MH episode, but subsequently experienced one.

One must obtain an ABG and switch to a nontriggering anesthetic. The result will most likely be consistent with mixed respiratory and metabolic acidosis in addition to hyperkalemia, hypercalcemia, and lactic acidemia. Further lab work will reveal an increase in serum CK and gross myoglobinuria

Essential Clinical Anesthesia Review: Keywords, Questions and Answers for the Boards, ed. Linda S. Aglio, Robert W. Lekowski, and Richard D. Urman. Published by Cambridge University Press. © Cambridge University Press 2015.

(urine dipstick positive for blood with absent RBCs). Cardiac arrest from ventricular fibrillation is the most common cause of death in MH due to the concurrent hyperkalemia and metabolic acidosis.

Differential diagnosis of MH includes pheochromocytoma, sepsis, thyrotoxicosis, mitochondrial myopathies, serotonin syndrome, and *neuroleptic malignant syndrome (NMS)*. NMS results from treatment with antipsychotic agents and has a clinical presentation similar to MH, including HTN, tachycardia, muscle rigidity, fever, and acidosis. Unlike MH, NMS occurs after long-term exposure to antipsychotics, is not inherited, and is caused by dopamine depletion in the CNS. A dopamine agonist, bromocriptine, is used to treat NMS.

Dantrolene is a lipophylic muscle relaxant that decreases the resting intracellular Ca^{2+} concentration of the myocyte to baseline levels and restores baseline muscle metabolism. Half-life of IV dantrolene is 12 hours, with therapeutic levels lasting four to six hours. One 20 mg vial of dantrolene (which also contains 3 g of mannitol) needs to be dissolved in 60 ml of sterile water prior to administration. Side effects include muscle weakness lasting up to 24 hours (100%), phlebitis (10%), GI discomfort (3%), and respiratory failure (3%).

Treatment of an acute MH episode:

1. Stop all inhalation agents, succinylcholine, and call for help.
2. Hyperventilate with 100% O_2 at >10 l/min.
3. Administer 2.5 mg/kg of IV dantrolene every 5 min up to a total of 10 mg/kg or until normalization of HR, body temperature, and $PaCO_2$.
4. In case of metabolic acidosis, administer sodium bicarbonate 2–4 mEq/kg along with intravenous fluid.
5. Actively cool patient with ice packs in axillae and groin, perform iced gastric and rectal lavage. Stop cooling when core temperature is 38°C to avoid hypothermia.
6. Hyperkalemia should be managed with insulin, glucose, hyperventilation, and sodium bicarbonate.
7. Cardiac arrhythmia usually responds to dantrolene therapy, correction of acidosis, and hyperventilation. **Calcium channel blockers should be avoided** during treatment of acute MH episode, because concurrent use of verapamil and dantrolene can cause myocardial depression and hyperkalemia.
8. Serial blood gases should be performed along with serum creatinine, myoglobin, CK, and coagulation profile.
9. Notify MH hotline 1–800–644–9737 and visit www.mhaus.org for further MH crisis resources.

Complications of MH include recurrence of it (in 20% of patients) within hours of first episode, which may require re-dosing of dantrolene every four to six hours; myogrobinuric renal failure requiring alkalinization of urine and administration of mannitol to maintain urine output >1 ml/kg/h; DIC; cerebral edema and CHF.

In the United States, the *caffeine halothane contracture test* is the gold standard for diagnosis of MH, with sensitivity of 97% and 78% specificity. During CHCT, a biopsy sample of vastus lateralis is exposed to different concentrations of caffeine, 3% halothane, and a combination of the two. **MH-susceptible** muscle will have an abnormal response (contracture) to caffeine, halothane, or the combination of both. Negative biopsies will have a normal response to halothane, caffeine, and their combination.

Management of the MH-susceptible patient: during the preoperative interview, one should gather information about family history of MH, previous MH episode, and its documentation. Vaporizers should be removed or disabled from the anesthesia machine, circuit should be changed, including CO_2 absorbent, and the machine must be flushed with O_2 at 10 l/min for 20 min or longer based on manufacturer recommendations. Ice and dantrolene must be available in the operating room or its vicinity. Patients should receive regional, local, or total intravenous anesthetic with nondepolarizing relaxants if necessary.

Questions

1. Use of which of the following agents can be a trigger for patients susceptible to MH?
   a. amide local anesthetics
   b. nitrous oxide
   c. sevoflurane
   d. propranolol

2. What is the first sign of MH in a patient under general anesthesia who is mechanically ventilated?
   a. tachycardia
   b. hyperthermia
   c. muscle rigidity
   d. increase in end-tidal CO_2

Answers

1. c. In patients susceptible to MH, all possible MH triggering agents must be avoided, including all volatile anesthetics. Nitrous oxide is not contraindicated.
2. d. Tachypnea may not be readily recognized in patients under general anesthesia who are mechanically ventilated. An increase in end-tidal CO_2 will ensue, despite aggressive hyperventilation. Tachycardia may be due to other causes.

Further reading

Vacanti, C. A., Sikka, P.K., Urman, R.D., et al. (2011) *Essential Clinical Anesthesia.* New York: Cambridge University Press, pp. 681–684.

Barash, P. G., Cullen, B. F., Stoelting, R. K., et al. (2006). *Clinical Anesthesia.* Philadelphia: Lippincott Williams Wilkins, pp. 598–613.

Miller, R. D. (2005). *Miller's Anesthesia,* 6th edn. Philadelphia: Elsevier Churchill-Livingstone, pp. 1180–1181.

Wappler, F. (2001). Malignant hyperthermia. *European Journal of Anesthesiology* 18, 632–652.

Lambert, C. et al. (1994). Malignant hyperthermia in a patient with hypokalemic periodic paralysis. *Anesthesia and Analgesia* 79, 1012.

Robinson, R. L. et al. (2003). Recent advances in the diagnosis of malignant hyperthermia susceptibility: how confident can we be of genetic testing? *European Journal of Human Genetics* 11, 342.

Hirshey Dirksen, S. J. et al. (2011). Special article: future directions in malignant hyperthermia research and patient care. *Anesthesia and Analgesia* 113(5), 1108–1119.

Hopkins, P. M. (2011). Malignant hyperthermia: pharmacology of triggering. *British Journal of Anaesthesia* 107(1), 48–56.

O'Flynn, R. P. et al. (1994). Masseter muscle rigidity and malignant hyperthermia susceptibility in pediatric patients: an update on management and diagnosis. *Anesthesiology* 80, 1228.

Chapter

110

Myasthenia gravis

Zinaida Chepurny and Alvaro A. Macias

Keywords

Myasthenia gravis (MG)
MG diagnosis
Myasthenia gravis (MG) preop risk evaluation
Anesthetic management of patient with MG
Neonatal MG
Myasthenic crisis vs. cholinergic crisis
Treatment of myasthenic crisis
NMB in myasthenia gravis
Predictive risk factors for postop ventilatory support
Lambert–Eaton myasthenic syndrome vs. myasthenia gravis
NMB in myasthenic syndrome

Myasthenia gravis is an autoimmune disorder caused by circulating antibodies against nicotinic acetylcholine receptors (AChRs) at the postsynaptic neuromuscular junction; leading to a decreased effective concentration of AChRs on postsynaptic membrane.

The patient demonstrates fatigue of skeletal muscle with repetitive use, affecting eyelids and extraocular muscles first. As the disease progresses it leads to respiratory involvement causing respiratory failure.

Diagnosis of MG is made with administration of 10 mg IV of edrophonium (a short-acting acetylcholinesterase inhibitor, which transiently increases the concentration of ACh at the NMJ) and causes improvement of symptoms in 45 seconds. A single-fiber EMG reveals more than a 10% decrease in muscle action potential during a 2 to 3 Hz stimulation. The most specific modality is presence of circulating autoantibodies.

Approximately, 85% of MG patients have an anti-AChR antibody. However, the remaining seronegative patients have an anti-MuSK IgG and present with bulbar (ptosis, diplopia, dysphagia) and respiratory weakness instead of limb weakness.

There are several types of MG: autoimmune, congenital, drug-induced, and neonatal. *Neonatal MG* is due to placental transfer of maternal anti-AChR antibodies. It manifests as generalized weakness in the neonate, placing them at risk of respiratory insufficiency. Symptoms typically resolve within three to four weeks.

Medical treatment: AChE inhibitors such as pyridostigmine are first-line therapy and result in the build up of ACh at the NMJ (neostigmine can be used as well, but has a shorter half-life of one to two hours). Pyridostigmine has fewer muscarinic side effects and half-life of three to six hours. Corticosteroids can be added to the above regimen and can contribute to already existing muscle weakness. Azathioprine is a purine analogue, which suppresses proliferation of T and B cells and is used in patients that do not tolerate high-dose corticosteroids (ADRs: myelosuppression, hepatotoxicity). Use of cyclophosphamide is limited due to its extensive side effect profile of delayed effect, myelosuppression, cardiotoxicity, leucopenia, and hemorrhagic cystitis.

Surgical treatment: thymectomy is recommended for post-puberty patients. Improvement of symptoms can take months to years following surgery.

Myasthenic crisis and *cholinergic crisis* can both present with respiratory failure. Myasthenic crisis can be precipitated by concurrent infection, disease exacerbation, surgery, pregnancy, tapering of immunosuppressive medications, or noncompliance with cholinesterase inhibitor. Cholinergic crisis is caused by increased vagal tone and excessive ACh stimulation of striated muscle, producing flaccid muscle paralysis from overdose of cholinesterase inhibitor. Increased vagal reflexes cause **SLUDGE** (salivation, lacrimation, urination, defecation, erection), hyperperistalsis, miosis, bradycardia, bronchoconstriction, and bronchial secretions.

Diagnosis: administer 2 mg IV of edrophonium initially and monitor patient closely for cholinergic side effects. If patient does not experience them, continue with additional 8 mg IV edrophonium. Muscle strength will improve in patients with myasthenic crisis and decrease in cholinergic crisis.

Treatment of myasthenic crisis includes a longer acting cholinesterase inhibitor, and on occasion plasma exchange

---

Essential Clinical Anesthesia Review: Keywords, Questions and Answers for the Boards, ed. Linda S. Aglio, Robert W. Lekowski, and Richard D. Urman. Published by Cambridge University Press. © Cambridge University Press 2015.

and IVIG. Plasma exchange decreases the patient's titer of anti-AChR antibodies by replacing the patient's plasma with albumin, saline, and plasma protein fraction. IVIG entails five-day long administration of pooled human IgG, which by unknown mechanism causes a decrease in native antibody production. Cholinergic crisis should be managed with respiratory support, discontinuation of ACh inhibitor, and symptomatic treatment of cholinergic effects.

Anesthetic management

The preoperative evaluation should include a thorough history, including recent course of disease, muscle groups involved, current and past drug therapy, and baseline PFTs. Patients with a weak cough or involvement of respiratory or bulbar muscles are at increased risk of aspiration and postoperative atelectasis.

Intraoperative management: MG patients are **resistant to succinylcholine** because of reduced number of AChR on the postsynaptic membrane. These patients require a higher concentration of succinylcholine to block a reduced number of AChRs in order to inhibit impulse transmission. It is important to note that the duration of action of succinylcholine can be prolonged if the patient is managed with AChE inhibitors for treatment.

NMB in myasthenia gravis: MG results in **increased sensitivity to nondepolarizing** NMBs, because of the decreased number of AChRs that need to be blocked at the NMJ. Baseline TOF ratio should be obtained prior to NMB administration. The dose of NMBs should be reduced to 40% and titrated to the effect. Patients with a decreased baseline TOF ratio are at an increased risk for postop weakness and possibility of prolonged mechanical ventilation.

Leventhal risk factors for postop ventilatory support (in patients undergoing transsternal thymectomy):

1. disease duration >6 years
2. peak inspiratory pressure <−20 cm H_2O
3. preoperative vital capacity <4 ml/kg or <2.9 l
4. pyridostigmine dose >750 mg/day
5. coexisting pulmonary disease

Medications that can exacerbate muscle weakness and should be avoided include lithium, phenytoin, aminoglycosides, clindamycin, ciprofloxacin, propranolol, magnesium, and procainamide.

Myasthenic syndrome (Lambert–Eaton myasthenic syndrome) is a paraneoplastic syndrome, which results from autoantibodies against presynaptic voltage-gated Ca^{2+} channels that reduce the amount of ACh released at the motor postsynaptic membrane. Presents as proximal muscle weakness of the lower extremities and can spread to involve upper extremities, respiratory, and bulbar muscle groups. The cardinal feature of LEMS is improvement of muscle strength with exercise and unresponsiveness of symptoms to steroids or AChE inhibitors, unlike in patients with MG.

Table 110.1 Comparison of MG and LEMS

Effect	LEMS	MG
Muscles	Proximal limb weakness (legs > arms) Exercise improves strength Muscle pain common Reflexes absent or decrease	Extraocular, bulbar, and facial muscle weakness Fatigue with exercise Muscle pain uncommon Reflexes normal
Gender	Male > female	Female > male
Coexisting pathology	Small cell carcinoma of the lung	Thymoma
Succinylcholine	Sensitive	Resistant
Nondepolarizing muscle relaxants	Sensitive	Sensitive
AChE agents	Decreased (poor) response	Good response

(Source: Vacanti, C. A., Sikka, P. K., Urman, R. D. et al. 2011. Essential Clinical Anesthesia. New York: Cambridge University Press, p. 688.)

LEMS patients have **increased sensitivity to both depolarizing and nondepolarizing NMBs**. Serious consideration should be given to neuromuscular blockade during surgery, as their reversal is often incomplete.

Questions

1. Which of the following agents can WORSEN muscular weakness in patients with myasthenia gravis?
   a. lithium
   b. ketamine
   c. propofol
   d. pyridostigmine

2. In patients with myasthenic syndrome, which of the following is TRUE?
   a. muscle weakness is exacerbated with exercise
   b. resistance to nondepolarizing NMBs
   c. resistance to succinylcholine
   d. absent or decreased reflexes

Answers

1. a. Medications such as glucocorticoids, lithium, aminoglycoside antibiotics, clindamycin, ciprofloxacin, propranolol, phenytoin, magnesium, and procainamide can exacerbate muscular weakness in patients with MG.
2. d. Unlike patients with myasthenia gravis, LEMS patients have decreased or absent reflexes (see Table 110.1).

Further reading

Vacanti, C. A., Sikka, P. K., Urman, R. D. et al. (2011). *Essential Clinical Anesthesia.* New York: Cambridge University Press, pp. 685–689.

Barash, P. G., Cullen, B. F., Stoelting, R. K. et al. (2009). *Clinical Anesthesia.* Philadelphia: Lippincott Williams & Wilkins, pp. 1064–1068.

Leventhal, S. R. et al. (1980). Predicting the need for postoperative mechanical ventilation in myasthenia gravis. *Anesthesiology* 53, 26–30.

Abel, M. et al. (2002). Anesthetic implications of myasthenia gravis. *Mount Sinai Journal of Medicine* 69, 31–37.

Miller, R. D. (2010). *Miller's Anesthesia,* 7th edn. Philadelphia: Elsevier Churchill-Livingstone, pp. 1876–1878.

Sanders, D. B. (2002). The Lambert–Eaton myasthenic syndrome. *Advances in Neurology* 88, 189–201.

Chapter 111

Muscular dystrophy and myotonic dystrophy

Zinaida Chepurny and Alvaro A. Macias

Keywords

- Duchenne muscular dystrophy (DMD)
- DMD cardiac implications
- Becker muscular dystrophy
- Emery–Dreifuss muscular dystrophy
- Limb-girdle muscular dystrophy
- Fascioscapulohumeral muscular dystrophy
- Congenital muscular dystrophy
- Muscular dystrophy anesthetic considerations
- Myotonic dystrophy
- Myotonia congenita
- Hyperkalemic periodic paralysis vs. hypokalemic periodic paralysis
- Central core disease

Duchenne muscular dystrophy (DMD) is the most common childhood muscular dystrophy. It is an X-linked recessive disorder in which the absence of dystrophin in the skeleton of myocytes' membranes causes muscle degeneration and atrophy (with leakage of intracellular proteins, including CPK). Atrophied myocytes are replaced by fibro-fatty infiltrates causing pseudohyperhtrophy of the muscle. Patients develop progressive proximal muscle weakness between ages two and five, with respiratory and cardiac muscle involvement eventually leading to death by the age of 30. Medical management consists of chronic steroids, which slow the progression of the disease by increasing insulin-like growth factor-I and stimulating muscle repair and regeneration.

Progressive **loss of cardiac muscle mass** (usually becomes significant after muscular disease develops) is reflected by a decrease in R-wave amplitude in the lateral precordial leads on EKG. Eventually, **dilated cardiomyopathy** ensues with fatty infiltration of the myocardium, involving posterobasal and lateral LV wall, ventricular dysrhythmia, and mitral regurgitation. Preoperative testing for patients with DMD should include EKG, echocardiography, PFTs, and cardiac MRI.

There is increased blood loss during scoliosis surgery, perhaps due to impaired vasoconstriction secondary to absence on dystrophin, platelet dysfunction, and reduced neuronal nitric oxide synthase.

Becker muscular dystrophy is an X-linked recessive disorder with a milder course of disease than DMD. These patients exhibit a reduced amount of partially functional dystrophin protein.

Emery–Dreifuss muscular dystrophy is characterized by contractures of the elbows, Achilles tendons, and humeropectoral muscle weakness. It can be either AD or X-linked recessive. Cardiac conduction defects are usually fatal and patients require **implantable defibrillators**.

Limb-girdle muscular dystrophy presents with shoulder and pelvic-girdle weakness; cardiomyopathy and AV conduction defects can also occur. This is a slow progressing disorder affecting families of North African descent.

Fascioscapulohumeral muscular dystrophy is an autosomal dominant disease. It has diverse manifestations, such as facial, scapulohumeral, anterior tibial, and pelvic-girdle weakness. In addition, patients may have deafness, retinal disease, and cardiac conduction defects.

Congenital muscular dystrophy is an AR disorder rarely seen outside of Japan. It carries a poor prognosis. Patients exhibit hypotonia at birth, respiratory and feeding difficulty, seizures, mental retardation, and death by ten years of age.

Anesthetic considerations in muscular dystrophy:

1. Succinylcholine should be avoided in these patients because hyperactive muscle membranes have been associated with rhabdomyolysis, hyperkalemia, and cardiac arrest secondary to release of intracellular contents. There is some speculation that inhalational agents cause a release of Ca^{2+} from the SR, which may cause damage to the myocyte cell membrane and result in rhabdomyolysis. Thus some experts believe that it is better to avoid volatile anesthetics.

2. Due to degeneration of alimentary smooth muscle, patients will have intestinal hypomotility and gastroparesis, causing increased risk of aspiration.

3. There is a reduced sensitivity of the nicotinic AChR to nondepolarizing muscle relaxants, with prolonged effect

Essential Clinical Anesthesia Review: Keywords, Questions and Answers for the Boards, ed. Linda S. Aglio, Robert W. Lekowski, and Richard D. Urman. Published by Cambridge University Press. © Cambridge University Press 2015.

due to patient's inability to mount enough contractile force from muscle wasting. NMB reversal should be avoided, as individual patient response is unpredictable.

Ion channel myotonias are a group of disorders with abnormal sodium, calcium, and chloride channels in muscle. **Myotonia** is the delayed relaxation of skeletal muscle following voluntary contraction, secondary to muscle membrane ion channels' dysfunction.

Myotonic dystrophy is the most common form of muscular dystrophy in adults. It is classified into two types based on the loci of gene mutation. Type 1 is the more common form and is further classified by age of onset.

Adult onset myotonic dystrophy is an AD disorder, which presents during the second or third decade of life, with myotonia, progressive myopathy, insulin resistance, DM, frontal balding, cataracts, thyroid dysfunction, adrenal insufficiency, and testicular atrophy. **AV conduction delay** (which can worsen with inhalational agents), atrial and ventricular dysrhythmias, along with LV systolic and diastolic dysfunction, comprise cardiac complications. Death in these patients is usually from respiratory or cardiac complications.

Succinylcholine produces an exaggerated contracture of skeletal muscle, which can make tracheal intubation and ventilation impossible. Therefore **succinylcholine should be avoided**. These patients also exhibit increased sensitivity to nondepolarizing NMBs, and reversal with neostigmine may provoke myotonia. Their response to respiratory-depressant effects of benzodiazepines, opioids, and inhaled anesthetics should be closely monitored.

Myotonia congenita: Thomsen (autosomal dominant) and Becker (autosomal recessive) both result from mutations in chloride ion channels, which decreases chloride conductance into the myocyte. Patients have difficulty initiating muscle movements, followed by impaired muscle relaxation. Muscle stiffness can be precipitated by succinylcholine, anticholinesterases, cold, and shivering. Anesthetic considerations are similar to myotonic dystrophy.

Hyperkalemic periodic paralysis vs. hypokalemic periodic paralysis: caused by distinct mutations of skeletal muscle, voltage-gated sodium channel in hyperkalemic periodic paralysis, and voltage-gated calcium channel in hypokalemic periodic paralysis. Both diseases have intermittent muscle weakness associated with hyperkalemia or hypokalemia, respectively, with different triggers.

A potassium-rich meal, rest after exercise, or stress can precipitate an episode of hyperkalemic periodic paralysis that can last up to an hour. **Succinylcholine, cholinesterase inhibitors, and potassium-containing IV fluids should be avoided during surgery.** Propofol administration may be beneficial due to inhibition of both normal and mutated voltage-gated sodium channels. Treatment includes administration of glucose, insulin, calcium, and epinephrine.

Hypokalemic periodic paralysis can be triggered by carbohydrate-rich meals, insulin, exercise, and stress. Associated voltage-gated calcium channel mutation commonly affects muscle groups in the arms and legs. General anesthesia, long-acting NMBs, and glucose-containing IV fluids can precipitate postoperative paralysis. Spinal and epidural anesthesia are safe in this population.

In acquired neuromyotonia, autoantibodies bind presynaptic voltage-gated potassium channels and cause inhibition of repolarization, rendering myocytes in a hyperexcitable state. Patients exhibit muscle cramps, twitching at rest, insomnia, mood changes, and hallucinations. Spontaneous muscle twitching can be inhibited by either a spinal or epidural anesthetic (not a peripheral nerve block). There is no contraindication to succinylcholine. NMBs can provide muscle relaxation.

Central core disease (CCD) is an autosomal dominant disorder caused by a ryanodine receptor mutation on chromosome 19, the location of which is responsible for genetic linkage of CCD to malignant hyperthermia. Biopsy of affected tissue contains central "cores" that are devoid of mitochondria in muscle fibers. Symptoms are variable but usually include hypotonia at birth and skeletal muscle weakness. During surgery, all of the MH precautions should be taken because patients are MH-susceptible.

Questions

1. Which of the following conditions is genetically linked with malignant hyperthermia?
   a. central core disease
   b. Duchenne muscular dystrophy
   c. acquired neuromyotonia
   d. hyperkalemic periodic paralysis

2. Which of the following agents can be used safely in patients with myotonic dystrophy?
   a. neostigmine
   b. propofol
   c. succinylcholine
   d. vecuronium

Answers

1. a. Ryanodine receptor mutation implicated in CCD is genetically linked to mutation in the ryanodine receptor implicated in MH; both of which are found on chromosome 19.
2. b. Succinylcholine and reversal agents may provoke myotonia. These patients also exhibit increased sensitivity to nondepolarizing NMBs. Propofol is the best answer choice.

Further reading

Vacanti, C. A., Sikka, P. K., Urman, R. D. et al. (2011). *Essential Clinical Anesthesia*. New York: Cambridge University Press, pp. 690–694.

Barash, P. G., Cullen, B. F., Stoelting, R. K. et al. (2009). *Clinical Anesthesia*. Philadelphia: Lippincott Williams & Wilkins, pp. 622–628.

Jurkat-Rott, K. et al. (2002). Skeletal muscle channelopathies. *Journal of Neurology* 249, 1493.

Klingler, W. et al. (2005). Complications of anaesthesia in neuromuscular disorders. *Neuromuscular Disorders* 15, 195.

Miller, R. D. (2010). *Miller's Anesthesia*, 7th edn. Philadelphia: Elsevier Churchill-Livingstone, pp. 1177–1182.

Hayes, J. et al. (2008). Duchenne muscular dystrophy: an old anesthesia problem revisited. *Paediatric Anaesthesia* 18(2), 100–106.

Ophthalmic procedures

Caryn Barnet and Dongdong Yao

Keywords

Intraocular pressure
Oculocardiac reflex
Intravitreal gas bubbles
Retrobulbar block
Peribulbar block
Open globe injury

Ocular neurovascular supply

- sensory innervation: ophthalmic branch of trigeminal nerve (cranial nerve V)
- vision: optic nerve (CN II)
- motor innervation: oculomotor nerve (CN III), trochlear nerve (CN IV), abducens nerve (CN VI)
- arterial supply: ophthalmic artery (from internal carotid artery)

There are six extraocular eye muscles: (1) superior rectus, innervated by oculomotor nerve, causes orbit elevation; (2) inferior rectus: innervated by oculomotor nerve, causes orbit depression; (3) lateral rectus: innervated by abducens nerve, causes orbit abduction; (4) medial rectus: innervated by oculomotor nerve, causes orbit adduction; (5) inferior oblique: innervated by oculomotor nerve, causes orbit external rotation, elevation, and abduction; (6) superior oblique: innervated by trochlear nerve, causes orbit internal rotation, depression, and abduction.

Oculomotor (CN III) palsy results in a characteristic "down and out" position of eye. This position is secondary to unopposed lateral rectus activity causing orbit abduction (CN VI) and superior oblique activity causing orbit depression (CN IV).

Intraocular perfusion pressure is the difference between the mean arterial pressure (MAP) and the *intraocular pressure (IOP)*.

Normal IOP is 10–20 mm Hg

Factors that raise IOP include coughing, bucking, or vomiting. Each of these can raise IOP by 10 to 20 mm Hg or more. Other factors that raise IOP include increased central venous pressure, elevated arterial carbon dioxide partial pressure, elevated blood pressure, low arterial oxygen partial pressure, and ketamine.

Succinylcholine transiently raises IOP by 6 to 8 mm Hg

Factors that lower IOP include benzodiazepines, barbiturates, inhalational agents, and glaucoma medications (anticholinesterase [echothiophate, *which of note can prolong the duration of action of succinylcholine and mivacurium*], beta-blocker [timolol], carbonic anhydrase inhibitor [acetazolamide, *which can cause a metabolic acidosis*]).

Opioids have little effect on IOP

The afferent limb of the *oculocardiac reflex* involves the trigeminal nerve, while the efferent limb involves the vagus nerve. This reflex is most often triggered by traction of the extraocular eye muscle (classic in strabismus surgery) but can also result from pressure on the globe. Oculocardiac reflex most commonly results in bradycardia, but may lead to asystole. To treat the oculocardiac reflex: (1) stop surgical manipulation/traction; (2) administer IV atropine or glycopyrrolate; and/or (3) deepen anesthesia.

As part of routine preoperative work-up, it is important to ask all patients about recent ophthalmologic procedures, as during these procedures *intravitreal gas bubbles* may be injected by the ophthalmologist. The gas injected is most often sulfur hexafluoride or perfluoropropane.

Avoid the use of nitrous oxide for any patient in whom an intravitreal gas bubble was injected (within a month for perfluoropropane gas or two weeks for sulfur hexafluoride gas), as nitrous oxide may result in increased IOP and central retinal artery occlusion.

A *retrobulbar block* provides both eye anesthesia and akinesia for surgery of the cornea, lens, or anterior chamber by blocking optic, oculomotor, nasociliary, and abducens nerves. Complications of retrobulbar block include retrobulbar hemorrhage, central retinal artery occlusion, globe perforation, intraneural injury, intrathecal injection from injection into the sheath of the optic nerve (or post retrobulbar apnea syndrome), arterial injection, and triggering of the oculocardiac reflex.

In comparison to retrobulbar block, a *peribulbar block* is easier to place, has a longer onset time, results in less complete eye akinesia, and carries a lower risk of complication. In addition, the block needle does not penetrate the muscle cone.

Surgery for *open globe injury* most often requires general anesthesia, as a retrobulbar block is contraindicated due to risk of extrusion of vitreous. Airway management decisions are clinically challenging for open globe injury given: (1) these patients often present emergently and full stomach precautions apply; (2) desire to avoid elevations in IOP.

Laryngoscopy and intubation can increase IOP, so it is important to maintain adequate anesthesia during induction. The anesthesiologist must weigh the benefits and risks of succinylcholine use. The importance of deep anesthesia and complete muscle relaxation as well as a rapid sequence intubation may make succinylcholine the preferred agent despite the impact on IOP.

Questions

1. Which of the following agents should be avoided in open globe injury because of its potential impact on intraocular pressure?
   a. fentanyl
   b. propofol
   c. succinylcholine
   d. ketamine
   e. acetazolamide

2. In comparison to retrobulbar block, which is TRUE of a peribulbar block?
   a. may cause incomplete akinesia of the globe
   b. has a longer time to onset of block
   c. needle does not penetrate the muscle cone
   d. has a lower risk of post block apnea syndrome
   e. all of the above are true

Answers

1. d. Factors that raise IOP include coughing, bucking, or vomiting. Each of these can raise IOP by 10 to 20 mm Hg or more. Other factors that raise IOP include increased central venous pressure, elevated arterial carbon dioxide partial pressure, elevated blood pressure, low arterial oxygen partial pressure, and ketamine. Ketamine should therefore be avoided as the anesthetic of choice in open globe injury. The anesthesiologist must weigh the benefits and risks of succinylcholine use. The importance of deep anesthesia and complete muscle relaxation as well as a rapid sequence intubation may make succinylcholine the preferred agent despite the impact on IOP. The other agents listed as answer choices (fentanyl, propofol, acetazolamide) do not increase IOP.

2. e. In comparison to retrobulbar block, a peribulbar block is easier to place, has a longer onset time, results in less complete eye akinesia, and carries a lower risk of complication. In addition, the block needle does not penetrate the muscle cone

Further reading

Matjucha, I. C. A. (2011). Cranial nerves III, IV, and VI: occulomotor, trochlear, and abducens nerves: ocular mobility and pupils. In Jones, H. R. et al. (eds) *Netter's Neurology*, 2nd edn. Elsevier.

Chapter

113

Common otolaryngology procedures

Caryn Barnet and Dongdong Yao

Keywords

Nitrous oxide in middle ear surgery
Complications of tracheotomy
Heliox
Laryngospasm
Obstructive sleep apnea

Review airway imaging, perform a complete airway examination, and review previous intubation history, as ENT patients have an increased risk of difficult mask ventilation and/or intubation. Have a back-up plan available and consider awake fiberoptic intubation or tracheotomy under local anesthesia where appropriate.

Nitrous oxide diffuses into air-filled cavities faster than nitrogen is absorbed into the blood. Gas expansion results in increased pressure in closed spaces. Gas pressure in the middle ear is normally relieved by an open Eustachian tube, but may not be relieved in cases of Eustachian tube obstruction. Therefore nitrous oxide is best avoided in cases of middle ear surgery.

Postoperative nausea and vomiting (PONV) is a common complication of middle ear surgery.

Many ENT cases involve nerve monitoring. Long-acting neuromuscular blocking agents should be avoided in these cases. Such cases may include radical neck dissection, parotidectomy, thyroidectomy, and acoustic neuroma surgery.

Early *complications of tracheotomy* include airway fire, bleeding, pneumothorax, subcutaneous emphysema, tube obstruction from impingement on posterior tracheal wall, mucus plugging, and inadvertent decanulation with inability to replace tube in true tracheal lumen. Late complications of tracheotomy include tracheal stenosis, tracheomalacia, and tracheoesophageal fistula.

If a fresh tracheotomy tube is inadvertently removed, there is a risk of inserting a replacement tube in a false passage rather than the true tracheal lumen. Intubation can be accomplished by direct laryngoscopy via the oropharynx.

Heliox is a mixture of helium and oxygen (usually 4:1 or 7:3 helium:oxygen) that is beneficial in cases of upper airway obstruction and in cases where small diameter endotracheal tubes are in place. The lower density of helium reduces airway resistance.

Some airway procedures can be accomplished with jet ventilation (bursts of 100% oxygen at pressure of 10 to 40 psi, risk of barotrauma) or apneic oxygenation (ventilate via LMA, mask, or ETT with 100% oxygen and then remove airway device and allow procedure to proceed with patient apnea for short period of time, and then reestablish ventilation).

Laryngospasm is a reflex of the glottis that may result in hypoxia and/or negative pressure pulmonary edema. It is associated with light anesthesia or irritation of the vocal cords. Treatment of laryngospasm includes: (1) jaw thrust, (2) positive pressure, (3) deepening anesthetic, and (4) muscle relaxation (10 to 20 mg succinylcholine may be given).

Obstructive sleep apnea (OSA) involves obstruction of the airway during sleep by the soft tissue of the oropharynx. Obesity is a risk factor. OSA may lead to hypertension, heart failure, pulmonary hypertension, arrhythmias, and vascular disease. OSA is associated with difficult ventilation after induction of anesthesia and may lead to difficult intubation. ENT procedures to treat OSA include uvulopalatopharyngoplasty (UPPP) and tonsillectomy. Limit opioid and sedating drugs as they can increase the risk of postoperative airway obstruction.

Prior to discharge from an outpatient procedure, *ASA Practice Guidelines for the Perioperative Management of Patients with Obstructive Sleep Apnea* indicate (based on consultant agreement) that room air oxygen saturation should return to baseline and the patient should not become hypoxemic when left undisturbed in the recovery room. The consultants indicated that patients with OSA should be monitored for three hours longer than their non-OSA counterparts before discharge, and that monitoring should occur for seven hours after the last episode of airway obstruction or hypoxemia while breathing room air in an unstimulated environment.

Essential Clinical Anesthesia Review: Keywords, Questions and Answers for the Boards, ed. Linda S. Aglio, Robert W. Lekowski, and Richard D. Urman. Published by Cambridge University Press. © Cambridge University Press 2015.

Question

1. Which of the following statements is false regarding the treatment of patients with OSA?
   a. Opioid medications may increase the risk of postoperative airway obstruction.
   b. ASA Practice Guidelines indicate that OSA patients who experience desaturation in the recovery room should remain in the hospital overnight.
   c. Patients with OSA should be monitored in the recovery room for three hours longer than their non-OSA counterparts.
   d. Patients with OSA are at increased risk for difficult ventilation after induction of anesthesia.

Answer

1. b. Prior to discharge from an outpatient procedure, *ASA Practice Guidelines for the Perioperative Management of* *Patients with Obstructive Sleep Apnea* indicate that room air oxygen saturation should return to baseline and patient should not become hypoxemic when left undisturbed in the recovery room. The consultants indicated that patients with OSA should be monitored for three hours longer than their non-OSA counterparts before discharge, and that monitoring should occur for seven hours after the last episode of airway obstruction or hypoxemia while breathing room air in an unstimulated environment. The guidelines do not list desaturation in the recovery room as a reason for the patient to remain in the hospital overnight.

Further reading

Gross, J. B., Bachenberg, K. L., Benumof, J. L. et al. (2006). Practice guidelines for the perioperative management of patients with obstructive sleep apnea: a report by the American Society of Anesthesiologists Task Force on Perioperative Management of Patients with Obstructive Sleep Apnea. *Anesthesiology* 104, 1081–1093.

Chapter

114

Lasers, airway surgery, and operating room fires

Caryn Barnet and Dongdong Yao

Keywords

LASER
Laser resistant endotracheal tubes
Airway fire
Operating room fire algorithm

LASER is "Light Amplification by Stimulated Emission of Radiation" and allows the surgeon to precisely resect tissue while minimizing bleeding by concentrating high levels of energy on a specific area.

A carbon dioxide laser is used as a tissue vaporizer or cutting instrument (soft tissue excision) by emitting a long wavelength (10,600 nm) infrared beam.

Neodymium-yttrium aluminum garnet (nd-YAG) laser is a pulsed near-infrared 1,064 nm beam, which can be transmitted fiberoptically and is used for excision of soft tissue.

Argon laser is a continuous 488 to 515 nm beam that is used primarily for photocoagulation.

For laser safety, notification should be placed on the operating room door that laser is in use, and the patient and operating room personnel should wear protective laser approved eyewear (goggles/glasses).

Laser resistant endotracheal tubes are less likely to ignite when exposed to intense heat in the setting of an oxygen-enriched environment. The only true laser resistant endotracheal tube (ETT) is a metal ETT. Polyvinyl chloride (PVC), red rubber, and silicone tubes are all combustible.

There exists an increased risk of *airway fire* during tracheotomy and laser surgery. Communication between the surgeon and anesthesiologist is key to reduce the risk of fire. The anesthesiologist should strive to reduce the FiO_2 to the minimum required to maintain oxygenation and should avoid nitrous oxide during high airway fire risk procedures.

All anesthesiologists should be familiar with the *American Society of Anesthesiologists (ASA) Operating Room Fires Algorithm*.

As per the ASA algorithm, in the event of an airway fire: (1) remove the endotracheal tube; (2) stop the flow of airway gases (*of note, steps (1) and (2) can and should occur simultaneously if possible to prevent a blow-torch effect*); (3) remove flammable material from the airway; (4) pour saline into the airway; (5) if fire not extinguished after preliminary steps, use a CO_2 fire extinguisher.

Essential Clinical Anesthesia Review: Keywords, Questions and Answers for the Boards, ed. Linda S. Aglio, Robert W. Lekowski, and Richard D. Urman. Published by Cambridge University Press. © Cambridge University Press 2015.

OPERATING ROOM FIRES ALGORITHM

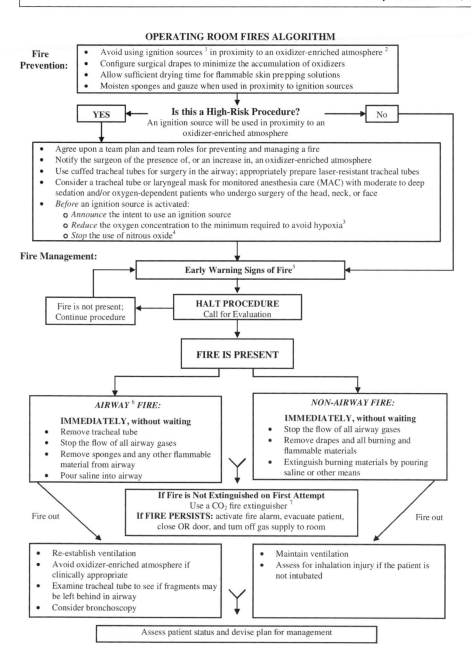

Figure 114.1 Current advice on operating room fires. Source: American Society of Anesthesiologists.

Fire Prevention:

- Avoid using ignition sources [1] in proximity to an oxidizer-enriched atmosphere [2]
- Configure surgical drapes to minimize the accumulation of oxidizers
- Allow sufficient drying time for flammable skin prepping solutions
- Moisten sponges and gauze when used in proximity to ignition sources

Is this a High-Risk Procedure?
An ignition source will be used in proximity to an oxidizer-enriched atmosphere

YES / No

- Agree upon a team plan and team roles for preventing and managing a fire
- Notify the surgeon of the presence of, or an increase in, an oxidizer-enriched atmosphere
- Use cuffed tracheal tubes for surgery in the airway; appropriately prepare laser-resistant tracheal tubes
- Consider a tracheal tube or laryngeal mask for monitored anesthesia care (MAC) with moderate to deep sedation and/or oxygen-dependent patients who undergo surgery of the head, neck, or face
- *Before* an ignition source is activated:
  o *Announce* the intent to use an ignition source
  o *Reduce* the oxygen concentration to the minimum required to avoid hypoxia [3]
  o *Stop* the use of nitrous oxide [4]

Fire Management:

Early Warning Signs of Fire [5]

Fire is not present; Continue procedure

HALT PROCEDURE
Call for Evaluation

FIRE IS PRESENT

AIRWAY [6] FIRE:

IMMEDIATELY, without waiting
- Remove tracheal tube
- Stop the flow of all airway gases
- Remove sponges and any other flammable material from airway
- Pour saline into airway

NON-AIRWAY FIRE:

IMMEDIATELY, without waiting
- Stop the flow of all airway gases
- Remove drapes and all burning and flammable materials
- Extinguish burning materials by pouring saline or other means

Fire out

If Fire is Not Extinguished on First Attempt
Use a CO_2 fire extinguisher [7]
If FIRE PERSISTS: activate fire alarm, evacuate patient, close OR door, and turn off gas supply to room

Fire out

- Re-establish ventilation
- Avoid oxidizer-enriched atmosphere if clinically appropriate
- Examine tracheal tube to see if fragments may be left behind in airway
- Consider bronchoscopy

- Maintain ventilation
- Assess for inhalation injury if the patient is not intubated

Assess patient status and devise plan for management

---

[1] Ignition sources include, but are not limited to, electrosurgery or electrocautery units and lasers.

[2] An oxidizer-enriched atmosphere occurs when there is any increase in oxygen concentration above room air level, and/or the presence of any concentration of nitrous oxide.

[3] After minimizing delivered oxygen, wait a period of time (*e.g.*, 1-3 min) before using an ignition source. For oxygen-dependent patients, *reduce* supplemental oxygen delivery to the minimum required to avoid hypoxia. Monitor oxygenation with pulse oximetry, and if feasible, inspired, exhaled, and/or delivered oxygen concentration.

[4] After stopping the delivery of nitrous oxide, wait a period of time (*e.g.*, 1-3 min) before using an ignition source.

[5] Unexpected flash, flame, smoke or heat, unusual sounds (*e.g.*, a "pop," snap, or "foomp") or odors, unexpected movement of drapes, discoloration of drapes or breathing circuit, unexpected patient movement or complaint.

[6] In this algorithm, airway fire refers to a fire in the airway or breathing circuit.

[7] A CO_2 fire extinguisher may be used on the patient if necessary.

Questions

1. Which of the following statements regarding tracheotomy surgery is TRUE?

   a. The anesthesiologist should provide 100% FiO_2 at all times because of the risk of airway loss and oxygen desaturation during tracheotomy tube placement.

   b. Nitrous oxide may be beneficial to decrease FiO_2 and therefore decrease risk of an airway fire.

   c. As long as you maintain FiO_2 less than 70%, the surgeon can use electrocautery to enter the trachea without an elevated risk of airway fire.

   d. According to the ASA algorithm, in the event of airway fire, the first step should be to remove the endotracheal tube.

   e. None of the above statements are true.

2. Which of the following endotracheal tubes (ETT) is laser resistant?

   a. Norton steel ETT

   b. PVC ETT

   c. red rubber ETT

   d. silicone ETT

Answers

1. d According to the ASA "Operating Room Fires" algorithm: in the event of an airway fire, the first step is to remove the endotracheal tube. Simultaneously, all airway gases should be turned off.

2. a. The only true laser resistant endotracheal tube (ETT) is a metal ETT. Polyvinyl chloride (PVC), red rubber, and silicone tubes are all combustible.

Further reading

Apfelbaum, J. L. et al. (2013). Practice advisory for the prevention and management of operating room fires: an updated report by the American Society of Anesthesiologists Task Force on Operating Room Fires. *Anesthesiology* 118(2), 271–290.

Hermens, J. M. et al. (1983). Anesthesia for laser surgery. *Anesthesia and Analgesia* 62, 218–229.

Chapter

115

Anesthesia for common orthopedic procedures

Christopher Voscopoulos and David Janfaza

Keywords

- ASRA guidelines
- Brachial plexus anatomy and blockade
- Interscalene nerve block
- Supraclavicular nerve block
- Infraclavicular nerve block
- Axillary nerve block
- Femoral nerve block
- Sciatic nerve block
- Lumbar plexus block
- Tourniquets and regional anesthesia techniques
- Tourniquet risk factors
- Venous thrombosis-associated pulmonary embolism
- Bone cement implantation syndrome

ASRA guidelines address the concern of performing neuraxial or regional anesthesia techniques in patients on anticoagulant or antiplatelet medications, or other primary anticoagulation abnormalities.

Brachial plexus anatomy and blockade: a common mnemonic describing the anatomy of the brachial plexus is "Robert Taylor Drinks Cold Beer". The "R" stands for the Roots, the "T" Trunks, the "D" Divisions, the "C" Cords, and the "B" Branches. It consists of the dermatomes C5–T1 (see Figure 115.1). Common blocks at each of the levels described in the mnemonic are listed below.

Interscalene nerve block: this block takes place at the level of the roots and trunks. At the level of C6 the roots lie between the anterior and middle scalene muscles. Common uses for this block are for anesthesia and postoperative pain control after shoulder surgery. This block commonly has incomplete block of the lower dermatomes of C8 and T1. Blockade of the phrenic nerve nears 100%.

Supraclavicular nerve block: this block takes place at the level of the trunks or divisions of the brachial plexus. Under ultrasound guidance, the trunks and divisions are found just superior to the clavicle, between the anterior and middle

scalene muscles, just lateral to the subclavian artery. The nerves at this level are hyperechoic and resemble "a bunch of grapes" (divisions) or circles like a "stop light" (trunks). This block is useful for surgery of the arm and hand, but may not be effective for surgery of the shoulder without high volumes of local anesthetic. Blockade of the phrenic nerve may be volume dependent, but still occurs in at least 50% of patients. The dome of the lung is in close proximity, and as a result pneumothorax is a risk with this block.

Infraclavicular nerve block: this block takes place at the level of the cords below the clavicle in proximity to the coracoid process. At this level the musculocutaneous nerve has not divided off and will be blocked. This block is commonly used for lower arm and hand surgeries.

Axillary nerve block: this block takes place at the level of branches of the brachial plexus. At this level the musculocutaneous nerve has already divided off the brachial plexus and needs to be blocked separately. This block is commonly used for lower arm and hand surgeries.

Femoral nerve block: the femoral nerve is formed from lumbar nerve roots L2 to L4. The surface landmarks for this block are the ASIS, pubic tubercle, inguinal ligament, inguinal crease, and femoral artery pulse. Under ultrasound guidance the femoral nerve is located lateral to the femoral vein and artery below the fascia iliaca (see Figure 115.2). This block is useful for surgery and postoperative recovery of surgery of the knee and thigh. For complete anesthesia of knee, a sciatic nerve block may be performed.

Sciatic nerve block: this nerve originates from the lumbosacral plexus (L4–S3). Common locations for this block are at the level of the gluteal muscles (traditional Labat approach), sub gluteal approach, or a distal popliteal approach (see Figure 115.4). Ultrasound can be more easily used for both the popliteal and subgluteal approach, due to the nerve being in a more superficial manner; however, for the deeper Labat approach, it is still common to combine this approach with the use of a nerve stimulator for further nerve localization confirmation.

Essential Clinical Anesthesia Review: Keywords, Questions and Answers for the Boards, ed. Linda S. Aglio, Robert W. Lekowski, and Richard D. Urman. Published by Cambridge University Press. © Cambridge University Press 2015.

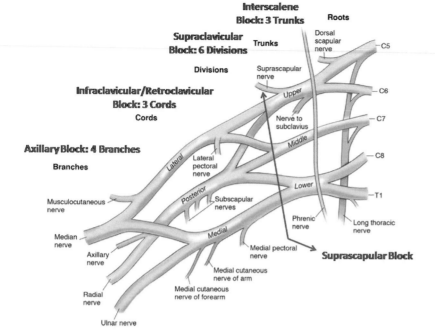

Figure 115.1 Schematic brachial plexus anatomy for upper extremity blocks. (Adapted from Vacanti et al. 2011. *Essential Clinical Anesthesia*, Cambridge University Press, Figure 60.1.)

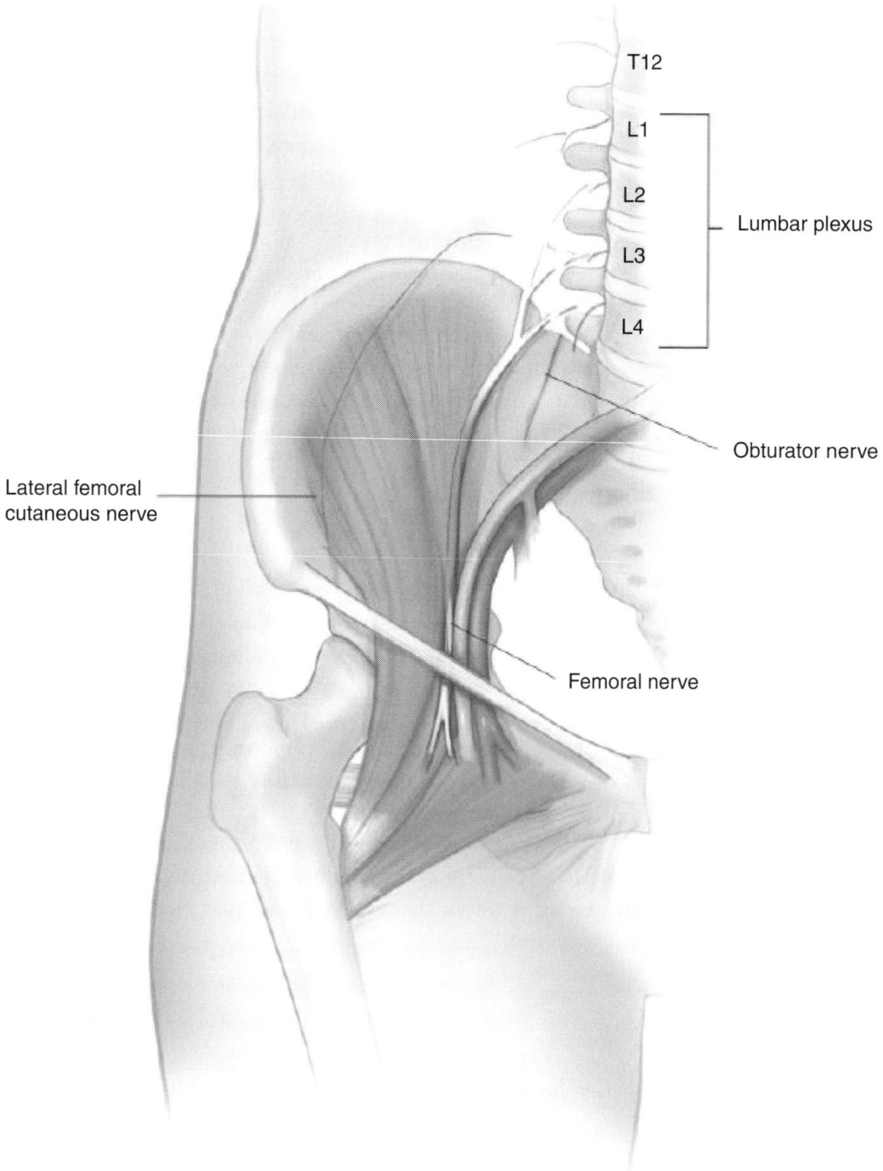

Interscalene Block: 3 Trunks

Supraclavicular Block: 6 Divisions

Infraclavicular/Retroclavicular Block: 3 Cords

Axillary Block: 4 Branches

Roots

Trunks

Divisions

Cords

Branches

Dorsal scapular nerve

C5

C6

C7

C8

T1

Suprascapular nerve

Upper

Nerve to subclavius

Middle

Lower

Phrenic nerve

Long thoracic nerve

Lateral

Lateral pectoral nerve

Posterior

Subscapular nerves

Medial

Medial pectoral nerve

Suprascapular Block

Musculocutaneous nerve

Median nerve

Axillary nerve

Radial nerve

Ulnar nerve

Medial cutaneous nerve of arm

Medial cutaneous nerve of forearm

Figure 115.2 Schematic lumbosacral anatomy for femoral nerve blocks. (From Vacanti et al. 2011. *Essential Clinical Anesthesia*, Cambridge University Press, Figure 61.1.)

T12

L1

L2

L3

L4

Lumbar plexus

Obturator nerve

Lateral femoral cutaneous nerve

Femoral nerve

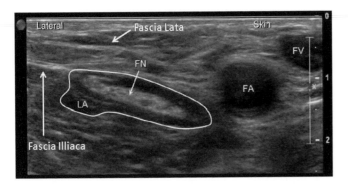

Figure 115.3 Ultrasonographic femoral nerve anatomy for femoral nerve blocks. FN, femoral nerve; LA, local anesthestic; FA, femoral artery; FV, femoral nerve. (Adapted from Vacanti et al. 2011. *Essential Clinical Anesthesia*, Cambridge University Press, Figure 61.6.)

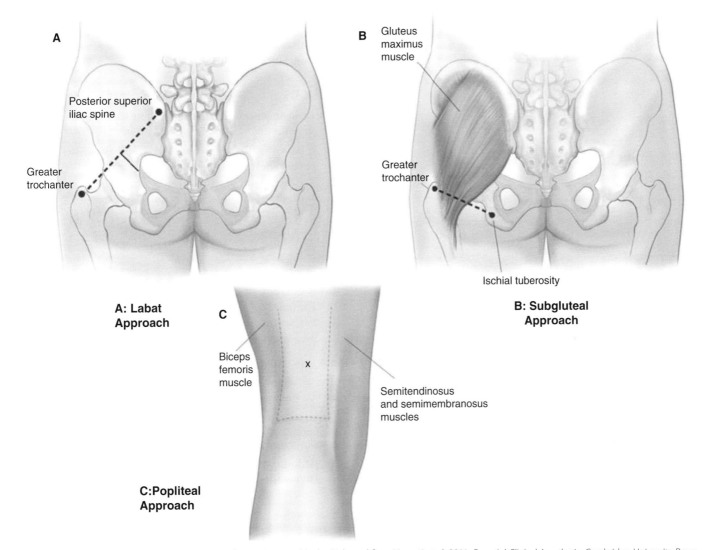

Figure 115.4 Schematic sciatic nerve anatomy for sciatic nerve blocks. (Adapted from Vacanti et al. 2011. *Essential Clinical Anesthesia*, Cambridge University Press, Figures 61.9, 61.11, and 61.12.)

Lumbar plexus block: the two most reliable methods to block the lumbar plexus are the lumbar paravertebral or psoas compartment block. It has been shown that this block provides equal analgesia as compared to an epidural block; however, the reported complication rates are relatively high.

Tourniquets and regional anesthesia techniques: if a thigh tourniquet is applied for lower extremity surgery, a neuraxial technique is often utilized to ensure complete analgesia of the leg to control tourniquet pain. If a tourniquet is applied at the level of the humerus for lower arm surgery, the

Table 115.1 Effects of tourniquet deflation

Hemodynamic	↓ MAP, SVR ↑ Venous capacitance ↓ PVR ↑ CO
Metabolic	Mixed acidosis Hypoxemia/hypoxia ↑ CO_2 production
Embolism	Thrombus Fat Air Cement (methacrylate) Bone marrow debris

MAP, mean arterial pressure; SVR, systemic vascular resistance; PVR, pulmonary vascular resistance; CO, cardiac output; CO_2, carbon dioxide. (Used with permission from *Essential Clinical Anesthesia*, 1st edn. 2011. Cambridge University Press, p. 718, Table 116.2.)

Table 115.2 Diagnostic criteria for fat embolism (two major or one major and four minor criteria are necessary for diagnosis)

Major criteria	Minor criteria
Petechial rash	Fever
Cerebral involvement	Tachycardia (>120 bpm)
Respiratory distress	Retinal changes (fat or petechiae)
Arterial blood gas abnormalities	Renal changes
PaO_2 <60 mm Hg breathing room air	Jaundice
$PaCO_2$ >55 or a pH <7.3	Fat macroglobulinemia Hemolytic anemia (a drop of more than 20% of the admission hemoglobin value)

(Adapted from Gurd, A. R. and Wilson, R. I. 1974. The fat embolism syndrome. *Journal of Bone and Joint Surgery* 566, 408–416; used with permission from *Essential Clinical Anesthesia*, 1st edn. 2011. Cambridge University Press, p. 715.)

musculocutaneous nerve, as well as intercostal brachial nerve, would need to be blocked to fully control for tourniquet pain.

Tourniquet risk factors: may cause systemic effects owing to ischemia and reperfusion effects (see Table 115.1) when released. Long torniquet time, or improper positioning, has been implicated in peroneal and tibial nerve palsies after total knee arthoplasty, with an incidence of tourniquet-induced palsy of 1 in 8,000 operations. Risk factors include pressurization above 400 mm Hg and time up of 145 min +/-25 min. However, complete recovery is seen in most cases. It has also been suggested that long-acting sciatic nerve blocks may delay the diagnosis of nerve injuries. As such, in those patients at risk for injury these blocks should likely be avoided. It is noteworthy that when giving perioperative antibiotic

prophylaxis, the full dose of antibiotic should be given prior to the inflation of the tourniquet.

Thrombosis-associated pulmonary embolism: venous thrombosis-associated pulmonary embolism is the third most common cause of death in hip fracture patients, accounting for 18% of perioperative deaths. As such, perioperative thrombo-prophylactic therapy is a cornerstone of comprehensive perioperative medicine in this patient population. Fat, air, or methyl methacrylate are also embolic risks (see Table 115.2).

Bone cement implantation syndrome: fat particles and other debris can be dislodged and enter the bloodstream, leading to bone cement implantation syndrome. This is a risk because of the high pressures reached inside the femoral canal during the insertion of the cemented femoral component, as a result of the manipulation and reaming that take place, leading to peak pressures as high as 680 mm Hg.

Questions

1. Interscalene block would be an absolute contraindication in which patient?
   a. A patient with, contralateral from the block site, phrenic nerve palsy.
   b. A patient with obstructive sleep apnea.
   c. A patient status total gastrectomy.
   d. A patient with a lumbar intrathecal pain pump.

2. The risk of nerve palsy with tourniquet use can be lessened by limiting the tourniquet to which?
   a. A pressure of 200 mm Hg above systolic.
   b. A duration of 90 to 120 minutes maximum.
   c. The use of epidural or other regional anesthesia techniques.
   d. Performing regional anesthesia techniques in the post-anesthesia phase of care.

3. All of the following are advantages of regional anesthesia over general anesthesia for total knee arthoscopy except which?
   a. Decreased incidence of postoperative nausea and vomiting.
   b. Detter pain control in the immediate post-anesthesia period.
   c. High patient satisfaction.
   d. Quicker discharge from the post-anesthesia care unit.

Answers

1. a. The incidence of phrenic nerve palsy from interscalene nerve block approaches 100%. As such, bilateral blocks, or blocks opposite a body side in which the nerve is already paralyzed, would be contraindicated.
2. b. A retrospective study suggests that patients with mean total tourniquet time of 145 +/- 25 minutes have a 7.7% incidence of nerve injury, recovering completely in 89% of the cases. This finding suggests that tourniquet time should

not exceed 90 to 120 minutes and tourniquet pressure should not be higher than 150 mm Hg above systolic blood pressure.

3. d. General anesthesia prolongs emergence time (time from the end of surgery until exit from the operating room), in most cases requires a post-anesthesia care unit (PACU) stay, and is associated with higher incidence of nausea and vomiting and lower overall patient satisfaction. Femoral nerve and lumbar plexus blocks are both suitable techniques for knee arthroscopy.

Further reading

Eagle, K. A., Berger, P. B., Calkins, H. et al. (2002). ACC/AHA guideline update for perioperative cardiovascular evaluation for noncardiac surgery-executive summary: a report of the American College of Cardiology/American Heart Association Task Force on Practice Guidelines (Committee to update the 1996 guidelines on perioperative cardiovascular evaluation for noncardiac surgery). *Anesthesia and Analgesia* 94(5), 1052–1064.

Hadzic, A., Karaca, P. E., Hobeika, P. et al. (2005). Peripheral nerve blocks result in superior recovery profile compared with general anesthesia in outpatient knee arthroscopy. *Anesthesia and Analgesia* 100(4), 976–981.

Horlocker, T. T., Hebl, J. R., Gali, B. et al. (2006). Anesthetic, patient, and surgical risk factors for neurologic complications after prolonged total tourniquet time during total knee arthroplasty. *Anesthesia and Analgesia* 102(3), 950–955.

Mauermann, W. J., Shilling, A. M., and Zuo, Z. (2006). A comparision of neuraxial block versus general anesthesia for elective total hip replacement: a meta-analysis. *Anesthesia and Analgesia* 103(4), 1018–1025.

Tziavrangos, E. and Schug, S. A. (2006) Regional anaesthesia and perioperative outcome. *Current Opinion in Anaesthesiology* 19(5), 521–525.

Vacanti, C. A., Sikka, P. K., Urman, R. D., et al. (2011). *Essential Clinical Anesthesia.* New York: Cambridge University Press.

Chapter

116

Rheumatoid arthritis and scoliosis

Christopher Voscopoulos and David Janfaza

Keywords

Rheumatoid arthritis (RA)
Vascular access
Atlanto-axial (C1–2) subluxation
Temporomandibular joint
Cricoarytenoiditis
Scoliosis
Preoperative assessment in scoliosis
Cardiorespiratory disease in scoliosis
Intraoperative hemodynamic management
Challenges in intraoperative management of patients
   with scoliosis
Hemodynamic management in scoliosis surgery
Intraoperative ventilation management in patients
   with scoliosis
Intraoperative spinal cord monitoring in patients with
   scoliosis

Rheumatoid arthritis is a chronic autoimmune disease of unknown etiology, characterized by symmetric polyarthropathy and systemic involvement (see Table 116.1), typically presenting between 30 and 50 years of age with a female predominance.

Vascular access: in indivudals that suffer with RA, peripheral veins are often small and brittle making intravenous access difficult, radial arteries are often calcified making arterial line difficult, and cervical vertebrae fusions can cause limited neck movement making internal jugular access for central line placement difficult.

Atlanto-axial (C1–2) subluxation can occur in patients with RA. Lateral neck radiographs or MRI studies revealing a greater than 3 mm gap between the anterior arch of the atlas and the odontoid process can confirm the presence of anterior subluxation. If present, care must be taken during movement of the neck, particularly during endotracheal intubation in which manual in-line stabilization must be achieved via numerous techniques.

Temporomandibular joint (TMJ): disease of the TMJ can be present in patients with RA, and present difficulties with

Table 116.1 Effects of rheumatoid arthritis on the organ systems

Organ systems	Presentation	Evaluation
Cardiac	Constrictive pericarditis	EKG
	Pericardial effusion	Consider echocardiography or stress test if cardiac history is significant
	Aortic root dilatation	
	Aortic insufficiency	
	Cardiac conduction abnormalities	
	Myocarditis	
	Coronary arteriitis	
	CAD (chronic steroid use implicated)	
Respiratory	Pleural effusion	Chest radiograph
	Pulmonary fibrosis	Consider spirometry or arterial blood gas if history is significant
	Pulmonary vasculitis	
	Pulmonary nodules	
	Obliterative bronchiolitis	
Neurologic	Nerve compression (cervical, peripheral)	Assess for neuropathies
	Muscle weakness due to mononeuritis	
Renal	Vasculitis	Baseline BUN and creatinine
	Amyloidosis	
	Autoimmune nephropathy	

Table 116.1 (*cont.*)

Organ systems	Presentation	Evaluation
Hematologic	Mild anemia (iron deficiency) Chronic use of COX inhibitors	Check preop CBC Anticipate variable platelet dysfunction
Endocrine	Adrenal insufficiency from chronic steroid use	Stress-dose steroids may be warranted in case of chronic use

(Used with permission from *Essential Clinical Anesthesia*, Cambridge University Press, 1st edn. 2011, p. 722, Table 117.1.)

Table 116.2 Summary of preoperative planning for scoliosis surgery

Airway	Potentially difficult C-spine movement may be limited Double-lumen ETT may be necessary
Respiratory	Chest radiography Arterial blood gas: usually low PaO_2 with normal $PaCO_2$
Cardiovascular	EKG Echocardiogram: LVEF and PA pressures Dobutamine stress echocardiogram considered in patients with limited exercise tolerance
Laboratory tests	CBC Coagulation profile Cross-matched blood
IV access	Large-bore IVs (possibly central line) Arterial line
Planned monitors	Standard Spinal cord monitoring Wake-up test Arterial line TEE (preferable to CVP or PAC)

(Used with permission from *Essential Clinical Anesthesia*, Cambridge University Press, 1st edn. 2011, p. 723, Table 117.2.)

endotracheal intubation by limiting the opening of the mouth. Patients may also present with micrognathia and obstructive sleep apnea.

Cricoarytenoiditis: due to the inflammatory nature of RA affecting several joint groups, cricoarytenoiditis can be present in patients with RA. If only mild, a smaller ETT should be considered for use; however, if severe, consideration of not undertaking oral tracheal intubation may be prudent as there is a risk for dislodgement of the arytenoids. Care must also be taken in the postoperative period, as the risk of supraglottic obstruction is higher if endotracheal intubation took place.

Scoliosis is a complex lateral and rotational deformity of the thoracolumbar spine. If there is thoracic involvement, ribcage deformity can also be present. The disease has a male to female

Table 116.3 Summary of intraoperative care for scoliosis surgery

Premedication	Anxiolytics Bronchodilators may be helpful
Introduction	Guided by patient's condition Avoid succinylcholine in patients with muscular dystrophy
Intubation	Direct versus fiberoptic laryngoscopy Double-lumen ETT, depending on surgical approach
Maintenance	Maintain stable depth so that spinal cord monitoring can be interpreted reliably Isoflurane <0.5 MAC with 60% nitrous oxide is compatible with SSEPs Total intravenous anesthesia (preferably with propofol and opioid infusions), especially when MEPs are monitored (avoidance of muscle relaxants preferred)
Positioning	Often prone; slight reverse Trendelenburg if possible Assess baseline neurologic deficits, including range of motion
Muscle relaxation	Continuous IV infusion of muscle relaxant Minimal or no muscle relaxants if MEPs monitored
Spinal cord monitoring	Commonly recommended methods include SSEPs, MEPs, or a wake-up test With wake-up test, use short-acting agents (e.g., remifentanil, propofol, desflurane)
Blood preservation	Antifibrinolytics Cell salvage Controlled hypotension

(Used with permission from *Essential Clinical Anesthesia*, Cambridge University Press, 1st edn. 2011, p. 724, Table 117.3.)

ratio of 1:4. Surgery is usually indicated when the Cobb's angle (lateral curvature) exceeds 50% in the thoracic spine, or 40% in the lumbar spine. If surgical correction is not sought when indicated, severe respiratory and cardiovascular compromise can result due to the restrictive anatomic pathology.

Preoperative assessment in scoliosis: see Table 116.2.

Cardiorespiratory disease in scoliosis: due to the anatomic restrictive pathology that ensues in the thoracic cavity, vital capacity and total lung capacity are often reduced, and ventilation/perfusion mismatch is common. As is common in restrictive lung pathology, cor pulmonale with right heart strain or failure is common, with resulttant pulmonary hypertension and chronic hypoxemia.

Challenges in intraoperative management of patients with scoliosis: (1) significant blood loss, (2) one-lung ventilation, (3) prone positioning, and (4) the wake-up test (see Table 116.3.).

Hemodynamic management in scoliosis surgery: since there may be significant blood loss, the use of antifibrinolytics, such as aminocaproic acid or tranexamic acid, intraoperative cell salvage, or transfusion of fresh frozen plasma, platelets, and/or cryoprecipitate may be needed, as well as the possible use of controlled hypotension.

Intraoperative ventilation management in patients with scoliosis: single-lung ventilation may be needed for surgical access to the spine. With underlying restrictive lung pathophysiology being common in patients with scolosis, high peak inspiratory pressures, as well as plateau pressures, may be an issue. As such, lowering inspiratory flow rates on volume-controlled ventilation, or switching to pressure-controlled ventilation, may be useful.

Intraoperative spinal cord monitoring in patients with scoliosis: to minimize the risk of postoperative neurologic deficits, including paraplegia, three monitoring techniques can be used: (1) somatosensory evoked potentials (SSEPs), (2) motor evoked potential (MEPs), or (3) the intraoperative wake-up test. The use of total intravenous anesthesia (TIVA) alone or in combination with minimal inhalational agents is needed for effective monitoring. Muscle relaxation should be avoided when monitoring MEP.

Questions

1. In a rheumatoid arthritis patient with a 3 mm gap, or greater, between the anterior arch of the atlas and the odontoid process, methods of securing the airway include all of the following EXCEPT for which?
   a. fiberoptic intubation
   b. direct larygnoscopy
   c. direct larygnoscopy with in-line C-spine stabilization
   d. fast track LMA

2. If peak pressures are high in a patient with restrictive lung disease because of scoliosis and prone positioning intraop, which is the best method of mechanical ventilation?
   a. volume-controlled ventilation
   b. assist-controlled ventilation
   c. pressure-support ventilation
   d. pressure-controlled ventilation

3. The best test to minimize the risk of motor neuron lesioning in scoliosis surgery is which?
   a. somatosensory evoked potentials
   b. motor evoked potentials
   c. a wake-up test
   d. postoperative magnetic resonance imaging of the spine

Answers

1. b. In securing the airway in a rheumatoid arthritis patient with a 3 mm gap, or greater, between the anterior arch of the atlas and the odontoid process, one must take great care to not flex or extend the neck from the neutral plane. Any method that accomplishes this goal can be used. Attempting to secure the airway with direct larygnoscopy without in-line C-spine stabilization could possibly cause overextension of the cervical spine.

2. d. Pressure-controlled ventilation is the only option listed that will stop the inspiratory flow of the ventilator once a set pressure is reached. An adequate or targeted tidal volume may not be reached, but barotrauma can be avoided or minimized.

3. c. Numerous devices have been created to help guide the safe care of the patient under anesthesia; however, the wake-up test is still the best test to minimize the risk of motor neuron lesioning in scoliosis surgery. After the patient is awoken and motor function documented, reinduction with general anesthesia can resume.

Further reading

Fleisher, L. (2005). *Anesthesia and Uncommon Diseases*, 5th edn. Philadelphia: Saunders, pp. 144–145.

Miller, R. D. (2005). *Miller's Anesthesia*, 6th edn. Philadelphia: Elsevier/Churchill-Livingstone, pp. 2418–2419.

Stoelting, R. and Dierdorf, S. (1993). *Anesthesia and Co-Existing Disease*, 3rd edn. New York: Churchill-Livingstone.

Vacanti, C. A., Sikka, P. K., Urman, R. D. et al. (2011). *Essential Clinical Anesthesia*. New York: Cambridge University Press.

Chapter

117

Anesthetic management in spine surgery

Christopher Voscopoulos and David Janfaza

Keywords

- Airway assessment in cervical or high thoracic spine surgery
- Unstable cervical spine below the second cervical vertebrae
- Unstable cervical spine above the second cervical vertebrae
- Respiratory assessment in spinal surgery
- Cardiovascular assessment in spinal surgery
- Neurologic assessment in spinal surgery
- Anesthetic techniques in spinal surgery: premedication
- Anesthetic techniques in spinal surgery: induction
- Indications for awake intubation
- Direct vs. fiberoptic laryngoscopy (FOB)
- Sematosensory evoked potentials (SSEPs)
- Motor evoked potentials (MEP)
- Maintenance of anesthesia in spinal surgery
- Prevention of blood loss in spinal surgery
- Venous air embolism
- Postoperative visual loss

Airway assessment in cervical or high thoracic spine surgery: must include assessment of stability of the spine. Stability of the cervical spine after injury is dependent on ligamentous and vertebral elements, and, as a result, may not be detectable by plain radiographs alone and may need magnetic resonance imaging if suspicion is high. Mobility of the neck may be limited by pain or require immobilization for instability with the use of cervical spine collars. In addition, patients with prior radiation therapy to the head and neck, because of the fibrosis of the tissues that occurs, can present with difficulties in mouth opening and range of motion of the neck. In addition to the determination of the route and method of intubation in patients with spine-related concerns, the decision to intubate awake vs. asleep needs to be made.

Unstable cervical spine below the second cervical vertebrae occurs when one of the following conditions are met: (1) all the anterior or all the posterior elements are destroyed, (2) there is >3.5 mm horizontal displacement of one vertebra in relation to an adjacent one on lateral radiograph, (3) there is more than 11 degrees of rotation of one vertebra relative to an adjacent one.

Unstable cervical spine above the second cervical vertebrae occurs when: (1) disruption of the transverse ligament of the atlas, (2) Jefferson burst fracture of the atlas following axial loading, (3) disruption of the tectorial and alar ligaments, (4) some occipital condylar fractures.

Respiratory assessment in spinal surgery: patients may have impaired respiratory function due to restrictive pulmonary processes that can occur with kyphotic deformities, scoliosis, or burst, or acute or chronic compression fractures. As such, pulmonary function studies may be helpful. Older studies have reported that if preoperative vital capacity is less than 30 +/– 35% of predicted, postoperative ventilation is likely to be required.

Cardiovascular assessment in spinal surgery: minimum investigations should include electrocardiography and echocardiography to assess left and right ventricular function and pulmonary arterial pressures. Since spinal deformities can cause restrictive pulmonary processes, pulmonary arterial pressures can be negatively affected, leading to right heart strain patterns. In patients that cannot have their cardiac function assessed with physical exertion due to limited exercise tolerance, dobutamine stress echocardiography may be useful.

Neurologic assessment in spinal surgery should be documented for the following reasons: (1) in cervical spine surgery to ensure minimization of neck motion; (2) muscular dystrophies that may predispose to perioperative aspiration; (3) in spinal cord injury patients there is the risk of spinal shock within the first three weeks after the injury, and the risk of autonomic dysreflexia later (especially injuries above the mid-thoracic level); and (4) to document the preoperative neurological function as a baseline for postoperative assessment in surgeries that may carry the risk of intraoperative spinal cord complications.

Anesthetic techniques in spinal surgery: premedication. In patients requiring fiberoptic intubation, administration of anticholinergic agents, such as glycopyrrolate, should be

Essential Clinical Anesthesia Review: Keywords, Questions and Answers for the Boards, ed. Linda S. Aglio, Robert W. Lekowski, and Richard D. Urman. Published by Cambridge University Press. © Cambridge University Press 2015.

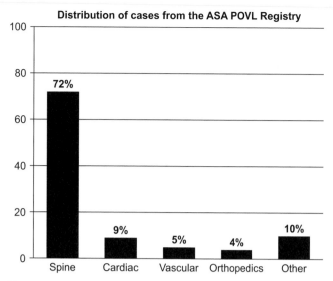

Figure 117.1 Distribution of cases from the ASA POVL Registry. Data were obtained from the study by Lee et al. The American Society of Anesthesiologists Postoperative Visual Loss Registry. *Anesthesiology*, 2006; 105: 652–9. (Figure with permission from Baig, M., Lubow, M., Immesoete, P. et al. 2007. Vision after spine surgery: review of the literature and recommendations. *Neurosurgery Focus*, 23(5): 15.)

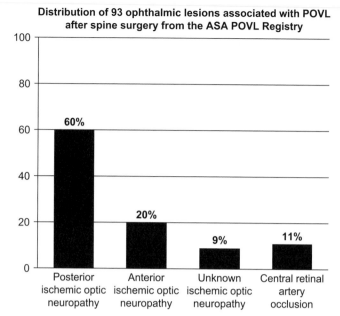

Figure 117.2 Distribution of 93 ophthalmic lesions associated with POVL after spine surgery from the ASA POVL Registry. Data were obtained from the study by Lee et al. The American Society of Anesthesiologists Postoperative Visual Loss Registry. *Anesthesiology*, 2006; 105: 652–9. (Figure with permission from Biag, M., Lubow, M., Immesoets, P. et al. 2007. Vision loss after spine surgery: review of the literature and recommendations. *Neurosurgery Focus*, 23(5), 15.)

considered to minimize secretions. Topicalization of the airway can be achieved with several techniques. It is recommended that both nasal and oral topicalization occur to allow for the anesthesiologist to change intubation methods if difficulty is encountered with the first route of attempt. As an alternative to topicalization, needle-block techniques can be used for the nasal, oral, and subglottic dermatomes that require blockade. Common sedation techniques focus on maintaining spontaneous respirations, and include the use of ketamine, dexmedetomidate, and midazolam.

Anesthetic techniques in spinal surgery: induction. The use of succinylcholine in patients with muscular dystrophies or spinal cord lesions resulting in denervation, may cause an increase in the number of extrajunctional acetylcholine receptors and place a patient at risk to succinycholine-induced hyperkalemia. These extrajunctional acetylcholine receptors can present themselves in as little as 24 hours post a neurologic injury. In addition to denervative trauma injury, this same phenomena can occur in critical illness myopathy or burn patients.

Indications for awake intubation should be considered if there is: (1) the need for neurologic assessment after airway management, (2) the risk of aspiration, (3) a potentially difficult airway, and (4) the presence of a neck stabilization device (such as halo traction) that could present a risk for a difficult airway due to airway access issues or cervical spine range of motion issues.

Direct vs. fiberoptic laryngoscopy (FOB): in general, no movement of the C-spine is the goal in a cervical spine which is clinically unstable. This can be achieved with either flexible fiberoptic techniques or direct laryngoscopy with manual in-line stabilization. Additionally, instead of manual in-line

stabilization, intubation with the use of a hard collar is also an accepted method that limits neck movement.

Sematosensory evoked potentials (SSEPs): monitoring of an electrical stimuli within the periphery of the body and recorded within the sematosensory cortex.

Motor evoked potentials (MEP): monitoring of an electric stimuli from the motor cortex to the peripheral muscles.

Maintenance of anesthesia in spinal surgery: in general, total intravenous anesthesia techniques are preferred when SSEP and MEPs are being used. Inhalational techniques with combined levels of less than 0.5 MAC are also compatible with SSEP and MEP monitoring. Long-acting or intermediate non-depolarizers should be avoided when monitoring MEP.

Prevention of blood loss in spinal surgery: blood loss in spinal surgery can vary between 10 to 30 ml/kg. Methods that can be used to reduce intraoperative blood loss include the use of a cell saver device, induced hypotension, intraoperative hemodilution, or the use of antifibrinolytic agents (tranexamic acid or aminocaproic acid).

Venous air embolism: the incidence of venous air embolism in patients undergoing neurosurgical procedures in the sitting, supine, prone, and lateral positions are 25%, 18%, 10%, and 8%, respectively. The presenting sign is usually hypotension with a raise in the end-tidal nitrogen concentration (anesthetic gas circuits do not contain nitrogen, but room air does). If detected, the wound should be immediately flooded to decrease the entry from the room air source, nitrous oxide should be discontinued to prevent the expansion of the air embolism, and vasopressors and fluid boluses administered to immediately support hemodynamic function in the face of possible acute right-sided heart failure.

Postoperative visual loss: the occurrence of ophthalmic complications after spine surgery is reported to be less than 0.2%. However, of the 131 cases of postoperative visual loss reported in a 2006, a review showed that 93 patients had undergone spine surgery (see Figure 117.2). The distribution of the source of the injury in the 93 patients can be found in this figure. Risk factors appear to be hypertension, carotid artery disease, smoking, obesity, diabetes, prolonged surgical procedures greater than 6.5 hours, and substantial blood loss.

Questions

1. CVP values in spinal surgery in the prone position can be which?
   a. falsely low
   b. falsely high
   c. correlate well with transesophageal assessment of ventricular filing
   d. correlate well with pulmonary artery occlusion pressure

2. The incidence of motor deficit or paraplegia after surgery to correct scoliosis in the absence of spinal cord monitoring has been quoted to vary between 3.7% and 6.9%. With the use of intraoperative neurophysiological monitoring this percentage can be reduced to:
   a. 0.5%
   b. 1%
   c. 2%
   d. 2.5%

3. The time from change in electrophysiologic recordings in SSEPs or MEPs from the spinal cord after overdistraction to the onset of irreversible ischemic damage in animal studies is:
   a. 2 to 3 minutes
   b. 5 to 6 minutes
   c. 8 to 9 minutes
   d. 11 to 12 minutes

Answers

1. d. In the prone position, CVP values can be falsely high. The changes are probably a result of raised intrathoracic pressure causing reduced ventricular compliance and compression of the inferior vena cava. The dependent position of the lower limbs results in reduced venous return to the heart.

2. a. The incidence of motor deficit or paraplegia after surgery to correct scoliosis in the absence of spinal cord monitoring has been quoted to vary between 3.7% and 6.9%. By using intraoperative neurophysiological monitoring (IONM), this percentage can be reduced to 0.5%. The American Academy of Neurology had published guidelines on IONM, concluding that considerable evidence favors the use of neurological monitoring as a safe and efficacious tool in clinical situations in which a significant risk for nervous system injury exists.

3. b. The time between change in the electrophysiologic recordings from the cord after overdistraction and the onset of irreversible ischemic damage is in the order of only five to six minutes in animal studies. The IONM ideally detects perturbations in spinal cord function early, allowing the surgeon to take appropriate corrective steps before irreversible damage occurs.

Further reading

Baig, M., Lubow, M., Immesoete, P. et al. (2007). Vision loss after spine surgery: review of the literature and recommendations. *Neurosurgery Focus* 23(5), 15.

Kearon, C., Viviani, G. R., Kirklet, A., and Killian, K. J. (1993). Factors determining pulmonary function in adolescent idiopathic thoracic scoliosis. *American Review of Respiratory Disease* 148, 288–294.

Yalda, S., Maltenfort, M. G., Ratliff, J. K., and Harrop, J. S. (2010). Adult scoliosis surgery outcomes: a systemic review. *Neurosurgery Focus* 28(3), E3.

Vacanti, C. A., Sikka, P. K., Urman, R. D. et al. (2011). *Essential Clinical Anesthesia*. New York: Cambridge University Press.

Chapter

118

Anesthesia for trauma

Christopher Voscopoulos and David Janfaza

Keywords

Unintentional injuries
Homicide
Guiding principles in the care of trauma patients
Advanced trauma life support (ATLS)
ATLS – airway
ATLS – breathing
ATLS – circulation
ATLS – disability
ATLS – exposure and environmental control
Focused assessment with sonography in trauma (FAST) examination
Secondary survey
Blunt aortic injuries
Blunt cardiac injuries
Blunt pulmonary injuries
Blunt abdominal injuries
Crush injuries in blunt trauma
Fat embolism syndrome
Blast injury
Trauma-specific indications for intubation
Full stomach precautions in trauma patients
Causes of hypotension in trauma patients
Classes of hemorrhage in trauma patients
Hypotensive resuscitation
Management goals in traumatic brain injury

Table 118.1 Indications for definitive airway

Airway protection, e.g., GCS <8 (or vomitus)
Inadequate ventilation, e.g., apnea, hypoxia, hypercarbia, airway bleeding, severe carboxyhemoglobinemia
Severe maxillofacial injury
Impending airway obstruction, e.g., inhalational injury, pulsatile neck mass
Need for hyperventilation

GCS, Glasgow Coma Scale.
(Used with permission from *Essential Clinical Anesthesia*, Cambridge University Press, 2011, p. 732.)

- Treatment should ensue immediately based on clinical diagnosis instead of waiting to establishing a definitive diagnosis.
- Prevent secondary injuries.

Advanced trauma life support (ATLS) was developed in the 1970s to create an algorithmic approach to the resuscitation of trauma victims. The algorithmic approach is based on the "ABCDE" mnemonic (airway, breathing, circulation [and hemorrhage control], disability, exposure/environmental control). However, it is noteworthy that when faced with trauma that is an operative emergency associated with massive and continuous blood loss, delaying operative treatment in order to further resuscitate or diagnose leads to worsened outcomes.

ATLS – airway: options for establishing a definitive airway in trauma include oral or nasal endotracheal intubation, cricothyroidotomy, or tracheostomy. The choice of airway is dependent on the amount of facial trauma limiting access to the airway. Table 118.1 illustrates the indications for a definitive airway.

ATLS – breathing: the goal of the examination is to rule out tension pneumothorax, open pneumothorax, flail chest, and massive hemothorax.

Chronic illness usually not manifesting until later years, unintentional injuries, the majority being motor vehicle accidents and blunt trauma, continue to be the leading cause of morbidity and mortality in the United States for people aged 1 to 44 years.

Homicide is the second most frequent cause of death in young adults.

Guiding principles in the care of trauma patients:
- With life-threatening conditions, prioritization for treatment should be given in the order of severity.

Essential Clinical Anesthesia Review: Keywords, Questions and Answers for the Boards, ed. Linda S. Aglio, Robert W. Lekowski, and Richard D. Urman. Published by Cambridge University Press. © Cambridge University Press 2015.

Table 118.2 The Glasgow Coma Scale (GCS)

Eye opening	Spontaneous 4 To speech 3 To pain 2 None 1
Verbal response	Oriented 5 Confused 4 Inappropriate 3 Incomprehensible 2 None 1
Best motor response	Obeys verbal commands 6 Localizes painful stimulus 5 Withdraws from painful stimulus 4 Decorticate posturing (upper extremity flexion) 3 Decerebrate posturing (upper extremity extension) 2 No movement 1

(*Source*: Teasdale, G. and Jennett, B. 1974. Assessment of coma and impaired consciousness. A practical scale. *Lancet*, 2: 81–84.)

ATLS – circulation: the working assumption for hypotension must be exsanguinating hemorrhage until proven otherwise. Exsanguinating hemorrhage may occur into five locations; the outside environment, the peritoneum, the retroperitoneal space, the thorax, and fractured long bones and their surrounding tissues. This means that if hemorrhage is suspected based on clinical grounds or laboratory evidence, if no source is obvious, imaging is needed of the chest, abdomen, pelvis, and femurs. Large-bore IV access should be established as soon as possible, and resuscitation initiated with warmed lactated Ringer's solution.

ATLS – disability: the neurological status of the patient is assessed by evaluating the patient's best pre-hospital mental status. This is assessed by the use of the Glasgow Coma Scale (GCS) score (see Table 118.2), the ability to move the four extremities, and the pupil size and reactivity.

ATLS – exposure and environmental control: the patient is undressed and briefly examined from head to toe, and obvious exposures to ingested and environmental toxins are identified.

Focused assessment with sonography in trauma (FAST) examination is meant to rapidly diagnose hemorrhage by using ultrasonography on four primary views – right upper quadrant, subxiphoid, left upper quadrant, and suprapubic.

Secondary survey begins when the primary survey is complete and resuscitation efforts are established. It includes a head-to-toe evaluation, a complete history and physical examination, and any further laboratory tests and imaging studies deemed necessary by the information gathered.

Blunt aortic injuries are thought to occur from torsion, deceleration with traction, or "osseous pinch", i.e., compression between bony structures. Predictors include age greater than 60 years due to the aorta being less likely to be mobile, high-energy collision as evidenced by chest wall deformity(ies),

multiple rib fractures, pneumothorax, or hemothorax, or radiographic abnormalities. If suspected, imaging evidence should be sought in the form of either computed tomography, transesophageal echocardiography, or angiography. Imaging evidence includes a widened mediastinum, abnormal aortic contour, large hemothorax, or rightward tracheal or esophageal deviation. If discovered, surgical consultation should be sought, and medical management initiated aimed at reducing the wall stress by lowering the heart rate below 100 bpm, and reducing the SBP below 100 mm Hg.

Blunt cardiac injuries may include contusion, infarction, or myocardial rupture.

Blunt pulmonary injuries may include pneumothorax, hemothorax, pulmonary contusion, tracheobronchial injuries, diaphragmatic rupture, and lung parenchymal injuries. Pulmonary contusions are usually not apparent at presentation. Evidence of contusion typically develop over the first 24 hours. Due to the injured lung parenchyma, contusion may be complicated by pneumonia and acute respiratory distress syndrome. These findings are especially prevalent in the elderly population with three or more rib fractures. Several studies have demonstrated significant reduction in the incidence of pneumonia and ventilator times in such patients when epidural or paravertebral analgesia is provided.

Blunt abdominal injuries occur via direct transmission of energy, with splenic injuries outnumbering hepatic. Increasingly, nonoperative management is favored.

Crush injuries in blunt trauma of the extremities may be associated with compartment syndrome, rhabdomyolysis, myoglobinuria, and fat embolism syndrome.

Fat embolism syndrome has a classic triad of petechiae, hypoxia, and neurologic manifestations occurring up to 24 to 72 hours after the fracture.

Blast injury by explosions causes four patterns of damage. Primary blast injury is the direct interaction of the blast wave with the body tissue. Secondary blast injury is the interaction of debris energized by the blast with the victim. Tertiary blast injury is the injury sustained by the physical displacement of the body by the blast wind, including tumbling and crush injury. Quaternary includes all other types, including burn injury.

Trauma-specific indications for intubation may be needed to: (1) decrease elevated intracranial pressure, (2) deliver 100% oxygen in patients with carbon monoxide poisoning, or (3) allow sedation for combative patients unable to comply with urgent diagnostic testing.

Full stomach precautions in trauma patients should occur as the associated catecholamine surge causes significant delay in gastric emptying. This means that even though eight hours may have elapsed since a patient's last meal, the delayed gastric emptying in trauma could still render a full stomach.

Causes of hypotension in trauma patients, see Table 118.3. Large-bore IV access should be established in the emergency department, defined by IV bore size of at least 18 gauge to allow for adequate speed of resuscitation efforts, followed by infusion of two liters of lactated Ringer's solution, or 20 ml/kg

Table 118.3 Causes of hypotension in the trauma patient

Hypovolemia (e.g., hemorrhage, "third-space" losses from burns, neurogenic)
Loss of sympathetic tone (high spinal cord injury)
Impaired venous return (tension pneumothorax, pericardial tamponade)
Myocardial dysfunction (myocardial infarction, myocardial contusion, fat or air embolism)
Medications, including ingestions or environmental toxins

(Used with permission from *Essential Clinical Anesthesia*, Cambridge University Press, 2011, p. 736, Table 119.3.)

Table 118.4 Classes of hemorrhage in trauma patients

	Heart rate	Blood pressure	Pulse pressure	Respiratory
Class I: <15% blood volume	—	—/▲	—	—
Class II: 15–30%	▲	—	▼	▲
Class III: 30–40%	▲	▼	▼	▲
Class IV: >40%	▲	▼	▼	▲

(Used with permission from *Essential Clinical Anesthesia*, Cambridge University Press, 2011, p. 736, Table 119.4.)

Table 118.5 Traumatic brain injury management goals

Maintain SBP >90 mm Hg
Maintain O$_2$ Sat >90%
Mannitol 0.25–1 g/kg
No evidence of benefit from hypothermia
ICP monitoring if GCS 3 to 8 and CT abnormalities
Maintain ICP <20 mm Hg
Maintain CPP (MAP-ICP) 50 to 70 mm Hg
Use of barbiturates only for surgically refractory elevated ICP
Use of anticonvulsants to prevent early post-traumatic seizures (<7 d)
Avoidance of hyperventilation – used only as a temporizing measure
No evidence of benefit from glucocorticoids

ICP, intracranial pressure; CPP, cerebral perfusion pressure; MAP, mean arterial pressure; SPB, systolic blood pressure; GCS, Glasgow Coma Scale. (Used with permission from *Essential Clinical Anesthesia*, Cambridge University Press, 2011, p. 737.)

in children. If the hypotension persists and there is strong clinical evidence of hemorrhage, transfusion of uncrossmatched type O blood should be considered.

Classes of hemorrhage in trauma patients: see Table 118.4.

Hypotensive resuscitation, or permitting hypotension until definitive hemorrhage control can be obtained, may reduce mortality in humans in certain cases, but specifically not head trauma. Patients with head trauma carry a high risk of increased intracranial hypertension with resultant risk of a decrease in cerebral perfusion pressure (cerebral perfusion pressure is defined as mean arterial pressure minus intracranial pressure). Patients with a single episode of hypotension, defined as an SBP <90 mm Hg, in the setting of cerebral trauma have 40% higher mortality.

Management goals in traumatic brain injury: see Table 118.5.

Questions

1. Hypotensive resuscitation may reduce morbidity and mortality in all patients EXCEPT which?
   a. head trauma and patients with a history of uncontrolled hypertension
   b. head trauma and patients with a history of kidney disease
   c. patients with a history of heart failure and kidney diease
   d. patients with a history of heart failure and COPD
   e. patients with a history of heart failure and uncontrolled hypertension

2. Primary blast injury affects which most severely?
   a. the brain as it is the most sensitive organ
   b. the lungs because they are mostly air filled
   c. the blood vessels as they are fluid filled
   d. the borders between substances of different densities
   e. the adipose tissue–visceral interface

3. The lowest score on the Glasgow Coma Scale (GCS) is which?
   a. 0
   b. 1
   c. 2
   d. 3

Answers

1. a. In patients with head trauma, hypotension is clearly associated with significantly increased mortality. Similarly, data on hypotension resuscitation in patients with impaired autoregulation, such as uncontrolled hypertension, are lacking.
2. d. Primary blast injury affects most severely the borders between substances of different densities, for example, at air tissue junctions in the ear, or air–fluid surfaces in the colon.
3. d. The GCS measures eye opening on a 1 to 4 rating scale, verbal response on a 1 to 5 rating scale, and best motor response on a 1 to 6 rating scale. The lowest score a person can receive on each scale is 1, making the lowest possible score a 3.

Further reading

American College of Surgeons Committee on Trauma (2004). *ATLS: Advanced Trauma Life Support for Doctors: Student Course Manual*, 7th edn. Chicago: American College of Surgeons.

The Brain Trauma Foundation (2007). Guidelines for the management of severe traumatic brain injury, 3rd edn. *Neurotrauma* 24(Suppl.).

Bickell, W. H., Wall, M. J., Pepe, P. E. et al. (1994). Immediate versus delayed fluid resuscitation for hypotensive patients with penetrating torso injuries. *New England Journal of Medicine* 331, 1105–1109.

Garner, J. and Brett, S. J. (2007). Mechanisms of injury by explosive devices. *Anesthesiology Clinics* 25, 147–160.

Shults, C., Sailhamer, E. A., Li, Y. et al. (2008). Surviving blood loss without fluid resuscitation. *Journal of Trauma* 64, 629–640.

Vacanti, C. A., Sikka, P. K., Urman, R. D. et al. (2011). *Essential Clinical Anesthesia*. New York: Cambridge University Press.

Physiologic changes during pregnancy

Brendan McGinn and Jie Zhou

Keywords

Increased CO with decreased SVR
Aortocaval compression
Left uterine displacement
Physiologic anemia
Autotransfusion
Vasopressors following a regional anesthetic
Upper airway changes
Respiratory mechanics changes
Increased sensitivity to anesthetics
Human placental lactogen
Lower esophageal sphincter tone
Increased GFR
Hypercoagulable state
Lumbar lordosis

Table 119.1 Cardiovascular changes in pregnancy

Increase
Heart rate
Stroke volume
Cardiac output
Blood, red blood cell, and plasma volume

Decrease
Systemic vascular resistance
Systolic, diastolic, and mean arterial pressure

Unchanged
Central venous pressure
Pulmonary capillary wedge pressure
Left ventricular ejection fraction
Left ventricular diastolic function
Troponin I
Brain natriuretic peptide

(Taken from *Essential Clinical Anesthesia*, p. 739.)

- Increased oxygen demand due to the fetoplacental unit causes an *increased cardiac output with decreased SVR* (CO increases at five weeks, peaks immediately postpartum; SVR decreases 20% due to the placental intervillous space and vasodilation from prostacyclin, estrogen, and progesterone).

- At approximately 20 weeks gestation the gravid uterus causes *aortocaval compression*. Near term there is an approximately 15% incidence of "supine-hypotension syndrome" (tachy > brady, hypotension, N/V, ΔMS) due to decreased venous return from IVC compression (*left uterine displacement* 15 to 30° generally improves symptoms).

- There is an increase in RBC volume by 30% with an increase in plasma volume by 50% (total blood volume increases 50%) causing a *physiologic anemia*.

- CO increases from baseline during labor stages: 1st = >15%, 2nd = >30%, 3rd = >45% (returns to prelabor values two to three days postpartum and prepregnant values at three to six months postpartum). The greatest increase in circulating blood volume occurs immediately after delivery (*autotransfusion*) due to the contracted uterus and relief of aortocaval compression.

- In terms of *vasopressors following a regional anesthetic*, there is no difference in neonatal condition with either ephedrine or phenylephrine (umbilical cord blood gases have been shown to be slightly better with phenylephrine).

- *Upper airway changes* are defined by naso- and oropharyngeal mucosal engorgement, increased Mallampati score (more during labor), decreased pharyngeal volume, and increased false vocal cord size, leading to failed ET intubation reported between 1:200 and 1:750, or 10× that of the general population.

- In terms of *respiratory mechanics changes*, both tidal volumes and minute ventilation increase leading to decreased $PaCO_2$ and increased PaO_2. The diaphragm pushing up the lung bases results in decreased ERV, RV, and FRC. With FRC reduced to 80% of nonpregnant values and increased O_2 consumption, falls in PaO_2 with resultant hypoxemia develop more rapidly during apnea compared to nonpregnant women (139 mm Hg/min vs. 58 mm Hg/min).

- Due to increased progesterone, central serotonergic activity, and endorphin system activity, pregnant women

Essential Clinical Anesthesia Review: Keywords, Questions and Answers for the Boards, ed. Linda S. Aglio, Robert W. Lekowski, and Richard D. Urman. Published by Cambridge University Press. © Cambridge University Press 2015.

Table 119.2 Pulmonary changes in pregnancy

Increase
Diaphragmatic excursion
Tidal volume
Minute ventilation
Alveolar ventilation
Inspiratory capacity
PaO_2
pH
Oxygen consumption
Mallampati score
Rate of induction of inhaled anesthetics

Decrease
Chest wall excursion
FRC
Expiratory reserve volume
Residual volume
Physiologic dead space
$PaCO_2$
HCO_3
Time to become hypoxemic

Unchanged
Respiratory rate
Vital capacity
Small airway resistance
FEV_1
FEV_1/FVC
Closing capacity
Flow–volume loop
Anatomic dead space

(Taken from *Essential Clinical Anesthesia*, p. 741, Table 120.2.)

have *increased sensitivity to anesthetics*. The MAC of volatile agents decreases by 30% and induction dose of thiopental decreases by 35%. Sensitivity of peripheral nerves to local anesthetics is also enhanced.

- *Human placental lactogen* secreted by the placenta causes insulin resistance, with maternal hyperglycemia associated with fetal hyperglycemia as glucose but not insulin crosses the placenta.

- *Lower esophageal sphincter tone* decreases due to an anatomic shift in the angle of the stomach but can be increased by metoclopramide, which also increases GI motility (which is markedly slowed during labor but not during pregnancy itself). A nonparticulate antacid (e.g., sodium citrate) administered before any anesthetic can minimize damage to respiratory epithelium if aspiration of gastric contents occurs.

- *Increased GFR* by 50% results in decreases in BUN and serum creatinine.

- All coagulation factor levels increase with the exception of II and V, which stay the same, and XI and XIII, which decrease, making pregnancy a *hypercoagulable state* (although pregnancy-induced thrombocytopenia has an 8% occurrence).

- As the uterus enlarges, *lumbar lordosis* is enhanced, which is the primary contributor to the low back pain that occurs in 50% of pregnant women.

Questions

1. All of the following cardiovascular parameters increase during pregnancy EXCEPT for which?
   a. stroke volume
   b. plasma volume
   c. central venous pressure
   d. heart rate

2. All of the following respiratory parameters are unchanged during pregnancy EXCEPT for which?
   a. tidal volume
   b. vital capacity
   c. anatomic dead space
   d. respiratory rate

3. The following statements are all true EXCEPT for which?
   a. Pregnancy is a hypercoagulable state.
   b. Factors II and V decrease during pregnancy.
   c. Pregnancy-induced thrombocytopenia has an incidence of 8%.
   d. Factors XI and XIII decrease during pregnancy.

4. The following statements concerning pregnancy are all false EXCEPT for which?
   a. Fetal hyperglycemia is prevented by maternal insulin crossing the placenta.
   b. Decreased GFR results in an increased BUN and creatinine.
   c. GI motility is slowed throughout pregnancy.
   d. There is an increase in Mallampati score and false vocal cord size.

Answers

1. a. Central venous pressure does not change during pregnancy, whereas both stroke volume and heart rate increase (therefore leading to an increased cardiac output), as well as plasma volume, which increases more than RBC volume, leading to a physiologic anemia.
2. a. Tidal volume and therefore minute ventilation increase due to an unchanged respiratory rate, leading to a respiratory alkalosis and increased PaO_2. Vital capacity and anatomic dead space remain unchanged.
3. b. Levels of factors II and V remain unchanged during pregnancy, with levels of XI and XIII decreasing but all other factor levels increasing, therefore making pregnancy a hypercoagulable state.
4. c. Lower esophageal sphincter tone is decreased during pregnancy, but gastric motility is not. Gastric motility is decreased during labor itself, but not before.

Further reading

Vacanti, C. A., Sikka, P. K., Urman, R. D. et al. (2011). *Essential Clinical Anesthesia.* New York: Cambridge University Press, pp. 739–743.

Gaiser, R. (2009). Physiologic changes of pregnancy. In Chestnut, D. H., Polley, L. S., Tsen, L. C., and Wong, C. A. (eds) *Obstetric Anesthesia: Principles and Practice*, 4th edn. Philadelphia: Mosby, pp. 15–36.

Kodali, B. S., Chandrasekhar, S., Bulich, L. N. et al. (2008). Airway changes during labor and delivery. *Anesthesiology* 108, 1–6.

Chapter

120

Analgesia for labor

Brendan McGinn and Jie Zhou

Keywords

Fetal heart rate decelerations
Labor pains
Tuffier's line
Epidural test dose
Local anesthetic for labor analgesia
Adjuncts
CEI and PCEA
Labor progression
Intrapartum fever
Postdural puncture headache
Epidural blood patch

Fetal heart rate decelerations have three classifications: (1) early, which is normal and caused by fetal head compression; (2) late, which occur with any cause compromising uteroplacental blood flow (hypotension, acidosis, preeclampsia); and (3) variable, which occur with compression of the umbilical cord (persistence can lead to fetal acidosis).

Labor pains during the different stages of labor have different pathways. The first stage (uterine pain) comes from sensory fibers accompanying sympathetic nerves that end in the dorsal horns of T10–L1. The second stage (perineal/vaginal pain) comes from afferent fibers of the pudendal nerve.

When administering a neuraxial anesthetic, anterior rotation of the pelvis causes *Tuffier's line* (the line connecting the interiliac crests) to cross the lumbar spine at a higher level than L4–L5. There is also a decrease in the physical dimensions of the lumbar intervertebral space due to increased lordosis and an engorgement of the epidural venous plexus, which increases the likelihood of a vascular cannulation.

An *epidural test dose* of local anesthetic (lidocaine 45–60 mg) and epinephrine (15 µg) is often used to assess whether an epidural catheter is intrathecal or intravascular (motor block within five minutes suggests intrathecal and an increase in HR from baseline by 25 to 30 bpm within 20 to 40 seconds suggests intravascular).

Table 120.1 Labor analgesic techniques.

Non-regional techniques
Pharmacologic:
Inhalational analgesia
Systemic opioids, including PCA
Nonpharmacologic:
Acupuncture
Transcutaneous electrical nerve stimulation (TENS)
Hypnotherapy
Prepared childbirth techniques
Hydrotherapy
Regional techniques
Neuraxial:
Lumbar epidural
CSE
Continuous spinal
Nonneuraxial:
Paracervical nerve block
Pudendal nerve block

(From Vacanti, et al., 2011, p. 744.)

The ideal *local anesthetic for labor analgesia* should provide excellent pain relief, minimize motor block, have a rapid onset and long duration of action, and cause no disruption in maternal–fetal physiology. Bupivicaine has an excellent sensorimotor differential blockade at low concentrations, long duration of action, and minimal transplacental transfer.

Adjuncts include: opioids → synergism with LAs with reduction in total LA dose; clonidine → prolongs duration of analgesia but causes sedation and hypotension; epinephrine → prolongs duration of analgesia by decreasing clearance of LAs and opioids through vasoconstriction with direct effects through alpha2-agonism.

Continuous epidural infusions (*CEI*) of dilute local anesthetics can provide a stable level of analgesia and hemodynamics but usually require top ups during labor progression. Patient-controlled epidural analgesia (*PCEA*) provides better maternal satisfaction and decreases the total dose of drug administered.

Essential Clinical Anesthesia Review: Keywords, Questions and Answers for the Boards, ed. Linda S. Aglio, Robert W. Lekowski, and Richard D. Urman. Published by Cambridge University Press. © Cambridge University Press 2015.

Table 120.2 Conduct of epidural analgesia for labor

Monitors	On
Position of patient	Supine (usually/lateral)
Back preparation	Povidone-iodine (Becadine, Purdue Pharma LP. Stamford, CT) × 3 times and draped
Lumbar space	L3–L4/L2–L3
Local infiltration	1–2 ml of 1% lidocaine
Needle	17 G or higher gauge Tuohy
Technique	Loss of resistance to air/saline
Wet tap	Remove needle and go one space above
Epidural catheter insertion	2–4 cm into epidural space
Aspiration of catheter	Negative for heme and CSF
Test dose	3 ml of 1.5% lidocaine with 1:200,000 epinephrine
Agent	0.25% bupivacaine 5–10 ml bolus
Desirable level of anesthesia	T10

(From Vacanti et al., *Essential Clinical Anesthesia*, 2011, p. 746.)

Table 120.3 Examples of suggested PCEA regimens

Anesthetic mixture	Infusion rate, ml/h	Bolus dose, ml	Lockout interval, min	Hourly maximum, ml
Bupivacaine 0.125%	6	6	15	30
Bupivacaine 0.125% with 2 µg/ml tentanyl	4–6	6	15	30
Bupivacaine 0.0625% with 2 µg/ml tentanyl	10–15	5	10	45
Bupivacaine 0.08% with 2 µg/ml tentanyl	10	5	15	30
Bupivacaine 0.125% with 1 µg/ml sufentanil	5	5	15	25

(From Vacanti et al., *Essential Clinical Anesthesia*, 2011, p. 747.)

Epidural analgesia does not increase the incidence of C-sections, but may prolong the second stage of *labor progression*, especially in nulliparous women.

Randomized studies have confirmed an association between epidurals and *intrapartum fever*, which leads to increased maternal antibiotic exposure and neonatal sepsis evaluations.

Table 120.4 Complications of epidural catheter placement for labor analgesia

Hypotension	Pruritus
Inadequate analgesia	Excessive motor block
Urinary retention	FHR abnormalities
Intrapartum fever	Back pain
PDPH	Subdural block
High or total spinal anesthesia	Epidural hematoma or abscess
Accidental IV injection of local anesthetics	

(From Vacanti et al., *Essential Clinical Anesthesia*, 2011, p. 748.)

Postdural puncture headache following a wet tap during attempted epidural placement manifests within 24 hours, is described as a severe fronto-occipital headache, sometimes with neck pain, is made worse with sitting or standing/better in the supine position, and may be accompanied by N/V, diplopia, or tinnitus.

If conservative measures do not resolve a PDPH (bed rest, fluids, analgesics, and caffeine) an *epidural blood patch* may be indicated, which relieves 85% to 90% of PDPHs after one blood patch (the remainder may require a second after 24 hours).

Questions

1. Labor epidurals are associated with all of the following EXCEPT for which?
   a. increased maternal antibiotic exposure due to intrapartum fever
   b. an increase in the incidence of C-sections
   c. an increase in the second stage of labor progression
   d. an incidence of postdural puncture headache of approximately 1:100

2. All of the following statements concerning fetal heart rate decelerations are true EXCEPT for which?
   a. Late decelerations are caused by fetal head compression.
   b. Variable decelerations are caused by compression of the umbilical cord.
   c. Early decelerations are normal and not a cause for concern.
   d. Persistent variable decelerations can lead to fetal acidosis.

3. None of the following statements associated with pregnancy are true EXCEPT for which?
   a. Pain from the first stage of labor is associated with somatic sensory fibers that end in the dorsal horns of T10–L1.

b. Decreased lordosis leads to an increase in the size of lumbar intervertebral spaces.

c. Postdural puncture headaches are generally parietotemporal in nature.

d. Engorgement of the epidural venous plexus increases the likelihood of vascular cannulation when placing an epidural catheter.

4. All of the following statements concerning neuraxial labor analgesia are true EXCEPT for which?

a. Epinephrine has direct analgesic effects via alpha2-agonism.

b. PCEA is associated with a decrease in total dose of drug administered.

c. Due to the dilute concentration of bupivicaine administered, cardiotoxicity is rare.

d. Clonidine prolongs duration of analgesia via indirect alpha-1 agonism.

Answers

1. b. Although labor epidurals may prolong the second stage of labor, they are not associated with an increased rate of C-sections.

2. a. Late decelerations are caused by anything leading to a decrease in uteroplacental blood flow, including hypotension, acidosis, and preeclampsia. Early decelerations, which are normal, are caused by fetal head compression.

3. d. Because the risk of intravascular cannulation with epidural catheters increases due to engorgement of the epidural venous plexus in parturients, the use of epinephrine in an epidural test dose to detect an increase in heart rate from baseline by 25 to 30 bpm within 20 to 40 seconds should be used before bolusing larger volumes of local anesthetic through the catheter.

4. d. Clonidine prolongs the duration of analgesia via direct alpha2-receptor agonism and can also cause sedation and hypotension, which are two things you would like to avoid in the laboring parturient.

Further reading

Vacanti, C. A., Sikka, P. K. Urman, R. D., et al. (2011). *Essential Clinical Anesthesia*. New York: Cambridge University Press, pp. 744–750.

Leighton, B. L. and Halpern, S. H. (2002). The effects of epidural analgesia on labor, maternal, and neonatal outcomes: a systematic review. *American Journal of Obstetric Gynecology* 186(5 Suppl Nature), S69–S77.

Chapter

121

Anesthesia for cesarean delivery

Brendan McGinn and Jie Zhou

Keywords

Neuraxial technique
T4 dermatome
3% 2-chloroprocaine
Alkalinization
Failed intubation
High spinal

A *neuraxial technique* (spinal, epidural, or a combination of both) is the preferred method of anesthesia for both elective and emergent C-sections, with contraindications being localized infection or sepsis, uncorrected coagulation disorders, severe hypovolemia, or cardiac pathologies that are most severe during hypotension (severe antepartum hemorrhage or preeclampsia may complicate further).

Spinal anesthesia is the most common technique used for elective C-section, with the goal of obtaining a *T4 dermatome*

Table 121.1 Advantages/disadvantages of neuraxial anesthesia

Advantages:
Minimal fetal exposure to drugs
Decreased incidence of maternal pulmonary aspiration
An awake mother with greater bonding with the neonate

Disadvantages:
Greater incidence of hypotension
Exposure to risk of neuraxial anesthesia

(From Vacanti et al., 2011, *Essential Clinical Anesthesia*, p. 752.)

Table 121.2 Advantages/disadvantages of general anesthesia.

Advantages:
Rapid onset and reliability
Airway control
Less hypotension than neuraxial anesthesia

Disadvantages:
Increased risk of pulmonary aspiration
Drug-induced fetal cardiorespiratory depression
Difficult airway management

(From Vacanti et al., 2011, *Essential Clinical Anesthesia*, p. 752.)

Table 121.3 Conduct of spinal anesthesia

Monitors	BP measurement every 2 min after spinal administration for 15 to 20 min, electrocardiogram pulse oximetry
Patient position	Sitting or lateral recumbent
Back preparation	Betadine or chlorhexidine × 3 times
Lumbar space	L3–4/L4–5
Local infiltration	1 to 2 ml of 1 % lidocaine
Needle	25 G or higher (need an introducer)
CSF flow	Free flow, typically no herne or paresthesia
Agent	10 to 12 mg of hyperbaric (8.25% dextrose) bupivacaine [0.75%]
Additives	Fentanyl 10 to 25 µg/morphine 0.2 to 0.3 mg. epinephrine 1: 200,000
Desirable level of anesthesia	T4
Patient position	Supine with left uterine displacement (tilt table toward left and/or put a blanket roll under right hip)
Oxygen supplementation	Nasal cannula/face mask
Hypotension	Phenylephrine 40 µg, ephedrine 5 to 10 mg, epinephrine if life-threatening, fluid supplementation, uterine tilt
Nausea	Check BP (usually due to impending hypotension), metoclopramide, ondansetron

(From Vacanti et al., 2011, *Essential Clinical Anesthesia*, page 752.)

level (despite a low abdominal incision) in order to prevent referred pain from traction on the peritoneum and uterus.

When a labor epidural is in place, *3% 2-chloroprocaine* is the local anesthetic of choice when an emergent C-section is required due, to its rapid onset and rapid maternal and fetal metabolism (fetal accumulation during acidosis is minimized).

Essential Clinical Anesthesia Review: Keywords, Questions and Answers for the Boards, ed. Linda S. Aglio, Robert W. Lekowski, and Richard D. Urman. Published by Cambridge University Press. © Cambridge University Press 2015.

Table 121.4 Conduct of general anesthesia

Aspiration prophylaxis	Sodium citrate 30 ml, within 30 min of induction, if possible Metoclopramide 10 mg IV, preferably 30 min prior to induction to avoid rapid IV push
Position	Supine with left uterine displacement
Preoxygenation	3 min/4–8 deep breaths of 100% oxygen
Induction	Rapid sequence with criticoid pressure, thiopental 3–5 mg/kg, succinylcholine at 1–2 mg/kg
Incision	If emergent, CD as soon as patient is intubated
Intubation	Usually a smaller size endotracheal tube (6 to 6.5 mm diameter), orogastric tube
Maintenance	Oxygen, inhalational agent (low concentration), muscle relaxant
After baby is delivered	Antibiotics, oxytocin, opioids
Reversal of muscle paralysis	Neostigmine and glycopyrrolate
Extubation	Awake

(From Vacanti et al., 2011, *Essential Clinical Anesthesia*, p. 753.)

It is not used in non-urgent C-sections due to the need for frequent re-dosing, due to its short duration of action, and may interfere with epidural opioid analgesia as well as increase the incidence of back pain with large volumes.

Alkalinization of local anesthetic with sodium bicarbonate (1 cc 8.4% solution to 10 cc 2% lidocaine or 3% 2-chloroprocaine) hastens the onset and increases the intensity of the epidural blockade when anesthesia for C-section is needed urgently.

General anesthesia for C-section is avoided if possible due to the four to five times increased risk of *failed intubation* and pulmonary aspiration than the general population.

After a failed, but partial, spinal or epidural attempt, the use of a repeat spinal technique may result in a *high spinal* when more than 10 mg of bupivicaine is used. Using a semi-sitting (Fowler's) position to limit cephalad spread or a CSE technique with a small initial intrathecal dose may help avoid this complication. If a C-section has already commenced,

sedation with IV fentanyl and/or midazolam, N_2O, or ketamine in the presence of severe pain can all be used before converting to GA.

A *high spinal* may manifest as mild dyspnea with a T2 level and more severely with MSΔs and respiratory depression at higher levels, at which point conversion to GA should occur.

Questions

1. Spinal anesthesia for C-section:
   a. Requires only a T10 level due to the low abdominal incision involved.
   b. May be repeated after a failed but partial attempt with a larger dose of local anesthetic without concern for a high spinal.
   c. Has a lower incidence of hypotension than GA in the parturient.
   d. Has a decreased incidence of pulmonary aspiration than GA in the parturient.

2. All of the following concerning 3% 2-chloroprocaine are true EXCEPT for which?
   a. Fetal accumulation during acidosis is minimal.
   b. A short duration of action makes use outside emergent C-sections impractical.
   c. It demonstrates synergism with epidural opioids.
   d. Large volumes may increase the incidence of back pain.

Answers

1. d. Spinal anesthesia provides an awake and comfortable patient with minimal risks for aspiration during a C-section, with the goal of obtaining a T4 level to prevent referred pain from traction on the peritoneum and uterus.
2. c. Along with being a short-acting local anesthetic with a very rapid onset, 3% 2-chloroprocaine can affect the efficacy of subsequent epidural opioid analgesia negatively, making its use impractical outside urgent or emergent situations.

Further reading

Vacanti, C. A., Sikka, P. K., Urman, R. D. et al. (2011). *Essential Clinical Anesthesia*. New York: Cambridge University Press, pp. 751–755.

Chapter

122

Obstetric hemorrhage

Benjamin Kloesel and Michaela K. Farber

Keywords

Uterine blood flow
Antepartum hemorrhage
Postpartum hemorrhage
Oxytocin
Ergot alkaloids
Prostaglandins

Antepartum hemorrhage refers to bleeding after 20 weeks of gestation that is not related to delivery. Common causes include placenta previa and placental abruption. Less common causes are vasa previa with velamentous cord insertion, uterine rupture, and genital tract lesions.

Postpartum hemorrhage is defined as blood loss greater than 500 ml or 1,000 ml within 24 hours of vaginal or cesarean delivery, respectively. Causes include uterine atony, retained products of conception, placenta accreta/percreta/increta, uterine inversion, genital tract laceration, and coagulopathy.

Uterine blood flow (UBF) increases during pregnancy from a baseline of 50 to 100 ml/min (<5% of CO) to 500 to 800 ml/min at term (12% of CO). It is defined as mean arterial pressure (MAP) minus central venous pressure (CVP) divided by uterine vascular resistance. The uterus cannot autoregulate blood flow, therefore uteroplacental perfusion is largely dependent on MAP. Main factors that reduce UBF are maternal hypotension, aortocaval compression, and uterine contractions, which increase uterine vascular resistance.

Placenta previa occurs in 1/200 pregnancies and presents as painless vaginal bleeding in the second or third trimester. Placenta previa is defined as a placenta that has implanted in advance of the fetal presenting part. Depending on how much of the cervical os is covered by the placenta, a subdivision into total (completely covering os), partial (involving part of the os), and marginal (only covering a margin of the os) can be made. The condition is diagnosed by ultrasound and managed with cesarean delivery. Five percent of cases are associated with placenta accreta; the risk of placenta accreta in conjunction with placenta previa increases with increasing number of prior cesarean deliveries. Neuraxial anesthesia is an option for cesarean delivery in a hemodynamically stable patient. Anesthetic management includes adequate IV access and cross-matched blood availability.

Placental abruption occurs in 3.4–7.9/1,000 pregnancies and presents as painful vaginal bleeding in the third trimester. It occurs when the placental bed prematurely separates from the decidua basalis; the immediate escape of blood from the implantation site through the vagina is referred to as the Duncan mechanism. Occasionally, the bleeding can be concealed and up to 1 to 2 liters can accumulate between the uterus and placenta, known as the Schultze mechanism. Ten percent of cases are associated with consumptive coagulopathy; risk increases to 50% in the presence of fetal demise. The condition is managed either expectantly (limited/chronic abruption) or by vaginal or cesarean delivery. Neuraxial anesthesia can be provided in a hemodynamically stable patient with normal coagulation tests.

Velamentous cord insertion with vasa previa is diagnosed when fetal vessels lie over the cervical os ahead of the fetal presenting part. This position predisposes them to tear during rupture of membranes, which can quickly lead to fetal exsanguination. Diagnosis should be suspected when fetal distress occurs with minimal maternal blood loss. Treatment includes expeditious delivery, typically under general anesthesia.

Uterine rupture usually occurs during attempted vaginal delivery and typically involves sudden onset, unexplained fetal distress. Induction of labor increases the risk ten-fold. The parturient may present with persistent abdominal pain but can also be asymptomatic. Fetal bradycardia is a leading sign. The condition is life-threatening and must be managed with emergent cesarean delivery. An urgent induction of anesthesia using an in-dwelling epidural catheter or general anesthesia is required. The concern that an epidural catheter for spontaneous vaginal deliveries in high-risk patients might mask early warning signs is unfounded. Only very dense epidural analgesia can mask uterine rupture pain, and fetal distress is the most reliable sign.

Essential Clinical Anesthesia Review: Keywords, Questions and Answers for the Boards, ed. Linda S. Aglio, Robert W. Lekowski, and Richard D. Urman. Published by Cambridge University Press. © Cambridge University Press 2015.

Genital tract lacerations can occur after direct trauma and require perineal repair under neuraxial or general anesthesia.

Uterine atony is the most common cause of postpartum hemorrhage, and is diagnosed clinically by a boggy uterus, absence of adequate contractions, and continued bleeding. Step-wise management begins with uterine massage and administration of oxytocin with second-line agents, including ergot alkaloids, prostaglandin E_1, and prostaglandin $F_2\alpha$. If preliminary maneuvers fail, further interventions include uterine artery embolization, uterine compression sutures (e.g., B-Lynch suture), tamponade devices (e.g., Bakri balloon), or hysterectomy.

Retained products of conception cause postpartum bleeding that can result from incomplete separation of the placenta after cord traction. It is treated by manual or surgical extraction of the retained fragments. Uterine relaxation may be required for manual extraction, and can be achieved using nitroglcyerin (100–250 μg IV) or deep inhalational anesthesia.

Placenta accreta describes an abnormal adherence of the placenta to the uterine myometrium due to the disruption of the decidua basalis layer. The most common variant is placenta accreta vera (placental adherence to the myometrium, 78% of cases); placenta increta (extension into myometrium, 17% of cases); and placenta percreta (extension through myometrium with neighboring organ invasion, predominantly the bladder, 5% of cases) are less common. Bleeding during the third stage of labor is caused by the inability to separate the placenta from the myometrium. Treatment to preserve fertility is possible in patients with limited or focal placenta accreta and includes uterotonic agents, excision of involved myometrium, uterine artery ligation/embolization, uterine sutures, or methotrexate. More severe cases require a hysterectomy, sometimes preceded by selective arterial embolization. Anesthetic management requires volume resuscitation with adequate IV access, cross-matched blood products in the operating room, and monitoring of coagulation parameters. General or neuraxial anesthesia can be employed.

Uterine inversion can occur after excessive traction on the umbilical cord in the third stage of labor and may herald a diagnosis of placenta accreta. Uterine inversion can lead to significant blood loss and cause vagally mediated bradycardia with hypotension. Treatment includes timely reduction facilitated by uterine relaxation using nitroglycerin or inhalational agents. After reduction is achieved, oxytocin is required to restore uterine tone.

Uterine relaxants include beta-agonists (Ritodrine®, Salbutamol®, Terbutaline®), inhaled amyl nitrate, magnesium sulfate, nitroglycerin, and volatile anesthetics.

Oxytocin (Pitocin®) is an ADH-related polypeptide that causes uterine contraction by activating G-protein-mediated calcium release from the sarcoplasmic reticulum in myocytes. Oxytocin is given intravenously, although intramuscular and intrauterine administration are also possible. Side effects include hyponatremia, due to structural similarity to vasopressin, pulmonary hypertension, hypotension, tachycardia, and flushing.

Ergonovine (Ergometrine®) and *methylergometrine maleate (Methergine®)* are *ergot alkaloids* that cause serotonin and α_1 receptor-mediated uterine contraction. Given intramuscularly, side effects of the ergot alkaloids include systemic and pulmonary hypertension, coronary artery vasospasm, bronchospasm, headache, nausea, and vomiting. These medications are contraindicated in patients with preeclampsia, chronic hypertension, cardiovascular, or cerebrovascular disease.

Carboprost tromethamine (Hemabate®), 15-methyl prostaglandin $F_2\alpha$, causes uterine contraction by increasing calcium levels in myometrial cells. Intramuscular or intrauterine administration of this medication can be associated with bronchospasm, and should be avoided in asthmatics.

Misoprostol is a prostaglandin E_1 analog with uterotonic and cervical ripening effects.

Recombinant activated Factor VIIa (NovoSeven®) is a precursor for the extrinsic clotting cascade that can be considered in massive coagulopathy. A major adverse effect is hypercoagulability. Use of rFVIIa for obstetric hemorrhage is controversial and safety is unknown.

Fibrinogen concentrate (RiaSTAP) can be helpful in obstetric hemorrhage with suspected disseminated intravascular coagulopathy (DIC) or other conditions of hyperfibrinolysis.

Questions

1. Uterine blood flow:
    a. is constant due to autoregulation at mean arterial blood pressures of 50 to 100 mm Hg
    b. decreases from the first to the third trimester
    c. decreases during uterine contractions
    d. is not affected by spinal anesthesia

2. The first agent of choice to treat uterine atony is which?
    a. magnesium sulfate
    b. vasopressin
    c. oxytocin
    d. carboprost tromethamine

3. Which condition requires a cesarean section for delivery?
    a. total placenta previa
    b. placental abruption
    c. velamentous insertion
    d. preeclampsia

Answers

1. c. Uterine contractions compress uterine blood vessels and cause a decrease in uterine blood flow, which is directly dependent on mean arterial pressures as the placenta lacks autoregulation. With increasing gestational age, the increasing placental mass leads to an increase in blood flow.

2. c. Oxytocin is the first-line treatment for atony; second-line agents, including ergot alkaloids and prostaglandins, are chosen based on patient comorbidities and side effect profile.

3. a While the other choices allow a vaginal delivery, a total placenta previa anatomically prohibits the passage of the fetus through the cervical os.

Further reading

Guaran, C. and Leffert, L. R. (2011). Chapter 123. Obstetric hemorrhage. In Vacanti, C. A., Sikka, P. J., Urman, R. D., Dershwitz, M., and Segal, B. S. (eds) *Essential Clinical Anesthesia*. Cambridge: Cambridge University Press.

Snegovskikh, D. and Braveman, F. R. (2012). Chapter 26: Pregnancy-associated disease. In *Stoelting's Anesthesia and Co-Existing Disease*, 6th edn. Philadelphia, PA: Saunders, Elsevier Inc.

Snegovskikh, D. et al. (2011). Anesthetic management of patients with placenta accreta and resuscitation strategies for associated massive hemorrhage. *Current Opinion in Anaesthesiology* 24(3), 274–281.

Wise, A. et al. (2008). Strategies to manage major obstetric haemorrhage. *Current Opinion in Anaesthesiology* 21(3), 281–287.

Chapter

123

Preeclampsia

Benjamin Kloesel and Michaela K. Farber

Gestational hypertension
Chronic hypertension
Chronic hypertension with superimposed
    preeclampsia
Preeclampsia
HELLP syndrome
Eclamptic seizures
Uteroplacental blood flow

Preeclampsia is defined as persistent hypertension (≥ 140 systolic and/or ≥ 90 diastolic) after 20 weeks of gestation in the presence of proteinuria (>300 mg in 24 hours) and occurs in 3% to 5% of all pregnancies (predominantly in nulliparous women). *Severe preeclampsia* requires the diagnosis of an organ dysfunction (e.g., CNS involvement, oliguria, pulmonary edema), proteinuria of ≥ 5 g in 24 hours or blood pressure of ≥ 160 systolic or ≥ 110 diastolic on two occasions at least six hours apart. It needs to be distinguished from *chronic hypertension* (present before and during pregnancy) and *gestational hypertension* (occurs after 20 weeks of gestation without organ system involvement).

Antihypertensive drugs considered safe during pregnancy include methyldopa, hydralazine, labetalol, nifedipine, isradipine, low-dose diazoxide, and selected beta-blockers (metoprolol, pindolol, propranolol).

Drugs to avoid during pregnancy include atenolol, which can cause fetal growth restriction, and ACE inhibitors/angiotensin type-2 receptor blockers, which have renal teratogenicity.

Patients with preeclampsia experience a variety of *pathophysiologic changes*. Increased peripheral vascular resistance, increased cardiac output, and increased sympathetic nervous system activity lead to systemic hypertension despite a decreased blood volume. Sensitivity to catecholamines is increased. Platelet activation can predispose to bleeding and hypercoagulability can increase clotting risk. Proteinuria leads to decreased oncotic pressure, increased vascular permeability,

Table 123.1 Physiologic changes in preeclampsia

Physiologic change	Normal pregnancy	Preeclampsia
Blood pressure	Decreased or normal	Increased
Cardiac output	Increased	Decreased to increased
PVR	Decreased	Increased
Intravascular volume	Increased	Decreased
CVP and PCWP	Normal	Normal

PVR, pulmonary vascular resistance; CVP, central venous pressure; PCWP, pulmonary capillary wedge pressure.
Form: Vacanti et al., 2011, p. 762.

and upper airway and pulmonary edema risk. Decreased glomerular filtration rate and oliguria can occur in addition to cerebral edema and CNS excitability. Uteroplacental perfusion is often compromised.

Definitive management of preeclampsia is delivery of the fetus. Timing of delivery is dependent on severity of disease and fetal lung maturity. Neuraxial techniques for labor analgesia or cesarean delivery are beneficial to reduce sympathetic tone and circulating catecholamines. Decreased circulating intravascular volume should be recognized. Sensitivity to vasopressors requires careful titration when treating hypotension after a neuraxial block. If general anesthesia is provided, an enhanced sympathetic response to laryngoscopy should be anticipated and prevented.

HELLP (Hemolysis, Elevated Liver enzymes, and Low Platelets) syndrome is a subset of severe preeclampsia, but can occur in the absence of hypertension. The only effective treatment is prompt delivery. All anesthetic techniques can be used, although progressive thrombocytopenia may preclude neuraxial techniques.

Administration of *corticosteroids* increases platelet count. Corticosteroids have not been shown to reduce fetal or maternal mortality but may be clinically useful to increase platelet count when neuraxial anesthesia is anticipated.

Table 123.2 Criteria for diagnosis of HELLP syndrome

Hemolysis: abnormal peripheral blood smear – schistocytes and helmet cells from microangiopathic hemolysis; increased total bilirubin >1.2 mg/dl

Elevated liver enzymes: AST >2 times normal; increased lactic dehydrogenase >600 U/L

Low platelets: platelet count <100,000/mm^3

Form: Vacanti et al., 2011, p. 762.

Magnesium sulfate is the medication of choice for prevention and treatment of eclamptic seizures. It is administered during labor, delivery, and up to 48 hours postpartum. Magnesium acts as a calcium antagonist in vascular smooth muscle cells, inhibits the release of catecholamines from the adrenal medulla and postganglionic sympathetic synapses, stimulates prostacyclin and nitric oxide release from vascular endothelium, and decreases uterine tone by relaxation of uterine blood vessels and smooth muscles. It potentiates the effects of nondepolarizing neuromuscular blockers. Therapeutic range of serum magnesium levels is 4 to 8 mEq/l. Symptoms of *hypermagnesemia* include hyporeflexia, respiratory depression, altered AV conduction, and complete heart block. On EKG, a prolonged QT interval is seen. Treatment of choice is administration of calcium gluconate. Magnesium antagonizes alpha-adrenergic agonists, therefore ephedrine is the vasopressor of choice for magnesium-related hypotension. Magnesium has an NMDA-antagonistic effect. Magnesium crosses the placenta; fetal effects of maternal magnesium administration include decreased beat-to-beat variability in fetal heart rate, hyporeflexia, and decreased respiratory efforts.

Eclamptic seizures are usually self-limited and last one to ten minutes. Treatment is supportive and includes supplemental oxygen, magnesium sulfate, protection from additional trauma, and, in rare cases, termination of seizure with benzodiazepines or barbiturates.

Due to endothelial dysfunction, increased vascular resistance in the placental blood vessels, and lack of autoregulation, the patient with preeclampsia is at high risk for impaired *uteroplacental perfusion* during episodes of hypotension.

The most frequent complication of preeclampsia is *pulmonary edema*. Management includes supplemental oxygen, glyceroltrinitrate, furosemide, and morphine. Other causes of maternal death include intracranial hemorrhage, cerebral infarction, respiratory failure, and hepatic failure/rupture.

Labetalol is a mixed α- and β-antagonist that can be administered orally or intravenously. It is a mixture of four stereoisomers. The α- to β-antagonism ratio is 1 to 5–10.

α-Methyldopa is a pro-drug that is metabolized in central adrenergic neurons to α-methylnorepinephrine, which is stored in synaptic vesicles. When released into the synapse, α-methylnorepinephrine acts as an α_2-agonist and inhibits adrenergic outflow, resulting in decreased norepinephrine release. Serious side effects include hepatotoxicity and hemolytic anemia.

Hydralazine is a direct arteriolar smooth muscle relaxant that has no effect on the venous system. Profound arteriolar smooth muscle relaxation and the ensuing hypotension stimulate the sympathetic nervous system, resulting in tachycardia, augmented inotropy, and increase in renin activity. Co-administration with β-blockers and diuretics may be beneficial.

Questions

1. In the setting of severe preeclampsia with a blood pressure of 230/120, which of the following statements is CORRECT?
   a. The blood pressure should be expeditiously corrected to prelabor values.
   b. Labetalol or hydralazine should be used as first-line agents.
   c. Intravenous atenolol is preferred over labetalol.
   d. The patient should be closely monitored; an intervention is not required at this point.

2. Which organ is the main driving factor of pathogenesis in preeclampsia?
   a. kidneys
   b. adrenal gland
   c. brain
   d. placenta

3. Which of the following statements about preeclampsia is INCORRECT?
   a. Studies have shown magnesium sulfate to be the better agent to prevent seizures in preeclamptic patients as compared to phenytoin and diazepam.
   b. The risk for eclamptic seizures stops after delivery of the fetus.
   c. An eclamptic seizure is not necessarily an indicator for urgent/emergent delivery.
   d. Eclampsia in pregnancy increases the risk for preeclampsia/eclampsia in subsequent pregnancies.

4. Which finding in a patient with preeclampsia at 29 weeks of gestation requires immediate delivery of the fetus?
   a. RUQ pain with AST of 560 and ALT of 450
   b. bilateral ankle edema
   c. blood pressure of 210/95
   d. platelet count of 142,000/l

Answers

1. b. Labetalol, hydralazine, and alpha-methyldopa are first-line agents for blood pressure control in pregnancy.
2. d. Preeclampsia requires the presence of a placenta; an imbalance of placental angiogenic and antiangiogenic growth factors lead to a shift in favor of antiangiogenesis;

multiple processes finally lead to endothelial damage and dysfunction.

3. b. Occurrence of eclamptic seizures has been reported during the third trimester as well as several weeks postpartum.

4. a. Presence of RUQ pain and liver function test elevation are consistent with HELLP syndrome; the other listed findings require treatment and/or monitoring but not immediate delivery.

Further reading

Ortman, A. and Leffert, L. R. (2011). Chapter 124. Preeclampsia. In Vacanti, C. A., Sikka, P. J., Urman, R. D., Dershwitz, M., and Segal, B. S. (eds) *Essential Clinical Anesthesia*. Cambridge, UK: Cambridge University Press.

Snegovskikh, D. and Braveman, F. R. (2012). Chapter 26. Pregnancy-associated disease. *Stoelting's Anesthesia and Co-Existing Disease*, 6th edn. Philadelphia, PA: Saunders, Elsevier Inc.

Gogarten, W. (2009). Preeclampsia and anaesthesia. *Current Opinion in Anaesthesiology* 22(3), 347–351.

Dennis, A. T. (2013). Management of pre-eclampsia: issues for anaesthetists. *Anaesthesia* 67(9), 1009–1020.

Chapter

124

Pregnant patients with comorbid diseases

Benjamin Kloesel and Michaela K. Farber

Keywords

Chronic hypertension
Valvular lesions
Pulmonary hypertension
Asthma
Diabetes mellitus
Rheumatoid arthritis
Systemic lupus erythematosus
Multiple sclerosis
Idiopathic thrombocytopenic purpura
von Willebrand disease

Neuraxial anesthesia is often beneficial for parturients with cardiovascular disease through blunting of the catecholamine stress response to labor pain.

Chronic hypertension often improves during pregnancy due to hormonal influences on maternal vasculature that have a vasodilatory effect. Many antihypertensive agents are contraindicated during pregnancy (atenolol, ACEI, ARB). Anesthetic management is typically unaffected.

Regurgitant valvular lesions are generally well tolerated during pregnancy, due to increased preload from an increase in plasma volume and decreased afterload due to decreased systemic vascular resistance. *Stenotic valvular lesions* are poorly tolerated since the parturient cannot sufficiently increase cardiac output.

Mitral stenosis is the most common and difficult to manage lesion in pregnancy. A decrease in mitral valve area results in obstruction of left ventricular filling and fixed cardiac output. Aggressively treating atrial fibrillation (beta-blockers, digoxin, cardioversion) and keeping the heart rate normal allows LV filling. Beta-blockers are the cornerstone of treatment. Triggers that can increase pulmonary vascular resistance, including hypoxia, hypercarbia, and pain, should be avoided. Situations that cause tachycardia, including fast-onset spinal anesthesia, laryngoscopy without beta-blockade, or anesthesia that is either too light or too deep, should also be avoided. There is a high risk for pulmonary edema, especially during autotransfusion in the immediate postpartum period.

Aortic stenosis worsens during pregnancy when increasing blood volume and decreased systemic vascular resistance increase the transvalvular gradient. Anesthetic goals are to optimize LV perfusion by maintaining sinus rhythm and maintaining high systemic vascular resistance. Tachycardia and bradycardia should be avoided. The parturient is dependent on preload and atrial kick to fill a stiff left ventricle.

Mitral regurgitation is the second most prevalent valvular lesion in pregnancy. An anesthetic goal is to avoid increases in systemic vascular resistance, including labor pain, uterine contractions, or surgical stimulation, which can increase the regurgitant fraction and lead to left ventricular failure and acute pulmonary edema.

Aortic insufficiency causes chronic volume overload of the left ventricle, resulting in left ventricular hypertrophy with worsening myocardial oxygen supply–demand mismatch. Anesthetic goals include avoidance of bradycardia (limits time for regurgitant flow), avoidance of increases in systemic vascular resistance, and avoidance of myocardial depression.

Pulmonary hypertension is a life-threatening condition in pregnancy, with maternal mortality of greater than 60%. Triggers that increase pulmonary vascular resistance, such as hypoxia, hypercarbia, pain, stress, and acidosis, should be avoided. Systemic vascular resistance and preload should be maintained.

Asthma is prevalent in women of childbearing age and has a highly variable course, improving in one-third, worsening in one-third, and remaining unchanged in one-third of patients. Oral corticosteroids in the first trimester may increase the risk of preterm delivery and preeclampsia. During labor, good pain control may prevent asthma triggered by vagal stimulus or stress. Providing neuraxial anesthesia over general anesthesia avoids the risk of bronchospasm with airway manipulation. In some asthmatics, attacks can be triggered by NSAIDs.

Diabetes mellitus in the pregnant patient increases the risk for gestational hypertensive disorders, intrauterine growth restriction, preterm labor, polyhydramnios, macrosomia, shoulder dystocia, fetal abnormalities, and fetal asphyxia. The risk for *DKA* increases during pregnancy and can be

Essential Clinical Anesthesia Review: Keywords, Questions and Answers for the Boards, ed. Linda S. Aglio, Robert W. Lekowski, and Richard D. Urman. Published by Cambridge University Press. © Cambridge University Press 2015.

Table 124.1 Optimal cardiovascular physiologic parameters in valvular lesions

	HR	Preload	SVR	Contractility
Mitral stenosis	Avoid tachycardia to allow LV filling; treat atrial fibrillation aggressively (cardioversion)	At risk for pulmonary edema. Keep PCWP ~15; avoid hypoxia, hypercarbia, pain (↑ PVR)	Keep normal to high	Normal
Aortic stenosis	Avoid extremes of HR; atrial "kick" necessary for LV filling	High pressures are needed to fill noncompliant LV, risk for pulmonary edema	Keep high to maintain LV perfusion pressure (decrease causes hypotension and possibly cardiac ischemia)	Keep normal to high to maintain CO; low if dynamic subvalvular lesion
Mitral regurgitaion	↑ HR (decreases regurgitant flow)	Keep normal to low; LV at risk for volume overload	Low SVR augments forward flow	Normal
Aortic insufficiency	↑ HR (decreases regurgitant fraction)	Keep normal to low; LV at risk for volume overload	Low SVR augments forward flow	Normal

LV, left ventricle; PCWP, pulmonary capillary wedge pressure; PVR, pulmonary vascular resistance; HR, heart rate; SVR, systemic vascular resistance; CO, cardiac output. (From, Vacanti, C.A., et al. (eds) 2011. *Essential Clinical Anesthesia*. New York, NY: Cambridge University Press, p. 767.)

compounded by hyperemesis, infections, steroid therapy, and poor medication compliance.

Gastroparesis in diabetic patients increases the risk of aspiration before and after general anesthesia; consider the use of a nonparticulate antacid such as sodium citrate and a prokinetic agent such as metoclopramide.

Severe retinopathy is a contraindication to vigorous maternal Valsalva during the second stage of labor. A dense epidural for operative vaginal delivery or a spinal anesthesia for cesarean delivery can be provided.

Peripheral neuropathy needs to be evaluated and documented, but does not preclude neuraxial techniques. *Autonomic neuropathy* can predispose to significant hemodynamic changes during neuraxial and general anesthesia.

Rheumatoid arthritis usually improves during pregnancy. Methotrexate, chlorambucil, and cyclophosphamide are contraindicated due to their teratogenic potential. Airway problems include *cervical spine instability* with risk of spinal cord injury from excessive flexion or extension, *TMJ ankylosis* causing limited mouth opening, and *cricoarytenoid joint involvement*, which may manifest as dysphonia, dysphagia, dyspnea, pharyngeal fullness, wheezing, sore throat, or ear pain. Positioning, IV access, and invasive monitoring can be complicated by lumbar or thoracic kyphoscoliosis, joint deformity, and polyarthritis. Severe skeletal deformities may impede neuraxial anesthesia and vaginal delivery.

Systemic lupus erythematosus infrequently flares during pregnancy; the flare risk is increased in the postpartum period due to increases in proinflammatory hormones. Due to risk for worsening of lupus nephritis, nephrotoxins and NSAIDs are best avoided. Patients have increased risk of miscarriage and thromboembolic events. Antiphospholipid antibodies (lupus anticoagulant, anti-cardiolipin antibodies) are present and falsely prolong aPTT. Neonatal lupus is related to antibodies (SSA/antiRo and SSB/antiLa) and may present as congenital heart block or rash.

Patients with *multiple sclerosis* experience fewer exacerbations during pregnancy but are at increased risk of relapse after delivery. While MS is not a contraindication to neuraxial techniques, local anesthetics can produce increased conduction blocks on demyelinated nerves and unmask symptoms. Triggering factors for exacerbations, including hyperthermia and physiologic stress, should be avoided. Document the neurological exam preoperatively.

Idiopathic thrombocytopenic purpura is characterized by thrombocytopenia secondary to circulating IgG antibodies against platelets. Treatment options include corticosteroids, intravenous immunoglobulin, plasmapheresis, and splenectomy. Platelet transfusion is usually not indicated because platelets are often hyperfunctional and severe bleeding rarely occurs, but can be considered in life-threatening hemorrhage. Antibodies cross the placenta and can cause fetal thrombocytopenia. Neuraxial anesthesia can be considered.

von Willebrand disease is an autosomal dominant disorder divided into quantitative (type 1 and 3) and qualitative (type 2) defects in von Willebrand factor. Typical presentation includes mucocutaneous bleeding, epistaxis, menorrhagia, and postpartum/postoperative bleeding. Treatment includes desmopressin for mild to moderate disease, but is not effective for type 2B, in which desmopressin can exacerbate thrombocytopenia. Cryoprecipitate, fresh frozen plasma, or factor VIII concentrates can be used for factor replacement. There can be increased risk for epidural hematoma and mucosal bleeding after airway instrumentation.

Medications used in comorbid diseases

Ergot alkaloids and 15-methyl prostaglandin $F_2\alpha$ are contraindicated in asthma patients due to the side effect of bronchospasm.

Steroids can be used during pregnancy and breastfeeding. Oral corticosteroids in the first trimester may increase the risk for preterm delivery and preeclampsia. Inhaled corticosteroids are generally considered safe.

Cytotoxic drugs such as azathioprine, mycophenolate, cyclophosphamide, and cyclosporine should be avoided.

Several antihypertensive agents (atenolol, ACEI, ARB) are contraindicated during pregnancy. Methyldopa, hydralazine, labetalol, nifedipine, isradipine, low-dose diazoxide, and some beta-blockers (metoprolol, pindolol, propranolol) are safe.

Questions

1. Which of the following statements is INCORRECT?
   a. Confirmation of asthma by spirometry includes an improvement of FEV_1 by >12% with albuterol use.
   b. During general anesthesia, atracurium, and mivacurium should be avoided in asthmatic patients.
   c. Carboprost, methylergonovine, and ergonovine can trigger bronchospasm.
   d. Asthma in pregnant patients should be managed with short- and long-acting beta-agonists and leukotriene modifiers. Inhaled steroids need to be discontinued.

2. In a parturient with multiple sclerosis that is being prepared for surgical delivery, which of the following considerations is CORRECT?
   a. Some studies found that spinal anesthesia can lead to postoperative symptom exacerbations; epidural anesthesia has not been found to cause problems.
   b. Hypothermia must be avoided and patients should be kept well above 37°C.
   c. Patients taking steroids should discontinue the medication perioperatively.

   d. The risk for disease exacerbation is greatly diminished after delivery.

3. Which of the following statements is CORRECT regarding the diabetic parturient?
   a. Insulin crosses the placenta, hence larger doses can lead to fetal hypoglycemia.
   b. Fetal macrosomia, which might necessitate cesarean delivery, is less common in diabetic as compared to healthy parturients.
   c. Insulin requirements remain unchanged during pregnancy.
   d. Fetal hypoglycemia often occurs after delivery, as umbilical cord clamping prevents placental passage of glucose.

Answers

1. d. Inhaled steroids have not been shown to exert any detrimental effects on the fetus; in contrast, suboptimal control of asthma is more likely to jeopardize the health of mother and fetus.

2. a. Multiple sclerosis causes demyelination of nerves, which increases the susceptibility to local anesthetics; studies have found a disease-exacerbating effect with spinal anesthesia, but not with epidural anesthesia or peripheral nerve blocks.

3. d. Clamping of the umbilical cord blocks transfer of glucose from mother to fetus; the newborn's metabolic pathways are immature and have to adapt to the extrauterine life; glucose levels reach a nadir after about one hour.

Further reading

Vasudevan, A. and Pratt, S. D. (2011). Chapter 125. Pregnant patients with comorbid diseases. In Vacanti, C. A., Sikka, P. J., Urman, R. D., Dershwitz, M., and Segal, B. S. (eds) *Essential Clinical Anesthesia*. Cambridge, UK: Cambridge University Press.

Snegovskikh, D. and Braveman, F. R. (2012). Chapter 26. Pregnancy-associated disease. In *Stoelting's Anesthesia and Co-Existing Disease*, 6th edn. Philadelphia, PA: Saunders, Elsevier Inc.

Gaiser, R. (2012). Chapter 22. Evaluation of the pregnant patient. In *Longnecker's Anesthesiology*, 2nd edn. Columbus, OH: McGraw-Hill.

Traill, T. A. (2012). Valvular heart disease and pregnancy. *Cardiology Clinics* 30(3), 369–381.

Chapter

125

Anesthesia for fetal intervention

Benjamin Kloesel and Michaela K. Farber

Keywords

Ex utero intrapartum treatment (EXIT)
Ex utero intrapartum treatment-to-extracorporeal
    membrane oxygenation (EXIT-to-ECMO)
Operations on placental support (OOPS)
Minimally invasive fetal procedures
Fetal monitoring

Three types of *fetal intervention* exist: (1) open midgestational, hysterotomy-based surgery between 18 and 26 weeks of gestation involving exteriorization of the affected fetal body part; (2) ex utero intrapartum treatment (EXIT) procedures, also called operations on placental support (OOPS), performed on term or near-term fetuses before umbilical cord clamping; and (3) minimally invasive fetal procedures performed throughout gestation.

The *EXIT procedure* involves partial delivery of the fetus to correct potentially life-threatening conditions. For the duration of the procedure, the fetus is left connected to the uteroplacental system. At the conclusion, the cord is clamped and the fetus is delivered. Initially, the goal is maximal uterine relaxation to improve placental perfusion; this is usually achieved by 2 to 3 MAC of volatile anesthetics, which also causes maternal and fetal anesthesia. After cord clamping, volatile agents are reduced and uterotonic agents given to optimize uterine tone. The major risk to the mother is hemorrhage from uterine atony.

Volatile anesthetics at >2 MAC produce maternal anesthesia and tocolysis while maintaining uterine relaxation and fetal perfusion. Major side effects include hypotension that is managed with fluid supplementation and vasopressors to maintain maternal blood pressures within 10% of baseline.

Maternal hypocapnia reduces umbilical blood flow, causes metabolic acidosis, can lead to fetal hypoxia, and should be avoided.

Amniotic fluid volume requires close monitoring after hysterotomy. Excessive fluid loss can result in umbilical cord compression or kinking and fetal distress. The fluid volume can be maintained by infusion of warmed saline or amniotic fluid.

The *main vulnerabilities of the fetus during interventions* are listed below:

1. Hypoxemia: optimizing uteroplacental perfusion minimizes this risk.
2. Myocardial depression: volatile anesthetics have this effect, and the newborn heart is unable to increase its contractility; therefore, relies on heart rate alone to augment cardiac output.
3. Anemia: small fetal blood volume of 100 to 110 ml/kg imparts risk for significant blood loss with surgical intervention.
4. Blood loss: immaturity of fetal hepatic and hematologic function may impair hemostasis and increase risk.
5. Hypothermia: the fetus is unable to compensate for heat loss by shivering and nonshivering mechanisms that develop after delivery.

The fetus is able to mount a *physicochemical stress response* to pain starting around 18 weeks of gestation. It becomes capable of experiencing *pain* between 20 and 30 weeks of gestation.

Intraoperative fetal monitoring is limited. If a body part is exposed, pulse oximetry should be employed, and SaO_2 levels of greater than 40% are acceptable. Transesophageal, transmyometrial, or transthoracic echocardiography can evaluate cardiac function. Doppler ultrasonography and near-infrared spectroscopy are useful to monitor adequacy of cerebral blood flow and oxygenation.

Fetal resuscitation includes maternal oxygen administration at an FiO_2 of 100%, left lateral decubitus position to relieve aortocaval compression, intravenous fluid supplementation, vasopressors, and tocolysis if uterine contractions are evident. In open procedures, direct access to the fetus enables cardiac compression and IV, IM, and intracardiac administration of medication and blood products. Special care should be given to avoid hypothermia or electrolyte imbalance. The greatest risk to the fetus in the postoperative period is *preterm labor*. Tocolytic agents are frequently administered.

Essential Clinical Anesthesia Review: Keywords, Questions and Answers for the Boards, ed. Linda S. Aglio, Robert W. Lekowski, and Richard D. Urman. Published by Cambridge University Press. © Cambridge University Press 2015.

Table 125.1 Diseases eligible for fetal intervention

Disease	Intervention type(s)
CCAM (cystic adenomatoid malformation)	EXIT, EXIT-to-ECMO (if significant airway obstruction)
CDH	EXIT, EXIT-to-ECMO, or minimally invasive (ultrasound-or fetoscopically guided tracheal plug placement and removal)
Cervical teratoma	EXIT, EXIT-to-ECMO (if significant airway obstruction)
CHAOS (congenital high airway obstruction syndrome)	EXIT, EXIT-to-ECMO (if significant airway obstruction)
Congenital goiter	EXIT, EXIT-to-ECMO (if significant airway obstruction)
Cystic hygroma	EXIT, EXIT-to-ECMO (if significant airway obstruction or high-output cardiac failure)
HLHS (hypoplastic left heart syndrome)	Minimally invasive (ultrasound-guided percutaneous aortic valve dilatation)
Hydronephrosis and bladder outlet obstruction	Minimally invasive (ultrasound-or fetoscopically guided shunt placement)
MMC (myelomeningocele)	EXIT, minimally invasive (fetoscopic patch application)
Pulmonary sequestration, bronchogenic cysts, and mixed or hybrid pulmonary lesions	EXIT
SCT (sacrococcygeal teratoma)	EXIT, EXIT-to-ECMO (for high-output cardiac failure)
TRAP (twin reversed arterial perfusion sequence)	Minimally invasive (fetoscopic laser/photoablation of aberrant vasculature)
TTTS (twin–twin transfusion syndrome)	Minimally invasive (fetoscopic laser/photoablation of aberrant vasculature)

(From Vacanti, C. A., et al. 2011. (eds) *Essential Clinical Anesthesia*. New York, NY: Cambridge University Press, p. 773.)

Questions

1. The EXIT procedure can be employed to do which?

   a. Deliver a fetus before 24 weeks of gestation.
   b. Treat hydronephrosis due to bladder outlet obstruction.
   c. Secure an airway prior to delivery in congenital high airway obstruction syndrome.
   d. Obtain a tissue sample for genetic testing prior to delivery of the fetus.

2. What is an important intervention after an EXIT procedure?

   a. Initiation of oxytocin to prevent uterine atony.
   b. Fetal ultrasound to confirm viability.
   c. Transfusion to keep maternal hematocrit above 30%.
   d. Initiation of nitroglycerine to avoid hypertension.

Answers

1. c. Congenital high airway obstruction includes a spectrum of diseases leading to compression of the airways; fetal reliance on the respiratory system can be fatal in this situation. An EXIT procedure allows establishment of a secure airway while the fetal circulation is supported by the placenta.
2. a. The EXIT procedure involves adequate uterine relaxation, which needs to be reversed at the conclusion to avoid postpartum hemorrhage.

Further reading

Brusseau, R. and Bulich, L. A. (2011). Chapter 126. Anesthesia for fetal intervention. In Vacanti, C. A., Sikka, P. J., Urman, R. D., Dershwitz, M., and Segal, B. S. (eds) *Essential Clinical Anesthesia*. Cambridge, UK: Cambridge University Press.

Tran, K. and Cohen, D. E. (2011). Chapter 19. Anesthesia for fetal surgery. In *Smith's Anesthesia for Infants and Children*, 8th edn. Burlington, MA: Elsevier Inc.

126

Basic considerations for pediatric anesthesia

Laura Westfall and Susan L. Sager

Keywords

Infant vs. adult respiratory function
Neonatal airway anatomy/epiglottis and airway
    dynamics
Pediatric breathing circuits
Fetal and neonatal circulatory system
Factors causing persistent fetal circulation
Pediatric fluid management
Pediatric blood transfusion
Intraoperative hypothermia in infants
Neonatal pharmacology
Succinylcholine-induced bradycardia
Neuromuscular reversal in infants
MAC: pediatric inhalational agents

Table 126.1 ETT size guidelines for patients less than two years old

Age	Weight, kg	ETT ID, n
Premature	<2	2.5–3.0
Term	3–4	3.0–3.5
0–6 months	3–5	3.5
6–12 months	5–10	4.0
1–2 years	10–14	4.5

The modified Cole's formula for ETT size: (internal diameter in mm) = age
(years) +16/4.
(Source: Vacanti, C., et al. (eds) 2011. *Essential Clinical Anesthesia*. New York,
NY: Cambridge University Press, Chapter 127.)

Infant vs. adult respiratory function:

- Tidal volumes and FRC approximate adult (ml/kg) values,
  but the infant's highly compliant chest wall predisposes
  to early airway closure and reduced FRC.
- Greater oxygen consumption and metabolic rate in infancy
  must be matched with faster respiratory rates; infants
  desaturate faster with hypoventilation or apnea.
- Faster emergence and induction with volatile anesthetic
  agents is a result of the infant's increased minute
  ventilation to FRC ratio.

Neonatal airway anatomy/epiglottis and airway dynamics:

- Infants' larynx is more cephalad (C3–4 vs. adult C6) and
  more cylindrical-shaped than adults, with the narrowest
  portion at the cricoid ring.
- Tongue is larger.
- *Epiglottis* is stiffer, shorter, and omega-shaped compared
  to an older child or adult.
- Vocal cords are more angulated, such that an ETT may
  easily catch in the anterior commisure.

Pediatric breathing circuits are designed to minimize dead
space, and reduce work of breathing. The Mapleson system is

most commonly used in pediatric practice, and is characterized
as a semi-closed, rebreathing system (without CO_2 absorption), with an absence of valves between the patient and fresh
gas flow. The main disadvantage to these designs is their
requirement for high fresh gas flows to prevent rebreathing,
especially in larger children (>15 kg).

- Mapleson D and the Jackson-Rees modification of Ayer's
  T-piece (Mapleson E) are the most well known. Mapleson
  D has the lowest fresh gas flow rates of all the
  configurations.
- The Bain circuit, in which the fresh gas flow line is within
  the expiratory limb in a coaxial arrangement, is
  functionally identical to the Mapleson D.
- Pediatric circle systems are closed, nonrebreathing circuits
  designed with low resistance valves, smaller connectors,
  and less compliant tubing, and confer the same advantages
  as adult circle systems of low fresh gas flow and
  conservation of heat, moisture, and volatile agent.

The fetal circulatory system undergoes dramatic changes
as the newborn adapts to extrauterine life. Expansion of the
lungs and removal of the placenta from circulation reduces
PVR while increasing SVR. Increased systemic pressures
and PaO_2 cause functional closure of the foramen ovale and
ductus arteriosus, completing the transition to the *neonatal*

Essential Clinical Anesthesia Review: Keywords, Questions and Answers for the Boards, ed. Linda S. Aglio, Robert W. Lekowski, and Richard
D. Urman. Published by Cambridge University Press. © Cambridge University Press 2015.

circulatory system. Anatomic closure occurs over the next few months. Until anatomic closure of these aforementioned shunts takes place, persistence of (or reversion to) fetal circulation may occur.

Factors causing persistent fetal circulation include hypoxemia, acidosis, or elevated PA pressure. Newborns are uniquely susceptible to these changes due to:

- noncompliant myocardium and limited cardiac reserve; dependence on heart rate as the primary mechanism to maintain cardiac output
- the parasympathetic nervous system is more developed than the sympathetic system; exaggerated bradycardic response to vagal stimuli (i.e., airway manipulation, hypoxia)

Pediatric fluid management: neonates are highly sensitive to fluid and electrolyte imbalances due to low renal blood flow, glomerular filtration rate, and urine-concentrating and diluting capacities at birth. While nephrogenesis is complete at term, renal function does not reach maturity until early childhood.

Guidelines for the calculation of hourly maintenance fluids for children must account for the newborn's higher metabolic rates, greater ratio of surface area to weight, larger V_d, and larger insensible losses. In general, maintenance fluids are calculated as follows:

- 4 ml/kg for the first 10 kg
- 2 ml/kg for the next 10 kg
- 1 ml/kg thereafter

Intraoperative glucose supplementation may be warranted, especially in preterm infants or term newborns. The neonatal liver (responsible for glycogen storage, protein synthesis, and drug metabolism) is not mature until one year of age. All neonates are given a single prophylactic dose of vitamin K at birth.

Pediatric blood transfusion: at birth, nearly 80% of newborn hemoglobin concentration is HbF. Hemoglobin concentrations transition to the predominant HbA during the first six months of life. To compensate for the high oxygen-affinity of HbF and allow oxygen unloading at tissues, neonates have higher levels of 2,3-DPG. Hemoglobin levels reach their physiological nadir (10–11 g/dl) at two to three months of age.

Most children can tolerate hematocrits in the low 20% range, except those who are premature, newborn, and patients with respiratory failure or cyanotic CHD. Intraoperatively, if the maximum allowable blood loss has been reached at a Hct of 20% and more EBL is anticipated, then a *blood transfusion* should be given. (See Table 126.3 for estimated blood volumes by age.)

The maximum allowable blood loss (MABL) prior to transfusion is calculated as follows:

MABL = EBV (Starting HCT − Allowed HCT)

Where EBV = estimated blood volume.

Intraoperative hypothermia: infants and young children are more susceptible than adults to *hypothermia* in the operating room due to greater surface area to volume ratio, thinner subcutaneous fat layer, less keratinized skin, and high minute

Table 126.2 Simplified pediatric transfusion guidelines

Component	Indication	Volume to transfuse	Change in parameter expected from transfusion
Packed RBCs	Hb <7–8 g/dl with symptoms Acute blood loss ≥15% of total blood volume Hb <12 g/dl with severe cardiopulmonary diseases (<15 g/dl for neonates and premature infants)	10–15 ml/kg	Hb increase of 2–3 g/dl
Platelets	<10,000 per μl <50,000 per μl if active bleeding or major surgery planned <100,000 per μl with CNS bleeding or planned CNS surgery or in sick, premature infant with active bleeding	5–10 ml/kg	Platelet increase of 50,000–100,000 per μl
FFP	Emergency reversal of warfarin PT >1.5 × midrange of normal value of PTT >1.5 × top range of normal value Replacement for specific factors when their concentrates are unavailable	10–15 ml/kg	Factor activity increase of 15–20%
Cryoprecipitate	Hypofibrinogenemia or dysfibrinogenemia with active bleeding or invasive procedure If DDAVP or factor VIII is unavailable; in a patient with von Willebrand disease with active bleeding or invasive procedure	1–2 U per 10 kg of patient weight	Fibrinogen increase of 60–100 mg/dl

PT, prothrombin time; PTT, partial thromboplastin time; FFP, fresh frozen plasma.
(Modified from Roseff, S. D. (ed) 2003. *Pediatric Transfusion: A Physician's Handbook*, 1st edn. Bethesda, MD: American Association of Blood Banks.)
(Source: Vacanti, C., et al., ed 2011. *Essential Clinical Anesthesia.* New York, NY: Cambridge University Press, Chapter 127.)

Table 126.3 Estimated circulating blood volume

Patient age	Estimated blood volume, ml/kg
Premature neonate	90–100
Full-term neonate	80–90
3–12 months	75–80
1–6 years	70–75
>6 years	65–70

(Source: Vacanti, C. et al. (ed) 2011. *Essential Clinical Anesthesia*. New York, NY: Cambridge University Press, p. 778.)

Table 126.4 Intubating doses of neuromuscular blockers in children[a]

Drug	Dose, mg/kg	Minutes to intubation	Minutes to recovery, T_{25}[b]
Succinylcholine	IV: 2.0 IM: 4.0	<10 3.0	3–5 20
Vecuronium	IV:0.1	2.0	73 (infants) 35 (children) 53 (adults)
Rocuronium	IV: 0.6 IV: 1.2	1.0 0.5	10–30 40–75
Cisatracurium	IV: 0.2	1.5	43 (infants) 36 (children)
Pancuronium	IV: 0.1	2.5	45–60

[a] Maintenance doses (one-fourth of the intubating dose) may be given when one twitch is present.
[b] T_{25} is the time from injection to recovery of 25% of baseline neuromuscular transmission of three to four twitches to a train-of-four stimulus.
(Source: Vacanti, C. et al. (eds) 2011. *Essential Clinical Anesthesia*. New York, NY: Cambridge University Press, Chapter 127.)

Table 126.5 MAC value (%) and age

	Sevoflurane	Isoflurane	Desflurane	Halothane
Neonate	3.3	1.3–1.7	9.2	0.87
Infant	3.3	1.7	9.4	1.1
Child	2.5	1.6	8.0	0.9
Adult	2.0	1.2	6.0	0.75

(Source: Vacanti, C. et al. (eds) 2011. *Essential Clinical Anesthesia*. New York, NY: Cambridge University Press, Chapter 127.)

ventilation. Neonates employ nonshivering thermogenesis (metabolism of brown fat) for heat production until age two. Covering the head, warming the operating room, thermal blankets, humidified inspired gases, and radiant warmers/incubators for transportation minimize heat loss.

Neonatal pharmacology: clinically significant differences exist between neonatal and adult pharmacokinetics and pharmacodynamics:

- greater total body water content and thus larger V_d
- decreased GFR
- decreased hepatic metabolism, delayed clearance and excretion
- increased fraction of unbound drug – lower levels of albumin and displacement due to elevated bilirubin in newborns

Succinylcholine-induced bradycardia, junctional rhythm, and sinus arrest following IV administration can occur due to cholinergic stimulation of autonomic receptors. Bradycardia can be mitigated by a concurrent dose of atropine. Side effects of succinylcholine limit its routine use in infants and children, and

include hyperkalemia, malignant hyperthermia, masseter spasm, and rhabdomyolysis. Succinylcholine is only recommended for emergency control of the airway in infants and children.

High-dose rocuronium may be used for rapid sequence induction when an alternative to succinylcholine is needed. Neonates require higher doses of succinylcholine and appear more resistant due to their higher V_d; however, quicker recovery may be observed given their high cardiac output. Conversely, neonates are more sensitive to nondepolarizing muscle relaxants (lower ED_{95}, due to reduced hepatic/renal function; a prolonged effect may be seen).

Neuromuscular reversal in infants is strongly recommended due to the variable effect of NMBs and the difficulty assessing return of neuromuscular function in neonates. This may be achieved with neostigmine (0.07 mg/kg) and concurrent atropine (0.02 mg/kg) or glycopyrrolate (0.01 mg/kg) to prevent bradycardia.

MAC: pediatric inhalational agents. The MAC of inhalational agents varies with age. In general, infants require the greatest MACs, with neonates (especially preterm neonates) and older children requiring less. An exception to this is the MAC of sevoflurane, which is nearly identical for neonates and infants.

Due to their lack of pungency, both sevoflurane and halothane can be used for inhalation inductions. While sevoflurane causes less myocardial depression than halothane, high levels of any volatile agent may cause bradycardia, hypotension, or cardiac arrest in infants and young children.

Questions

1. Which is the estimated blood volume of a 5 kg neonate?
   a. 300 cc
   b. 425 cc
   c. 550 cc
   d. 600 cc

2. A four-month-old is undergoing hypospadias repair under general anesthesia. All of the following cause loss of body heat EXCEPT for which?
   a. metabolism of brown fat
   b. high fresh gas flow
   c. conduction through the operating room table
   d. evaporation after preparation of surgical field

3. Which of the following statements about the pediatric airway is FALSE?

   a. The cricoid cartilage in infants is located at the level of the 4th cervical vertebrae.
   b. The adult epiglottis is more angled into the lumen of the airway than the infant epiglottis.
   c. The expected ETT size for an average six-year-old is 5.5 mm.
   d. The narrowest portion of the infant airway is the thyroid cartilage.

Answers

1. b. With a blood volume of approximately 80 to 90 cc/kg, a 5 kg neonate has an estimated blood volume of 425 cc.

2. a. Conduction, evaporation, and high fresh gas flows cause heat loss in infants. Nonshivering thermogenesis via brown fat metabolism is one way in which infants produce heat.

3. b. The infant epiglottis is more angled into the lumen of the airway than the adult epiglottis.

Further reading

Cote, C. J., Lerman, J., and Anderson B. J. (2013). *A Practice of Anesthesia for Infants and Children*, 5th edn. Philadelphia, PA: Saunders, Chapters 6 and 51.

Miller, R. D. (2009). *Miller's Anesthesia*, 7th edn. Orlando, FL: Churchill-Livingstone, Chapter 82.

Chapter

127

Preoperative evaluation of the pediatric patient and coexisting diseases

Laura Westfall and Susan L. Sager

Keywords

Infant preoperative fasting
Pierre Robin syndrome
Neonates and postoperative apnea
Child with a URI
Cystic fibrosis
Cerebral palsy
Myotonic dystrophy
Trisomy 21
HbSS causes of sickling

The anesthetic plan must take into account the child's age and developmental stage, medical history, anatomy, and requirements of the surgical procedure.

Infant preoperative fasting may be challenging as infants and younger children are more prone to hypoglycemia due to smaller glycogen stores. To minimize the risk of aspiration, the NPO guidelines recommended by the ASA are: two hours for clear liquids, four hours for breast milk, six hours for nonhuman milk or formula, and eight hours for solids.

Neonates and postoperative apnea: due to CNS immaturity and abnormal responses to hypercapnia and hypoxia, preterm infants <34 weeks gestation may exhibit apnea of prematurity, defined as respiratory pauses less than 15 seconds and/or hypoxia or bradycardia. When preterm or former preterm infants are anesthesized during the first few months of life, they have a higher incidence of life-threatening apneic episodes after anesthesia than older infants. Newborn postoperative apnea is a mixed apnea with both central and obstructive components. Excessive forward flexion of the neck due to large occiput, low tone of pharyngeal muscles, and relatively large tongue predispose to airway obstruction. Immature brainstem response to hypercarbia and hypoxia, and early fatigue of diaphragmatic and intercostal muscles make neonates more susceptible to postoperative apneic episodes. Infants at greatest risk for postoperative apnea are premature infants, and sick infants who required ICU care, those with CNS deficits, anemia, or apnea at home. Importantly, both postconceptual age (PCA) and gestational age strongly correlate with apnea. For this reason, it is recommended that infants less than 60 weeks PCA should be admitted and monitored following surgery, regardless of anesthetic technique.

A child with a URI is at increased risk of laryngospasm, bronchospasm, oxygen desaturation, postextubation croup, and postoperative atelectasis. Bronchial and small airway hyperreactivity may persist for up to seven weeks after resolution of a lower airway infection; thus controversy exists as to appropriate rescheduling of procedures. Use of a mask airway or LMA instead of ETT may reduce the risk of airway complications.

Patients presenting with craniofacial anomalies have challenging airways that require advance planning and specialized techniques for airway management.

Pierre Robin malformation sequence is characterized by a small mandible (micrognathia), a posteriorly displaced or retracted tongue (glossoptosis), and frequently a u-shaped cleft palate. PRS patients are prone to airway obstruction in the supine position, and visualizing the trachea can be difficult without specialized equipment. Placement of an LMA and fiberoptic intubation may be needed to ventilate the patient and secure the airway. These patients frequently have associated congenital heart disease.

Newborns and children with *cystic fibrosis* require anesthesia for treatment of meconium ileus, intestinal atresia, bronchial obstruction, nasal polyps, and vascular access. Associated conditions include malnutrition, increased secretions, chronic airway inflammation, electrolyte imbalance, and pancreatic insufficiency. Preoperative PFTs and SaO_2 help establish baseline function. Patients may be admitted early to optimize pulmonary function prior to elective surgery, in consultation with the patient's pulmonologist. Regional anesthesia techniques should be considered whenever possible. Postoperative atelectasis and hypoventilation should be anticipated; opioid-sparing systemic analgesics, local anesthetic wound infiltration, and regional analgesia should be used as part of a multimodal analgesic approach to postoperative pain management.

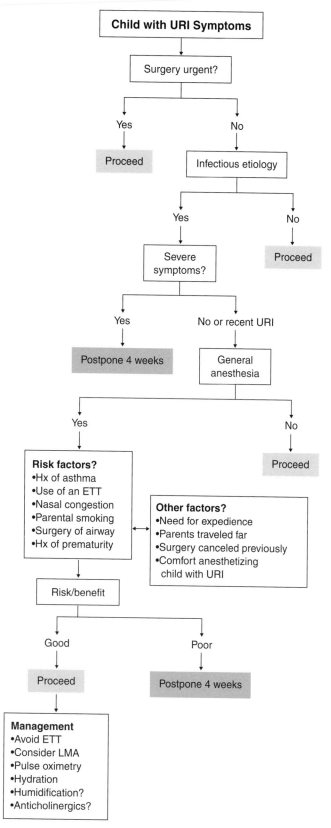

Figure 127.1 Suggested algorithm for the assessment and anesthetic management of the child with a URI. Hx, history; ETT, endotracheal tube. (Reproduced with permission from Tait, A. R. et al. 2005. Anesthesia for the child with an upper respiratory tract infection: still a dilemma? *Anesthesia and Analgesia*, 100: 59–65.)

Cerebral palsy is a complex CNS disorder that most commonly manifests as skeletal muscle spasticity and quadriplegia. Patients also frequently exhibit cerebellar ataxia, seizure disorders, varying degrees of developmental delay, excessive secretions, and speech defects. Preoperatively, medical management of these conditions should be optimized. Spasticity can be associated with contractures of the limbs, making IV access and intraoperative positioning challenging. Patients with severe GERD or heavy secretions may require RSI. Despite skeletal muscle spasticity, succinylcholine does not cause excessive potassium release.

Patients with *muscular dystrophies* may have cardiac and respiratory muscle involvement with associated arrhythmias and cardiomyopathies as well as decreased respiratory effort. Both succinylcholine and inhalational agents are generally avoided in this patient population due to potential life-threatening rhabdomyolysis and hyperkalemia that may ensue. Patients with muscular dystrophy may have variable response to nondepolarizing NMBs.

Anesthetic concerns for patients with *Trisomy 21* include atlanto-axial instability and possible airway difficulty secondary to macroglossia, mandibular hypoplasia, enlarged tonsils, subglottic stenosis, and hypotonia. Underlying congenital heart disease is present in 40% of patients with Trisomy 21, most commonly atroventricular canal defects. Patients have the potential to develop pulmonary hypertension, and are more prone to bradycardia under anesthesia.

Sickle cell disease usually does not manifest until HbSS production outpaces the decline of HbF, usually around six months of age. *HbSS sickling* and ensuing vaso-occlusive crises are more likely to occur during hypoxia, acidosis, dehydration, and hypothermia; thus perioperative management should focus on avoidance of these conditions. Patients should receive IV fluids during the preoperative fasting period. Perioperative transfusion should be discussed with the patient's hematology team prior to planned surgeries. Postoperatively, patients should be observed for vaso-occlusive crises, stroke, and acute chest syndrome. Perioperative pain management may be challenging as treatment of frequent painful crises may lead to chronic opioid use, opioid tolerance, or withdrawal symptoms.

Questions

1. You are doing a preoperative evaluation of a 15-year-old patient with Trisomy 21, who is having a port-a-cath placed prior to chemotherapy for ALL. Which of the following is LEAST likely to be part of his past medical and surgical history?

   a. hypothyroidism
   b. prior repair of VSD
   c. smaller ETT (than expected) required for past intubations
   d. prior posterior cervical spine fusion
   e. all of the above are likely

2. A healthy 12-month-old presents for an elective surgical procedure. Which of the following statements is TRUE?
   a. The patient should have fasted for two hours after drinking cow's milk.
   b. The patient should have fasted six hours after drinking apple juice.
   c. NPO guidelines do not apply to healthy children undergoing a regional anesthetic (no sedation).
   d. The patient should have fasted for four hours after drinking breast milk.

Answers

1. e. There are many conditions associated with Trisomy 21 that may affect the anesthetic management. Among them are potential congenital cardiac defects, atlanto-axial instability (potential for cord compression should be ruled out), choanal atresia, subglottic stenosis, duodenal atresia (intestinal obstruction), and hypothyroidism. These patients are also more prone to bradycardia during induction of anesthesia.

2. d. Pediatric patients should fast for six hours after cow's milk (or formula), four hours after breast milk, and two hours after clear liquids (such as apple juice). NPO guidelines apply to any type of anesthesia (regional or general) for any elective procedure.

Further reading

Vacanti, C. A., Sikka, P. K., Urman, R. U., Dershwitz, M., and Segal, B. S. (2011). *Essential Clinical Anesthesia*. New York: Cambridge University Press.

Barash, P. G., Cullen, B. F., and Stoelting, R. K. (2009). *Clinical Anesthesia*, 6th edn. Philadelphia, PA: Lippincott Williams & Wilkins, Chapter 45.

Hines, R. L. and Marschall, K. E. (2008). *Stoelting's Anesthesia and Co-Existing Disease*, 5th edn. Philadelphia, PA: Churchill-Livingstone, Chapter 24.

Cote, C. J., Lerman, J., and Anderson, B. J. (2013). *A Practice of Anesthesia for Infants and Children*, 5th edn. Philadelphia, PA: Saunders, Chapters 11 and 14.

Chapter 128

Anesthetic considerations for common procedures in children

Laura Westfall and Susan L. Sager

Keywords

Spinal anesthesia for hernia repair
OSA
Post-tonsillectomy hemorrhage
Croup vs. epiglottitis
Foreign body aspiration
PONV in the pediatric patient

Children and infants are more prone to airway obstruction in the operating rooms. Choice of anesthetic technique will depend on the patient's history of prematurity, apnea of prematurity, obstructive sleep apnea, recent URI, and history of reactive airways, as well as other medical issues that impact anesthetic care.

Spinal anesthesia for hernia repair: premature infants are more prone to develop inguinal hernias. Repair of inguinal hernias, hydrocele, and other lower abdominal and GU surgical procedures in young infants can be performed under general or regional anesthesia. General anesthesia may be necessary for emergency cases such as strangulated or incarcerated hernias. Spinal anesthesia may be preferred for premature and former premature infants to reduce the risk of postoperative apnea. Infants who have continuing apnea at home, or a hematocrit of less than 30%, are at particular risk for postoperative apnea, and may require postoperative monitoring regardless of which technique is used.

Differences in hepatic maturity, and local amide anesthetic binding to alpha-1 glycoprotein and the infant's ability to metabolize amide anesthetics must be taken into consideration when chosing a local anesthetic.

Amides should be used carefully in newborns, infants, and children due to decreased ability to metabolize these drugs in the liver. Amide anesthetics (bupivacaine, ropivacaine), are 90% bound to two plasma proteins, alpha-1 acid glycoprotein and albumin. Infants under six months of age have fewer plasma proteins and, as a result, a larger fraction of free unbound drug. Elevated levels of bilirubin can further displace these drugs from protein binding and cause even

Table 128.1 Advantages and disadvantages of regional and general anesthesia for infant hernia

Regional anesthesia	General anesthesia
Advantages:	*Advantages:*
Minimal infant exposure to general anesthetics	Rapid onset and reliability
Minimal disruption in feeding schedule	Airway control
Disadvantages:	*Disadvantages:*
Limited duration (spinal)	Postoperative apnea and bradycardia in preterm or former preterm infants
Failure rate in infants ranges from 5% to 30% (spinal)	Risk of pulmonary complications (e.g., atelectasis)

(From: Vacanti, C. et al. (eds) 2011. *Essential Clinical Anesthesia.* New York, NY: Cambridge University Press, Chapter 129.)

higher levels of free drug and greater toxicity. By one year of age, the infant liver matures, and the ability to bind and metabolize amides reaches adult levels.

Ester anesthetics (tetracaine, chloroprocaine) are metabolized by plasma cholinesterase and have fewer age-related differences. Although infants have lower serum esterases, this has little clinical impact.

OSA: pediatric ORL procedures encompass a variety of challenges to airway management. Routine tonsillectomy and adenoidectomy are often performed for obstructive sleep apnea (OSA), which affects 2% to 3% of the pediatric population. Patients with enlarged tonsils and those who suffer from OSA may have an airway obstruction on induction, altered response to CO_2, and increased sensitivity to opioids and sedatives. Opioid-sparing analgesics should be optimized; IV acetaminophen has been shown to reduce morphine requirements postoperatively. Codeine is not recommended for children undergoing tonsillectomy and adenoidectomy. Unintended high levels of its metabolite, morphine, have led to death in

Table 128.2 Common conditions causing airway obstruction in children

Diagnosis	Onset	Breathing on examination	Miscellaneous	Typical presenting age
Croup (laryngotracheobronchitis)	Insidious with prodrome of URI; also seen postoperatively after traumatic intubation	Inspiratory stridor, barky cough, slow inspiratory phase	Stridor and respiratory compromise worsened with increased respiratory rate	Infants, children younger than 3 years
Epiglottitis, acute supraglottitis	Rapid, fulminant onset with sore throat and dysphagia	Sitting up, drooling, dysphonia or aphonia, dysphagia with inspiratory obstruction	Limited airflow from the obstruction can muffle or obviate the inspiratory stridor	Children 2–7 years
Subglottic stenosis	Congenital, post-trauma, or prolonged intubation	Respiratory distress, notable retractions, biphasis stridor	Most common cause is prolonged intubation	Neonates, infants, or children of any age after prolonged intubation
Foreign body	Insidious or rapid	Decreased air exchange and/or wheezing	Organic foreign bodies cause more inflammation; small, inert foreign bodies may cause chronic wheeze or cough	Toddler

(From: Vacanti, C. et al. (eds) 2011. *Essential Clinical Anesthesia.* New York, NY: Cambridge University Press, Chapter 129.)

patient populations who are rapid metabolizers of codeine, due to a genetic variability. Children with severe OSA, especially those under the age of three years, should be observed overnight postoperatively.

Post-tonsillectomy hemorrhage most often occurs within six hours postoperatively, if not within the first 24 hours. Patients returning to the OR for hemostasis should be considered to have a full stomach. Establishing IV access and fluid resuscitation should be achieved prior to induction.

Croup vs. epiglottitis: among airway emergencies seen in the pediatric population, croup and epiglottitis are two common conditions that must be differentiated (see Table 123.2). With development of the haemophilis influenza type B (HiB) vaccine in 1992, epiglottitis is less common.

Foreign body aspiration can create a partial fixed obstruction or a dynamic (ball-valve) obstruction of airflow. Dislodging a foreign body may lead to complete airway obstruction. Foreign body retrieval is a surgical emergency and should be considered in any child with intractable wheeze or stridor. The most common site of obstruction is the right mainstem bronchus and 90% of foreign bodies are radiolucent. A mask induction with spontaneous ventilation may be preferred depending on the history and type of obstruction present.

PONV: pediatric patients have a higher incidence of postoperative nausea and vomiting than adults. Children at greatest risk are those undergoing adenotonsillectomy, strabismus repair, orchidopexy, herniorrhaphy, middle ear surgery, dental procedures, laparotomy, and long procedures. Four

Table 128.3 Strategies to reduce baseline PONV risk

Perioperative period	Strategy	Evidence
Preoperative	Premedication (clonidine or midazolam)	Weak
Intraoperative	Avoidance of general anesthesia through use of regional anesthesia	Strong
	Use of propofol for induction and maintenance of anesthesia	Strong
	Avoidance of nitrous oxide	Strong
	Avoidance of volatile anesthetics	Strong
	Minimization of opioids	Weak
	Minimization of neostigmine	Weak
	Adequate hydration	Strong
Postoperative	Minimization of opioids	Strong
	Minimization of movement	Weak
	Timing of oral intake	Weak
	Adequate hydration	Strong

(From: Vacanti, C. et al. (eds) 2011. *Essential Clinical Anesthesia.* New York, NY: Cambridge University Press, Chapetr 129.)

independent risk factors for increased PONV that have been identified are: surgical duration >30 minutes, age three or older, strabismus surgery, and history of PONV in the patient or immediate family member. (See Tables 128.3 and 128.4).

Table 128.4 Properties of antiemetic drugs

Class	Drug	Receptor antagonism	Dose, mg/kg	Antiemetic efficacy	Relative cost	Timing of administration
Corticosteroids	Dexamethasone	?	0.1–0.25	√√√√	$$	At induction
Anti-serotonins	Dolasetron	5-HT₃	0.035	√√√√	$$$$	Timing not important
	Granisetron	5-HT₃	0.04	√√√√	$$$$$	End of surgery
	Ondansetron	5-HT₃	0.05–0.1	√√√√	$$$$	End of surgery
	Tropisetron	5-HT₃	0.1	√√√√	$$$$	End of surgery
Antihistamines	Dimenhydrinate	Histamine	0.5	√√√√	$	End of surgery
	Diphenhydramine	Histamine	1.0–1.25	√√	$	End of surgery
	Hydroxyzine	Histamine	1.0	√√√	$	End of surgery
Butyrophenones	Droperidol	Dopamine	0.025–0.075	√√√√	$$	End of surgery
Phenothiazines	Prochlorperazine	Dopamine	0.125	√√√	$	End of surgery
	Promethazine	Dopamine	0.25–0.5	√√√	$	At induction
	Perphenazine	Dopamine	0.025–0.07	√√√	$	End of surgery
Anticholinergics	Scopolamine	Muscarinic acetylcholine	0.006	√√	$$$	Prior evening or 4 h before
Benzamides	Metoclopramide	Dopamine	0.1–0.25	√	$$	End of surgery

(From: Vacanti, C. et al. (eds) 2011. *Essential Clinical Anesthesia*. New York, NY: Cambridge University Press, Chapter 129.)

Questions

1. A worried mother brings her five-year-old daughter to the Emergency Department with a history of fever (38.5°C) and a sore throat that developed suddenly over the last 24 hours. On examination the child appears flushed, is sitting in tripod position, and drooling. The most likely diagnosis is?

   a. foreign body aspiration
   b. croup
   c. epiglottitis
   d. streptococcal throat infection
   e. obstructive laryngeal papillomatosis

2. Which of following surgeries is LEAST likely to cause PONV?

   a. tonsillectomy in a seven-year-old
   b. orchidopexy in a two-year-old
   c. bilateral myringotomy in an 18-month-old
   d. open splenectomy in a five-year-old

Answers

1. c. This patient has epiglottitis. Croup is characterized by inspiratory stridor, "barking cough," mild temperature elevation in children less than three years old. Children with epiglottitis, in contrast, develop symptoms acutely, and often present with high fever, odynophagia, drooling, tachypnea, and tend to lean forward with mouth open to maintain their airway. Foreign body aspiration may cause wheezing; however, fever is not consistent with the clinical picture described. Laryngeal papillomatosis can cause upper airway obstruction but typically presents with *chronic* hoarseness and wheezing, and would not cause fever.

2. c. Children less than three years old are less prone than older children to suffer from PONV.

Further reading

Vacanti, C. A., Sikka, P. K., Urman, R. U., Dershwitz, M., and Segal, B. S. eds. (2011). *Essential Clinical Anesthesia*. New York, NY: Cambridge University Press, Chapter 129.

Barash, P. G., Cullen, B. F., and Stoelting, R. K. (2009). *Clinical Anesthesia*, 6th edn. Philadelphia, PA: Lippincott Williams & Wilkins, Chapter 50.

Hines, R. L. and Marschall, K.E., (2008). *Stoelting's Anesthesia and Co-Existing Disease*, 5th edn. Philadelphia, PA: Churchill-Livingstone, Chapter 24.

Chapter

129

Neonatal surgical emergencies

Jonathan R. Meserve and Susan L. Sager

Keywords

Retinopathy of prematurity
Pediatric maintenance fluid requirements
Gastroschisis
Omphalocele
Congenital diaphragmatic hernia (CDH)
Tracheoesophageal fistula (TEF) and esophageal
  atresia (EA)
Necrotizing enterocolitis (NEC)
Spina bifida/meningocele/meningomyelocele
Pyloric stenosis (PS)

Retinopathy of prematurity is the progressive vascular overgrowth of retinal vessels resulting in intraocular hemorrhage, retinal detachment, and eventual blindness. Risk factors include prematurity and high FiO_2 exposure. FiO_2 should be minimized in all infants less that 44 weeks gestational age to target a SpO_2 of 92% to 96%.

Pediatric maintenance fluid requirements are higher than adults in the first year of life due to the infant's higher metabolic rate and increased caloric expenditure. Total body water decreases slowly over the first year of life from 80% in the newborn period to 60% at one year of age. Calculation of maintenance fluids takes into consideration insensible losses from perspiration and respiration, and sensible losses from urine and stool. Reduced GFR and immature kidneys make the infant more susceptible to hyponatriema.

Maintenance fluids can be quickly calculated as 4 ml/h for the first 10 kg, 2 ml/kg for the next 10 kg, and 1 ml/kg for the remaining kg weight.

Factors increasing maintenance fluid requirements in infants and children include higher surface area to weight in babies (more water loss from skin), faster respiratory rates, and congenital defects in the abdominal wall (larger evaporative losses), as well as fever, pain, and hypermetabolic states in hospitalized infants.

Gastroschisis is caused by a right-sided abdominal wall defect resulting in extruded bowel without a peritoneal covering. Typically gastroschisis is not associated with other congenital malformations, but 10% of children suffer intestinal atresia due to vascular compromise by the restrictive fascial defect.

Omphalocele is caused by failure of abdominal wall muscles to close, resulting in the herniation of abdominal viscera from the base of the umbilical stalk with a peritoneal covering. Omphalocele is associated with cardiac anomalies (20%), hypoglycemia, Beckwith–Wiedemann syndrome, and macroglossia. Abdominal wall closure may increase intra-abdominal pressures, thereby compromising respiratory mechanics.

Gastroschisis/omphalocele: preoperative management includes fluid resuscitation, treatment of sepsis, prevention of heat loss, decompressing the stomach to prevent aspiration, and protection of the abdominal wall defect. Intraoperatively, primary closure is aborted if bladder pressures are greater than 20 mm Hg or if PIPs are greater than 35 mm Hg.

Congenital diaphragmatic hernia occurs when the pleuroperitoneal canal fails to close at eight weeks gestation leaving a posterolateral diaphragmmatic defect (foramen of Bochdalek). Consequently, abdominal viscera herniate into the pleural space disrupting normal pulmonary development, and resulting in pulmonary hypoplasia. Ninety percent of CDHs are left sided, and 5% right, with included hepatic herniation.

A *tracheoesophageal fistula (TEF) and/or esophageal atresia (EA)* is due to failure of the esophagus to separate from the trachea, resulting in five possible anatomic outcomes. EA with a distal TEF is the most common (85%). Fifty percent of cases are associated with other anomalies, particularly VACTERL (Vertebral, Anal atresia, Cardiac, Renal, Limb malformations) associations and trisomy 21. TEF/EA is diagnosed by the inability to pass a nasogastric tube with gastric bubble on KUB.

Necrotizing enterocolitis results from ischemia and inflammation of the GI tract. Risk factors include prematurity, umbilical artery catheterization, cardiac disease, enteral formula feeding. May be medically managed, but may progress to necrosis, ulceration, or stricture, requiring bowel resection and stoma formation.

Spina bifida is a result of failed closure of the neural tube in the fourth week of fetal life. A *meningocele* is a fluid-filled

Essential Clinical Anesthesia Review: Keywords, Questions and Answers for the Boards, ed. Linda S. Aglio, Robert W. Lekowski, and Richard D. Urman. Published by Cambridge University Press. © Cambridge University Press 2015.

Table 129.1 Anesthetic considerations for neonatal surgical urgencies and emergencies

Surgical diagnosis	Surgical emergency?	Preanesthetic considerations	Intraoperative considerations	Post-anesthetic considerations
Gastroschisis/ omphalocele	Yes	Full stomach precautions Hypovolemia Hypoglycemia Sepsis Difficult airway (macroglossia with omphalocele)	Hypothermia Hypovolemia Respiratory compromise with abdominal wall closure	Analgesia (opioid or epidural) Bowel ischemia Renal failure Oxygenation/ ventilation problems
Congenital diaphragmatic hernia (CDH)	No – some require ECMO preoperatively	Decompress stomach Avoid BMV Hypoplastic ipsilateral lung	Permissive hypercarbia Minimize airway pressures Highly sensitive PVR Aggressive ventilation can cause contralateral pneumothorax Hypothermia	Analgesia (opioid or epidural) Pneumothorax/ barotrauma Pulmonary HTN R to L shunting May require HFOV or ECMO 24–48 h after repair
Tracheoesophageal fistula (TEF) and esophageal atresia (EA)	Yes – often staged repair	Aspiration risk, VACTERL associations Gastric distension decreases pulmonary compliance	Pneumothorax Place ETT past fistula to prevent gastric distension Extubate in OR to reduce pressure on suture Hypothermia	Analgesia (typically epidural) Pneumothorax RLN injury Tracheal leak
Necrotizing enterocolitis (NEC)	Yes	Full stomach precautions ROP with high FiO_2 Sepsis DIC Hypovolemia	Hypovolemia Hypothermia Hypocalcemia Hypoglycemia Preductal arterial line Respiratory compromise with abdominal wall closure	Analgesia (opioid) Sepsis Postoperative intubation Pulmonary edema ROP with high FiO_2
Meningomyelocele	Yes (within 48 h of life)	Maintain sac integrity Cardiac defects Hydrocephalus Meningitis	Hypovolemia Hypothermia Prone positioning Latex allergy risk	Analgesia (opioid) CSF leak Hydrocephalus Prone positioning Bladder dysfunction
Pyloric stenosis	No	Full stomach precautions Metabolic alkalosis Hypoglycemia Hypothermia Hypovolemia	RSI or awake intubation Hypovolemia Hypothermia Muscle relaxation	Analgesia (opioid and local) Increased apnea risk Hypoglycemia Hypothermia

(Source: Adapted from Table 130.4. Vacanti, C. et al. (eds) 2011. *Essential Clinical Anesthesia*. New York, NY: Cambridge University Press, Chapter 130, p. 810.)

sac that contains skin and meninges. The most severe form is a *meningomyelocele*, which is a fluid-filled sac containing neural elements. Often associated with cardiac defects, orthopedic abnormalities, and Arnold–Chiari-2 malformations, which require shunting for hydrocephalus. The integrity of the sac must be maintained until surgery.

Pyloric stenosis (PS) is an idiopathic hypertrophy of antral muscles and the pylorus, causing frequent emesis and resulting electrolyte abnormalities in the second to eighth weeks of life. PS is a medical emergency to correct a hypovolemic,

hypochloremic metabolic alkalosis, with surgical intervention occurring after stabilization. In severe cases metabolic alkalosis is confounded by metabolic acidosis due to profound hypovolemia. Pyloromyotomy is performed either as an open procedure or laparoscopically.

Questions

1. Which is the most critical lab test prior to pyloromyotomy?
   a. CBC with differential

b. chemistry (Na, K, Cl, CO_2, BUN, Cr, Gluc, Ca, Mg, Phos)

c. coagulation studies (Pt, INR, PTT, fibrinogen)

d. G 6PD deficiency testing

2. Prior to emergent cesarean delivery of an infant, the obstetrician mentions the infant has an abdominal wall defect but is unsure if it is an omphalocele or gastroschisis. A gastroschisis is more likely to:

a. be associated with congenital heart disease

b. have facial abnormalities making intubation difficult

c. be associated with atretic portions of bowel

d. be associated with karytope abnormalities

3. You are called to the NICU to assess a four-hour-old infant with suspected congenital diaphragmatic hernia for emergent surgical intervention. The infant is breathing 40 times a minute with a SpO_2 of 94%. Which of the following should be prioritized?

a. umbilical artery catheter

b. umbilical vein catheter

c. endotracheal tube

d. orogastric tube

Answers

1. b. Management of pyloric stenosis, an idiopathic hypertrophy of the antral muscles at the second to eighth week of life is a medical emergency. Due to recurrent emesis and hypovolemia, infants typically present with hypochloremic metabolic alkalosis with compensatory hypokalemia due to increased aldosterone upregulation. A basic chemistry is the most important lab study to be obtained to evaluate the extent of metabolic and electrolyte derangement, which should be corrected prior to surgical intervention.

2. c. Gastroschisis is a right-sided abdominal wall defect resulting in extruded bowel without a peritoneal covering. Typically gastroschisis is not associated with other congenital malformations, but 10% of children suffer intestinal atresia due to vascular compromise by the restrictive fascial defect. Conversely, omphalocele is associated with cardiac lesions, macroglossia, hypoglycemia, Trisomy 13 (Patau syndrome), and Trisomy 18 (Edward's syndrome).)

3. d. The newborn with a congenital diaphragmatic hernia is a delivery room and surgical emergency. While initial management includes umbilical and arterial access, the most pressing intervention is gastric decompression. Visceral contents in the thorax may become distended with resuscitation (especially with PPV in the distressed infant), thus expanding abdominal content and further compressing the minimal pulmonary tissue. Following OG placement, further vascular access may be pursued along with endotracheal intubation.

Further reading

Vacanti, C. A., Sikka, P. K., Urman, R. U., Dershwitz, M., and Segal, B. S. eds. (2011). *Essential Clinical Anesthesia*. New York, NY: Cambridge University Press, Chapter 130.

Cote, C. ed.(2009). *A Practice of Anesthesia for Infants and Children*, 4th edn. Philadelphia, Pennsylvania: Saunders/ Elsevier, Chapter 36.

Morgan, G. E. ed. (2006). *Clinical Anesthesiology*, 4th edn. New York: Lange

Medical Books/McGraw-Hill Medical Publishing Division, Chapter 33.

Chapter

130

Congenital heart disease

Jonathan R. Meserve and Susan L. Sager

Epidemiology of congenital heart disease (CHD): CHD affects 4 to 9 per 1,000 live births. There are 1.2 million people in the United States with CHD, 300,000 of whom are under 21 years old.

Cyanotic vs. acyanotic heart disease: a heart defect is considered cyanotic if deoxygenated blood bypasses the lungs and enters the systemic circulation. These heart defects include those with right-to-left or bidirectional shunting, or malposition of the great arteries. Shunting may be the result of anatomic lesions including right-sided obstructive lesions. Acyanotic lesions include heart defects with net left-to-right shunts and left-sided obstructive lesions without shunt.

Obstructive lesions increase resistance and thus reduce blood flow from the respective ventricle. The resulting increased work and O_2 consumption lead to ventricular hypertrophy and eventual heart failure. A *patent ductus-arteriosis* may allow mixing and shunting of blood in the presence of obstructive lesions and lesions that create parallel circulation.

Manipulation of pulmonary vascular resistance (PVR) and systemic vascular resistance (SVR): blood flow from the

Table 130.1 Classification of CHD (incidence of lesion as percentage of all CHD)

Cyanotic	Acyanotic
Right-to-left-shunts	**Left-to-right shunts**
Tetralogy of Fallot (10%)	VSD (20%–25%)
Pulmonary atresia (1%)	ASD (5%–10%)
Tricuspid atresia (<1%)	Endocardial cushion defect (AV canal) (4%–5%)
	PDA (5%–10%)
Complex "mixing" lesions	
Transposition of the great vessels (5%)	
Total anomalous pulmonary venous return (1%)	
Truncus arteriosus (1%)	
HLHS (1%)	
Double-outlet RV (<1%)	
Obstructive lesions (right-sided)	**Obstructive lesions (left-sided)**
Pulmonary stenosis (5%–8%)	Coarctation of the aorta (8%–10%)
	Aortic stenosis (5%)

(Source: Vacanti, C., et al. (eds) 2011. *Essential Clinical Anesthesia*. New York, NY: Cambridge University Press, Chapter 131, p. 813.)

ventricles is determined by the relative resistance of the outflow pathways available. Flow will preferentially follow the path of least resistance. Venous return is determined by the relative compliance of the downstream chambers available. Blood flow will preferentially fill high-compliance chambers.

Pulmonary vascular obstructive disease (PVOD): increased pulmonary blood flow results in pulmonary arteriole hypertrophy, vasoconstriction, the development of pulmonary hypertension (PH), increased PVR, and eventual RV hypertrophy.

Eisenmenger syndrome occurs when increased PVR exceeds SVR causing a right-to-left shunt and cyanosis. Chronic hypoxia associated with right-to-left-sided lesions

Essential Clinical Anesthesia Review: Keywords, Questions and Answers for the Boards, ed. Linda S. Aglio, Robert W. Lekowski, and Richard D. Urman. Published by Cambridge University Press. © Cambridge University Press 2015.

Table 130.2 Manipulation of PVR

Factors increasing PVR	Factors decreasing PVR
• PEEP	• No PEEP
• High airway pressure	• Low airway pressure
• Atelectasis	• Normal FRC
• Low FiO$_2$	• High FiO$_2$
• Acidosis and hypercapnia	• Alkalosis and hypocapnia
• Increased hematocrit	• Low hematocrit
• Sympathetic stimulation	• Blunted stress response
• Pain and agitation	• Nitric oxide
• Epinephrine, dopamine	• Vasodilators (milrinone)
• Direct surgical manipulation	

PEEP, positive end-expiratory pressure.
(*Source*: Vacanti, C. et al. (eds) 2011. *Essential Clinical Anesthesia*. New York, NY: Cambridge University Press, Chapter 131, p. 814.)

Table 130.3 Manipulation of SVR

Factors increasing SVR	Factors decreasing SVR
• Sympathetic stimulation – pain and agitation – epinephrine, dopamine – norepinephrine – ketamine	• Adequate sedation and analgesia • Vasodilators – milrinone, dobutamine – nitroprusside – ACE inhibitors
• Negative intrathoracic pressure	• Positive pressure ventilation
• Hypothermia	• Fever, sepsis

(From Vacanti et al. 2011. *Essential Clinical Anesthesia*, Cambridge University Press, Chapter 131, p. 813.)

causes polycythemia and an increased risk of thrombosis and ischemic stroke.

Ventricular septal defects (VSD) are the most common form of CHD. The degree of left-to-right shunt is determined by PVR/SVR ratios. Uncorrected VSDs lead to LA dilation and eventual CHF, though many VSDs close spontaneously. Infants can present with signs of CHF (tachypnic, feeding difficulty, diaphoretic) at six to eight weeks of age when the physiologic drop in pulmonary resistance results in left-to-right shunting. Medical treatment includes diuresis and afterload reduction. Surgical or interventional closure is indicated in children with congestive heart failure (CHF), failure to thrive (FTT), or a pulmonary/systemic flow ratio (Qp/Qs) >2:1. Alternate procedures include pulmonary artery banding.

Atrial septal defects (ASD) are left-to-right shunts that may lead to progressive RA/RV dilation and eventual pulmonary hypertension. ASDs often occur with more complex cardiac defects. Closure may be performed at two to five years of life by interventional procedures; surgical closure may be indicated in children with CHF or FTT. Introduction of air into venous lines may cause paradoxical air embolus and air filters should be used routinely.

Patent ductus arteriosis (PDA) is fetal structure connecting the main pulmonary artery to the descending aorta. Functional closure normally occurs at birth secondary to increased PaO$_2$ and decreased prostaglandins. When the PDA fails to close, shunting between the pulmonary and systemic circulations can occur; a "machine-like murmur" may be heard at the LSB. Shunt physiology is determined by the PDA size and the PVR/SVR ratio. Medical treatment includes indomethacin, but PDA ligation has the highest success rate. Measurement of pre- and postductal SpO$_2$ is important in ensuring ligation of the proper vessel has occurred, as is auscultating the quieting of the murmur after ligation.

Coarctation of the aorta (COA) causes a left outflow track obstruction, which may be mitigated by collateral circulation. Over time, COA can cause LVH and systemic hypertension. When stenosis is severe, newborns may be dependent on flow through the patent ductus arteriosus and require prostglandin E to maintain ductal patency and blood flow distal to the coarct. The origin of the PDA (just distal to the origin of the left subclavian artery) is the most common location of a coarct. Coarct of the aorta is frequently diagnosed by noting difference in upper and lower extremity blood pressures. Preductal (right radial) arterial lines are necessary as the left subclavian artery (left radial) may be clamped during repair. Anesthetic goals include ensuring adequate perfusion to descending aorta strutures, including the spinal cord, by decreasing oxygen consumption (passive cooling), supporting cardiac output and blood pressure while the aorta is cross-clamped. This is usually well tolerated with short cross-clamp times – longer times may require correction of a metabolic acidosis following clamp removal.

Tetralogy of Fallot (TOF) is characterized by right ventricular outflow tract obstruction (RVOT), nonrestrictive VSD, an overriding aorta, and RV hypertrophy. Decreased preload, tachycardia, and inotropes may acutely worsen right ventricular outflow obstruction, resulting in worsening cyanosis "tet spell." TOF is associated with Trisomy 13, 18, and 21, as well as CHARGE and VACTERL syndromes. Historically, neonates with TOF underwent a staged repair with the creation of an arterial–pulmonary shunt (Blalock–Taussig shunt), followed by a definitive repair of the right ventricular outflow tract later in infancy. Now, neonates with TOF typically undergo a complete repair at age three to four months. Complete single-stage repair involves relief of right ventricular outflow obstruction with repair of the pulmonary valve, excision of RVOT muscle mass, and VSD closure. An RV–PA conduit is created in those patients where a coronary artery passes over the RVOT. TOF with pulmonary stenosis is most common, though the pulmonary artery may be atretic, necessitating an RV–PA conduit. Introduction of air into venous lines may cause paradoxical air embolus via the VSD and air filters should be used routinely.

Transposition of the great arteries (TGA) is the most common CHD cause of cyanosis in the newborn period and is fatal unless the PDA remains patent or a second mixing lesion (ASD, VSD) exists. Prostaglandin E is used to maintain PDA patency. Balloon atrial septostomy may be performed as a bridge to definitive surgical repair. TGA repairs include atrial switching via baffling, or arterial switch with transfer of the coronary arteries. Anesthetic goals include balancing PVR and SVR to maintain CO and adequate systemic oxygenation.

Hypoplastic left heart syndrome (HLHS) occurs when the left ventricle fails to develop, thus preventing blood flow from the heart to the systemic circulation. HLHS is characterized by variable degree of mitral and pulmonary valve stenosis, and hypoplasia of the LV and ascending aorta. Newborn survival depends on PDA patency and the presence of an atrial level shunt ASD/PFO. Babies born without an ASD often require emergent atrial septostomy to ensure adequate mixing. Prostaglandin E is used to maintain PDA patency; however, HLHS is fatal without surgical intervention. The goal of surgical palliation is to create a single ventricle series circulation. Systemic venous blood is routed to the pulmonary circulation by staged palliations as the pulmonary arterial pressures decrease from birth to toddler.

Stage I: the *Norwood procedure* (first week of life) provides systemic circulation by creating a neo-aorta from the pulmonary artery; the PDA is closed, and pulmonary perfusion is then provided by creation of a Blalock–Taussig shunt (subclavian to PA) or Sano modification (RV to PA shunt). Anesthetic goals include balancing PVR/SVR, which is often reflected in an SpO$_2$ of 80% to 85%.

Stage II: A *bidirectional Glenn* shunt (three to six months) redirects SVC drainage into the right PA, so that deoxygenated blood from the SVC enters the pulmonary circulation and the heart via the common atrium. Balancing the PVR and SVR is critical to providing adequate flow to the lungs.

Stage III: definitive *Fontan procedure* (two years of life) connects the IVC to the pulmonary artery, thus establishing a complete series circulation.

Table 130.4 Anesthetic considerations for patients with repaired CHD

VSD	Dysrhythmias and conduction delays (RBBB) Ventricular dysfunction
ASD	Dysrhythmias and conduction delays (RBBB) RV dilation and PH if repair delayed
PDA	Recurrent laryngeal nerve damage may occur LV dilation and PH if repair delayed
COA	Recoarctation may occur LVH and diastolic dysfunction if corrected late Increased risk of CAD if uncorrected
TOF	Endocarditis prophylaxis needed long term Dysrhythmias and RV dysfunction Anomalous CAs may cause LV ischemia/dysfunction
TGA	Baffle obstruction following the atrial switch may result in RV dysfunction and SVC syndrome Supravalvular pulmonary stenosis or regurgitation in the neo-aorta after arterial switch
HLHS	Pulmonary blood flow and CO are dependent on the transpulmonary pressure gradient following the Fontan procedure Higher incidence of thrombosis and strokes

Questions

1. A two-year-old boy newly diagnosed with a VSD presents with heart failure and pulmonary edema. His heart rate is 90, blood pressure 110/50, breathing 20 times a minute and he has an SpO$_2$ of 94%. Besides diuretics, which of the following medications is likely to improve his symptoms?
   a. norepinephrine
   b. oxygen
   c. enalapril
   d. esmolol

2. Which of the following syndromes is associated with supravalvular aortic stenosis that may cause sudden cardiovascular collapse following induction of anesthesia?
   a. Beckwith–Wiedemann syndrome
   b. Williams syndrome
   c. Down's syndrome
   d. Klippel–Trenauny syndrome

Answers

1. c. Symptomatic VSDs are associated with left-to-right shunting, increased pulmonary blood flow, pulmonary edema, and right ventricular dilatation. Untreated, pulmonary hypertension will occur and the patient will eventually develop Eisenmenger syndrome. Therapeutic goals include diuresis, afterload reduction, and surgical closure. This patient's symptoms are likely to improve with enalapril to reduce afterload. Oxygen, while necessary to maintain O$_2$ saturation, will cause pulmonary dilation and may worsen pulmonary edema and gas exchange. Beta-blockers are not routinely used in pediatric patients as cardiac output is highly dependent on HR.

2. b. William's syndrome is characterized by elfin features, developmental delay, and supravalvular aortic stenosis. Undiagnosed children may have sudden cardiovascular collapse after induction of anesthesia. Beckwith–Wiedemann syndrome is associated with hemihypertrophy, renal disorders, and cardiac anomalies, as is Down's syndrome, though neither are specifically associated with supravalvular aortic stenosis. Klippel–Trenauny syndrome is associated with vascular and lymphatic malformations, but is not associated with cardiac lesions.

Further reading

Vacanti, C. A., Sikka, P. K., Urman, R. U., Dershwitz, M., and Segal, B. S. eds. (2011). *Essential Clinical Anesthesia*. New York, NY: Cambridge University Press, Chapter 131.

Cote, C. ed (2009). *A Practice of Anesthesia for Infants and Children*, 4th edn. Philadelphia, PA: Saunders/Elsevier, Chapter 23.

Morgan, G. E. ed. (2006). *Clinical Anesthesiology*, 4th edn. New York, NY: Lange Medical Books/McGraw-Hill Medical Publishing Division, Chapter 26.

Chapter

131

Management of postoperative pain in children

Jonathan R. Meserve and Susan L. Sager

Keywords

Pain assessment
Cognitive–behavioral therapy
Volume of distribution
Decreased hepatic metabolism
Delayed enzymatic maturation
Opioids
Patient-controlled analgesia
Nurse-controlled analgesia/parent-controlled analgesia
NSAIDS
Regional anesthesia
Narrow therapeutic index
Caudal analgesia
Continuous lumbar and thoracic epidurals

Pediatric postoperative pain has historically been undertreated, though nerve pathways for pain transmission and perception are functioning by 24 weeks gestation. Safe analgesia requires knowledge of age-related differences in drug action. Developmental changes are most prominent during the first year of life:

- Anatomically, infants have a *larger volume of distribution* with lower initial plasma concentrations due to their greater TBW and higher water/adipose tissue ratio.
- *Decreased hepatic metabolism* and *delayed enzymatic maturation* of Phase I (cytochrome P450) and Phase II (glucuronidation) enzymes contribute to delayed clearance.
- Lower albumin and alpha-1 glycoprotein levels result in increased unbound fraction of drugs.
- Elevated bilirubin in neonates may displace drugs from albumin causing higher levels of benzodiazepines and local anesthetics.

Pediatric postoperative analgesia is best achieved with a multimodal approach that optimizes opiate-sparing analgesics (acetaminophen, NSAIDS) and regional techniques, such as wound infiltration and peripheral and neuraxial blocks. While opioids are an integral part of postoperative analgesia, opioid side effects (nausea, pruritis, constipation, respiratory depression, cognitive changes) can slow postoperative recovery. Increasingly, opiates are used for rescue and not as sole or primary analgesia.

Acetaminophen and COX-1 and COX-2 inhibitor *NSAIDs* are non-opioid analgesics and antipyretics that are widely used in the pediatric population. Acetaminophen is the most commonly used antipyretic and analgesic in children and can be administered orally, rectally, or intravenously. In combination with opioids, these analgesics have an opioid-sparing effect, unlike opioids, they do not affect ventilation or produce physical dependence. In general, acetaminophen and NSAIDS are safe for short-term pediatric postoperative use and significant side effects are rare in this setting.

NSAIDs prevent the synthesis of prostaglandins and thromboxane from arachidonic acid by blocking the cyclo-oxygenase (COX) pathway. Accordingly, arachadonic acid is shunted toward the production of leukotrienes. In the postoperative setting, NSAID side effects such as platelet dysfunction, gastritis, renal impairment, and bronchospasm rarely occur in children. NSAIDS should be used cautiously in children with asthma.

Opioids can be administered via IV, PO, intrathecal, epidural/caudal, transdermal, and transmucosal routes; IM injections should be avoided whenever possible.

Use of opioids in infants and premature babies requires special expertise and continuous monitoring of cardiorespiratory status, oxygen saturation, and sedation.

Opioids are more likely to cause sedation, apnea, and bradycardia in infants <2 months, due to increased permeability of the blood–brain barrier, hepatic immaturity (reduced clearance, greater fraction of unbound drug), immature respiratory responses to hypoxemia and hypercarbia, and greater risk of upper airway obstruction. Reversal agents and resuscitation equipment to treat opiate side effects of nausea, pruritis, sedation, hypoventilation, oxygen desaturation, and bradycardia should be immediately available.

Morphine is the most commonly used opiate in pediatrics. It is metabolized by the liver to an active and inactive form,

Essential Clinical Anesthesia Review: Keywords, Questions and Answers for the Boards, ed. Linda S. Aglio, Robert W. Lekowski, and Richard D. Urman. Published by Cambridge University Press. © Cambridge University Press 2015.

both cleared by renal excretion. Accumulation of the active metabolite, morphine-6-glucuronide, can cause toxic side effects in the young infant. Disadvantages include histamine release and vasodilation.

Methadone has the longest half-life of any opioid and can provide 12 to 36 hours of analgesia after a single dose, though is usually titrated up over three doses. Methadone is most commonly used in pediatrics to treat neonatal abstinence syndrome and opioid dependence after long-term analgesia. Methadone can also provide additional pain relief for patients with chronic neuropathic pain due to its antagonist actions at the NMDA receptor. Disadvantages include accumulation over time, tendency for oversedation, and prolongation of the QT interval.

Fentanyl is a synthetic, rapidly acting opioid used for short procedures or as a continuous infusion. It is 100 times more potent than morphine and more lipophilic. Fentanyl blocks pulmonary and systemic hemodynamic responses to pain and therefore is ideally suited for the intensive care setting, trauma, or cardiac surgery. Disadvantages include chest wall rigidity with rapid boluses, and bradycardia.

Hydromorphone is a morphine derivative and is five times more potent and ten times more lipid-soluble than morphine.

Oxycodone is the most commonly prescribed opiate for relief of postoperative pain. It comes in immediate and extended release formulations.

Codeine is no longer recommended due to potential unexpected high levels of its active metabolite, morphine, in some populations. Codeine is metabolized in the liver to morphine via a pathway dependent on the P450 enzyme CYP2D6. In "rapid metabolizers," this enzyme is more active due to genetic variations, causing higher than normal levels of morphine in the blood and unintended overdose. Deaths have been reported in children with obstructive sleep apnea who received codeine for postoperative pain relief after tonsillectomy and adenoidectomy.

Patient-controlled analgesia (PCA) is an intravenous method for self-titration of opioid analgesia. PCA requires developmental maturity (typically >6 years), and physical ability to push the button.

Nurse-controlled analgesia (NCA) can be used in infants, younger children, and children with developmental disabilities. *Parent-controlled analgesia* is an established method of opioid titration in home palliative care, though remains controversial when used in opioid-naive children after surgery. When a nurse or parent administers opioids, the inherent safety feature relying on the patient being alert enough to push the button is removed. Individualized dosing parameters, and protocols for pain assessment and treatment of side effects, are needed for implementing PCA/NCA safely.

Pediatric *regional anesthesia* consists of peripheral and neuraxial approaches as well as local infiltration, and is used for intraoperative, postoperative, and post-traumatic pain management. The majority of nerve blocks in children are performed after induction of GA and aided by ultrasound guidance. Regional techniques have a role in routine surgeries to reduce PONV, in premature infants with a history of apnea, and other patients who cannot tolerate opioid-induced ventilatory depression, or in patients who have become tolerant to opioids.

Local anesthetics have a *narrow therapeutic index* because they are relatively weak drugs with a low margin of safety between the effective dose and the toxic dose. Accordingly, dosing adjusted for weight and age is important for their safe administration. Newborns <3 months are more susceptible to local amide toxicity due to immature hepatic metabolism and greater free unbound fraction of local anesthetic, due to reduced albumin and alpha-1 glycoprotein levels.

Chloroprocaine is a short-acting ester local anesthetic with rapid onset used in continuous epidural analgesia in neonates. Chloroprocaine is rapidly metabolized by plasma cholinesterase and toxicity is rare.

Prilocaine is an amide local anesthetic that is present in the topical anesthetic EMLA cream in a 1:1 mixture with lidocaine. Rarely, prilocaine metabolism results in production of oxidants that can lead to the development of methemoglobinemia. Infants are more susceptible to methemoglobinemia due to their decreased level of methemoglobin reductase, and the fact that fetal hemoglobin is oxidized relatively easier than adult hemoglobin.

The *caudal* approach is the most common regional technique in pediatric anesthesia for accessing the epidural space. It is easy to perform and has decreased risk of trauma to the spinal cord. The epidural space is accessed through the uncalcified sacrococcygeal ligament palpated below the sacral hiatus, and local anesthetic is deposited in the epidural space. Complications of a caudal approach include sacral and rectal puncture, and inadvertent dural puncture. Patients should be examined for sacral anomalies, looking for sacral dimples, hair patches, and pigmented lesions.

Clonidine and opioids are used as adjuncts to local anesthetics in neuraxial blocks. Advantages are additive effects, increased duration of action, and reduced systemic side effects. Opioids have varying rates of diffusion across the CNS membranes due to differences in lipid solubility. Morphine may have a delayed peak effect. Patients must be monitored for sedation and respiratory depression.

Continuous lumbar and thoracic epidurals may be placed at the desired spinal level or by advancing a caudal catheter. Placement may be confirmed via fluoroscopy, epidurography, Tsui's technique, or ultrasound in infants. Complications include catheter tip migration, epidural hematoma, abscess, nerve root damage, and retained catheter fragment. The infant spinal cord ends at L3 and is at a greater risk of injury during lumbar punctures at L3–4.

Questions

1. All of the following are appropriate pain management strategies in a three-year-old EXCEPT?

    a. opioids

    b. NSAIDS

    c. cognitive–behavioral therapy

    d. distraction and redirection

2. Which of the following medications may be contraindicated in a child with severe atopy and asthma?

    a. fentanyl

    b. ketorolac

    c. acetaminophen

    d. ketamine

Answers

1. c. Opioids, NSAIDs, and acetaminophen are part of a multimodal approach to pain management. Distraction techniques may help divert attention from the painful experience and decrease distress. CBT requires developmental maturity that may not be present under the age of six years.

2. b. NSAIDs should be used cautiously in patients with asthma. NSAIDS inhibit cyclooxygenase and shunt the arachadonic acid pathway to produce more leukotrienes, which are mediators in IgE-induced asthma.

Further reading

Vacanti, C. A., Sikka, P. K., Urman, R. U., Dershwitz, M., and Segal, B. S. (eds) (2011). *Essential Clinical Anesthesia*. New York, NY: Cambridge University Press, Chapter 132.

Cote, C. ed. (2009). *A Practice of Anesthesia for Infants and Children*, 4th edn. Philadelphia, PA: Saunders/Elsevier, Chapters 42 and 44.

Schechter, N. L., Berde, C. B., and Yaster, M. (eds) (2003). *Pain in Infants, Children, and Adolescents*, 2nd edn. Philadelphia, PA: Lippincott Williams & Wilkins.

Chapter

132

Neonatal resuscitation: clinical and practical considerations

Jonathan R. Meserve and Susan L. Sager

Keywords

Initial assessment
Supplemental oxygen
Meconium
Target neonatal preductal saturations
Positive pressure ventilation
Chest compressions
Epinephrine
Volume resuscitation
Apgar score

Prior to delivery, it is important to know the gestational age (term versus preterm), presence of meconium, and fetal history including known gestational or labor complications. Maternal history of preeclampsia, placental rupture, and medications given during labor can help anticipate resuscitative needs.

The *initial assessment* of a neonate should be completed within the first few seconds of life. Asking the following can help quickly determine the need for *neonatal resuscitation*:

1. Term gestation?
2. Breathing or crying?
3. Good muscle tone?

Management in the first 30 seconds. Initial management for each newborn should include:

- warming under radiant heat
- clearing the airway if necessary
- placing infant in "sniffing" position
- stimulating the infant while continuously assessing respiration, HR, and color.

Routine suctioning of the vigorous newborn is no longer indicated and may cause bradycardia. Preventing heat loss is vital to maintaining neonatal homeostasis, as hypothermia can increase oxygen consumption.

When *meconium* is present, no intervention is necessary if the infant is vigorous. If the infant emerges limp and unresponsive, the infant should be intubated with an endotracheal tube (ETT) affixed with a meconium aspirator, and the trachea suctioned while removing the ETT. In the event of thick meconium, this may be repeated a second time. Repeated or prolonged attempts at intubation risks trauma, bradycardia, and hypoxemia. Following deep suctioning, the infant should be stimulated per routine initial care.

At 30 seconds: initiate positive pressure ventilation. If apneic or HR <100 and attempts at clearing the airway have not led to improvement, *positive pressure ventilation (PPV)* should be initiated. PIPs of 30 to 40 cm H_2O are often needed at first to expand the newborn lungs, but then require only 15 to 20 cm H_2O. Excessive pressures may cause a pneumothorax.

In healthy term infants, blood oxygen levels do not reach extrauterine values until approximately ten minutes of life. *Supplemental oxygen* use should be limited to the newborn via use of an oxygen blender. Contrary to previous recommendations for using an FiO_2 of 100% during resuscitations, oxygenation should begin at an FiO_2 of 21%, increasing as needed to *target neonatal preductal saturations*. The neonatal-targeted preductal saturation varies with time and reflects changes in oxygenation associated with transitional circulation in healthy term babies.

Table 132.1 Targeted preductal saturation varies with time

Time	Target neonatal preductal saturation
1 minute	65%
2 minutes	70%
3 minutes	75%
4 minutes	80%
5 minutes	90%
10 minutes	90–95%

(*Source*: data extrapolated from: Omar, C., Kamlin, K., O'Donnell, C., Davis, P., and Morley, C. 2006. Oxygen saturation in healthy infants immediately after birth. *Journal of Pediatrics*, 148(5): 590–594.)

Table 132.2 Apgar score

Physical examination	0	1	2
Heart rate	None	<100/minute	100/minute
Respiratory effort	Apnea	Irregular, slow	Crying, good effort
Muscle tone	Limp	Flexed extremities	Actively moving
Irritability	No response	Facial grimace	Cough, cry
Color	Blue or pale	Peripheral cyanosis	All pink

(*Source*: Vacanti, C. A. et al. (eds) 2011. *Essential Clinical Anesthesia*. New York: Cambridge University Press, Chapter 133, p. 834.)

At 60 seconds: further airway interventions. If the HR is still <100 at 60 seconds of life, additional interventions should be initiated, such as repositioning the mask, ventilation with an oral airway, or suctioning prior to continuing PPV.

At 90 seconds: chest compressions. If at 90 seconds of life the HR is <60 bpm, *chest compressions* should be started at a rate of 90 compressions per minute. Intubation should be considered at any of the above steps.

More than 90 seconds: *epinephrine*. If HR remains <60 bpm after 30 seconds of chest compressions and 90 seconds of PPV, consider administering *epinephrine* via IV (umbilical vein or PIV: 0.1–0.3 ml/kg of 1:10,000) or via ETT (0.5–1 ml/kg of 1:10,000)

Chest compressions should continue until HR >60 and PPV should continue until HR is >100.

Volume resuscitation may be initiated if the infant is not responding to resuscitation and acute maternal blood loss is suspected. Volume may be given as normal saline (0.9% NaCl), Ringer's lactate, or O negative blood (10ml/kg).

The routine use of sodium bicarbonate, naloxone, atropine, or calcium in neonatal resuscitation is no longer indicated, though may play a role in post-resuscitative care.

The *Apgar score* helps determine the need for further interventions or continued resuscitation of the neonate. It does not predict developmental outcome. It is scored at 1, 5, and 10 minutes.

Questions

1. An infant is born via vaginal delivery with a thick meconium, crying, with appropriate tone. Initial management should include all of the following EXCEPT for which?
   a. bulb suctioning
   b. intubation and suctioning beyond the vocal cords with a meconium aspirator

c. drying and stimulation
d. assessment of HR and respiratory effort at 30 seconds of life

2. You are asked to assist in the resuscitation of a term newborn via cesarean delivery to a preeclamptic woman. At one minute of life the infant is grunting, centrally cyanotic, with minimally flexed extremities, mild grimace, and with HR of 110. The Apgar score is?
   a. 4
   b. 5
   c. 6
   d. 7

3. Following cesarean delivery of a preterm infant for placental abruption, the pediatrician requests your help during resuscitation. The infant is 90 seconds old, has an HR of 45 and is unresponsive. The pediatrician has been giving PPV effectively for 60 seconds. You begin chest compressions at 100/min. After 30 seconds there is no change in the infant's condition. Which is the next step to take?
   a. umbilical artery cannulation
   b. umbilical venous cannulation and administration of 10 cc/kg pRBC
   c. umbilical venous cannulation and administration of epinephrine 1:10,000, at 1 ml/kg
   d. endotracheal administration of epinephrine 1:10,000, at 1 ml/kg while obtaining IV access

4. Administration of epinephrine to the newborn during resuscitation is associated with which of the following?
   a. intracranial bleeding
   b. bronchopulmonary dysplasia
   c. retinopathy of prematurity
   d. pyloric stenosis

Answers

1. b. Routine intubation and suctioning of the vigorous infant born with meconium are no longer indicated. Bulb suctioning may be performed at the discretion of the provider to clear meconium from the oropharynx. All infants must be dried, stimulated, and warmed, with routine evaluation of respirations and HR by 30 seconds of life.

2. b. Using the Apgar score, the infant receives 2 for HR >100, 1 for poor respiratory effort, 1 for flexed extremities, 1 for grimace, and 0 for color.

3. d. After 60 seconds of PPV and 30 seconds of effective chest compressions, any infant with an HR <60 should receive epinephrine. If IV access has been obtained, administration of epinephrine should be given at a dose of 0.1 to 0.3 ml/kg of 1:10:000. More often, umbilical access has not been obtained and endotracheal

administration of 1 ml/kg 1:10,000 epinephrine is indicated until IV access is established.

4. a Administration of epinephrine is associated with intracranial bleeding in the newborn, yet its use in resuscitation greatly outweighs this possible complication. Oxygen and prematurity are the primary risk factors for ROP. Mechanical ventilation and oxygen exposure may cause bronchopulmonary dysplasia. Newborn erythromycin exposure is associated with pyloric stenosis.

Further reading

Vacanti, C. A., Sikka, P. K., Urman, R. U., Dershwitz, M., and Segal, B. S. (eds) (2011). *Essential Clinical Anesthesia*. New York, NY: Cambridge University Press, Chapter 133.

Cote, C. (ed) (2009). *A Practice of Anesthesia for Infants and Children*, 4th edn. Philadelphia, Pennsylvania: Saunders/Elsevier, Chapter 35.

Kattwinkel, J. (ed) (2011). *Textbook of Neonatal Resuscitation*, 6th edn. American Academy of Pediatrics and American Heart Association.

Section 25 — Ambulatory and remote location anesthesia

Chapter 133: Introduction to ambulatory anesthesia

Jonathan R. Meserve and Richard D. Urman

Keywords

Patient selection
General anesthesia: TIVA versus inhalational agents
Apfel score
Ambulatory antiemetics
Discharge criteria
Phase I recovery
Phase II recovery
Fast tracking

Ambulatory surgery offers improved efficiency, decreased costs, and better resource allocation. Anesthetic goals include rapid induction and emergence with minimal postoperative complications.

Institutions should create guidelines on eligible patient populations for ambulatory surgery. *Patient selection* should be tailored to each institution and the resources available.

Special consideration should be given to patients with significant comorbidities, including elderly patients, morbid obesity, obstructive sleep apnea, pulmonary and cardiovascular disease. Eligibility for ambulatory anesthesia depends on individual symptomatology and the surgery proposed.

General anesthesia can be performed via short-acting inhalational agents or total intravenous anesthetics (TIVA).

Desflurane and sevoflurane provide fast onset and fast recovery, but are risk factors for postoperative nausea and vomiting (PONV). Adjunct nitrous oxide may additionally increase PONV, which may delay discharge. Recover indices for inhalational agents are faster than for propofol-based TIVA.

Propofol is the primary anesthetic for a TIVA approach. The addition of a quick recovery opioid (remifentanil/sufentanil) increases risk for PONV. There is no reduction in rates of PONV from use of remifentanil versus longer acting opioid analgesics.

The *Apfel score* is a simplified PONV risk score. One point is assigned for: (1) female gender, (2) nonsmoker, (3) history of PONV, (4) use of postoperative opioids. Score of 0 implies 10% risk PONV, 1: 20%, 2: 40%, 3: 60%, and 4: 80%.

Ambulatory antiemetic options include 5-HT3 receptor antagonists (ondansetron), steroids (dexamethasone), anticholinergics (scopolamine), and butyrophenones (droperidol). If one agent is unsuccessful, adding a second-line agent instead of increasing dosages yields improved efficacy

Institutional *discharge criteria* are established algorithms with predetermined protocols used by PACU nursing to ensure a patient is stable and safe for discharge. There are three phases of recovery for ambulatory patients.

Phase I recovery refers to the period immediately following surgery. The patient is observed closely to ensure they are maintaining their airway, hemodynamically stable, and returning to baseline mental status. Once these criteria are met the patient is moved to the second phase.

In *phase II* of recovery, monitors can be judiciously weaned, family can visit, and the patient should be observed ambulating. Voiding is encouraged, but not required except in some urologic procedures. PO should be offered but limited to reduce the risk of PONV. Analgesia should be ideally achieved with OTC non-opioid analgesics. Once criteria are met, the patient is discharged home.

Fast tracking refers to those patients who are alert enough following recovery to bypass phase I recovery.

Questions

1. According to the Apfel scoring system, what is the likelihood that a 30-year-old, nonsmoking female undergoing a hernia repair will develop PONV if she receives oxycodone for postoperative pain control?

   a. 20%
   b. 40%
   c. 60%
   d. 80%

2. Which of the following is NOT a requirement for a patient undergoing ambulatory anesthesia?

   a. anesthetic consent
   b. onsite preoperative evaluation prior to day of surgery
   c. transportation home
   d. appropriate patient selection

Essential Clinical Anesthesia Review: Keywords, Questions and Answers for the Boards, ed. Linda S. Aglio, Robert W. Lekowski, and Richard D. Urman. Published by Cambridge University Press. © Cambridge University Press 2015.

3. Which of the following anesthetic techniques is NOT appropriate for ambulatory anesthesia?
    a. propofol/short-acting opioid TIVA
    b. spinal anesthesia
    c. continuous peripheral nerve block
    d. none of the above

Answers

1. c. Risk factors for PONV according to the Apfel score include: female gender, nonsmoker, history of PONV, use of postoperative opioids. A single risk factor carries 20% chance of PONV, with each additional risk factor increasing the risk by 20%. The baseline risk for PONV is 10%.

2. b. All patients require a preoperative evaluation, though many ambulatory patients may be evaluated via phone-screen and patient questionnaires. Institutional criteria should be established to determine which patients may be safely phone-screened versus those that require in-person preoperative evaluation in the preoperative clinic.

3. d. All of the above anesthetics can be safely utilized in ambulatory patients, with some institutions even managing continuous peripheral nerve blocks following discharge. Anesthetic technique should be patient-specific to yield the safest, most cost-efficient anesthetic, minimizing recovery times and PONV risk.

Further reading

Vacanti, C. A., Sikka, P. K., Urman, R. U., Dershwitz, M., and Segal, B. S. (eds) (2011). *Essential Clinical Anesthesia*. New York, NY: Cambridge University Press, Chapter 134.

Stoelting, R. (ed) (2007). *Basics of Anesthesia*, 5th edn. Philadelphia, PA: Churchill-Livingstone Elsevier, Chapter 36.

Gan, T. J., Meyer, T. A., Apfel, C. C. et al. (2007). Society for Ambulatory Anesthesia guidelines for the management of post-operative nausea and vomiting. *Anesthesia and Analgesia* 105, 1615–1628.

Chapter

134

Anesthesia outside the operating room

Jonathan R. Meserve and Richard D. Urman

Keywords

Non-OR standards of care
Radiation intensity
Maximum annual occupational radiation dose
Computed tomography considerations
Magnetic resonance imaging considerations
Missile injury
Angiography/interventional radiology considerations
Electroconvulsive therapy considerations
Endoscopy considerations
Radiation oncology considerations
Dental surgery considerations

New diagnostic and therapeutic modalities require specialized equipment that has resulted in an increasing volume of anesthetic cases occurring outside the operating room.

The *non–OR standards of care* guidelines by the American Society of Anesthesiologists (ASA) require the OR model of care to extend to "remote locations." These guidelines include: (1) preprocedure assessment, (2) standard ASA monitors, (3) readily available emergency equipment, (4) adequate back-up, (5) available PACU care, and (6) a clear understanding of the planned procedure and proposed anesthetic.

Many out-of-OR (OOR) locations rely on therapeutic and diagnostic radiation that can pose health risks to the anesthesiologist. Anesthesiologists should take steps to protect themselves from radiation, including lead glass screens, and lead aprons with thyroid shields. *Radiation intensity* decreases with the inverse square of the distance from the emitting source. Personnel should be at least one to two meters from any emitting source of radiation.

100 rem = 1 sievert (Sv). Radiation exposure should be monitored with exposure film badges. Average annual public radiation exposure is 3 mSv (300 mrem). A chest X-ray provides 0.02 mSv. A CT scan can provide from 2 to 22 mSv of exposure. OSHA guidelines limit the *maximum annual occupational radiation dose* at 5 rem (50 mSv).

Computed tomography considerations

Diagnostic CT scans are quick and rarely require sedation except in children and patients unable to remain immobile or lie supine. CT-guided cryoablations of solid tumors requires sedation and analgesia. Ablation of chest lesions near bronchi may require double-lumen tubes, and the team should expect pneumothoraces.

Magnetic resonance (MR) imaging considerations

Scanning times for MR vary from 25 minutes to three hours, and the necessity of sedation is determined by the patient's ability to remain still and supine. All anesthesia equipment must be MRI compatible (nonmagnetic: devoid of iron, nickel, cobalt). Unrestrained magnetic equipment risks *missile injury*: injury sustained from projectile magnetic objects when brought into an MRI's magnetic field. Machine noise is a risk to staff and patients, with increasing noise for increasing MRI strength (Tesla). Current exposure limits are 140 decibels. Remote monitoring is required if staff are to remain outside the MRI. EKG monitoring, though improved, remains inaccurate during MRI scanning. In the event of emergent magnet shut down (due to patient complication, missile injury, or malfunction), the patient should first be removed from the MRI, as magnetic quenching causes severe heat loss and patients are at risk for hypothermia.

Angiography/interventional radiology considerations

Up to 70% of angiography/interventional radiology cases are emergent. Patient comorbidities and the scope of the procedure determine analgesia/anesthesia, though most cases require the patient to be supine, which may exacerbate pulmonary processes or be infeasible in the noncompliant patient. In addition to radiation exposure, hypothermia is a severe risk for patients, as some equipment functions best at lower environmental temperatures (60°F).

Essential Clinical Anesthesia Review: Keywords, Questions and Answers for the Boards, ed. Linda S. Aglio, Robert W. Lekowski, and Richard D. Urman. Published by Cambridge University Press. © Cambridge University Press 2015.

Electroconvulsive therapy considerations

The therapeutic effects of ECT for depression, bipolar disorder, and schizophrenia are due to neurotransmitter release following electrically induced grand mal seizures. Anesthesia goals include: (1) motor blockade to prevent limb injury during convulsion, and (2) unconsciousness during the stimulus. Seizure duration must exceed 20 seconds to be therapeutic. Propofol may shorten seizure duration. Etomidate may prolong seizure duration, but myoclonus and fasciculations with concurrent succinycholine may worsen muscle myalgia. Adrenocortical suppression with repeat doses of etomidate should be taken into consideration.

Endoscopy considerations

Endoscopic procedures typically require minimal IV sedation. Patient comorbidities and lengthy procedures (ERCP, gastric bypass repair, balloon enteroscopy, and laser treatment of Barrett's esophagus) have increased the number of cases performed by anesthesiologists. Anesthesia may be provided in ICU settings for patients unstable to transport. ETT dislodgement remains a concern with EGD manipultation, as does laryngospasm in the unsecured airway.

Radiation oncology considerations

Patient immobility (typically with GA) is required to accurately deliver radiation therapy. Prolonged radiation therapy in cases of interstitial implants may require continuous epidural analgesia during the three-day therapy. Stereotactic radiation (GammaKnife or CyberKnife) generates scattered gamma radiation, which necessitates health care providers be outside treatment rooms. Physiologic monitoring during GA/sedation requires remote data monitoring.

Dental surgery considerations

Many children and developmentally delayed patients require GA for dental procedures. Induction can be achieved though IM, IV, or inhalational methods. Cuffed nasal endotracheal tubes are the optimal method for securing the airway.

Questions

1. Which of the following carries potential risk for burn injury to a patient undergoing a sedated MRI procedure?
   a. arterial catheter
   b. pulse oximeter
   c. titanium knee joint replacement
   d. EKG leads

2. Following the cleaning of a CT scanning room, you notice the anesthesia machine is half the distance to the radiation source as previously arranged. The radiation intensity at the anesthesia machine is how many times greater than the previous configuration?
   a. 2
   b. 4
   c. 8
   d. 16

3. The non-OR standards of care require all of the following EXCEPT for which?
   a. temperature probe
   b. available PACU care
   c. IV access
   d. variable pitch and low threshold alarm pulse oximeter

4. Which of the following metals does not pose missile injury risk if brought into an MRI suite?
   a. cobalt
   b. copper
   c. nickel
   d. all pose missile injury risk

Answers

1. d. EKG leads contain magnetic metals (iron, nickel, cobalt) that may result in thermal injury during MRI. Specially designed nonferrous EKG leads minimize burn risk. To additionally minimize risk, all cable must be off the patient and cannot be coiled.
2. b. Radiation intensity decreases with the inverse square of the distance from the emitting source, thus decreasing the distance by half will increase the radiation exposure by four times.
3. c. The non-OR standards of care include a preprocedure assessment, standard ASA monitors, readily available emergency equipment, adequate back-up, available PACU care, and a clear understanding of the planned procedure and proposed anesthetic.
4. b. Ferromagentic metals include iron, nickel and cobalt. Paramagnetic metals include aluminum, titanium, copper, and silver, which do not pose missile danger.

Further reading

Vacanti, C. A., Sikka, P. K., Urman, R. U., Dershwitz, M., and Segal, B. S. (eds) (2011). *Essential Clinical Anesthesia*. New York, NY: Cambridge University Press, Chapter 135.

Stoelting, R. (ed) (2007). *Basics of Anesthesia*, 5th edn. Philadelphia, PA: Churchill-Livingstone Elsevier, Chapter 37.

ASA Standards for Basic Anesthesiology Monitoring. (2011). www.asahq.org/For-Members/Standards-Guidelines-and-Statements.aspx.

Chapter

135

Office-based anesthesia

Jonathan R. Meserve and Richard D. Urman

Keywords

Office-based anesthesia
Classification of surgical facilities
Office-based surgery accreditation
Patient selection
Procedure selection
Standards for basic anesthetic monitoring

Office-based anesthesia (OBA) is the practice of ambulatory anesthesia in an office-based setting operating under three principles: (1) safe, (2) pleasant, and (3) comfortable delivery of surgical care for the patient and staff.

It is approximated that 80% of surgeries are currently performed in an outpatient facility and 10% of surgeries are office based.

The most common procedures in office-based surgery (OBS) are endoscopies, cosmetic surgeries, and ophthalmic procedures, though there are increasing numbers of orthopedic, urologic, gynecologic, cardiac, and even neurosurgical procedures.

The American College of Surgeons (ACS) *classification of surgical facilities* delineates office-based practices by degree of anesthetic required for the procedures performed:

- Class A (level I): minor surgical procedures with local anesthetic with or without oral or IM sedation.
- Class B (level II): minor or major surgical procedures with oral, parenteral, or IV sedation, or under analgesic or dissociative drugs.
- Class C (level III): major surgical procedures requiring general anesthetic or regional block anesthesia.

Office-based surgery accreditation is performed by: (1) the American Association for Accreditation of Ambulatory Surgery Facilities (AAAASF), (2) the Accreditation Association for Ambulatory Health Care (AAAHC), and (3) the Joint Commission (TJC).

In the United States, guidelines and regulations for OBS are developed by the individual states (though about half of

50 states have regulations) and must meet minimum criteria as defined by the ASA.

ASA facility and safety requirements include:

1. Adherence to federal, state, and local law regarding fire, occupancy, waste disposal, building design, and occupational safety.
2. Adherence to laws and regulations regarding controlled substances administration and storage.

The anesthesiologist is responsible for proper *patient selection*, ensuring the patient is an appropriate candidate for the proposed procedure.

The anesthesiologist is additionally responsible for proper *procedure selection*, ensuring the procedure is appropriate for an office-based setting.

OBS requires adherence to the ASA *standards for basic anesthetic monitoring* including: (1) the presence of qualified anesthesia practitioners, and (2) monitoring of patient's oxygenation (pulse oximeter, oxygen analyzer and alarm, adequate exposure and light to observe patient), ventilation (capnography), temperature, and circulation (continuous EKG, BP, and HR minimum every 5 minutes).

At least one practitioner is required to be credentialed in advanced resuscitative techniques (e.g., ATLS, ACLS, PALS).

Discharging the patient is a physician responsibility and should be documented in the medical record as such.

Questions

1. Which of the following is NOT true regarding safety guidelines and accreditation for office-based anesthesia?
   a. The Joint Commission with the AAAASF and AAAHC performs accreditation.
   b. Every state has local and statewide regulations dictating OBA safety requirements.
   c. Physicians are encouraged to select patients for OBA by specified criteria (including the ASA Physical Status Classification System).
   d. AMA and ASA recommend that all physicians in an OBA setting should be board certified.

Essential Clinical Anesthesia Review: Keywords, Questions and Answers for the Boards, ed. Linda S. Aglio, Robert W. Lekowski, and Richard D. Urman. Published by Cambridge University Press. © Cambridge University Press 2015.

2. The urologist in your practice books a cystoscopy under local anesthesia, but during the procedure requests additional anesthesia and sedation. An LMA is required to ensure adequate ventilation. At a minimum, the American College of Surgeon requires this degree of anesthesia to be performed in which type of facility?

   a. Class A facility
   b. Class B facility
   c. Class C facility
   d. inpatient facility

3. Examination of the Closed Claims Database since 1990 revealed that 40% of claims associated with monitored anesthesia care involved death or permanent brain damage. Which of following is NOT true?

   a. Rates were similar to general anesthesia claims.
   b. Equipment failure was the most common mechanism of injury.
   c. Approximately half of claims could have been prevented by improved monitoring (capnography, audible alarms, improved vigilance).

   d. Data pertains to office-based, ambulatory, and acute care anesthesia settings.

Answers

1. b. Currently, only 22 of 50 US states have created guidelines and regulations specific to the office-based anesthetic practice. It is true that the Joint Commission with the AAAASF and AAAHC performs OBA accreditation, and that the AMA and ASA recommends that all physicians in an OBA setting be board certified.

2. c. Procedures that require general anesthesia are performed in a Class C facility as determined by the American College of Surgeons (ACS) classification of surgical facilities.

3. b. Although analysis of the Closed Claims Database since 1990 includes case reporting from office-based, ambulatory, and acute care anesthesia settings, the incidence of brain injury or mortality in MAC cases were similar to general anesthetics. The conclusion of the study revealed that over half of all mortality/brain injury cases (20% total CCD) could have been prevented with improved monitoring.

Further reading

Vacanti, C. A., Sikka, P. K., Urman, R. U., Dershwitz, M., and Segal, B. S. (eds) (2011). *Essential Clinical Anesthesia.* New York, NY: Cambridge University Press, Chapter 136.

Stoelting, R. (ed) (2007). *Basics of Anesthesia*, 5th edn. Philadelphia, PA: Churchill-Livingstone Elsevier, Chapter 37.

ASA Standards for Basic Anesthesiology Monitoring. (2011). www.asahq.org/For-Members/Standards-Guidelines-and-Statements.aspx.

ASA Guidelines for Office-Based Anesthesia. (2009). www.asahq.org/For-Members/Standards-Guidelines-and-Statements.aspx.

Bhananker, S. M., Posner, K. L., Cheney, F. W. et al. (2006). Injury and liability associated with monitored anesthesia care: a closed claims analysis. *Anesthesiology* 104(2), 228–234.

136

Patient safety, quality assurance, and risk management

Jaida Fitzgerald and Robert W. Lekowski

Keywords

Quality
Anesthesia Patient Safety Foundation (APSF)
Adverse events
Anesthesia crisis resource management (ACRM)
Risk management
Reporting adverse events

Quality, as defined by the Institute of Medicine (IOM), is the "extent to which health services for individuals and populations increase the likelihood of desired health outcomes and are consistent with current professional knowledge."

There are three major components to *quality* of health care:

- Structure – facilities and environment in which care is delivered.
- Process – how care is being delivered.
- Outcome – measuring results of medical care.

It is the *patient's* perspective on the quality of care that is the most important.

The *Anesthesia Patient Safety Foundation* (APSF) is an organization whose goal is to ensure that no patient is harmed by the administration of anesthesia. The APSF provides research grants to investigate preventable anesthetic injuries.

- Difficult airway management is perceived by anesthesiologists as the greatest patient safety issue.

An *adverse event* is defined as an accident or complication related to the administration of anesthesia. Examples of adverse events include, but are not limited to:

- peripheral nerve injury
- brain damage
- airway trauma
- intraoperative awareness
- eye injury
- aspiration

The cause of adverse events is almost always *multifactorial*; however, poor communication is often involved.

Guidelines for safe, quality care

- Teamwork – effective teamwork and open communication has been shown to improve safety.
- Preparation of equipment and medication – ensuring equipment is functional and emergency drugs are available.
- Preoperative assessment and planning – thorough medical evaluation, formulated anesthetic plan, with communication of plan to both the patient and surgeon.
- Monitors – standard ASA monitors plus additional monitoring, if necessary, based on the case and comorbidities of the patient.

Safety in transitions of care – handoffs are a vulnerable time for adverse events to occur as information can be lost in the transition of care. Anesthesia care providers should implement a standardized way of conducting handoffs to decrease the risk of failing to communicate vital patient information.

Anesthesia crisis resource management (ACRM) is an organized set of principles for managing crisis situations. It consists of five main concepts:

- Call for additional help as soon as unusual circumstances are recognized.
- Identify an event leader and establish clear roles for every individual involved.
- Use closed-loop communication.
- Use resources effectively and identify what additional resources are needed.
- Maintain situational awareness and avoid fixation.

Critical events involved in the administration of anesthesia are relatively rare, as a result many practitioners do not have clinical experience in managing such events. Over the last several years in an attempt to address this issue, simulation has become increasingly utilized for crisis training and in some specialties has already become part of the evaluation process of accrediting agencies.

Essential Clinical Anesthesia Review: Keywords, Questions and Answers for the Boards, ed. Linda S. Aglio, Robert W. Lekowski, and Richard D. Urman. Published by Cambridge University Press. © Cambridge University Press 2015.

Risk management

The risk management team within an anesthesiology department is responsible for predicting, preventing (when possible), and managing adverse events that can cause harm to an anesthesia practice. This usually involves:

- quality improvement initiatives
- conducting analyses of adverse events
- managing litigation
- performing risk analysis of policy and procedure

It is crucial that a risk management program has a user-friendly, non-threatening reporting system to ensure cooperation with employees.

Reporting of an adverse event

Any incident should be reported immediately to supervisors, the risk management department of the institution where the incident occurred, as well as the company that provides professional liability insurance to all parties involved. It is important to tell the patient and family what happened as soon as possible. The details surrounding adverse events as well as all conversations that take place should be documented in the patient's chart. The actual mandates for reporting differ between states and types of anesthesia practice, so it is the responsibility of the anesthesia care provider to be aware of the requirements of these external regulatory agencies within their area (department of public health, FDA, etc.).

Questions

1. All of the following are examples of adverse events EXCEPT for which?
    a. peripheral nerve injury
    b. airway trauma
    c. aspiration
    d. postoperative nausea and vomiting
    e. medication overdose

2. All of the following are components of anesthesia crisis resource management except for which?
    a. closed-loop communication
    b. avoiding fixation
    c. calling for help once exact diagnosis of the problem has been made
    d. assigning an event leader
    e. utilizing all resources available

Answers

1. d. Postoperative nausea and vomiting is a potential side effect of anesthesia and surgery, but is not considered to be an adverse event. All the other options are examples of adverse events associated with the administration of anesthesia.

2. c. It is important to call for help as soon as the practitioner recognizes something unusual is occurring; you should not delay calling for help in order to obtain an exact diagnosis.

Further reading

Institute of Medicine (2001). *Crossing the Quality Chasm.* Washington, DC: National Academies Press.

Vacanti, C. A., Sikka, P. K., Urman, R. U., Dershwitz, M., and Segal, B. S. (eds)

(2011). Chapter 137. Patient safety, quality assurance, and risk management. In *Essential Clinical Anesthesia.* New York, NY: Cambridge University Press.

Stoelting, R. and Miller, R. D. (eds) (2007). Chapter 4. Anesthesia risk, quality improvement and liability. In *Basics of Anesthesia*, 5th edn. Philadelphia, PA: Churchill-Livingstone Elsevier.

Chapter

137

Operating room management: core principles

Jaida Fitzgerald and Robert W. Lekowski

Keywords

OR manager
Block scheduling
Open scheduling
Release time
Resource hours
Adjusted OR utilization
Raw OR utilization
Block time
Block utilization
Surgical controlled time
Anesthesia controlled time
First case starts
Turnover time

Due to a recent emphasis on cost containment in health care and the need for accountability to both federal and state governments, there has been a dramatic shift in the way operating rooms are run over the last 20 years. Previously, ORs were run with a great deal of autonomy; however, they were often inefficient and expensive. Now there is a role for an effective OR management team whose purpose is to increase productivity while decreasing cost.

An effective *OR manager* must take into account four distinct groups that play a role in the day-to-day activity of an operating room:

- anesthesiologists
- surgeons
- nurses
- hospital administration

One of the most important roles of operating room management is efficient scheduling, as the amount of revenue that is made is proportional to the number of cases performed.

Most institutions use *block scheduling*, *open scheduling*, or a combination of both in creating the daily operating room schedule. With *block scheduling*, guaranteed OR time is given to a surgeon or surgical service to schedule cases prior to an agreed-upon cut-off time (i.e., 24 or 48 hours before surgery); whereas *open scheduling* is a "first come, first served" system.

With the increasing complexity of surgical cases and equipment over the last 20 years, *block scheduling* has become the strategy of choice, as it allows greater predictability in daily OR function and tends to be more efficient. With this type of system, certain ORs are designated as only being available for certain cases (i.e., cardiac ORs, vascular ORs, ambulatory ORs), which prevents unnecessary movement of equipment and staff.

There must be rules in place to regulate how OR time is allocated to different surgeons when utilizing the *block scheduling* strategy. One of these regulations is *release time*, which is defined as the number of hours before the scheduled time of surgery when a block of time must be either booked or released for use by others.

Measurements of operating room efficiency

- *Resource hours*: total time in which the OR is staffed and available for performance of procedures.
- *Adjusted OR utilization* = (in-OR time + turnover time) × 100/resource hours.

  The amount of time the OR is used divided by the total amount of time that the OR is staffed and ready for use. This number reflects how much of the day has been filled with scheduled OR time.

- *Raw OR utilization* = (in-OR time/resource hours) × 100.

  This excludes turnover time and reflects the ratio of billable to total OR hours. Unbooked time and excessive turnover time will drive this value down.

- *Block time* = total amount of time that a surgeon/service has been given for procedure.
- *Block utilization* = (in-OR time + turnover time) × 100/block time.
- *Surgical controlled time* = time from induction complete to when last dressing is placed.
- *Anesthesia controlled time* = induction time + emergence time.

Essential Clinical Anesthesia Review: Keywords, Questions and Answers for the Boards, ed. Linda S. Aglio, Robert W. Lekowski, and Richard D. Urman. Published by Cambridge University Press. © Cambridge University Press 2015.

- *First case starts* = percentage of ORs in which the first scheduled patient arrives into the OR prior to or at the scheduled start time.

A major focus of improving efficiency within the OR system has been decreasing *turnover time*, which is defined as the time from when one patient leaves the OR until the next patient arrives into the OR. Multiple studies have shown that even a maximal reduction in *turnover time* does not typically save enough time to allow additional cases to be booked later in the day; however, it may decrease "overtime," which is a significant cost to the system.

Another responsibility of the OR management team is to ensure that all surgeons and anesthesiologists working within their system remain current with credentialing and re-certification.

Questions

1. The term "resource hours" is defined as which of the following?
   a. total amount of time the OR is in use
   b. total amount of time the OR is staffed and ready for use
   c. cumulative turnover time per day
   d. total amount of time that a surgeon has been given for a procedure
   e. total amount of time spent allocating resources throughout the OR

2. All of the following are responsibilities of OR management EXCEPT for which?
   a. OR scheduling
   b. managing urgent and add-on cases
   c. ensuring proper credentialing of all surgeons and anesthesiologists
   d. managing the preanesthesia testing center
   e. managing communication between the four groups within the OR system: nurses, anesthesiologists, surgeons, and hospital administration

Answers

1. b. Resource hours is defined as the total time in which the OR is staffed and available for performance of procedures.
2. d. OR management may or may not be involved in the preanesthesia testing center.

Further reading

Vacanti, C. A., Sikka, P. K., Urman, R. U., Dershwitz, M., and Segal, B. S. (eds) (2011). Chapter 138. Operating room management: core principles. In *Essential Clinical Anesthesia*. New York, NY: Cambridge University Press.

Stoelting, R. and Miller, R. D. (eds) (2007). Chapter 2. Scope of practice. In *Basics of Anesthesia*, 5th edn. Philadelphia, PA: Churchill-Livingstone Elsevier.

Chapter

138

Practice management

Jaida Fitzgerald and Robert W. Lekowski

Keywords

Contracting
CPT codes
ICD-9-CM codes
ASA codes
Human resources department
Finance department
Cash-based accounting
Accrual-based accounting

Practice management refers to the business, financial, and clinical operations that maintain an anesthesia practice.

Contracting is the process in which formal agreements are made between two parties. Anesthesia practices must typically negotiate contracts with three distinct groups: (1) health care facilities, (2) insurers, and (3) employees. It is in the best interests of the practice to utilize legal counsel with specific expertise in contracts and negotiations to ensure the practice is protected.

Billing and coding

Every practice must have a billing and collections department whose purpose is to collect revenue associated with physician services. Anesthesia records that are created at the time of service act as the basis for charges that are submitted to third-party payers. The diagnoses and procedures obtained from the anesthetic record will then be "coded" by converting them into:

- *CPT codes* (Current Procedural Terminology).
- *ICD-9-CM codes* (International Classification of Diseases, 9th Revision, Clinical Modification).
- *ASA codes* (American Society of Anesthesiologists).
- *CPT codes* describe the medical, surgical, and diagnostic services that are performed by physicians and other health care providers.
- *ICD-9-CM codes* describe signs, symptoms, injuries, diseases, and conditions.

- *ICD-9-CM codes* must support the medical necessity of the procedures defined by the *CPT code*.
- All time-based billing requires that the *CPT code* be converted to a corresponding *ASA code*. Any inaccurate coding can result in delayed reimbursement.

Once coding has been completed, processing of claims can begin. This involves the transfer of coding and billing documents to third-party insurers. All reimbursements should be matched against contracted rates to ensure that there are no under- or overpayments. Once a correct payment has been received, the claim is closed. If a payment is not received within a reasonable amount of time, the claim is submitted to the collections department. A short collection period is desirable, as the older the claim, the more difficult it is to collect.

It is very important that the financial department of an anesthesia practice is aware of the demographics of the patient population that they are treating (e.g., government vs. nongovernmental payers) as this has a direct impact on the practice's profitability and budgeting.

Scheduling

Scheduling involves creating the day-to-day work schedule, on-call schedule, as well as the vacation schedule. The larger the practice, the more complicated the scheduling process becomes. There are a variety of ways of implementing a work schedule; however, the most important issue is to ensure fairness throughout the process in order to maintain employee satisfaction.

Human resources

The goal of a *human resources department* within an anesthesia practice is to recruit, employ, and retain the most competitive and qualified individuals, thus making the practice as successful as possible. Given the current shortage of anesthesiologists and nurse anesthetists, recruiting and hiring has taken on a more important role in recent years. The *HR department* must implement an objective evaluation process for current

Essential Clinical Anesthesia Review: Keywords, Questions and Answers for the Boards, ed. Linda S. Aglio, Robert W. Lekowski, and Richard D. Urman. Published by Cambridge University Press. © Cambridge University Press 2015.

employees, which allows for appeal in the event of a negative evaluation. When an employee is to be terminated, the *HR department* must ensure that the employee is treated fairly and that the practice follows all current employment laws in order to avoid litigation.

Finance

There are many responsibilities of a *finance department* within an anesthesia practice, some of which include: payroll, accounts payable, expense reimbursement, revenue and expense tracking, creation of financial reports, and preparation of tax documents. There are typically two types of accounting that an anesthesia practice may implement: *cash-based and accrual-based accounting*. With *cash-based accounting*, revenue is recognized when money is received, and expenses are recognized when payment is made (i.e., when money actually changes hands). This is in contrast to *accrual-based accounting*, in which revenue is recognized at the time the service is provided, and expenses are recognized when they are incurred. Larger anesthesia practices will typically use *accrual-based accounting* because it gives a more accurate picture of practice performance at any given time.

Financial reports should be drafted and reviewed on a regular basis. The three most commonly reviewed financial reports are: (1) the balance sheet, (2) the income statement, and (3) the statement of cash flows. The balance sheet is prepared on a single date and gives the reader a glimpse of the financial condition of the practice in a single moment in time. The income statement reports revenue, expenses, and net income over a defined time period. The statement of cash flows reports the sources and uses of cash over a defined time period and describes the change in cash balance during that time period.

Risk management

Concepts of risk management were discussed in Chapter 137; however, some of these issues are pertinent when discussing anesthesia practice. It is the responsibility of the risk management department to predict, prevent, and manage adverse events that have the potential to cause harm to the practice. This typically involves quality improvement initiatives, conducting analyses of adverse events, managing litigation, and performing risk analysis of policy and procedure. The risk management team should also be involved in securing malpractice insurance for the practice and its employees.

Questions

1. With reference to coding, which of the following statements is TRUE?
   a. All time-based billing requires that the CPT code be converted to a corresponding ASA code.
   b. ICD-9-CM codes reflect the medical, surgical, and diagnostic services that are rendered by physicians and health care professionals.
   c. "CPT" stands for Current Procedural Technology.
   d. Claims processing begins before coding has been completed.
   e. Reimbursement is typically not delayed by inaccurate coding.

2. The term "accrual-based accounting" refers to which of the following?
   a. recognizing revenue at the time payment is made
   b. recognizing revenue at the time service is provided
   c. recognizing revenue at the time the claim is presented to the insurance company
   d. recognizing all revenue accrued over a defined time period
   e. none of the above

Answers

1. a. (a) is a true statement; (b) is false because it describes CPT codes rather than ICD-9-CM codes; (c) is false because "CPT" stands for Current Procedural Terminology; (d) is false because claims processing starts after coding has been completed; (e) is false because reimbursement *is* delayed by inaccurate coding.
2. b. (a) refers to "cash-based accounting"; (b) is correct.

Further reading

Vacanti, C. A., Sikka, P. K., Urman, R. U., Dershwitz, M., and Segal, B. S. (eds) (2011). Chapter 139. Practice management. In *Essential Clinical Anesthesia*. New York, NY: Cambridge University Press.

139

Principles of medical ethics

Christian Peccora and Richard D. Urman

Keywords

Autonomy
Informed consent
Capacity
Proxy
Durable power of attorney for health care
Advance directive
DNR orders
Comfort measures
Doctrine of double effect
Futility
Brain death
Donation after cardiac death (DCD)
Health Insurance Portability and Accountability
    Act (HIPAA)
Protected health information
Anesthesia Patient Safety Foundation

Autonomy and informed consent

The principle of *autonomy* dictates that patients must consent to a procedure, including anesthesia, and have the right to refuse it. *Informed consent* requires a patient to understand the risks, benefits, and alternatives to the procedure, as well as have *capacity* to make the decision. The patient should be provided with all the information a "reasonable person" would expect to make an informed decision, save for emergency circumstances where delaying medical services to obtain consent would cause permanent harm to the patient. If a person is not able to make a decision because they lack capacity, one should determine whether they executed a *durable power of attorney for health care*, wherein a *proxy* was designated to make decisions on their behalf. The patient may also have an *advance directive* that provides instructions regarding his or her health care. Whether the surrogate decision maker be a proxy or the patient's next of kin, he or she must be guided by what the patient would have wanted based on an advance

directive or previously expressed wishes. Persons with partial capacity (such as children or patients with developmental delay) may participate in decision making, but consent for the procedure is provided by a parent or legal guardian. One should be aware of and sensitive to religious beliefs that can influence decision making (e.g., Jehovah's Witnesses may refuse blood products), as well as cultural determinants of the appropriateness of family involvement in decision making.

Do not resuscitate orders (DNR) and comfort care

There are a variety of approaches for a patient for whom *DNR orders* are active yet requires resuscitation because of an anesthetic or surgical procedure. One option is to rescind the order for the operative and perioperative period. Another option is to have a detailed discussion with the patient as to the resuscitative efforts he or she would want (e.g., endotracheal intubation is acceptable for the surgery but chest compressions are not). Yet another alternative requires the anesthesiologist to intervene to alter reversible circumstances to meet clearly defined goals. For example, if a patient does not desire pressor support, but the effects of an anesthetic have caused hypotension easily treatable by phenylephrine, the anesthesiologist may provide pressor support to achieve a goal blood pressure. Regardless of which strategy is chosen, a detailed conversation with the patient about benefits, risks, and goals should be conducted. In situations where it is very unlikely that any intervention will result a meaningful recovery, *comfort measures* can be provided per the patient's wishes. Opiates, hypnotics, and other anesthetic interventions make a patient more comfortable but usually do not hasten death. The *doctrine of double effect* states that the intention of the treatment (relief of pain) makes a treatment permissible even if it may cause harm (hasten death). Treatments that will not achieve goals of therapy are deemed *futile* and do not have to be provided.

Essential Clinical Anesthesia Review: Keywords, Questions and Answers for the Boards, ed. Linda S. Aglio, Robert W. Lekowski, and Richard D. Urman. Published by Cambridge University Press. © Cambridge University Press 2015.

Organ donation

Organ donation can occur after *brain death* (irreversible loss of all brain and brainstem function), which is legally equivalent to death, even if the heart continues to beat. If a patient sustains injury that makes meaningful recovery extremely unlikely, life-sustaining interventions can be ceased, and organ donation can occur after irreversible cessation of respiratory and circulatory function (*donation after cardiac death [DCD]*). DCD can occur without assessing whether brain death has occurred. Careful coordination between surgeons and anesthesiologists is required for organ harvest soon after asystolic death.

Patient privacy

The *Health Insurance Portability and Accountability Act (HIPAA)* applies to any health care provider that transmits patient information and works to ensure information remains private and is only accessed or amended by those authorized to do so. *Protected health information* is any information created in the process of caring for a patient that can be matched to a patient, including records related to research. Adequate security must be in place to ensure that data is not accessed by an unauthorized individual.

Patient safety

In many ways, anesthesiology has been at the forefront of advances in patient safety. In 1983, the British Royal Society of Medicine and Department of Anesthesiology at Harvard Medical School jointly held a symposium to study deaths and injuries caused by anesthesia. By 1984, the American Society of Anesthesiology had founded the *Anesthesia Patient Safety Foundation (APSF)*. The standards for quality and safety in anesthesia have coincided with impressive decreases in untoward events due to anesthesia. The National Patient Safety Foundation was founded in 1997 by the American Medical Association and was largely modeled after the APSF. The ASA established a repository of legal cases derived from adverse outcomes called the Closed Claims Project to help identify and prevent mistakes. An intense focus on patient safety and quality have significantly reduced malpractice claims and premiums over the last 20 years.

The Institute of Medicine estimates that medication errors harm 1.5 million Americans per year, and drug errors have been the most common cause of morbidity, mortality, and legal claims related to anesthesia services in some studies. Systematic review of the literature suggests that drug errors can be decreased if the labels of ampules are checked (and double checked) before a medication is drawn up, syringes are clearly and consistently labeled, and working areas are neatly organized.

When errors do occur, the patient and family should be told what happened (though details regarding how and why require careful review and should be reserved until the circumstances surrounding the error have been investigated). The anesthesiologist should take responsibility for what happened and apologize, even when there were factors that might have significantly contributed to the error outside of the doctor's control. Communication of remorse and addressing how such errors will be prevented in the future are helpful to families and patients. There should be proper reporting to agencies, hospital departments, and risk management personnel in order to improve processes and address the legal ramifications of errors.

Training and licensure

After obtaining a doctor of medicine or doctor of osteopathy degree, four years of training under an approved postgraduate program must be completed to be eligible for certification with the American Board of Anesthesiology (ABA). Diplomates must pass an oral and written board examination. Starting in 2000, diplomates are required to re-certify every ten years (Maintenance of Certification in Anesthesiology, or MOCA).

Physician impairment or disability

American Medical Association House Policy H-95.955 defines impairment as "any physical, mental, or behavioral disorder that interferes with ability to engage safely in professional activities." Impairment is therefore almost inevitable. Fatigue from the hours of stressful work, the auditory and visual decline that accompanies aging, and the disability caused by injury or forces external to a physician's control can cause impairment. A physician should be cognizant of his limitations, and AMA Opinion 0.031 states that physicians "have an ethical obligation to report impaired, incompetent, and/or unethical colleagues." Rehabilitation and appropriate assistance should be sought to remove impairment and allow the physician to continue practicing medicine if he or she desires.

Though the contention that anesthesiologists have increased rates of chronic chemical dependence compared to other professions has been disproven, unique access to controlled substances is inherent in anesthesia practice. Warning signs that a colleague is misusing substances include overadministration of controlled medicines, volunteering for extra shifts or other changes in work habits, frequent absences, loss of interest in activities, and problems at home. These are obviously nonspecific indicators, and irrefutable evidence should be gathered before an intervention is conducted in a formal setting by an expert. Addiction is a disability, and, according to the Americans with Disabilities Act, former addicts cannot be denied employment based on a history of addiction. A history of addiction does increase the likelihood of substance abuse, however, and long-term remission should be maintained by adhering to a detailed recovery program in the short term and with the support and accountability of colleagues in the long term.

Questions

1. A 55-year-old patient presents to the emergency room with high fever and altered mental status. A partial work-up strongly suggests a perforated sigmoid colon. The decision is made to immediately take him to the operating room. He adamantly refuses the operation to both the anesthesiologist and the surgeon. Other expressions are illogical and he is not oriented to place or time. However, his next of kin states that he has always been very careful with his health, takes all his vitamins and medications, and exercises regularly. His next of kin insists he have the operation. There is no durable power of attorney for health care. What should be done?

   a. The patient has clearly expressed that he does not want the procedure. Under the principle of autonomy, the procedure should not be done.
   b. His next of kin should make the decision.
   c. The patient should be treated with antibiotics and supportive measures, and once he has regained capacity, the decision regarding operative intervention can be made.
   d. If two attending physicians agree, the patient should proceed to the OR without consent.

2. Which of the following is required to be a board-certified anesthesiologist in the United States of America?

   a. passage of written and oral board examinations
   b. a doctorate of medicine or osteopathy
   c. completion of an accredited four-year residency program
   d. if it has been more than ten years since certification, passage of MOCA.
   e. (a), (b), and (c)
   f. all of the above

3. What is the doctrine of double effect?

   a. DNR orders have the dual effect of prohibiting both intubation and chest compressions.
   b. Doctors cannot discuss private health information without a patient's consent unless its effect is to both address an emergency and coordinate care among the patient's health care providers.
   c. An intervention with a primary intention of providing comfort is permissible even if its secondary effect is hastening of death.
   d. In order to be eligible for coverage under the ADA, you must be both a US citizen and have a disability confirmed by a physician.

Answers

1. b. The patient does not have the capacity to make the decision since evidence suggests that his mental status is significantly altered, and thus he cannot sufficiently understand the procedure or its associated risks and benefits. Capacity can be assessed by a physician. If a person lacks capacity and there is no durable power of attorney or other directive, his or her next of kin must decide in accordance with what the patient's wishes would be if he or she had capacity.

2. f. All of these are requirements to become a board-certified anesthesiologist.

3. c. An intervention may simultaneously have desired, ethically acceptable effects (decreasing pain) and undesired effects (hastens death). The doctrine of double effect states that the primary effects and intent of an intervention should be of primary importance when this intervention could also have adverse effects. Even if some of the secondary effects are considered harmful, if the primary and overriding intent is beneficial, the intervention may be performed.

Further reading

Vacanti, C. A., Sikka, P. K., Urman, R. U., Dershwitz, M., and Segal, B. S. (eds) (2011). Chapter 140. Principles of medical ethics. In *Essential Clinical Anesthesia*. New York, NY: Cambridge University Press.

Vacanti, C. A., Sikka, P. K., Urman, R. U., Dershwitz, M., and Segal, B. S. (eds) (2011). Chapter 137: Patient safety, quality assurance, and risk management. In *Essential Clinical Anesthesia*. New York, NY: Cambridge University Press.

Miller, R. (2011). Chapter 2. Scope of anesthesia practice. In *Basics of Anesthesia*, 6th edn. Philadelphia: Elsevier.

Meyer, R. (2007). Medication error: a leading cause of anesthesia-related morbidity and mortality. *Anesthesiology* 107(6), 1033.

Hove, L. D. (2007). Analysis of deaths related to anesthesia in the period 1996–2004 from closed claims registered by the Danish Patient Insurance Association. *Anesthesiology* 106(4), 675–680.

Stabile, M., Webster, C., and Merry. A. (2007). Medication administration in anesthesia. *APSF Newsletter*. www.apsf.org/newsletters/html/2007/fall/02_medical_administration.htm

American Medical Association (n.d.). Opinion 9.031: Reporting impaired, incompetent, or unethical colleagues. www.ama-assn.org/ama/pub/physician-resources/medical-ethics/code-medical-ethics/opinion9031.page.

Urman, R. et. al. (2009). Ethical issues in anesthesia. In *Pocket Anesthesia*. Philadelphia: Lipincott Williams & Wilkins.

Chapter

140

Risks in the operating room

Jaida Fitzgerald and Robert W. Lekowski

Keywords

Needle safety
Waste anesthetic gases (WAGs)
Fire triad
Ionizing radiation
Non-ionizing radiation

Needle safety

- There are approximately 384,000 sharps-related injuries that occur in hospitals each year.
- It has been estimated that 23% of these injuries occur in the surgical setting, which means that the majority are occurring during other procedures that anesthesia providers may be involved in.
- Hollow-bore devices are more dangerous because they are more likely to transmit disease.
- The three most common diseases transmitted via needle-stick injury are:
  - hepatitis B (HBV)
  - hepatitis C (HCV)
  - HIV.
- The likelihood of transmission from an infected person to a noninfected person as a result of a needle-stick injury is:
  - 6% to 30% with HBV
  - 0% to 7% with HCV
  - 0.3% with HIV.
- It has been estimated that the management of a single sharps-related injury can cost from US$376 to US$2,456 depending on the need for medical examination, medication prophylaxis, etc.
- Multiple organizations within the last several years have made sharps safety a priority, including the Centers for Disease Control (CDC) and the Occupational Safety and Health Administration (OSHA).

Waste anesthetic gases (WAGs)

WAGs are small amounts of volatile anesthetic gases that leak from the patient's anesthetic breathing circuit into the air of operating rooms during the delivery of anesthesia. Although there are known negative health consequences of exposure to anesthetic gases at *high* concentrations (headache, irritability, fatigue, etc.) there is no literature on the effects of exposure to anesthetic gases at *low* concentrations (i.e., WAGs). Given the potential side effects of unregulated anesthetic gas exposure, multiple organizations have published guidelines to ensure the safety of all OR personnel, including both the Occupational Safety and Health Administration (OSHA) as well as the National Institute for Occupational Safety and Health (NIOSH). The ASA also has a specific committee dedicated to this issue, deemed the Task Force on Trace Anesthetic Gases (TFTAG). Recently the TFTAG concluded that there is not sufficient evidence to prove any adverse health effects from *trace* amounts of *waste anesthetic gases*; however, they do promote the use of scavenging systems whenever anesthetic gas is being delivered, regardless of location.

Fire safety in the OR

Most operating room fires involve the airway, therefore it is essential that anesthesiologists are prepared to recognize and appropriately manage such an event. In order for a fire to occur, three components, known as the *fire triad* must be present:

- an oxidizer
- an ignition source
- a source of fuel

Oxidizers include:

- air
- oxygen
- nitrous oxide

Ignition sources include:

- electrocautery

Essential Clinical Anesthesia Review: Keywords, Questions and Answers for the Boards, ed. Linda S. Aglio, Robert W. Lekowski, and Richard D. Urman. Published by Cambridge University Press. © Cambridge University Press 2015.

- lasers
- fiberoptic light source

Fuel sources include:

- endotracheal tubes
- drapes, sponges, etc.

It is estimated that there are approximately 100 operating room fires yearly, with as many as 20% resulting in serious injury or death. In response to this potential risk, in 2008 the ASA released a Practice Advisory on the Prevention and Management of Operating Room Fires. The most common scenario in which a fire occurs in or on a patient, involves procedures in which an ignition source (electrocautery, laser) is used in an oxidizer-rich environment.

Common examples of this include:

- tonsillectomy
- tracheostomy
- other forms of head and neck surgery

See Table 140.1 for key principles for the prevention and management of airway fires.

Radiation safety

There are two types of radiation that anesthesia providers may be exposed to in the operating room: *ionizing radiation* and *non-ionizing radiation. Ionizing radiation* is composed of particles that individually carry enough energy to liberate an electron from an atom or molecule, thus ionizing it.

Common forms of *ionizing radiation* include:

- alpha rays
- beta rays
- gamma rays
- x-rays

Non-ionizing radiation includes:

- electromagnetic radiation ranging from extremely low frequency to ultraviolet

Ionizing radiation is carcinogenic at high doses. The amount of radiation exposure is determined by three factors:

- intensity and time of exposure
- distance between anesthesiologist and source of radiation
- use of shielding

Shielding should be used at all times when exposure is occurring and should consist of a lead body shield as well as additional protective equipment for the eyes and thyroid gland.

The laser is a form of *non-ionizing radiation* that is frequently used in the operating room. Laser is an acronym for "light amplification by stimulated emission of radiation." There are four types of lasers that are used clinically:

- carbon dioxide (CO_2) laser
- argon laser

Table 140.1 Recommendations for the prevention and management of operating room fires

Prevention
- Allow flammable skin preparations to dry before draping
- Configure surgical drapes to avoid build up of oxidizer
- Anesthesiologist collaborates with team throughout the procedure to minimize oxidizer-enriched environment near ignition source
  - Keep oxygen concentration as low as clinically possible
  - Avoid nitrous oxide
- Notify surgeon if oxidizer and ignition source are in proximity to each other
- Moisten gauze and sponges that are near an ignition source

Airway fire
- *Simultaneously* remove the endotracheal tube and stop gases/disconnect circuit
- Pour saline into airway
- Remove burning materials
- Mask-ventilate patient, assess injury, consider bronchoscopy, reintubate

(American Society of Anesthesiologists Task Force on Operating Room Fires. 2008. Practice advisory for the prevention and management of operating room fires. *Anesthesiology*, 108(5): 786–801.)

- neodymium-yttrium aluminum garnet (nd-YAG) laser
- potassium titanyl phosphate (KTP) laser (green laser)

There are significant risks associated with the use of lasers, including thermal burns, eye injuries, fires, explosions, and electrical hazards. Protective eyewear must be worn by all OR personnel whenever a laser is in use.

Ultraviolet rays represent another health risk to which anesthesiologists may be exposed. UVB (290–320 nm) radiation is more dangerous than UVA (320–400 nm) radiation, as it directly damages DNA and is highly mutagenic. There have been various recommendations published by both NIOSH and the International Commission on Non-Ionizing Radiation Protection (ICNIRP) regarding the limits of UV ray exposure.

Questions

1. In regards to needle-stick injury, which of the following lists the rate of transmissibility of infection from greatest to least?

   a. HBV > HIV > HCV
   b. HCV > HIV > HBV
   c. HBV = HCV > HIV
   d. HBV > HCV > HIV
   e. HIV > HCV > HBV

2. All of the following are effective strategies in preventing an OR fire EXCEPT for which?

   a. arranging surgical drapes to prevent build up of oxygen and nitrous oxide
   b. allowing flammable skin preparations to dry before draping

c. keeping gauze and sponges that are near an ignition source dry

d. maintaining open communication with surgeons regarding proximity of oxidizer and ignition source

e. keeping oxygen concentrations as low as clinically possible when oxidizer-enriched environment is close to ignition source

Answers

1. d. The likelihood of transmission from an infected person to a noninfected person as a result of a needle-stick injury is 6% to 30% with HBV, 0% to 7% with HCV, and 0.3% with HIV.

2. c. Gauze and sponges that are located near an ignition source should be moistened to decrease the likelihood of setting fire.

Further reading

American Society of Anesthesiologists Task Force on Operating Room Fires, et al. (2008). Practice advisory for the prevention and management of operating room fires. *Anesthesiology* 108(5), 786–801.

Vacanti, C. A., Sikka, P. K., Urman, R. U., Dershwitz, M., and Segal, B. S. (eds) (2011). Chapter 141. Risks in the operating room. In *Essential Clinical Anesthesia*. New York, NY: Cambridge University Press.

Stoelting, R. K. and Miller, R. D. (2007). Chapter 8. Electrical and fire safety. In *Basics of Anesthesia*, 5th edn. Philadelphia, PA: Churchill-Livingstone Elsevier.

FDA, NIOSH & OSHA Joint Safety Communication (May 2012). Blunt-tip surgical suture needles reduce needlestick injuries and the risk of subsequent bloodborne pathogen transmission to surgical personnel. www.fdo.gov/MedicalDevices/Safety/AlertsandNotices/ucm305757.htm.

CDC, NIOSH (September 2007). Waste anesthetic gases; occupational hazards in hospitals. www.cdc.gov/niosh/docs/2007–151/pdfs/2007–151.pdf.

141

Statistics for anesthesiologists and researchers

Jaida Fitzgerald and Robert W. Lekowski

Keywords

Sensitivity
Specificity
Positive predictive value
Negative predictive value
Interval data
Categorical data
Probability
p value
Type I (α) error
Type II (β) error
Mean, median, mode
Standard deviation
Statistical techniques: student's *t* test, ANOVA,
  chi-square test
Linear regression
Exponential functions
Odds ratio
Risk ratio

It is crucial that anesthesiologists from all types of practices have a basic understanding of statistics in order to objectively interpret the abundance of medical literature that is encountered in daily practice.

Basic definitions

Sensitivity represents the number of people who test positive for a disease divided by the number of people who have the disease (sensitivity = TP/TP + FN, where TP = true positive, FN = false negative). A highly sensitive test will essentially "rule out" those who do not have the disease, therefore sensitive tests are often used as screening tests.

Specificity represents the number of people who test negative for a disease divided by the number of people who do not have the disease (specificity = TN/TN + FP, where TN = true negative, FP = false positive). A highly specific test will help to "rule in" those who have the disease.

Table 141.1 Sensitivity, specificity, PPV, NPV

	Have disease	No disease	
Positive test	True positive (TP)	False positive (FP)	Positive predictive value (PPV) = TP/TP + FP
Negative test	False negative (FN)	True negative (TN)	Negative predictive value (NPV) = TN/TN + FN
	Sensitivity = TP/TP + FN	*Specificity* = TN/TN + FP	

Positive predictive value: the proportion of positive results that are true positives (PPV = TP/TP + FP).

Negative predictive value: the proportion of negative results that are true negatives (NPV = TN/TN + FN).

Classification of data: *interval data* describes *quantitative* variables, which can be discrete or continuous. *Categorical data* describes *qualitative* data, which can be dichotomous, nominal, or ordinal. See Table 141.2 for examples of each type of data.

Probability: the proportion of times an event is likely to occur in a long sequence of trials. Probabilities always lie between 0 and 1.

p value: a measure of the probability that a difference observed between two groups in an experiment is due to chance. $p = 0.05$ means that there is a 5 in 100 chance that the result occurred by chance. The lower the *p value*, the more likely it is that the difference between two groups was due to experimental intervention.

Type I (α) error: the probability that the experiment will show that a difference between groups exists, when none actually exists.

Type II (β) error: the probability that the experiment will not demonstrate a difference between two groups, when one actually does exist. Type II error is usually set at 0.2. The statistical *power* of a study is related to the β value,

Essential Clinical Anesthesia Review: Keywords, Questions and Answers for the Boards, ed. Linda S. Aglio, Robert W. Lekowski, and Richard D. Urman. Published by Cambridge University Press. © Cambridge University Press 2015.

Table 141.2 Examples of interval vs. categorical data

Type of data	Description	Example
Interval	Discrete: integer only	Number of toes
Interval	Continuous: constant scale interval	Temperature
Categorical	Dichotomous: binary data	Male/female
Categorical	Nominal: qualitative; cannot be ranked	Eye color (blue/brown/gray/green)
Categorical	Ordinal: ranked, but do not have consistent scale interval	ASA Class (I, II, III, IV)

(Adapted from Vacanti, C. A., Sikka, P. K., Urman, R. D., Dershwitz, M., and Segal, B.S. eds (2011) Chapter 142. Statistics for anesthesiologists and researchers. In *Essential Clinical Anesthesia*. New York: Cambridge University Press, p. 875.)

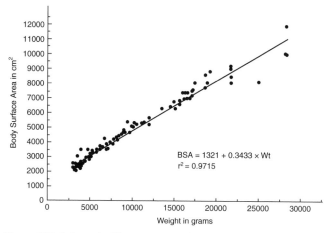

Figure 141.1 Example of linear regression. (From Vacanti et al. (2011). *Essential Clinical Anesthesia*, Cambridge University Press, p. 874.)

where power $= 1 - \beta$, if $\beta = 0.2$, the power $= 0.8$ or 80%. Conceptually, a statistical power of 80% means that there is an 80% chance of finding an effect if one is really there.

Mean is the average of all data values. This reflects the central tendency of the data.

Median: the central sample when the data are arranged in ascending or descending order. When there is an even number of data points, the average of the two central samples reflects the median.

Mode: the data value that occurs with the greatest frequency.

Range: the difference between the maximum and minimum values in a data set. The range reflects the dispersion of the sample.

Standard deviation (SD): a measure of the amount of dispersion there is from the mean within a given data set. With data of a normal distribution, 1, 2, and 3 standard deviations from the mean represent 68%, 95%, and 99% of the population, respectively.

Variance: equal to standard deviation squared.

Confidence intervals (CI) define a range of values within which the mean is likely to lie. If $p = 0.05$, the CI represents the range of values within which you can be 95% sure the true value lies.

Statistical techniques

In general there are two categories of statistical tests: parametric tests and nonparametric tests. Parametric tests should be used to evaluate data that is normally distributed, while nonparametric tests are used for data that is not normally distributed or is ordinal in nature (i.e., ASA score, VAS pain score).

Student's t test determines if the difference between the *means* of two data points are statistically significant relative to the spread or variability of their data. The *t* test is an example of a parametric test. There are two types of *t* test:

- One sample or *paired t* test.
  - Used when data from a *single patient* are paired. For example, in an experiment in which each patient has two measurements taken, one before and one after an intervention, the control measurement is paired with the measurement after intervention.
  - The pairing of measurements in the same patient reduces variability and increases statistical power.
- Two sample or *unpaired t* test.
  - Used to compare the means of *two different groups*. For example, one group receives lipid-lowering medication, which is compared to the second control group, which does not receive intervention.

Analysis of variance (ANOVA): a parametric test that is used to compare means between *more than two groups* or between several measurements in the same group. ANOVA puts all the data into one number (*F* statistic) that provides the probability of the null hypothesis. ANOVA should be used for independent *categorical* variables (i.e., male/female, blue/brown eyes).

Chi-square test: a type of nonparametric test that is used to compare the *frequencies* of two or more groups. It is often used to test nominal data.

Regression analysis

A statistical technique that is used to predict the value of one characteristic from knowledge of another characteristic. Depending on the number of variables, either *linear regression* or *multiple regression* should be used.

- *Linear regression*: analyzes the relationship between two variables, *x* and *y*. The goal is to find the line that best predicts *y* from the known value of *x*. In the simplest type, a straight line is assumed between the two variables, where *y*,

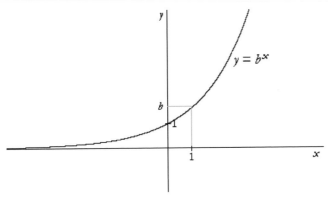

Figure 141.2 Exponential function. (From Vacanti et al. (2011). *Essential Clinical Anesthesia*, Cambridge University Press, p. 875.)

the dependent variable, is a function of x, the independent variable. This relationship is expressed with the linear regression equation, $y = a + bx$ (y, dependent variable; x, independent variable; a, intercept; b, slope of straight line relating a and b). See Figure 141.1, where $y =$ BSA; $a =$ 1,321; $b = 0.3433$; $x =$ weight.

- r^2 is a fraction between 0 and 1. When $r^2 = 0$, there is no linear relationship between x and y, and therefore knowing x does *not* help predict y. When $r^2 = 1$, all points lie exactly on a straight line, and therefore knowing x allows one to perfectly predict y.
- *Multiple regression* is used for data sets in which the dependent variable, y, is thought to be linearly related to many explanatory variables (i.e., not just x).

Exponential functions: depicted as hyperbolic or parabolic curves, which are used to determine the value of y when x is known, or vice versa. Exponential function equation, $y = b^x$. (See Figure 141.2.)

Odds ratio: the ratio of the odds of an event occurring in an experimental group compared to the odds of it occurring in the control group. If odds ratio = 1, this indicates that the odds of an event occurring are equally likely between two groups.

Risk ratio: the ratio of the experimental event rate to the control event rate. Risk ratios are typically used in randomized controlled trials and cohort studies.

Questions

1. Which of the following statistical tests should be used when two measurements from the same patient are paired?
   a. two sample, unpaired t test
   b. chi-square test
   c. one sample, paired t test
   d. analysis of variance (ANOVA)
   e. linear regression analysis

2. All of the following are true statements EXCEPT for which?
   a. Type I error refers to the probability that the experiment will show that a difference between groups exists, when none actually exists.
   b. ANOVA is a parametric test that is used to compare means between *more than two groups* or between several measurements in the same group.
   c. A test with a high specificity is best to rule out disease.
   d. ANOVA should only be used for categorical data.
   e. Standard deviation measures the amount of dispersion there is from the mean within a given data set.

Answers

1. c. A paired, one sample t test should be used when data from the same patient are compared.
2. c. A test with a high sensitivity (not specificity) should be used to rule out disease.

Further reading

Vacanti, C. A., Sikka, P. K., Urman, R. U., Dershwitz, M., and Segal, B. S. (eds) (2011). Chapter 142. Statistics for anesthesiologists and researchers. In *Essential Clinical Anesthesia*. New York, NY: Cambridge University Press.

Stoelting, R. K. and Miller, R. D. (2007). Chapter 9. Experimental design and statistics. In *Basics of Anesthesia*, 5th edn. Philadelphia, PA: Churchill-Livingstone Elsevier.

Chapter

142

Neurophysiology of pain

Christian Peccora and Jie Zhou

Keywords

Nociception
Pain
Spinothalamic tract
A-delta and C fibers
Periaqueductal gray
Reticular formation
Nucleus raphe magnus
Hyperalgesia
Allodynia
Wind up
Sensitization
Sympathetic nerve blocks
Pain perception variation with gender, age, and culture
Types of pain: nociceptive, inflammatory, neuropathic

The initial theories about pain perception contained numerous incorrect assumptions regarding the neuroanatomy and neurophysiology that underlie unpleasant sensation. They also ignored psychological, environmental, biological, genetic, and social contributors to pain. Because these theories went largely unquestioned for hundreds of years, treatment of pain was neither optimal nor evolving significantly until the 20th century. With the publication of the gate control theory of pain by Melzack and Wall in 1965, research was rekindled, and a greater understanding of pain led to better treatments.

Nociception vs. pain

Nociception indicates the activation of a nociceptive pathway by a noxious stimulus. It triggers *pain*, which is a consciously perceived unpleasant sensation accompanied by an emotional experience. Therefore nociception can occur in a patient whose cerebral cortical functions are not intact (such as a patient under general anesthesia), whereas pain requires conscious perception by the cerebral cortex. Pain is usually associated with tissue damage.

Pathways

Ascending pain sensory information is transmitted mostly by the *spinothalamic tract* to supraspinal processing centers. Sensation of cold and well-localized, quickly detected pain are mediated by larger, rapidly conducting *A-delta fibers* that are myelinated. Slower, smaller *C fibers* are unmyelinated and are stimulated by mechanical stimuli. Pain transmitted by C fibers is poorly localized. A-delta and C nociceptive fibers synapse with second-order neurons primarily on lamina I, II, and V of the dorsal horn of the spinal cord. Visceral and somatic nociception both converge on lamina V, which may help explain the phenomenon of referred pain. Opioids are believed to have much of their effect on lamina II (the substantia gelatinosa).

Second-order neurons cross the anterior white commissure and ascend the spinothalamic tract to synapse at the thalamus with third-order neurons that subserve the sensory cortex, namely the posterior central gyrus. Second-order neurons also send branches to the the limbic system and other subcortical areas, as well as the reticular formation and periaqueductal gray that are a part of descending inhibitory pathways.

The inhibitory pathways include supraspinal structures (such as the *periaqueductal gray, reticular formation*, and *nucleus raphe magnus*), from whence neurons descend to inhibit first- and second-order neurons. These descending neurons release noradrenergic, opioid, gamma-aminobutyric acid (GABA) and serotonergic neurotransmitters onto serotonergic, adrenergic (alpha2), and opiate receptors. Much of this activity occurs in lamina II of the dorsal horn. Of note, there are also descending pathways that facilitate pain via cholecystokinin, dynorphin, and excitatory amino acids.

Neurotransmitters, messengers, and inflammatory mediators

Excitatory chemicals and neurotransmitters include glutamate, aspartate, vasoactive intestinal peptide, ATP, and substance P. Enkephalins, endorphins, GABA, somatostatin, serotonin,

Essential Clinical Anesthesia Review: Keywords, Questions and Answers for the Boards, ed. Linda S. Aglio, Robert W. Lekowski, and Richard D. Urman. Published by Cambridge University Press. © Cambridge University Press 2015.

acetylcholine, and norepinephrine are inhibitory. All sensation involves a balance between excitatory and inhibitory pathways and neurotransmitters. When there is an imbalance between excitation and inhibition, sensation becomes abnormal. *Hyperalgesia* is an increased sensation of pain to a stimulus that is normally painful. *Allodynia* is the sensation of pain from a stimulus that is normally not painful (see Figure 142.1).

Increased pain sensation can occur from facilitation of peripheral nociceptive firing, increased activity of central nociceptive pathways, or decreased activity of descending inhibitory pathways. Persistent release of prostaglandins, histamine, bradykinin, lactic acid, hydrogen ions, and other inflammatory mediators sensitizes peripheral nociceptors. Persistent injury causes repeated C fiber stimulation, which leads to *wind up*, whereby neurons in the dorsal horn become more responsive to nociceptive input. This contributes to central *sensitization*. Central sensitization contributes to hyperalgesia and chronic pain. Persistent release of glutamate and aspartate activates N-methyl-D-asparte (NMDA) receptors, which induces and maintains central sensitization. Sensitization can be decreased by activation of inhibitory processes from higher centers, opioids, tricyclic antidepressants, NMDA antagonists, voltage-sensitive calcium channel blockers, nitric oxide synthetase inhibitors, transcutaneous electrical nerve stimulation (TENS), and spinal cord stimulators.

The sympathetic nervous system has cell bodies between T1 and L2, and it contributes to perception and maintenance of pain sensation. *Sympathetic nerve blocks* can significantly reduce sympathetically maintained pain and most commonly involve blockade of the stellate ganglion, the celiac plexus, lumbar sympathetics, and the ganglion impar. If a sympathetic nerve block is efficacious, there is an increased likelihood that spinal cord stimulator insertion would provide effective therapy for chronic pain.

Pain perception variation with gender, age, and culture

Pain perception may vary by gender, age, and culture. Women appear to have increased pain sensitivity and greater activation of autonomic and affective regions of the brain when exposed to noxious stimuli. Tolerance of pain is less and pain ratings of supra threshold stimuli are generally higher in women. As a patient ages, nerve degeneration alters the perception of pain. Initial perception of some types of pain may be decreased, and inhibitory mechanisms are also less robust. This means less pain may be perceived, but once the pain threshold is surpassed, it is more intense and difficult to treat. A patient's psychological

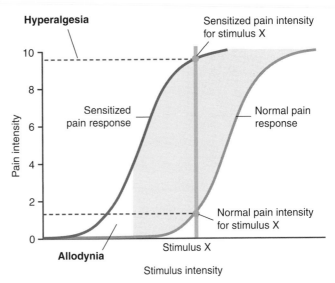

Figure 142.1 Sensitization leading to change in responsiveness to stimulus. (Adapted from Vacanti et al. 2011. *Essential Clinical Anesthesia*, Cambridge University Press, p. 881.)

state can also contribute to pain perception. Persons with personalities that are prone to catastrophizing are more prone to have increased postoperative pain. Some studies suggest pain perception varies among different cultures. Culture and ethnic background do not appear to change pain threshold, but they may influence pain tolerance. There may be increased pain sensitivity in Hispanic American and African American populations compared to White Americans. Investigators have found, however, that opioids are prescribed less and pain is undertreated in non-white populations. Recent studies have shown that a health care providers' preconceptions about pain perception by people of a certain age, gender, or ethnicity can influence how pain is assessed and treated. The psychosocial contributors to both pain perception and pain assessment make conducting and interpreting studies on pain perception differences among cultures and gender more complicated.

Types of pain

There are three major etiologies of pain (see Figure 142.2). *Nociceptive pain* is caused by temperature, mechanical force, or chemical irritant triggering a nociceptive neuron. It does not cause physiologic change to the nervous system. *Inflammatory pain* occurs with tissue damage and does lead to sensitization. *Neuropathic pain* is due to peripheral or central nervous system damage from unchecked sensitization or physical damage. It is commonly more severe, resistant to treatment, and irreversible.

A

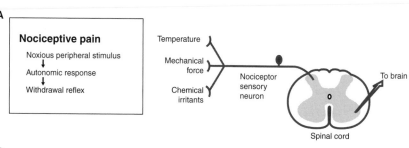

Figure 142.2 Types of pain. (Adapted from Vacanti et al. 2011. *Essential Clinical Anesthesia*, Cambridge University Press, p. 883.)

Nociceptive pain

Noxious peripheral stimulus
↓
Autonomic response
↓
Withdrawal reflex

B

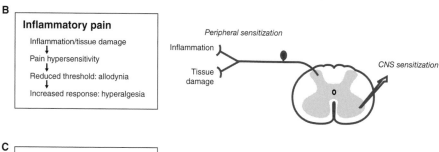

Inflammatory pain

Inflammation/tissue damage
↓
Pain hypersensitivity
↓
Reduced threshold: allodynia
↓
Increased response: hyperalgesia

C

Neuropathic pain

Nerve damage/CNS injury
↓
Spontaneous pain
↓
Pain hypersensitiviy

Questions

1. Which of the following is true of A-delta neurons?
   a. they are unmyelinated
   b. they play a role in the sensation of well-localized, sharp pain
   c. they synapse with second-order neurons of the spinothalamic tract
   d. (b) and (c)
   e. all of the above

2. Which of the following are components of inhibitory pathways?
   a. serotonin
   b. periaqueductal gray
   c. alpha2 receptors
   d. lamina II of the dorsal horn
   e. (a), (b), and (c)
   f. all of the above

3. You are following up a patient who has had arm pain and changes in sensation after a car accident. A few days ago, a pin prick test resulted in "3 out of 10" pain. Today, she states that the same test causes "9 out of 10" pain. What phenomenon is she exhibiting? Choose the one best answer.
   a. allodynia
   b. hyperalgesia
   c. neuropathic pain
   d. dorsal horn inhibition

Answers

1. e. A-delta fiber stimulation results in sensing sharp, well-localized pain via activation of the spinothalamic tract. These fibers are large and myelinated, unlike C fibers.

2. f. Neurons descend from the periaqueductal gray that influence neurons in lamina II of the dorsal horn. Serotonin release and activation of alpha2 receptors inhibit the activation of pain pathways.

3. b. Increased pain from a normally painful stimulus is hyperalgesia. Allodynia is when pain results from a normally nonpainful stimulus. Wind up phenomenon results in increased activity in the dorsal horn and contributes to hyperalgesia. More information is needed to determine whether there may be a neuropathic component to this patient's pain.

Further reading

Vacanti, C. A., Sikka, P. K., Urman, R. U., Dershwitz, M., and Segal, B. S. (eds) (2011). Chapter 143. Neurophysiology of pain. In *Essential Clinical Anesthesia*. New York, NY: Cambridge University Press, pp. 881–884.

Vacanti, C. A., Sikka, P. K., Urman, R. U., Dershwitz, M., and Segal, B. S. (eds) (2011). Chapter 148. Interventional pain management II. In *Essential Clinical Anesthesia*. New York, NY: Cambridge University Press, pp. 919–924.

Miller, R. (2011). Chapter 39. Acute postoperative pain management. In *Basics of Anesthesia*, 6th edn. Philadelphia: Elsevier.

Morgan, G. E. (2006). Chapter 18. Pain management. In *Clinical Anesthesiology*, 4th edn. New York: McGraw-Hill Companies, pp. 359–411.

Macintyre, P. E., Schug, S. A, Scott, D. A., Visser, E. J., and Walker, S. M. (2010). *APM:SE Working Group of the Australian and New Zealand College of Anaesthetists and Faculty of Pain Medicine, Acute Pain Management: Scientific Evidence*, 3rd edn. Melbourne: ANZCA & FPM, Chapter 11, pp. 385–437.

Hyungsuk, K. et. al. (2004). Genetic influence on variability in human acute experimental pain sensitivity associated with gender, ethnicity and psychological temperament. *Pain* 109, 488–496.

Gibson, S. J. et al. (2004). A review of age differences in the neurophysiology of nociception and the perceptual experience of pain. *Clinic Journal of Pain* 20(4), 227–239.

Wandner, L. D. et. al. (2012). The perception of pain in others: how gender, race, and age influence pain expectations. *Journal of Pain* 13(3), 220–227.

Chapter

143

Postoperative acute pain management

Christian Peccora and Jie Zhou

Keywords

- Somatic pain
- Visceral pain
- Neuropathic pain
- Nonpharmacologic interventions
- Pharmacodynamics and pharmacokinetics of opioids
- Active metabolites of opioids: morphine-6-glucoronide, normeperidine
- Cross-tolerance reduction
- Postoperative risk of ketorolac use
- Ketamine mechanism of action
- Hydrophilic vs. lipophilic epidural opioid use

Basic concepts

A patient's assessment of his or her pain is extremely important because pain is a subjective phenomenon. A multimodal approach to pain management is desirable, and there should be frequent assessment of the patient's response to interventions, as well as the location and intensity of the pain (using a numerical or face scale). If pain is expected to persist for an extended period of time, scheduled, long-acting agents should be used with PRN breakthrough immediate-release agents. If frequent breakthrough doses are being used, one should increase the sustained-release agent by 50% to 100% of the 24-hour total breakthrough dose. It is important to determine the analgesics that were previously efficacious for a patient. The adverse consequences of inadequately treated pain include hypertension, tachycardia, myocardial strain, atelectasis, hyperglycemia, fluid retention, ileus, urinary retention, and decreased immune function. Chronic pain patients are sometimes undertreated because they require opioid dosing that is higher than opioid-naïve patients, and doses are almost always more than simply a replacement of their home opioid regimen.

Analgesic modalities

Available analgesic modalities are numerous, and choosing the correct one requires the mechanism of pain to be assessed (see Table 143.1). *Somatic pain* is usually sharp and constant, *visceral pain* is not well localized and can be constant or intermittent, and *neuropathic pain* is usually burning or tingling pain that can be localized to a particular nerve distribution.

Nonpharmacologic interventions, such as acupuncture, heat or cold, transcutaneous electrical nerve stimulation, and hypnosis have varying and sometimes limited scientific underpinnings, but they are relatively low risk and exhibit potential benefits either in directly decreasing nociception and/or addressing the cognitive and affective nature of pain.

Pharmacologic interventions include opioid and non-opioid options. If one uses opioids, it is important to understand the agents' varying *pharmacokinetic* and *pharmacodynamic* profiles. The most stable pharmacokinetics are obtained via enteral administration. If the patient is NPO or more rapid analgesia is required, IV options can be employed. Transmucosal delivery of pain medication provides rapid onset of effect.

There are important characteristics of each opioid that are important to remember. Hydromorphone has a similar pharmacokinetic profile whether given subcutaneously or intravenously. Codeine is not metabolized to its active form (morphine) by 10% to 20% of the population because they lack the necessary cytochrome P450 2D6 enzyme. Morphine should be used with caution in patients with renal insufficiency because the metabolite *morphine-6-glucoronide* can accumulate and lead to respiratory depression. A metabolite of meperidine, *normeperidine*, can accumulate and cause nervous system excitation (e.g., tremors, seizures), especially in patients with renal failure. Meperidine should also be avoided in patients using an MAOI. Transdermal fentanyl has a black box warning regarding its use in the acute setting, given that its peak effect is delayed and may occur after pain has decreased. It should be used in patients who already have tolerance to opioids at equivalent potency. Methadone should

Table 143.1 Mechanisms of pain

Pain mechanism	Character	Examples	Treatment options
Somatic	• Usually well localized • Constant • Aching, sharp, stabbing	• Laceration • Fracture • Burn • Abrasion • Localized infection or inflammation	• Heat/cold • Acetaminophen • NSAIDs • Opioids • Local anesthetics (topical or infiltrate)
Visceral	• Not well localized • Constant or intermittent • Ache, pressure, cramping, sharp	• Muscle spasm • Colic or obstruction (GI or renal) • Sickle cell crisis • Internal organ infection or inflammation	• NSAIDs • Opioids • Muscle relaxants • Local anesthetics (nerve blocks)
Neuropathic	• Localized (i.e., dermatomal) radiating, can also be diffuse • Burning, tingling, electric shock, lancinating	• Trigeminal • Pastherpetic • Pastamputation • Peripheral neuropathy • Nerve infiltration	• Anticonvulsants • Antidepressants • NMDA receptor antagonists • Neural/neuraxial blockade

NSAIDS, nonsteroidal anti-inflammatory drugs; GI, gastrointestinal; NMDA, N-methyl-D-aspartate. (From Correll, D. (ed.) 2008. *Pain Management in Hospital Medicine: Just the Facts*, McKean Bennett, pp. 527–528. Halasyamani.)

Table 143.2 Recommended starting doses for adults over 50 kg who are opioid-naïve

Agonist	Oral	IV
Codeine	15–60 mg q 3–4 hours	N/A
Hydrocodone	5–10 mg q 3–6 hours	N/A
Tramadol	40–100 g q 4–6 hours (max 24 dose is 400 mg <75 years old, 300 mg >75 years old)	N/A
Oxycodone	50–10 mg q 3–4 hours	N/A
Morphine	10–30 mg q 3–4 hours	5–10 mg q 2–4 hours
Hydromorphone	2–6 mg q 3–4 hours	1–1.5 mg q 3–4 hours
Oxymorphone	10–20 mg q 4–6 hours	1 mg q 3–4 hours

(Adapted from Vacanti, C. et al. (eds) 2011. Postoperative acute pain management. In *Essential Clinical Anesthesia*. p. 887. Used with permission.)

not be used as a first-line agent in opioid-naïve patients because of its dose-dependent potency and the fact that it takes a few days to reach a stable plasma concentration. Table 143.2 provides recommendations for starting doses of opioids, but patients have significant variability in their responses to, and side effects from, these agents.

If a patient is having pain before the next dose of pain medication can be given, the frequency of administration should be increased, assuming the maximum dose of the drug itself or associated drugs used in combination pills (e.g., acetaminophen) is not surpassed. If pain is not adequately decreased by a given dose, it can be increased by 25% to 50%. Using a different opioid may be necessary when a patient does not respond or has become tolerant to a particular opioid.

Cross-tolerance is resistance to a drug when a patient has been exposed to a similar drug. Opioids exhibit incomplete cross-tolerance. When switching to a new opioid, therefore, the equianalgesic dose should be reduced by 25% to 75%.

Non-opioid analgesics (see Table 143.3) are effective and sometimes underutilized. Though they lack some of the side effects associated with opioids, they are not advisable in certain clinical situations. For example, *ketorolac* should not be used after surgeries where there is concern for hemostasis or in patients with active peptic ulcer disease or GI bleeding.

Central sensitization and hyperexcitability can increase the perception of postoperative pain. Therefore early and multimodal treatment of pain can decrease future perception of pain by avoiding central and peripheral sensitization. *Ketamine* decreases central sensitization and opioid tolerance via its *NMDA antagonism*. Preoperative NSAIDs, gabapentin, and pregabalin have been shown to decrease postoperative pain.

Analgesia can also be provided via epidural or spinal opioid and local anesthetic administration, intra-articular injections, intrapleural analgesia (mode of last resort), paravertebral blocks (especially for breast surgery), and peripheral nerve blockade.

IV patient-controlled analgesia (IV PCA)

PCA machines allow for individualization of demand dose (bolus the patient receives each time the machine is activated), lockout interval (the amount of time before which a patient may administer an additional demand dose), hourly limit (maximum amount of opioid allowed for a given time period), continuous infusion (especially useful in opioid-tolerant patients who are unable to take their home opioids enterally), and rescue doses (given by health care provider for breakthrough pain). Compared to nurse-administered PRN opioids, PCA is associated with increased patient satisfaction, slightly decreased pain scores, and no change in side effects, except for a higher incidence of

Table 143.3 Non-opioid analgesics

Agent	Adult dosing	Maximum dose	Comments
Acetaminophen	650–1,000 mg q 6 h PO/PR	4,000 mg	Single doses >1,000 mg do not improve analgesia
Choline magnesium trisalicylate	1,000–1,500 mg BID PO	3,000 mg	Caution in liver disease, avoid in severe liver disease
Diclofenac	50 mg BID-QID PO	200 mg	Low GI effect incidence, but possible increased renal effects; recent data suggest increased negative CV effects
Etodolac	200–400 mg q 6–8 h PO	1,000 mg	Low GI and renal effect incidence; safest NSAID in liver disease
Ibuprofen	400–600 mg q 4–6 h PO	3,000 mg	<1,500 mg QD has low risk of GI effects, possible increased renal effects, inhibits CV benefits of aspirin when given concomitantly
Ketorolac	30 mg q 6 h IV	120 mg	High risk of renal and GI complications; use no more than 5 days; 15 mg q 6 h in renal impairment, age >65 y, weight <50 kg
Naburnetone	750–1,500 mg QD or BID PO	1,500 mg	Low GI effects incidence
Naproxen	250–500 mg q 6–12 h PO	1,500 mg	Possible increased liver and renal effects, probably least negative CV effects
Celecoxib	100–200 mg QD PO	200 mg	Use 100 mg dose If possible; long-term use has increased negative CV effects

CV, cardiovascular; PO, oral; PR, rectal. (Adapted from Vacanti, C. et al. (eds) 2011. Postoperative acute pain management. In *Essential Clinical Anesthesia*. p. 886. Used with permission.)

Table 143.4 Usual PCA demand dose changes for inadequate analgesia

Opioid agonist	Demand dose increase
Morphine	0.5–1 mg
Fentanyl	5–10 μg
Hydromorphone	0.1 mg
Methadone	0.5–1 mg
Sufentanil	2 μg
Meperidine	5–10 mg

(Adapted from Vacanti, C. et al. (eds) 2011. Postoperative acute pain management. In *Essential Clinical Anesthesia*. p. 889. Used with permission.)

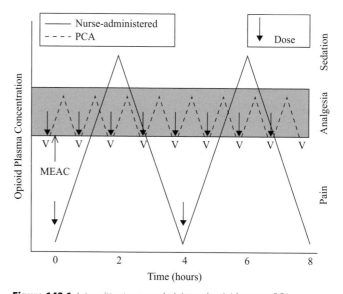

Figure 143.1 Intermittent nurse-administered opioids versus PCA-administered opioids. Shaded area: analgesic plasma concentration range. (Adapted from Vacanti et al. 2011. *Essential Clinical Anesthesia*, Cambridge University Press, p. 890.)

pruritis. There is a paucity of evidence that continuous infusions decrease pain scores, improve sleep, or lessen demand dose use. Continuous infusions should be used with caution in the elderly, persons with obstructive sleep apnea, opioid-naïve patients, and patients on other sedatives. PCA doses may need to be increased to achieve adequate pain relief (see Table 143.4).

It is theorized that PCA provides better pain control because the patient is better able to maintain the serum opioid concentrations at therapeutic levels (see Figure 143.1). The Anesthesia Patient Safety Foundation recommends constant monitoring of oxygenation and ventilation for patients on PCA.

Patient-controlled epidural analgesia (PCEA)

Just as with PCA, PCEA parameters include demand dose, lockout interval, hourly limit, continuous infusion, and rescue dose. Bupivicaine PCEA is commonly used because of its resistance to tachyphylaxis. *Lipophilic* opioids (e.g., fentanyl or sufentanil) in the epidural space likely exert their effect through systemic absorption and action. *Hydrophilic* opioids (e.g., morphine or hydromorphone) stay in the epidural space longer and thus act more directly on the spinal cord opioid receptors. Epidural adjuvants include neostigmine, clonidine, and epinephrine, though they are rarely used, given a lack of data for their effectiveness and associated side effects. There are data from several studies that PCEA analgesia is superior to that of PCA, pulmonary and cardiac complications are reduced in major vascular surgery and high-risk populations when thoracic epidurals are employed, and postoperative ileus after abdominal surgery is less frequent with PCEA. The epidural should be placed at the dermatome near the middle of the incision. Local anesthetic infusion at the thoracic level tends to spread caudally, while infusion at lumbar levels spreads in a cephalad manner.

PCEA complications include catheter dislodgement (6%), intrathecal or intravascular migration (0.2%), epidural abscess (0.05%), spinal hematoma (1:150,000 for epidurals, 1:220,000 for spinals), and permanent neurologic damage (extremely rare). Anticoagulation status, immunosuppressed states, and anatomic abnormalities can increase the aforementioned probabilities. The risk of spinal hematoma is highest not only on needle insertion, but also at the time of catheter removal. Epidural abscess risk theoretically increases the longer the catheter is in place.

Side effects of PCEA include hypotension, motor block, seizures with sufficient local anesthetic accumulation, and urinary retention (especially with lumbar epidurals). Hypotension is usually not seen unless greater than 14 dermatomes are affected. It is usually due to decreased preload as a result of venodilation from epidural-induced sympathectomy. Increasing intravascular volume can therefore mitigate this side effect. Opioid in the epidural space can cause pruritis, sedation, respiratory depression, and nausea. This pruritis is due to central mu-receptor activation, not histamine release. Nalbuphine, rather than an antihistamine, is a recommended treatment. Respiratory depression and sedation can be treated with naloxone. Nausea can be treated with metoclopramide, nalbuphine, or naloxone. Side effects can be mitigated by removing the opioid from the epidural solution. Neuraxial morphine is associated with reactivation of varicella zoster virus, not herpes simplex virus. In general, opioids should not be concomitantly administered via epidural and IV routes. Removing opioid from a neuraxial infusion and giving it intravenously is referred to as "splitting the epidural."

Troubleshooting an epidural includes assessing dermatome coverage using pin prick or cold stimulus. Pulling the catheter out in 0.5–1 cm increments can improve a one-sided block. If the block is not covering sufficient dermatomes, the rate or concentration can be increased (total milligrams of local anesthetic is what determines how many dermatomes are covered). The concentration of local anesthetic can be increased if the block is not sufficiently dense (though one should simultaneously decrease the rate if one does not want additional spread). The differential for complete motor block includes epidural hematoma or excessive local anesthetic blockade. Turning off the epidural and monitoring for return of motor function allows for differentiation between the two.

Questions

1. A 67-year-old lady presents to the emergency room with abdominal pain from a bowel obstruction. The pain is severe, dull, and achy. She points to her entire abdomen when asked where the pain is. What kind of pain is this patient likely experiencing, and which is an appropriate treatment modality?
   a. somatic pain: opioid
   b. neuropathic pain: duloxetine
   c. visceral pain: opioid
   d. somatic pain: nerve blockade
   e. visceral pain: anticonvulsant

2. You placed a thoracic epidural for a patient who received an extrapleural pneumonectomy for lung cancer who was otherwise healthy. The primary team calls you stating the patient's blood pressure is 92/60, which is greater than 20% below her baseline. Assuming the hypotension is related to the epidural, what is the appropriate next step in management?
   a. turn off the epidural for eight hours and reassess
   b. decrease the rate by 50%
   c. give the patient a bolus of IV fluid
   d. start low-dose vasopressin

3. Which of the following is TRUE of ketorolac?
   a. It is safe to use in patients with renal failure.
   b. Its mechanism of action includes NMDA antagonism.
   c. It is not optimal for patients with poor hemostasis.
   d. It is effective for treating somatic pain but not visceral pain.

4. A 54-year-old gentleman is status post exploratory laparotomy. He received an epidural preoperatively but has significant pain associated with his incision in the PACU. The level is checked and found to not cover the upper part of the incision. Which changes would increase the spread of the block?
   a. increase the concentration of the local anesthetic
   b. decrease the concentration of the local anesthetic
   c. increase the infusion rate
   d. split the epidural
   e. (a) and (c)
   f. (a) and (d)
   g. all of the above

Answers

1. c. Dull, poorly localized pain suggests visceral pain. NSAIDs, opioids, local anesthetics, and muscle relaxants can decrease this type of pain.
2. c. Hypotension due to an epidural is often because sympathectomy results in vasodilation, which decreases preload. A fluid bolus can mitigate these effects.
3. c. Ketorolac should be used with care or not at all in patients with poor hemostasis, peptic ulcer disease, GI bleeding, and decreased renal function.
4. e. The total milligrams of local anesthetic is what determines how many dermatomes are covered. Increasing the concentration and increasing the rate will provide a higher dose of local anesthetic.

Further reading

Vacanti, C. A., Sikka, P. K., Urman, R. U., Dershwitz, M., and Segal, B. S. (eds) (2011). Chapter 144. Postoperative acute pain management. In *Essential Clinical Anesthesia*. New York, NY: Cambridge University Press, pp. 885–893.

Miller, R. (2011). Chapter 40: Perioperative pain management. In *Basics of Anesthesia*, 6th edn. Philadelphia: Elsevier.

Urman, R., et. al. (2009). Acute pain management. In *Pocket Anesthesia*. Philadelphia: Lipincott Williams & Wilkins.

Hurley, R. W. et al. (2006). The analgesic effects of perioperative gabapentin on postoperative pain: a meta-analysis. *Regional Anesthesia and Pain Medicine* 31, 237–247.

Elia, N. et al. (2005). Does multimodal analgesia with acetaminophen, nonsteroidal antiinflammtory drugs, or selective cyclooxygenase-2 inhibitors and patient-controlled analgesia morphine offer advantages over morphine alone? Meta-analyses or randomized trials. *Anesthesiology* 103, 1296–1304.

Keywords

Chronic pain management
Pharmacologic management
Opioid analgesics
Adjunctive analgesics
Psychological approaches to chronic pain management
Behavioral therapy
Rehabilitation
Interventional pain management

As with the treatment of other chronic illnesses, chronic pain management is usually complex given the biological, psychological, and social influences on the development and persistence of chronic pain. A multimodality approach addressing these complex interrelated factors leads to the best possible outcome.

A treatment plan for a patient with chronic pain should consider each of the following components often offered concurrently:

- *pharmacologic management*
- *interventional pain management*
- evaluation and management of pain-related psychological symptoms along with *behavioral therapy*
- *rehabilitation* directed toward improving the patient's function and capacity to be physically active

Different classes of medications are often used in treatment of pain. An individualized treatment plan utilizing combinations of medications can lead to both synergistic analgesic effects as well as a reduction in individual medication side effects, due to dose reduction.

Nociceptive pain conditions typically respond to primary treatment with opioid or non-opioid drugs such as NSAIDs. Adjunctive medications can contribute to pain and symptom control, including anticonvulsants, antidepressants, N-methyl-D-aspartate (NMDA) antagonists, muscle relaxants, or topical medications. For neuropathic pain conditions, it is these medications that often serve as the primary medications

for pain control, and the opioid and non-opioid medications (such as NSAIDs) work as adjuvants.

Opioid analgesics are μ receptor agonists, which are the oldest class of medication used in management of both cancer and noncancer pain. Tolerance and dependence are common among all opioid medications. Analgesia due to tolerance may be improved by using different opioids in the same patient, a concept known as "opioid rotation."

Acetaminophen is a common analgesic drug that is now thought to work on a recently identified cyclooxygenase (COX)-3 receptor.

Typical side effects of opioid use may include: nausea, sedation, euphoria, constipation, loss of libido, low testosterone levels, osteoporosis, loss of appetite, dizziness, urinary retention, respiratory depression, and myoclonus.

Antidepressants are used in chronic pain management both to reduce pain and depression. For some patients, their use is limited by debilitating side effects, including: cardiovascular effects (hypotension and arrhythmias), sedation, anticholinergic effects, weight change, psychiatric complications (suicidal ideas, mania, and bipolar disorders) and withdrawal syndrome.

Anticonvulsants that are used for chronic pain management may also lead to intolerable side effects. Carbamazepine may produce bone marrow depression, phenytoin may cause gum hyperplasia, hirsutism, and ataxia at high doses, valproic acid may produce hepatotoxicity, and gabapentin may cause weight gain and sedation.

Muscle relaxants are a varied group of medications that have different types. The γ-aminobutyric acid (GABA) agonists and other CNS depressants have been shown to have analgesic effects in treating both chronic and acute pain. Benzodiazepines and carisoprodol have long-term dependency liability. Sedation is a common side effect with most of the muscle relaxants. Clonidine and tizanidine are α2-agonist drugs that act via an independent analgesic mechanism and by potentiating the effects of opioids. Clonidine is most commonly used intrathecally along with opioids.

Psychological approach: coexisting psychological problems, including depression, anxiety, personality disorders, anger,

---

Essential Clinical Anesthesia Review: Keywords, Questions and Answers for the Boards, ed. Linda S. Aglio, Robert W. Lekowski, and Richard D. Urman. Published by Cambridge University Press. © Cambridge University Press 2015.

Table 144.1 Behavioral theraphy for chronic pain

Therapy	Description
Hypnosis and visualization	The patient is taught to visualize relaxing mental images, such as a secluded beach or a peaceful meadow. This helps to decrease anxiety, and facilitates deep relaxation.
Guided imagery	Directed visualization focuses on specific psychological issues using pain-decreasing images.
Biofeedback	Relaxation technique measures a physiologic phenomenon, such as muscle tension, and provides audible or visual feedback indicating a state of relaxation.
Cognitive–behavioral therapy	This teaches various techniques, such as distraction training, cognitive restructuring, role-playing, or mental imagery.
Group therapies	When well planned and with appropriate patient dynamics, group therapy is helpful. The interaction is planned to share important breakthroughs in insight, discuss progress with treatment, and different strategies for overcoming everyday obstacles to improvement.
Family therapy	Patients and their families often feel angry at each other. The family can be a significant stressor but is an important source of support that is needed for progress. This approach attempts to bring insight into how to provide support without enabling continued disability.

(Vacanti C. et al., (eds) 2011. *Essential Clinical Anesthesia*, 1st edn. Cambridge University Press, Chapter 145 Table 8.)

and history of abuse are commonly associated with chronic pain.

Rehabilitation and physical therapy techniques are important in the treatment of chronic pain, along with pharmacologic and interventional approaches and psychological therapy. Patients are shown techniques to improve their strength and functionality to minimize the effect that pain has upon their level of activity. Patients are encouraged to maintain their strength and normal body mechanics, using rehabilitative techniques to minimize the level of pain. Given that physical therapy may be difficult in this patient population, maintaining motivation is crucial to a better outcome.

Questions

1. Which of the following statements is TRUE regarding pharmacologic management of chronic pain?

   a. Prescribing medications from different classes usually results in higher doses of individual medications being prescribed and increased side effects from individual medications.

   b. In neuropathic pain syndromes anticonvulsants, antidepressants or N-methyl-D-aspartate (NMDA) antagonist drugs are usually recommended as primary analgesic medications.

   c. Initial management of nociceptive pain is most often done by prescribing long-acting opioid drugs.

   d. For breakthrough pain, it is recommended to dose short-acting opioids at 50% of the daily total opioid dose.

2. What is the most appropriate management plan for a patient with a high risk of opioid overuse?

   a. Do not prescribe opioids under any conditions.

   b. Avoid the use of non-opioid pharmaceutical agents that enhance opioid analgesia and reduce side effects.

   c. Use treatment contracts for controlled substances and monitor effects of medication.

   d. Only use opioids if a patient has a nociceptive and not neuropathic pain condition.

3. "Relaxation techniques measuring a physiologic phenomenon such as muscle tension and providing visual feedback" defines which of the following types of behavioral therapy?

   a. hypnosis and visualization

   b. family therapy

   c. guided imagery

   d. biofeedback

Answers

1. b. Prescribing medications from different classes usually results in lower doses of individual medications being prescribed and reduces side effects from individual medications. In neuropathic pain syndromes anticonvulsants, antidepressants, or N-methyl-D-aspartate (NMDA) antagonist drugs are usually recommended as adjuvants. Initial management of nociceptive pain is most often done by prescribing short-acting opioid drugs.

2. c. Using treatment contracts for controlled substances and monitoring effects of medication are appropriate managements for patients with a high risk of opioid overuse.

3. d. Relaxation techniques measuring a physiologic phenomenon such as muscle tension and providing visual feedback is part of biofeedback treatment modality.

Further reading

Vacanti, C. A., Sikka, P. K., Urman, R. U., Dershwitz, M., and Segal, B. S. (eds) (2011). *Essential Clinical Anesthesia*. New York, NY: Cambridge University Press, Chapter 145.

Ross, E. L. (2003). *Pain Management. Hot Topics.* 1st edn. Philadelphia: Hanley & Belfus.

Chapter

145

Psychological evaluation and management of patients with chronic pain

Cyrus Ahmadi Yazdi and Srdjan S. Nedeljkovic

Keywords

Visual analogue scale (VAS)
Verbal rating scale
Psychological interventions
Cognitive–behavioral therapy
Group therapy
Vocational rehabilitation

The International Association for the Study of Pain defines pain as an "unpleasant sensory and emotional experience associated with actual or potential tissue damage or described in the terms of such damage." This definition recognizes that pain is a multifactorial phenomenon that includes a behavioral and a sensory component.

Patients who experience chronic pain frequently report depression, anxiety, irritability, sexual dysfunction, and decreased energy.

In evaluating a patient with chronic pain, it is important to conduct a psychological assessment that includes a description of pain intensity, functional capacity, mood and personality, coping and pain beliefs, and medication usage.

Each of the following categories should be assessed during the patient's assessment: (1) pain description; (2) aggravating factors; (3) daily activity level; (4) relevant medical history; (5) past and current treatment; (6) education and employment history; (7) compensation history; (8) history of drug or alcohol abuse; (9) history of psychiatric disturbance; (10) current emotional status.

Methods of measuring pain intensity include obtaining a quantitative numeric pain rating, administering the *visual analogue scale* (VAS), and utilizing a qualitative verbal rating scale.

In obtaining the VAS, the patient who is experiencing pain is instructed to place a mark at the point on a 10 cm line that best indicates their present pain severity. Scores are obtained by measuring the distance from the end labeled "no pain" to the mark provided by the patient. Disadvantages of using this method include that it is time consuming to score and that it has questionable validity for use in older patients.

The verbal rating scale for pain consists of words that are chosen by patients to describe their severity of pain from "no pain" to "excruciating pain." Using a verbal rating scale not only measures pain intensity but also assesses sensory and reactive dimensions of the pain experience. Verbal rating scales for pain can be used to measure the descriptive nature of pain; the patient chooses words from a list that best describes the pain experience (e.g., piercing, stabbing, shooting, burning, throbbing).

The McGill Pain Questionnaire (MPQ) is a frequently used comprehensive questionnaire that includes 20 subclasses of descriptors as well as a numeric pain intensity scale and dermatomal pain drawing. The MPQ exists in both a long and short format.

A number of self-reported measures can be used to assess activity level and function, and serve as an overall measure of patient health: the Sickness Impact Profile (SIP), the Short Form 36 Health Survey (SF-36), the Multidimensional Pain Inventory (MPI), and the Pain Disability Index. These devices should be used in conjunction with self-monitoring assessment techniques.

In patients who have experienced injuries that lead to decreased cognition (such as head injury) or in patients who have other causes of decreased cognitive functioning, *neuropsychological assessment* may be indicated.

The goals of *psychological interventions* for pain management are:

- reduction of pain intensity
- increased physical functioning
- control of medication use
- improvement in sleep, mood, and interaction with others
- return to work or to normal daily activities

Therapy with a *cognitive–behavioral* orientation is designed to help patients gain control of the emotional reaction associated with chronic pain. Cognitive–behavioral therapy (CBT) has three major objectives. First, CBT helps patient change their view of their problem from overwhelming to manageable. Second, CBT can help motivate patients that treatment is relevant to their problem and they need to be actively involved

Essential Clinical Anesthesia Review: Keywords, Questions and Answers for the Boards, ed. Linda S. Aglio, Robert W. Lekowski, and Richard D. Urman. Published by Cambridge University Press. © Cambridge University Press 2015.

in their own treatment and rehabilitation. Third, CBT is used to teach patients to monitor maladaptive thoughts and substitute them for positive thoughts that will aid in their management and rehabilitation.

Group therapy provides an opportunity for patients and clinicians to discuss concerns or problems that patients have in common.

The goal of *vocational rehabilitation* is a return to work or retraining to other forms of employment. Vocational rehabilitation counselors are specialists in the assessment of aptitudes and interests, transferable skills, skill training, and job readiness.

Chronic pain involves complex interaction of anatomic, physiologic, and psychological factors. Successful intervention requires the coordinated efforts of a treatment team with expertise in a variety of therapeutic disciplines.

Questions

1. Which of following "*pain rating scales*" is most appropriate to assess the sensory and reactive dimensions of a patient's pain experience?
   a. numeric pain rating
   b. visual analogue scale
   c. verbal rating scale
   d. faces scale

2. Which of the following outcomes can be expected when behavioral interventions are used to manage chronic pain?
   a. no change in physical functioning
   b. improved neuropsychological assessment
   c. improvement in sleep, mood, and interaction with others
   d. increased use of analgesic medications

3. Which of the following principles is used as part of cognitive–behavioral therapy for chronic pain?
   a. You will most likely be "cured."
   b. Your pain will likely remain chronic and severe.
   c. You need to stay out of work for those times when you have a flare up of pain.
   d. Rarely does pain intensity remain exactly the same over time.

4. Which of the following is considered as an objective of behavioral therapy?
   a. To educate a patient that their problem is overwhelming and difficult to manage.
   b. To help convince patient that treatments provided by health professionals are most important in their treatment and rehabilitation.
   c. To discuss the pharmacologic basis of medication use and their side effects.
   d. To teach patients to monitor maladaptive thoughts and substitute positive thoughts.

Answers

1. c. The verbal rating scale not only measures pain intensity but also assesses sensory and reactive dimensions of the pain experience.
2. c. Improvement in sleep, mood, and interaction with others are usually seen after behavioral interventions in chronic pain patients.
3. d. Therapy with a cognitive–behavioral orientation is designed to help patients gain control of the emotional reaction associated with chronic pain. Patients are taught the fact that pain intensity might vary over time.
4. d. One of the objectives of behavioral therapy is to teach patients to monitor maladaptive thoughts and substitute positive thoughts.

Further reading

Vacanti, C. A., Sikka, P. K., Urman, R. U., Dershwitz, M., and Segal, B. S. (eds) (2011). *Essential Clinical Anesthesia*. New York, NY: Cambridge University Press, Chapter 146.

Interventional pain management I
Epidural, sympathetic, and neural blockade procedures

Cyrus Ahmadi Yazdi and Srdjan S. Nedeljkovic

Keywords

Epidural steroid injection (ESI)
Transforaminal and paravertebral nerve blocks
Interlaminar ESI
Stellate ganglion block
Celiac plexus block
Cervical plexus block
Radicular pain
Superior hypogastric plexus block
Trigeminal nerve block

Patients who undergo interventional injection procedures for the treatment of pain, such as single-shot *epidural steroid injections* (ESIs), sympathetic ganglion or plexus blocks, or other nerve blocks, should be instructed about the potential risks and benefits for the procedure. Fasting is generally not necessary for routine injection therapies unless necessitated by the type of anesthesia provided for the procedure. For neuraxial procedures, it is important to assess the patient's anticoagulation status. If there are no medical contraindications, anticoagulation should be temporarily held according to established guidelines.

Procedures typically include an injection of local anesthetics and glucocorticoids. The most commonly used local anesthetics are bupivacaine 0.25% to 0.5% and lidocaine 0.5% to 2%. Bupivacaine should not be mixed with bicarbonate because of the risk of precipitation. Glucocorticoids reduce inflammation by stabilizing leukocytes, inhibiting macrophages, decreasing edema, and reducing scar formation. The most commonly used steroids are long-acting depot formulations such as triamcinolone or methylprednisolone. Glucocorticoids administered for pain treatment may have systemic effects, including fluid retention and hyperglycemia. However, the degree of systemic side effects from steroids given for neuraxial pain procedures is not well understood.

Neurolytic substances like alcohol 50% to 95% and phenol 6% to 10% may be appropriate for use in cancer pain. Phenol acts as an anesthetic at lower concentrations, is more viscous, and is considered less painful on injection than is alcohol.

Fluoroscopy may be used to enhance the accuracy of needle placement for certain procedures. Contrast dye may be injected under live fluoroscopy to visualize potential intravascular injections. Just aspirating and looking for blood return in a needle has an up to 50% false-negative rate.

Radicular pain is a neuropathic pain presentation in the distribution of spinal nerve roots, whereas radiculopathy is defined as a conduction block in the spinal nerve with findings of neurologic deficit. Radiculitis is defined as inflammation of the nerve root. Varieties of ESI include interlaminar, transforaminal, selective spinal nerve block, and caudal. Most evidence-based reviews show that ESI provides short-term benefit for pain radiating in the distribution of spinal nerves. Spinal stenosis symptoms and neurogenic claudication may also be treated with ESI. Interlaminar and transforaminal ESI are commonly used to treat cervical and lumbar radicular pain.

Interlaminar ESIs are performed in the cervical and lumbar spine using a loss of resistance (LOR) technique via a Tuohy needle. The patient is placed typically prone on a fluoroscopy table. As the tip of the Touhy needle nears the ligamentum flavum, lateral imaging is used to check the depth of the needle placement. Contrast may be used to assess epidural flow of injectate. Typically, a mixture of steroid and local anesthetic is injected upon proper localization of the needle. This technique may be difficult to perform if the patient has had a laminectomy at that level due to disruptions in the ligamentum flavum, scar tissue, and adherence of the dura. In such cases, transforaminal or caudal approaches for epidural steroid injection are a reasonable alternative.

Transforaminal ESIs are more commonly performed in lumbar spine, as there has been concern over complications from cervical transforaminal injections. The patient is placed prone and an oblique view is used to identify the pedicle over the target nerve. The tip of a spinal needle is directed to a position under the pedicle within the zone outlined by the inferior border of the pedicle, the spinal nerve itself, and the lateral border of vertebral body. Non-ionic contrast dye is used to confirm epidural flow. Typical injections consist of a combination of local anesthetics and steroids.

Essential Clinical Anesthesia Review: Keywords, Questions and Answers for the Boards, ed. Linda S. Aglio, Robert W. Lekowski, and Richard D. Urman. Published by Cambridge University Press. © Cambridge University Press 2015.

Sympathetic blocks have utility in the evaluation and treatment of pain that may be at least partially mediated by the sympathetic nervous system. The cervical sympathetic ganglia include the superior, middle, and inferior. The inferior is often fused with the first thoracic ganglion (82%) and is called the stellate ganglion. Sympathetic innervation of abdominal viscera from the distal third of the esophagus to the transverse colon, liver, biliary tract, and adrenal glands is supplied by celiac plexus. The preganglionic sympathetic nerves pass through the paravertebral sympathetic chain without synapsing. The gastrointestinal tract from the descending colon to the rectum, as well as the urogenital system, is supplied via the superior hypogastric plexus.

One of the methods to determine the success of a lumbar or cervical/stellate sympathetic block is temperature change in a peripheral extremity. After sympathetic block, the skin temperature should be increased by 1 to 2°C. Another method involves testing the galvanic skin response or sweat testing.

The *stellate ganglion* lies anterior to the neck of the first rib, anteromedial to the vertebral artery, and medial to the common carotid artery and jugular vein. The sympathetic innervation to the head and neck arises from preganglionic fibers at T1 and T2 and travels to the ganglia. The sympathetic innervation to the upper extremities arises from the preganglionic fibers T2 to T8.

Sympathetic innervation to the abdominal viscera is composed of preganglionic axons from the T5 through to the T12 level that leave the spinal cord, pass through the sympathetic chain, and synapse at distal sites. A network of ganglia, including the celiac ganglia, superior mesenteric ganglia, and the aortocorenal ganglia, compose the celiac plexus.

Celiac plexus blockade is indicated for the treatment and diagnosis of pain from visceral structures innervated by the celiac plexus. These structures include the pancreas, liver, gallbladder, omentum, and mesentery and alimentary tract from the stomach to the transverse colon. Neurolytic celiac plexus block is indicated as a palliative measure in upper abdominal malignancies such as pancreatic carcinoma. Celiac plexus neurolysis often results in diarrhea due to unopposed parasympathetic activity. It may, however, reduce nausea and vomiting symptoms in these patients.

Superior hypogastric plexus block is performed for the treatment of pain from pelvic viscera and for pain reduction from pelvic malignancies.

The ganglion impar block can be performed with local anesthetic and steroid for nonmalignant pain conditions, such as coccygodynia, or for the treatment of cancer-related perirectal pain from tumor involvement.

Peripheral nerve blocks that may be performed for chronic pain include trigeminal nerve block, cervical plexus block, and paravertebral nerve blocks.

Trigeminal nerve block can help reduce pain caused by trigeminal neuralgia. With the patient supine, a 22-gauge needle may be inserted 2.5 cm lateral to the corner of the mouth and directed to the pupil of the eye, into the foramen

Table 146.1 Stellate block indications

Pain	Vascular	Other
Complex regional pain syndrome type I or II	Vasospasm	Hyperhidrosis
Postherpetic neuralgia	Occlusive and embolic vascular disease	Ménière disease
Phantom limb pain	Scleroderma	Vascular headaches
Paget's disease		
Neoplasm of upper extremity		
Postradiation neuritis		
Intractable angina pectoris		

(Vacanti C. et al. (eds) 2011. *Essential Clinical Anesthesia*, 1st edn. Cambridge University Press, Chapter 147 Table 1–2.)

Table 146.2 Signs of a successful stellate ganglion block

Horner syndrome (ipsilateral)
Nasal congestion
Venodilation of the ipsilateral limb
Increase in temperature of the limb by at least 1–2°C

ovale. Alternately, the peripheral branches of the trigeminal nerve may be blocked, including the supraorbital nerve (V1), the maxillary nerve (V2), and the mandibular nerve (V3).

Cervical plexus injections may be used to provide analgesia to the head and neck region. Either the superficial or the deep cervical plexus can be blocked. A deep cervical plexus block can provide anesthesia for surgeries such as carotid endaterectomy and thyroid surgeries. These blocks may have a role in pain management of the upper extremity, including postoperative pain, pain from trauma, complex regional pain syndrome (CRPS), cancer-related pain, and neuropathic pain.

Paravertebral nerve block is an injection of local anesthetic adjacent to the vertebral body close to the exit of the spinal nerves from the intervertebral foramina. Indications include postoperative and surgical analgesia in breast, thoracic, renal, and abdominal surgeries.

Questions

1. Regarding epidural steroid injections (ESI) which of the following is TRUE?

   a. Using fluoroscopy is necessary for all injections.
   b. Interlaminar ESI is the preferred approach when a laminectomy has been performed at that level.
   c. The zone of proper placement of a needle for a transforaminal ESI is outlined by the inferior border of the pedicle, the spinal nerve, and the lateral border of the vertebral body.

d. For cervical interlaminar ESIs, a patient is typically placed in a lateral position.

2. Which of the following is considered as a sign of successful stellate ganglion block?
   a. ipsilateral Horner syndrome
   b. rhinnorhea
   c. vasoconstriction of the ipsilateral limb
   d. decrease in temperature of the ipsilateral limb by at least 1°C

3. Which of the following typically occurs following a celiac plexus block?
   a. constipation
   b. abdominal cramp
   c. diarrhea
   d. ileus

Answers

1. c. The zone of proper placement of a needle for a transforaminal ESI is outlined by the inferior border of the pedicle, the spinal nerve, and the lateral border of the vertebral body.
2. a. Ipsilateral Horner syndrome, nasal congestion, venodilation of ipsilateral limb, and increase in the temperature of the limb by at least 1 to 2°C are considered a sign of successful stellate ganglion block.
3. c. Celiac plexus neurolysis often results in diarrhea due to unopposed parasympathetic activity. It may, however, reduce nausea and vomiting symptoms in these patients.

Further reading

Vacanti, C. A., Sikka, P. K., Urman, R. U., Dershwitz, M., and Segal, B. S. (eds) (2011). *Essential Clinical Anesthesia*. New York, NY: Cambridge University Press, Chapter 147.

Section 27 Pain management

Chapter 147

Interventional pain management II
Implantable and other invasive therapies

Cyrus Ahmadi Yazdi and Srdjan S. Nedeljkovic

Keywords

Medial branch nerve block (MBB)
Radiofrequency lesioning (RFL)
Intra-articular facet injection
Vertebral body augmentation
Intrathecal infusion pump placement
Electrical stimulation techniques
Peripheral nerve stimulator

Medial branch nerve blocks (MBBs) also known as zygoapophyseal or facet joint injections are performed using local anesthetic, sometimes in combination with steroid, to the painful facet joints. If the patient experiences pain relief, they may be considered for *radiofrequency lesioning* (RFL) of the medial branch nerves. RFL is intended to result in longer lasting pain relief.

Intra-articular facet injections involve the deposition of medication inside the articular capsule of the facet joint. Potential side effects of performing these injections include those from the repetitive use of corticosteroids.

The sacroiliac (SI) joint may be a significant cause of low back pain, especially in elderly populations. Sacroiliac pain may be difficult to differentiate from other causes of low back pain, but tenderness to palpation over the SI joint may be the single most accurate examination to evaluate for this condition.

RFL is typically used for the treatment of axial back pain produced by facet arthropathy and SI joint arthropathy. After a positive diagnostic block (usually considered to be 50% pain relief), RFL is a reasonable option for treatment. This therapeutic procedure may provide pain relief for up to six months.

Indications for *vertebral body augmentation* therapy are recent compression fractures secondary to osteoporosis or malignancies. Osteoporosis is more common in women, with a 4:1 ratio of female to male prevalence. Patients often present with symptoms of acute back pain immediately after the fracture. Initially, patients are typically treated with systemic analgesics. If noninterventional treatment is inadequate, and if the patient experiences loss of function or is unable to tolerate

oral analgesics, then vertebral augmentation therapy may be recommended.

Contraindications for therapy include allergies, severe spinal stenosis, or retropulsion of fracture fragments. Two methods of augmentation are used: kyphoplasty or vertebroplasty. Kyphoplasty involves the use of a balloon to create a cavity in the collapsed vertebral body for cement injection. Vertebroplasty involves giving a cement injection directly into the fractured vertebral body without creating a cavity. Extravasation of cement outside of the vertebral body is thought to be less likely in kyphoplasty.

Discography is a procedure performed for the diagnosis of a suspected painful disc. Discography is typically used for patients with multiple abnormally appearing discs on an imaging study to determine which disc is causing painful symptoms. The procedure can also help identify whether a degenerated disc is the source of pain in patients who have already had lumbar spine surgery. A small amount of contrast is injected into a suspect disc to determine disc integrity and to evaluate whether pain provocation occurs.

Implantable therapies such as *intrathecal or epidural pumps* and catheters and spinal cord stimulation have long held a role in the treatment of the most refractory pain states. As with other interventional pain procedures, proper patient selection is important in determining who is an appropriate candidate for these types of therapies.

There are two types of implantable epidural catheter systems. One method involves the use of a post-a-cath subcutaneous reservoir system and the other utilizes a Hickman catheter style system. These techniques are typically used when patients need short- to medium-term analgesia. In both systems, a catheter is tunneled subcutaneously from the epidural space to a distance from the epidural insertion site.

A subcutaneous reservoir or port-a-cath system consists of two parts: (1) a subcutaneous port attached to (2) a catheter that either accesses the epidural or intrathecal space. A port-a-cath system is indicated for intermediate-length therapy especially for cancer patients with less than three months of life expectancy. Epidural port-a-cath systems may also be used to

Essential Clinical Anesthesia Review: Keywords, Questions and Answers for the Boards, ed. Linda S. Aglio, Robert W. Lekowski, and Richard D. Urman. Published by Cambridge University Press. © Cambridge University Press 2015.

treat patients with complex regional pain syndrome (CRPS). The port-a-cath reservoir can be accessed percutaneously for intermittent or continuous infusions of analgesics.

There are two common types of *intrathecal infusion pumps*: fixed flow systems and programmable pumps. Indications for implanting an intrathecal pump include refractory pain due to malignancy or chronic pain from nonmalignant causes in a patient who has not benefited from medications, other non-invasive approaches, and is not a candidate for primary surgical intervention. Implantation of an intrathecal pump also involves the surgical creation of a pocket in the anterior abdominal wall to hold the pump reservoir.

Electrical stimulation techniques of the central nervous system (CNS) are typically indicated for analgesia for patients who have neuropathic pain conditions. Epidural placement of multielectrode arrays can be effective for a variety of other conditions in addition to neuropathic pain, including chronic anginal pain and pain from vascular insufficiency. Deep brain stimulation is less commonly used as an analgesic technique, but it may be effective to treat certain central pain syndromes and symptoms of Parkinson's disease. In spinal cord stimulation, electrodes must be placed in the posterior epidural space adjacent to the level of the spinal cord that is intended for stimulation. Intrathecal or ventral epidural placement of electrodes may cause unwanted motor stimulations that can be painful.

Peripheral nerve stimulator placement requires visualization of the affected nerve. Either a percutaneous approach using a needle or a direct approach using a cut down to the nerve to allow placement of a lead is used. For epidural stimulation, insertion of the electrode is similar to insertion of an epidural catheter. Two common types of pulse generators exist: an external system that relies on radiofrequency current for providing power to the system or a battery-operated implantable pulse generator (IPG).

Questions

1. Regarding vertebral body augmentation, which of the following statements is TRUE?

   a. It is the first step in the management of vertebral compression fractures.
   b. It is indicated when a patient has severe spinal stenosis.
   c. Extravasation of cement is less common in kyphoplasty than in vertebroplasty.
   d. Recent studies have shown significant long-term improvement after vertebroplasty compared to a sham procedure.

2. Which of the following statements is TRUE regarding interventional pain management techniques?

   a. RFL of the facet joints may provide pain relief for six months or longer.
   b. Radiographic studies of the SI joint predict the results from SI joint injections.
   c. Port-a-cath implantable systems are indicated for long-term use of more than one year.
   d. Placement of spinal cord stimulation electrodes is usually performed under general anesthesia.

Answers

1. c. Vertebroplasty involves giving a cement injection directly into the fractured vertebral body without creating a cavity. Extravasation of cement outside the vertebral body is thought to be less likely in kyphoplasty.

2. a. RFL is typically used for the treatment of axial back pain produced by facet arthropathy and SI joint arthropathy. After a positive diagnostic block (usually considered to be 50% pain relief), RFL is a reasonable option for treatment. This therapeutic procedure may provide pain relief for up to six months.

Further reading

Vacanti, C. A., Sikka, P. K., Urman, R. U., Dershwitz, M., and Segal, B. S. (eds) (2011). *Essential Clinical Anesthesia*. New York, NY: Cambridge University Press, Chapter 148.

Chapter

148

Complications associated with interventions in pain medicine

J. Tasker Gundy and Elizabeth M. Rickerson

Serious complications resulting from common interventional techniques in pain medicine are *rare*. Nevertheless, there are potential complications attendant to any interventional treatment for acute or chronic pain conditions. Avoiding complication requires:

- detailed knowledge of the anatomy surrounding target structures
- meticulous use of radiographic guidance whenever possible (fluoroscopy has greatly increased the precision and safety of many techniques)
- adherence to published guidelines
- understanding of the technical aspects of procedures that were devised to minimize risk to target structures

An organized, thoughtful history and physical examination are essential prior to any planned intervention, in order to identify patient factors that may increase the risk for complications (e.g., diabetes, immunosuppression, coagulopathy, occult infection).

It is likewise essential that patients receive informed consent regarding common side effects and possible complications prior to any intervention, along with instruction to promptly report any neurologic changes, new or increasing pain, headache, or fever following the procedure. *Prompt recognition and treatment of complications will result in less catastrophic outcomes.*

Complications associated with steroid injections (epidural, facet, SI joint, etc.)

- **Neurotoxicity.** Despite widespread use, steroid preparations are not labeled for epidural administration by

the FDA; unintended intrathecal injection can result in *arachnoiditis* (inflammation of the leptomeninges and adjacent neural structures) or *cauda equina syndrome* (compression or injury to the nerve roots below the conus medullaris).

- **Neurologic injury.** Needle placement for injection risks direct mechanical *nerve injury*, including potential injury to the spinal cord itself during epidural injection. Factors increasing the risk of direct injury to the spinal cord include injecting at the high lumbar level or above, and performing injections under heavy sedation or general anesthesia, as patients are then unable to report symptoms such as parasthesias. *In ASA Closed Claims analysis, nerve injury was the most common complication associated with invasive pain management procedures.*

- **Vascular injury.** Unintended vascular injection of particulate steroid is possible with any approach, and is of particular concern during transforaminal injection. While intravenous penetration is innocuous, intra-arterial injection can be catastrophic, potentially resulting in infarction of the brain or spinal cord (e.g., anterior cord infarction from accidental injection into a low-lying artery of Adamkiewicz during lumbar transforaminal injection).

- **Bleeding complications.** Due to the risk of epidural or subdural bleeding, epidural steroid injections should be avoided in patients receiving systemic anticoagulation or antiplatelet agents (adhere to ASRA guidelines). NSAIDS and aspirin do not appear to increase the risk of epidural hematoma formation. Suspicion of epidural hematoma should prompt immediate MRI and surgical consultation (see Chapter 57, Epidural anesthesia), as compression of neural structures can result in paraplegia or quadriplegia if untreated.

- **Infectious complications.** With adherence to proper sterile technique, including use of an iodine-based skin preparation, infectious complications (tissue infection, meningitis, osteomyelitis, epidural abscess) are rare. Neuraxial infections, especially abscesses, can have severe neurologic consequences; if confirmed by MRI, an epidural

Essential Clinical Anesthesia Review: Keywords, Questions and Answers for the Boards, ed. Linda S. Aglio, Robert W. Lekowski, and Richard D. Urman. Published by Cambridge University Press. © Cambridge University Press 2015.

abscess will require immediate treatment with systemic antibiotics and surgical drainage.

- **Complications from steroids.** Sequelae of chronic oral steroid therapy may also emerge with continued exogenous steroid injection, including hypercortisolism, adrenal suppression, fluid retention/CHF, insulin resistance, weight gain, and Cushingoid features.

Complications associated with sympathetic or neurolytic nerve blocks also fall into the categories mentioned above (neurotoxicity, neurologic injury, vascular injury, and bleeding or infectious complications). Complications and side effects unique to the anatomic orientation of two blocks are worth noting.

Stellate ganglion block (SGB): complications

This sympathetic block is used for painful conditions of the head, neck, and upper extremity. *Side effects of SGB are actually signs of successful block, including Horner's syndrome, nasal congestion, and flushing/increased temperature of the ipsilateral limb.* Several complications owing to the location of the target ganglion (C6–7) are also possible. *Unintended block of the recurrent laryngeal nerve* can result in hoarseness/stridor, while the potential for *phrenic nerve block* discourages bilateral blockade. Intrathecal injection of local anesthetic at this level results in *high spinal* and the need for intubation/assisted ventilation. *Pneumothorax* can result from damage to the pleural dome above the first rib. Finally, there is a risk for occult bleeding in this highly vascular area, which may result in compressive *paratracheal hematoma*.

Celicac plexus block (CPB): complications

For patients with abdominal malignancies (especially pancreatic cancer), palliative neurolytic CPB is often performed. Once neurolysis of the celiac plexus is achieved, both *orthostatic hypotension and bowel hypermotility* may result from the sympathectomy and increased splanchnic parasympathetic tone. These are generally benign side effects that respond to supportive care and symptomatic treatment. *Neurologic complications*, including permanent lower extremity sensory/motor deficits, bowel/bladder dysfunction, and impotence in males, are rare but serious complications associated with

CPB. Prior to injection of neurolytic agent, a test injection with local anesthetic to confirm needle position is recommended. Further prudence includes intermittent injection and frequent aspiration, which protect against *accidental injection into the aorta or IVC*, both of which run proximal to the celiac plexus.

Questions

1. Adverse consequences of unintended dural puncture during lumbar epidural injection of 40 mg methylprednisolone acetate in 9 ml saline diluent may include all of the following EXCEPT for which?
   a. cauda equina syndrome
   b. headache
   c. total spinal anesthesia
   d. arachnoiditis
   e. direct mechanical injury to the spinal cord

2. Anterior cord infarction, a catastrophic complication that may occur during lumbar transforaminal injection, is LEAST LIKELY to be associated with which of the following?
   a. accidental injection of particulate steroid into the artery of Adamkiewicz
   b. preservation of fine touch/discrimination below the level of the lesion
   c. motor paralysis below the level of the lesion
   d. loss of proprioception and vibration sense below the level of the lesion
   e. loss of pain and temperature sensation at and below the level of the lesion

Answers

1. c. Total spinal anesthesia would not be an expected risk if the epidural steroid was diluted with normal saline rather than local anesthetic.
2. d. Proprioception and vibration sense are transmitted by afferent nerve fibers posteriorly in the dorsal column, where blood supply is provided by the two posterior spinal arteries.

Further reading

Fitzgibbon, D. R., Posner, K. L., Domino, K. B. et al. (2004). Chronic pain management: American Society of Anesthesiologists Closed Claims Project. *Anesthesiology* 100(1), 98–105.

Gilligan, C. J. and Rathmell, J. P. (2011). Complications associated with interventions in pain medicine. In Vacanti, C. A., Sikka, P. J., Urman, R. D., Dershwitz, M., and Segal, B. S. (eds) *Essential Clinical Anesthesia.* New

York: Cambridge University Press, pp. 925–932.

Neal, J. M. and Rathmell, J. P. (2006). *Complications in Regional Anesthesia and Pain Medicine.* Philadelphia: Saunders Elsevier.

Back pain

J. Tasker Gundy and Jie Zhou

Keywords

Back pain: differential diagnosis
Back pain: red flags
Low back pain: treatment
Low back pain and epidural steroids

Back pain (lumbosacral spinal pain) is among the most common and costly medical conditions, prompting millions of annual physician visits (in fact, as many as one-fifth of all physician visits are prompted by back pain). Between 50% and 80% of adults will experience significant low back pain in their lifetime, making this a leading cause of disability (25% of all workers compensation costs), absenteeism, and lost productivity.

Fortunately, the vast majority of cases will be self-limited, resolving without treatment in fewer than six weeks (70% of disabling episodes resolve in four to six weeks, 90% by 12 weeks).

Acute low back pain is defined as lumbosacral spinal pain present for less than four weeks' duration; *chronic* low back pain is present when pain has persisted for three months or longer.

Back pain is described relative to the perceived origin of the pain, as in *lumbar spinal pain* (T12→S1), *sacral spinal pain* (originating from the sacrum below S1), or *radicular pain* (perceived as lower extremity in origin, in a dermatomal distribution owing to ectopic compression, and subsequent inflammation of sensory fibers at a spinal root level). *Radiculopathy* describes a focal neurologic deficit in the distribution of the compressed nerve root(s), and *sciatica* is a colloquial term used to describe the radicular symptoms that result from compression of lumbosacral nerve roots contributing to the sciatic nerve. Unfortunately a patient's pain will often be nonspecific, and as many as 90% of patients with chronic lumbosacral pain will never find a precise anatomic source of their discomfort.

Back pain: differential diagnosis

In considering a differential diagnosis for back pain, clinicians must evaluate not only for etiologies intrinsic to the spine itself, but consider the possibility that systemic disease and/or referred pain (from the abdomen or pelvis) are responsible. The initial evaluation of back pain should always involve screening for *red flags* (see Table 149.1), which include *bowel/bladder dysfunction or saddle anesthesia* (concerning for cauda equina syndrome, which typically requires emergent surgical decompression), *unexplained weight loss or fever* (suggesting possible infection/malignancy), and *pain worse with recumbency* (suggesting possible spinal tumor).

After excluding red flags, a diagnostic algorithm begins with determining the pattern of pain (lumbosacral or radicular) and its chronicity (acute or chronic). Physical examination is paramount, and maneuvers that may aid in diagnosis include the straight leg raise (detects nerve root compression), facet loading tests (detect facet arthropathy), and the FABERE or "Patrick" test (flexion, abduction, and external rotation of the hip, detects sacroiliitis). Importantly, in the absence of red flags, *diagnostic imaging is not generally used during the first six weeks of an episode* of lumbosacral back pain.

The most common (identifiable) causes of low back pain include the following:

- **Lumbosacral strain/sprain.** Approximately 80% to 90% of low back pain injuries result from chronic "strain" or acute "sprain" of the paravertebral muscles/ligaments or the sacroiliac joint. Such injuries are typically associated with heavy lifting, falls, or sudden rotatory movements.

- **Degenerative disc disease.** Age-related changes to intervertebral discs (dehydration, height loss, and mechanical disruption from repetitive loading) predispose toward "herniated disc" (posterolateral bulging or extrusion of the nucleus pulposus into the spinal canal, most commonly at levels L4/5 or L5/S1) and osteophyte formation (spondylosis) that may progress to spinal stenosis, threatening the cauda equina. Disc herniation is suggested by radicular pain/radiculopathy; pain from spinal stenosis (characteristically radiating to the buttocks/thighs) worsens with exercise and is relieved by sitting or leaning forward.

Essential Clinical Anesthesia Review: Keywords, Questions and Answers for the Boards, ed. Linda S. Aglio, Robert W. Lekowski, and Richard D. Urman. Published by Cambridge University Press. © Cambridge University Press 2015.

- **Myofascial syndromes**. Characterized by pain reproducible at discrete trigger points (nondermatomal), which develop following an injury.

Table 149.1 The red flags of back pain

History
Gradual onset of back pain
Age <20 years or >50 years
Thoracic back pain
Pain lasting longer than six weeks
History of trauma
Fever/chills/night sweats
Unintentional weight loss
Pain worse with recumbency
Pain worse at night
Unrelenting pain despite supratherapeutic doses of analgesics
History of malignancy
History of immunosuppression
Recent procedure known to cause bacteremia
History of intravenous drug use
Physical examination
Fever
Hypotension
Extreme hypertension
Pale, ashen appearance
Pulsatile abdominal mass
Pulse amplitude differentials
Spinous process tenderness
Focal neurologic signs
Acute urinary retention

(Winters, M. E., Kluetz, P., and Zilberstein, J. 2006. Back pain emergencies. *Medical Clinics of North America*, 60(3): 505–523.)

Less common etiologies on the differential include *facet syndrome* (paramedian back pain radiating to the buttock and thigh, resulting from degenerative changes in the zygapophyseal joints), *congenital abnormalities* (i.e., sacralization of L5, lumbarization of S1), *arthridities* (i.e., ankylosing spondylitis, psoriatic arthritis), as well as *infection* or *tumor* presenting subacutely without the aforementioned red flags.

Low back pain: treatment

Acute lumbosacral or radicular pain may initially respond to a brief course of NSAID, acetaminophen, or muscle relaxant. Opioids are also commonly prescribed, though there is little evidence suggesting their superiority over more conservative analgesics.

The anti-inflammatory effect of lumbar *epidural steroid injection* ("ESI," see Chapter 146) is believed to speed resolution of acute radicular pain that is unresponsive to noninvasive therapy. *ESI is most effective when administered within the first two to six weeks* of symptoms, but is of little benefit in the absence of actual nerve root compression/irritation.

Patients with chronic radicular pain can benefit from the addition of adjuvant analgesics (anticonvulsants and TCAs) to their therapeutic regimen, and good outcomes evidence exists for a multidisciplinary treatment strategy that includes physical therapy and psychological counseling.

For facet and sacroiliac joint pain, diagnostic injections (medial branch nerve block, sacroiliac joint injection, see Chapter 147) are the gold standard for diagnosing problem joints as pain generators. "Positive" blocks that relieve pain are typically followed by radiofrequency lesioning at the same joints, providing longer lasting pain relief (three to six months).

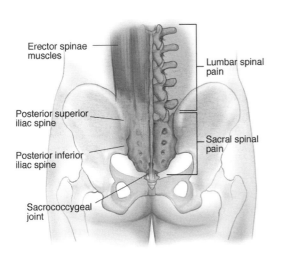

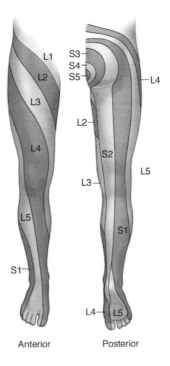

Figure 149.1 Lumbosacral spinal and radicular pain. (From Vacanti et al. 2011. *Essential Clinical Anesthesia*, Cambridge University Press, pp. 933–937.)

Indications for surgery are severe or progressing motor deficit, cauda equina syndrome, or motor deficit that persists despite six weeks of conservative management.

Questions

1. Following a thorough history and physical examination excluding potential "red flags," any of the following may be considered reasonable initial treatment strategies for nonspecific low back pain EXCEPT for which?

    a. a brief course of acetaminophen
    b. bed rest
    c. brief course of NSAID
    d. brief course of centrally acting muscle relaxant (i.e., benzodiazepine)
    e. noninvasive strategy emphasizing patient education and advice to resume normal everyday activities as soon as possible

2. Which of the following statements regarding radicular pain is MOST likely true?

    a. Pain is generally poorly responsive to NSAID therapy.
    b. Opioid therapy has been proven superior to NSAID therapy.
    c. The optimal time to consider epidural steroid injection is following three months of unsuccessful conservative treatment.
    d. It is commonly caused by annulous fibrosis herniation into the lumbar spinal canal.
    e. Pain is perceived as lower extremity in origin.

Answers

1. b. Each treatment strategy listed is a reasonable initial treatment strategy with the exception of bed rest, which is no longer recommended.
2. e. Radicular pain may be perceived as lower extremity in origin, and occurs in a dermatomal distribution. Each of the other statements are incorrect.

Further reading

Casazza, B. A. (2012). Diagnosis and treatment of acute low back pain. *American Family Physician* 85(4), 343–350.

Chou, R., Qaseem, A., Snow, V. et al. (2007). Diagnosis and treatment of low back pain: a joint clinical practice guideline from the American College of Physicians and the American Pain Society. *Annals of Internal Medicine* 147, 478–491.

Keel, J. C. (2011). Back pain. In Vacanti, C. A., Sikka, P. J., Urman, R. D., Dershwitz, M., and Segal, B. S. (eds) *Essential Clinical Anesthesia*. New York: Cambridge University Press, pp. 933–937.

Morgan, G. E., Mikhail, M. S., and Murray, M. J. (2006). *Clinical Anesthesiology*, 4th edn. New York: McGraw-Hill, pp. 401–405.

Winters, M. E., Kluetz, P., and Zilberstein, J. (2006). Back pain emergencies. *Medical Clinics of North America* 90(3), 505–523.

Chapter

150

Complex regional pain syndrome

J. Tasker Gundy and Elizabeth M. Rickerson

The complex regional pain syndromes (CRPS type I and type II, formerly known as "reflex sympathetic dystrophy" and "causalgia," respectively) are regional neuropathic pain conditions that may develop in one or multiple extremities in response to traumatic injury or surgery.

Characteristics and diagnosis

CRPS is subclassified into two types according to the presence or absence of an identifiable antecedent nerve injury. Cases lacking a culprit nerve injury are referred to as CRPS type I (formerly RSD), while cases that occur in the presence of distinct major nerve damage are classified as CRPS type II (formerly causalgia).

The hallmark characteristic of CRPS is continuous, intense, localized neuropathic *pain, which is disproportionate in severity to the inciting event*. The exact etiology of CRPS is yet to be determined, though accumulating evidence suggests that genetic predisposition does exist. CRPS appears to affect women (60–80% of cases) more often than men.

There is no single laboratory test to diagnose CRPS. Instead, the syndrome is suspected in the presence of:

1. disproportionate pain
2. allodynia or hyperalgesia
3. an antecedent noxious event

A set of further characteristic features have been used as arbitrary criteria to establish the diagnosis (though not all

criteria need to be met for a diagnosis, and symptoms may fluctuate over time). These features collectively suggest *autonomic nervous system dysfunction*, and include:

4. edema
5. changes in skin perfusion (e.g., asymmetric temperature abnormalities)
6. abnormal sudomotor activity (sweating abnormalities)
7. dystrophic tissue changes (e.g., focal skin atrophy, bone demineralization)

CPRS type I has historically been described as having three distinct stages (acute, dystrophic, and atrophic); however, this staging system has since been abandoned due to clinical inconsistency. In general, it may be said that *early signs* tend toward skin warmth and edema in the affected extremity, with skin cooling and cyanosis appearing later.

Treatment

The cornerstone of treatment for CRPS of either type is *use of the affected extremity as much as possible*. A multimodal, interdisciplinary approach emphasizing physical therapy and restoration of function through activity is most effective.

Early diagnosis and treatment are important, as CRPS can spread to all extremities if left untreated, placing the patient at risk for chronic pain and permanent deformity, and complicating the rehabilitation process. The speed with which therapy commences, including sympathetic nerve block (see below), has been correlated with outcomes.

As adjuncts to physical therapy, numerous analgesics have been shown to augment pain management, including NSAIDs, pulse corticosteroids, tramadol, anticonvulsants, TCAs, mild opioids, calcitonin, bisphosphonates, lidocaine infusion, clonidine, dextromethorphan, muscle relaxants (clonazepam, baclofen), and ketamine/midazolam in anesthetic doses for refractory cases. Cognitive–behavioral therapy techniques, as well as supportive psychotherapy, can teach skills for coping with chronic pain.

For patients whose mobility has been significantly impaired by CRPS, it becomes important to determine the

Essential Clinical Anesthesia Review: Keywords, Questions and Answers for the Boards, ed. Linda S. Aglio, Robert W. Lekowski, and Richard D. Urman. Published by Cambridge University Press. © Cambridge University Press 2015.

extent to which sympathetic nervous system dysfunction is contributing to the pain. This is commonly accomplished via *sympathetic nerve block to the affected extremity*, typically with a stellate ganglion block (for upper extremity involvement) or lumbar sympathetic block (for lower extremity involvement). Pain relief following a sympathetic block is usually considered diagnostic of sympathetically maintained pain (SMP), and subsequent therapy may be dictated based on the classification of pain as SMP or sympathetically independent (though mixed pain can also exist). For SMP, repeat sympathetic blocks may be appropriate in order for the patient to participate in physical therapy, and alpha-1 adrenoreceptor blockers (e.g., terazosin, phenoxybenzamine) may also be useful.

Interventional options for patients with refractory pain include isolated somatic nerve block, IV regional (Bier) block, spinal cord stimulation, peripheral nerve stimulation, intrathecal therapy, and, finally, palliative surgery, including sympathectomy or amputation.

Questions

1. Each of the following examples contain features that might suggest a diagnosis of CRPS type I (complex regional pain syndrome type I), EXCEPT for which?
   a. burning pain, thinning of the epidermis in the hand, and fingernail changes following ipsilateral shoulder arthroplasty
   b. lancinating pain and hyperhidrosis in the forearm following surgical fixation of an ipsilateral olecranon fracture
   c. severe pain, allodynia, edema, and hair loss at the foot following an ankle sprain

   d. continuing hyperalgesia, edema, and changes in skin blood flow in the ipsilateral hand following a stab wound to the arm injuring the median nerve
   e. unrelenting shooting pain and skin atrophy in the forearm following contusion to the upper arm

2. Regarding CRPS, all of the following statements are true EXCEPT for which?
   a. CRPS type II was formerly called "reflex sympathetic dystrophy."
   b. Three distinct stages of CRPS type I have been described.
   c. Clinicians lack a reliable test to diagnose CRPS.
   d. CRPS type II describes cases where an antecedent major nerve injury is identified.
   e. Therapy with alpha-1 blockers may be useful in sympathetically maintained pain.

Answers

1. d. CRPS is classified according to the presence or absence of an identifiable nerve injury. The case in example (d), with a culprit nerve injury identified, would be better classified as CRPS type II.
2. a. CRPS type II was formerly known as "causalgia," while CRPS type I was formerly called "reflex sympathetic dystrophy."

Further reading

Ghalambor, O. (2011). Complex regional pain syndrome. In Vacanti, C. A., Sikka, P. J., Urman, R. D., Dershwitz, M., and Segal, B. S. (eds) *Essential Clinical Anesthesia*. New York: Cambridge University Press, 938–939.

Stanton-Hicks, M. (2003). Complex regional pain syndrome. *Anesthesiology Clinics of North America* 21, 733–744.

Chapter 15

Cancer pain

J. Tasker Gundy and Elizabeth M. Rickerson

Pain attributable to cancer therapy, or to cancer itself, is a complex and significant concern for patients and their clinicians: 25% of cancer patients in active treatment and 90% of patients with advanced disease will suffer from pain. Alas, despite a multitude of available treatment options and the knowledge that successful treatment is possible, studies show that pain management is inadequate for as many as 50% of cancer patients.

Cancer pain: diagnosis

Essential elements in the initial assessment of the patient with cancer pain include the following:

1. A detailed *history* of the pain, focusing on duration, quality, temporal pattern, intensity (measured using a validated pain assessment tool such as numerical/visual analogue scale or face scale), inciting factors, previous therapies, and nonphysical factors contributing to pain (psychological, social, or existential components). If the patient notes more than one pain source, each should be considered independently.
2. Physical examination, including a complete neurologic exam.
3. Appropriate diagnostic testing, such as plain films and CT to determine fracture or visceral pathology, and MRI to evaluate soft tissue changes.
4. Development of a management plan, including a substitute strategy to be invoked if the initial plan proves ineffective.

Cancer pain, whether acute or chronic (present for more than three months), is generally classified into one of three types:

- **Somatic**: *sharp and well-localized* pain resulting from activation of nociceptors in cutaneous or deep tissues (bone, fascia). May be related to metastasis or may be postsurgical pain.
- **Visceral**: *dull, pressure-like, poorly localized* pain. Nociceptors activated involve internal structures such as thoracic, abdominal, or pelvic viscera.
- **Neuropathic**: *burning, tingling, electric-like* pain resulting from a directly injured or dysfunctional nervous system. Nerve damage may result from tumor compression or infiltration, as well as cancer treatments (e.g., chemotherapy or surgeries).

Within these broad categories, pain may be further classified into three basic subtypes, which include *pain associated with tumor* (e.g., metastases, bone lesions, visceral obstruction, organ capsule distention, neural compression), *pain associated with therapy* (e.g., postradiation enteritis, chemo-induced neuropathy, radiation fibrosis, mucositis), and *pain not specifically related to the malignancy*, including preexisting chronic pain syndromes, headaches, and muscle strains.

Cancer pain: management

The majority (70–80%) of cancer pain can be managed with appropriate pharmacologic and anticancer therapy, but some patients will require invasive interventions to relieve pain and improve quality of life.

From the pharmacologic perspective, oral analgesics, particularly opioids, are the mainstay of treatment for cancer pain; clinicians should be comfortable prescribing opioids for cancer pain at any stage of disease, without concern for life expectancy.

The best known algorithm for cancer pain management is the *World Health Organization (WHO) three-step analgesic ladder*, which provides a tiered approach to guide analgesic selection according to the severity of the patient's pain. Administering medications "by the ladder" rests on several additional principles:

Essential Clinical Anesthesia Review: Keywords, Questions and Answers for the Boards, ed. Linda S. Aglio, Robert W. Lekowski, and Richard D. Urman. Published by Cambridge University Press. © Cambridge University Press 2015.

Freedom from Cancer Pain

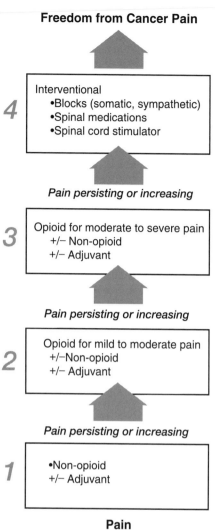

Figure 151.1 Modified analgesic ladder for cancer pain, including interventional management. (Adapted from World Health Organization. 1990. *WHO Technical Report Series 804*, pp. 1–73; Miguel, R. 2000. *Cancer Control 7*, 149–156; and Krames, E. 1999. *Medical Clinics of North America 83*, 787–808)

1. **By mouth.** Analgesics are given orally whenever possible.
2. **By the clock.** Analgesics should be given at regular intervals, with respect to the medication's duration of action, efficacy, and the level of the patient's pain.
3. **For the individual.** Analgesics should be given based on the pain intensity *as evaluated by the patient.* Dosing should be based on the individual's needs; i.e., there is no standard dose for every patient.
4. **Attention to detail.** Analgesics should be prescribed with an emphasis on taking medications at scheduled intervals in addition to PRN dosing. Ideally, each patient should receive written instructions including the name of each medication, the reason for use, the dose (number of mg and number of tablets), and the dosing interval.

The fourth step of the ladder, described below, is a proposed addition to the WHO ladder.

Step one = mild pain: medications include non-opioid analgesics including NSAIDS and other adjuvants (e.g., anticonvulsants, corticosteroids, tricyclic antidepressants, acetaminophen).

Step two = mild to moderate pain: second-tier medications include "weak opioids," which combine opioids with non-opioid analgesics (e.g., acetaminophen, ibuprofen, or ASA), with or without adjuvant therapy. These drugs have been labeled "weak" because ceiling dosages (attributable to the maximum 24 h dose of non-opioid component) limit their analgesic potential.

Step three = moderate to severe pain: the cornerstone of tier three are the pure agonist opioids (e.g., morphine, hydromorphone), usually given in sustained-release form every 8–12 hours (after daily dose requirements have been determined with a trial of short-acting formulation) in combination with PRN immediate-release preparation for breakthrough pain. There is no ceiling or upper limit dose, and these are titrated to the patient's pain relief. Transdermal fentanyl is an available alternative for patients unable to take oral medication.

Step four (a proposed addition to the WHO ladder) = severe to intractable pain: if escalating doses of step three analgesics fail to adequately treat persistent pain or are associated with intolerable side effects (see below), interventional techniques (e.g., nerve or neurolytic blocks, neuraxial opioid therapy, SCS) and conversion to parenteral opioid therapy may be warranted.

There are a multitude of criticisms of the WHO ladder; there are no recommendations for treatment-related adverse events, and there is no assessment of the patient's mental health. Ultimately, a patient may require more specialized therapy such as a PCA, chemotherapy, radiation, or interventional pain procedures. The proposed "fourth step" described above is one suggestion for incorporating additional procedures into the pain treatment process; however, it may be that a patient requires a procedure/intervention before progressing through steps one to three. A multidisciplinary approach to pain, anxiety, depression, and other symptoms can get us closer to a goal of treating 100% of cancer pain. A multidisciplinary team could include specialists from oncology, surgical oncology, radiation oncology, pain management, palliative care, social work, physical therapy, chaplaincy, psychiatry, and occupational therapy, among others.

Methadone is a synthetic opioid, which is a popular choice for cancer pain management due to its long half-life (15 to 60 hours) and its additional activity at non-opioid receptors (MAO reuptake inhibition and NMDA antagonism). Clinically, the duration of analgesia is similar to other sustained-release opioids (6–12 hours); caution must be taken when titrating the drug due to its unpredictable half-life. Resting EKG should be obtained prior to starting methadone therapy, as it can prolong the QTc interval (torsades de points has been reported with high doses).

While management goals should be to achieve adequate analgesia without significant side effects, proactive *side-effect management* is an integral part of any cancer pain treatment regimen that utilizes opioids. Nausea is the most common side effect and will be present in one-third of patients. Opioid-induced constipation is also common, and prophylaxis should be initiated concomitantly with the initiation of opioids (tolerance to constipation does *not* occur). Other side effects can include CNS effects (sedation, dysphoria, confusion, myoclonus), urinary retention, dry mouth, respiratory depression, pruritis, and miosis.

Anticipate *sequelae of chronic opioid use*, including:

- *Tolerance* to analgesic effect. Note that while opioid rotations are often necessary (for patients experiencing intolerable side effects or inadequate pain control with one agent), *incomplete cross-tolerance* renders it necessary to decrease the equianalgesic dose of a new drug by 30% to 50% when rotating.
- *Physical dependence*. Patients will exhibit withdrawal symptoms when an opioid is abruptly discontinued or an antagonist administered.
- *Psychological dependence (addiction)*. Distinct from tolerance and physical dependence, addiction is characterized by patterns of craving and compulsive drug-seeking behavior.
- *Pseudoaddiction*. Behavior that may suggest addiction, but instead results from undertreatment or progression of disease.

Interventional modalities that may be useful in managing pain include local anesthetic nerve blocks, neurolytic sympathetic nerve blocks, radiofrequency lesioning, and neuraxial opioid therapy (via an epidural, intrathecal, or intraventricular approach).

Questions

1. For the initial treatment of mild cancer-related pain, each of the following step-one analgesics (using the WHO analgesic ladder) might be considered, EXCEPT for which?
   a. oxycodone
   b. acetaminophen
   c. gabapentin
   d. amitriptilyne
   e. clonazepam

2. Which of the following would NOT be an expected side effect from opioid therapy for chronic cancer pain?
   a. pruritus
   b. nausea
   c. diarrhea
   d. dry mouth
   e. urinary retention

Answers

1. a. Step-one analgesics on the WHO analgesic ladder include non-opioids and other adjuvants; oxycodone is an opioid.
2. c. Each of the choices listed are common side effects of opioid therapy, with the exception of diarrhea. Constipation might be expected; diarrhea is not.

Further reading

American Pain Society (2008). *Principles of Analgesic Use in the Treatment of Acute Pain and Cancer Pain*, 6th edn. Skokie, IL: American Pain Society.

Morgan, G. E., Mikhail, M. S., and Murray, M. J. (2006). *Clinical Anesthesiology*, 4th edn. New York: McGraw-Hill, pp. 398–400.

Thomas, J. R., Ferris, F. D., and von Gunten, C. F. (2004). Approach to management of cancer pain. In Benzon, H. T., Raja, S. N., Molloy, R. E., Liu, S., and Fishman, S. M. (eds) *Essentials of Pain Medicine and Regional Anesthesia*, 2nd edn. Elsevier Science.

Valovska, A. and Klickovich, R. J. (2011). Cancer pain. In Vacanti, C. A., Sikka, P. J., Urman, R. D., Dershwitz, M., and Segal, B. S. (eds) *Essential Clinical Anesthesia*. New York: Cambridge University Press, pp. 941–946.

World Heath Organization (1996). *Cancer Pain Relief*, 2nd edn. Geneva: World Health Organization.

Chapter

152

Cardiopulmonary resuscitation

Christopher Voscopoulos and Joshua Vacanti

Keywords

2010 Cardiopulmonary Resuscitation Guidelines
Compression–ventilation ratio
Hyperventilation during CPR
Capnography during ACLS
Electrical defibrillation
Pharmacotherapy for ACLS
Neonatal resuscitation
ACLS algorithms

In contrast to the classically taught "Airway–Breathing–Circulation" sequence (ABC), the *2010 Cardiopulmonary Resuscitation Guidelines* recommend a "Circulation–Airway–Breathing" approach (CAB). As a result, emphasis is placed on early initiation of chest compressions to restore systemic circulation. Interruptions should be minimized, even at the expense of intubation, unless ventilation is assessed as inadequate.

Single rescuers of infant, child, and adult victims should maintain a *compression–ventilation ratio* of 30:2. For two-rescuer CPR in children and infants, the ratio should be 15:2. Compressions should occur at least 100 times a minute

Table 152.1 Pharmacologic agents for use in pulseless cardiac arrest

Drug	Initial dose	Frequency	Mechanism	Comment
Epinephrine	1 mg IV/IO for adults (0.01 mg/kg of 1:1,000 for children or 0.1 mg/kg 1:10,000)	Every 3–5 min	α- and β-adrenergic; increases cerebral and myocardial perfusion	High-dose epinephrine is no longer recommended
Vasopressin	40 Units IV/IO	One-time dose only	Nonadrenergic peripheral vasoconstrictor	One dose may replace either first or second dose of epinephrine
Atropine	1 mg IV/IO (0.02 mg/kg IV/IO for children, minimum dose 0.1mg)	Every 3–5 minutes; maximum dose 3.0 mg for adults, 1.0 mg for children	Reversal of cholinergic-mediated decreases in heart rate, systemic vascular resistance, and blood pressure	Only indicated in children with bradycardia, due to increased vagal tone or primary AV block
Amiodarone	300 mg IV/IO for arrest (5 mg/kg for children)	First dose can be followed by 150 mg	Sodium, potassium, calcium channel blocker; α- and β-adrenergic blocker	If successful, should be followed with a continuous infusion
Lidocaine	1.5 mg/kg first dose IV/IO (1 mg/kg for children)	1.0 mg/kg at 5 to 10 min intervals to maximum dose of 3 mg/kg	Sodium channel blocker	No proven short-term or long-term efficacy in cardiac arrest
Magnesium	1–2 g IV/IO (50 mg/kg IV/IO, maximum dose 2 g for torsades in children)	Give in 10 ml of D_5W over 5–10 min	Calcium channel blocker	Effective for termination of polymorphic VT (torsades de pointes)

AV, atrioventricular; D_5W, 5% dextrose in water; VT, ventricular tachycardia.
(From Essential Clinical Anesthesia, 1 edn. Cambridge University Press, p. 950, Table 153.2.)

Resuscitation of the Newborn

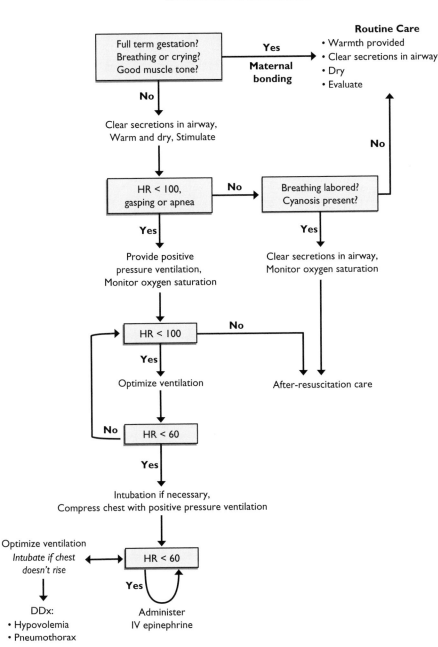

Figure 152.1 Resuscitation algorithm for neonates. (From Vacanti et al. 2011. *Essential Clinical Anesthesia*, Cambridge University Press, p. 954; Adapted from Katwinkel, J. 2006. *Neonatal Resuscitation Textbook*, T1, American Heart Association.)

and allow for complete chest recoil. Optimal circulatory blood flow is achieved when the chest is allowed to fully recoil. After securing an advanced airway, ventilation for adults, children, and infants should be achieved by administering eight to ten breaths a minute.

Hyperventilation during CPR has been shown to decrease venous return and cardiac output, decrease coronary perfusion pressure, increase gastric inflation, and worsen outcomes.

The ACLS guidelines recommend the use of quantitative waveform *capnography during ACLS* for confirmation of endotracheal tube placement. Capnography also provides a method to assess the effectiveness of chest compressions and restoration of circulation; end-tidal CO_2 values can provide evidence of pulmonary blood flow. Accordingly, capnography may also demonstrate the return of spontaneous circulation by an abrupt increase in the carbon dioxide reading.

Successful *electrical defibrillation* is most effective if performed within five minutes of arrest. Continuous CPR before and after shock delivery increases the chances of survival by nearly three-fold. Survival rates decrease by 10% without chest compressions, and by 4% with chest compressions, for every minute that passes between onset of

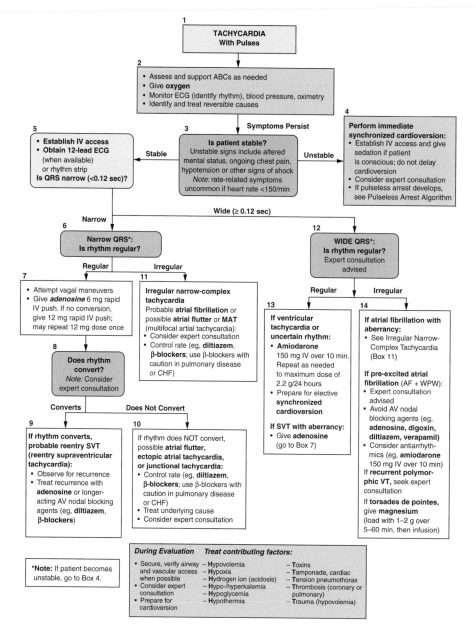

Figure 152.2 Adult tachycardia (with pulse). 2010 American Heart Association Guidelines for Cardiopulmonary Resuscitation and Emergency Cardiovascular Care, Part 8: Adult Advanced Cardiovascular Life Support. *Circulation*, 2010; 122 (Suppl 3): S751, Figure 4. Copyright 2010 American Heart Association, Inc.)

ventricular fibrillation and defibrillation. Defibrillation in pediatric patients should be attempted using two joules per kilogram.

Pharmacotherapy for ACLS can be administered during CPR in a CPR–Rhythm–CPR–Shock sequence (Table 152.1).

A fraction of newborns need some degree of *neonatal resuscitation*: 10% require assistance with breathing after birth, and 1% require initiation of the neonatal resuscitation algorithm (Figure 152.1).

ALCS algorithms: See Figures 152.2 and 152.3.

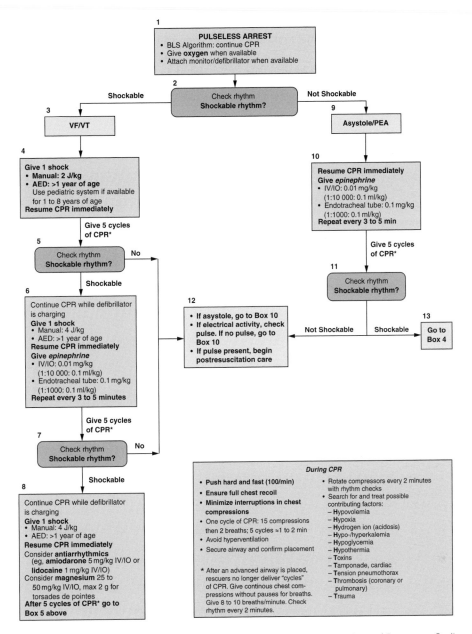

Figure 152.3 Pulseless arrest. 2010 American Heart Association Guidelines for Cardiopulmonary Resusciatation and Emergency Cardiovascular Care, Part 8: Adult Advanced Cardiovascular Life Support. *Circulation*, 2010; 122(Suppl 3): S749, Figure 3. Copyright 2010 American Heart Association, Inc.)

Questions

1. Hyperventilation in ACLS is associated with which?

   a. improved survival up to 20%
   b. increased morbidity
   c. improved coronary perfusion
   d. minimal changes in cardiac output

2. During ACLS, the primary purpose of epinephrine is to stimulate which of the following adrenergic receptors?

   a. β_1 receptors to increase cardiac inotropy and chronotropy
   b. β_2 receptors to reduce afterload on the heart
   c. α_1 receptors to increase venous return to the heart
   d. α_2 receptors to control sympathetic nervous system tone

3. Initial electrical shock dose in an unstable, wide-complex irregular heart rhythm is which?

   a. synchronized cardioversion 120–200 J biphasic
   b. synchronized cardioversion 200 J monophasic
   c. defibrillation 200 J
   d. defibrillation 50–100 J

Answers

1. b. Particularly during the initial phases of CPR, restoration of perfusion with chest compressions takes priority over ventilation and establishing a secured airway. Positive pressure ventilation can decrease systemic perfusion by

decreasing venous return. Once the airway is secured, avoidance of hyperventilation allows for optimal cardiac output during CPR.
2. c. Epinephrine's primary action in ACLS is via its α_1 effects acting to increase venous return to the heart and restore systemic perfusion.

3. c. The correct, initial electrical energy dose in an unstable wide-complex irregular heart rhythm is 200 J. Synchronized cardioversion is used in patients with a regular R wave to avoid an electrical impulse delivered on the R wave, which can result in ventricular fibrillation.

Further reading

American Heart Association (2010). American Heart Association guidelines for cardiopulmonary resuscitation and emergency cardiovascular care. *Circulation* 122 (Suppl 3), S729–S676.

Aufderheide, T. P., Sigurdsson, G., Pirrallo, R. G. et al. (2004). Hyperventilation-induced hypotension during cardiopulmonary resuscitation. *Circulation* 109, 1960–1965.

Sayre, M. R., Koster, R. W., Botha, M. et al. (2005). Part 5: Adult basic life support: 2010 International Consensus on Cardiopulmonary Resuscitation and Emergency Cardiovascular Care Science with Treatment Recommendations. *Circulation* 2010 Oct 19; 122(16 Suppl 2): S 298–324.

Stiell, I. G., Wells, G. A., Hebert, P. C. et al. (1995). Association of drug therapy with survival in cardiac arrest: limited role of

advanced cardiac life support drugs. *Academy of Emergency Medicine* 2, 264–273.

Young, K. D. and Seidel, J. S. (1999). Pediatric cardiopulmonary resuscitation: a collective review. *Annals of Emergency Medicine* 33, 195–205.

Vacanti, C. A., Sikka, P. K., Urman, R. U., Dershwitz, M., and Segal, B. S. (eds) (2011). *Essential Clinical Anesthesia.* New York, NY: Cambridge University Press.

Chapter 53

Multiorgan failure and its prevention

Timothy D. Quinn and Sujatha Pentakota

Keywords

Definition of multiorgan dysfunction syndrome and failure

Multiorgan dysfunction syndrome and failure: morbidity and mortality

Dysfunction of key organs

Assessing the severity of multiorgan dysfunction syndrome and failure

Conditions leading to multiorgan dysfunction syndrome failure

Prevention and management of multiorgan dysfunction syndrome failure

Table 153.1 ICU survival is related to the number of failing organ systems involved

Failing organ systems, *n*	Mortality, %
0	0.8
1	6.8
2	26.2
3	48.5
4	68.8
5	83.3

(Vacanti, C., Segal, S., Sikka, P., Urman, R. (eds) 2011. *Essential Clinical Anesthesia*. Cambridge University Press, p. 955.)

Multiorgan dysfunction syndrome (MODS) and *multiorgan failure (MOF)* are defined as the simultaneous presence of dysfunction or failure of two or more organs for more than 24 hours. The underlying pathophysiology is a systemic inflammatory response secondary to infectious (e.g., bacteremia, pneumonia) or noninfectious (e.g., burns, trauma, pancreatitis) causes. The lungs, kidney, liver, heart, and brain are the most likely organ systems to be affected.

Patient survival is inversely proportional to the number of organ systems failing. (See Table 153.1.) Early detection of impending organ failure is both crucial for good outcomes and challenging due to the lack of effective biomarkers or diagnostic tests to predict problems.

Lungs

Acute respiratory distress syndrome (ARDS) is divided into three categories: mild (PaO_2/FiO_2 ratio of 200–300), moderate (PaO_2/FiO_2 ratio of 100–200), and severe (PaO_2/FiO_2 ratio of <100) based on the "Berlin definition." Mortality rises with increasing severity of ARDS.

Cardiovascular

Cardiovascular failure manifests as hypotension due to low cardiac output resulting from a pump problem (e.g., intrinsic heart failure), or due to high cardiac output in the presence of low systemic vascular resistance (e.g., sepsis). Sometimes patients may be hypovolemic and in septic shock.

Kidneys

Acute kidney injury is defined as an increase in serum creatinine more than 0.3 mg/dl from the patient's baseline. The risk, injury, failure, loss, and end-stage (RIFLE) kidney criteria are shown in Table 153.2.

Liver

Evidence of liver dysfunction includes persistent elevation of aspartate aminotransferase (AST) and alanine aminotransferase (ALT), bilirubin and prothrombin time (PT). The Child–Turcotte–Pugh classification of liver failure (Table 153.3) is one common scoring system, which correlates with one year mortality.

Brain

Cognitive dysfunction can range from altered mental status and delirium to coma. Delirium is a *fluctuating* state of consciousness, ranging from disorientation to altered mental

Essential Clinical Anesthesia Review: Keywords, Questions and Answers for the Boards, ed. Linda S. Aglio, Robert W. Lekowski, and Richard D. Urman. Published by Cambridge University Press. © Cambridge University Press 2015.

Table 153.2 Risk, injury, failure, loss, and end-stage (RIFLE) kidney criteria

Class	Glomerular filtration rate criteria	Urine output criteria
Risk	Increase in serum creatinine × 1.5 from baseline	<0.5 ml/kg/h × 6 h
Injury	Increase in serum creatinine × 2 from baseline	<0.5 ml/kg/h × 12 h
Failure	Increase in serum creatinine × 3 from baseline, or serum creatinine ≥4 mg/dl with an acute rise >0.5 mg/dl	<0.3 ml/kg/h × 24 h, or anuria × 1
Loss	Persistent acute renal failure = complete loss of kidney function >4 weeks	
End-stage kidney disease	End-stage kidney disease >3 months	

(Adapted from Bellomo, R., Kellum, J. A., and Ronco, C. 2007. Defining and classifying acute renal failure: from advocacy to consensus and validation of the RIFLE criteria. *Intensive Care Medicine*, 33: 409–413. Vacanti, C., Segal, S., Sikka, P., Urman, R. et al. 2011. *Essential Clinical Anesthesia*. Cambridge University Press, p. 956.)

Table 153.3 Child–Turcotte–Pugh classification of liver failure

	Points (per variable)		
	1	2	3
Serum bilirubin (mg/dl)	<2	2–3	>3
Serum albumin (g/dl)	>3.5	2.8–3.5	<2.8
Prolongation of PT (sec/control)[a]	<4	4–6	6
Ascites	None	Mild	Moderate
Encephalopathy	None	Minimal	Advanced

Interpretation

Class	Points	Mortality risk, 3 months–1 year (%)
A	5–6	4–10
B	7–9	14–31
C	10–15	51–76

[a] Nutrition (excellent, good, poor) was replaced with prothrombin time by Pugh's modification of the Child–Turcotte classification.
(Modified from Rowe, P. and Mandell, M. S. 2002. Perioperative hepatic dysfunction. In *Anesthesia Secrets*. Philadelphia: Hanley and Belfus, pp. 289–290; and Garg, R. K. 2005. Anesthetic considerations in patients with hepatic failure. *International Anesthesia Clinics*, 43(4): 45–63; Vacanti, C., Segal, S., Sikka, P., Urman, R. et al. 2011. *Essential Clinical Anesthesia*. Cambridge University Press, p. 50.)

status, whereas dementia is a progressive and usually permanent loss of cognitive function. Occurrence of critical illness polyneuropathy hinders weaning from the ventilator and results in prolonged rehabilitation.

Table 153.4 MOD scores

	Score				
Organ system	0	1	2	3	4
Respiratory: PaO_2/FiO_2	>300	226–300	151–225	76–150	≤75
Renal: creatinine (μmol/l)	≤100	101–200	201–350	251–500	>500
Hepatic bilirubin (μmol/l)	≤20	21–60	61–120	121–240	>240
Cardiovascular: PAR[a]	<10.0	10.1–15	15.1–200	20.1–30.0	>30.0
Hematologic: platelet count	>120	81–120	51–80	21–50	≤20
Neurologic: Glasgow Coma Scale score	15	13–14	10–12	7–9	≤6

[a] PAR (pressure-adjusted heart rate) is the product of the heart rate and the ratio of the right atrial pressure to the mean arterial pressure.
(Adapted from Marshall, J. C., Cook, D. J., Christou, N. V. et al. 1995. Multiple organ dysfunction score: a reliable descriptor of a complex clinical outcome. *Critical Care Medicine*, 23: 1638–1652; Vacanti, C., Segal, S., Sikka, P., Urman, R. et al. 2011. *Essential Clinical Anesthesia*. Cambridge University Press, p. 956.)

Hematopoietic system

Thrombocytopenia and elevation of prothrombin time (PT) and international normalized ratio (INR) are common during sepsis. Leukocytosis is common, but leukopenia can also be seen in severe sepsis.

The MOD score (Table 153.4) *and SOFA score* (Table 153.5) *are two scoring system designed to quantify multiorgan failure.* Both scores correlate with survival. The SOFA score looks at the most abnormal value over a 24-hour period whereas the MOD score looks at values at the same time point each day.

Systemic inflammatory response syndrome (SIRS)

SIRS is a *common cause of organ failure*, defined as two or more of the following:

- temperature >38°C or <36°C
- heart rate >90 beats per minute
- respiratory rate >20 breaths per minute or $PaCO_2$ <32 mm Hg
- white blood cell count >12,000 cells/mm^3 or <4,000 cells/mm^3 or >10% bands

Conditions associated with SIRS and MOF

Sepsis, burns, pancreatitis, cardiac arrest, congestive heart failure, gastrointestinal bleeding, surgery, inadequate resuscitation, persistent inflammation, prior organ dysfunction, steroid use, and chronic comorbidities.

Table 153.5 SOFA scores

Organ system	Score				
	0	1	2	3	4
Respiratory: PaO$_2$/FiO$_2$	400	≤400	≤300	≤200	≤100
Renal: creatinine (μmol/l)	≤110	101–170	171–299	300–440; urine output ≤500 ml/d	>440; urine output <200
Hepatic bilirubin (μmol/l)	≤20	20–32	33–101	102–204	>240
Cardiovascular: hypotension	No hypotension	MAP <70 mm Hg	Dopamine ≤5[a] or dobutamine (any dose)	Dopamine >5[a] or epinephrine ≤0.1[a] or norepinephrine ≤0.1[a]	Dopamine >15[a] or epinephrine >0.1[a] or norepinephrine >01[a]
Hematologic: platelet count	150	≤150	≤100	≤50	≤20
Neurologic: Glasgow Coma Scale score	15	13–14	10–12	7–9	<6

[a] Adrenergic agents administered for at least h (doses given are in μg/kg/min). MAP. mean arterial pressure.
(Vacanti, C., Segal, S., Sikka, P., Urman, R. et al. 2011. *Essential Clinical Anesthesia*. Cambridge University Press, p. 957.)

Surgical procedures associated with SIRS and MOF

Surgery for head trauma, elective abdominal aortic aneurysm repair, aortic dissection or rupture, cardiac surgery involving cardiopulmonary bypass, and gastrointestinal surgery for perforation, inflammatory disease, or carcinoma.

Since SIRS is most likely a result of sepsis, the prevention of MOF can best be achieved by early, evidence-based management of underlying infection. Key steps include early administration of empiric broad spectrum antibiotics, elimination of the infectious source, and appropriate fluid resuscitation.

For ARDS, low tidal volume ventilation (6 to 8 ml/kg based on ideal body weight), with permissive hypercapnia if necessary, and maintaining airway plateau pressures less than 30 cm H$_2$O have been shown to decrease mortality.

Questions

1. Which of the following is not a component of the Child–Turcotte–Pugh classification of liver failure?
   a. creatinine
   b. serum albumin
   c. serum bilirubin
   d. presence of ascites

2. Which of the following meets one of the criteria of the systemic inflammatory response syndrome (SIRS)?
   a. heart rate of 40
   b. temperature of 36.1°C
   c. white blood cell count of 11,000 cells/mm^3
   d. respiratory rate of 24 breaths/min

Answers

1. a. The Child–Turcotte–Pugh classification of liver failure includes scoring of bilirubin, albumin, prothrombin time, ascites, and encephalopathy.

2. d. SIRS is defined as two or more of the following: temperature >38°C or <36°C, heart rate >90 beats per minute, respiratory rate >20 breaths per minute, PaCO$_2$ <32 mm Hg and white blood cell count >12,000 cells/mm^3 or <4,000 cells/mm^3 or >10% bands.

Further reading

Vacanti, C. A., Sikka, P. K., Urman, R. U., Dershwitz, M., and Segal, B. S. eds. (2011). *Essential Clinical Anesthesia*. New York, NY: Cambridge University Press, pp. 955–959.

ARDS Definition Task Force. (2012). Acute respiratory distress syndrome: the Berlin Definition. *Journal of the American Medical Association* 307(23), 2526–2533.

Rivers, E., Nguyen, B., Havstad, S. et al. (2001). Early goal-directed therapy in the treatment of severe sepsis and septic shock. *New England Journal of Medicine* 345, 1368–1377.

Dellinger, R., Levy, M., Rhodes, A. et al. (2013). Surviving sepsis campaign: international guidelines for management of severe sepsis and septic shock: 2012. *Critical Care Medicine* 41(2), 580–637.

Supraventricular arrhythmias

Timothy D. Quinn and Sujatha Pentakota

Keywords

Common supraventricular tachyarrhythmias: irregular and regular

Atrial fibrillation: clinical implications and risk factors

Acute intraoperative atrial fibrillation in mitral stenosis: treatment

Postoperative atrial fibrillation

Stable atrial fibrillation: management

Atrial flutter

Multifocal atrial tachycardia

Sinus tachycardia

Atrioventricular nodal reciprocating tachycardia (AVNRT)

Atrioventricular reentry tachycardia (AVRT)

Wolff–Parkinson–White (WPW): definition

Supraventricular tachyarrhythmias: management

Supraventricular tachyarrhythmias (SVT) originate above the His bundle and usually result in a narrow-complex QRS (<0.12 s); however, a wide-complex QRS (>0.12 s) SVT can be seen with aberrant conduction into the ventricles via accessory bundles and rate-responsive bundle blocks.

Irregular supraventricular tachyarrhythmias include atrial fibrillation, atrial flutter with variable atrioventricular block, and multifocal atrial tachycardia (MAT).

Regular supraventricular tachyarrhythmias include sinus tachycardia, atrial flutter with consistent atrioventricular block (e.g., 2:1, 3:1), atrioventricular nodal reciprocating tachycardia (AVNRT), and atrioventricular reentry tachycardia (AVRT).

Figure 154.1 below depicts the mechanism of common pathologic *supraventricular tachyarrhythmias*.

Atrial fibrillation is caused by multiple activation foci in the atria with absence of P waves and irregularly spaced QRS complexes. The ventricular rate depends on the conduction of the irregular atrial depolarizations across the AV node and through the His bundle. It is the *most common* dysrhythmia in the surgical ICU.

Risk factors for atrial fibrillation include electrolyte disturbances (hypokalemia, hypomagnesemia), hyperadrenergic state, beta-adrenergic drugs such as dopamine, withdrawal of beta-blockade, atrial manipulation (cardiac or thoracic surgery), COPD, obesity, atrial enlargement (e.g., mitral stenosis), advanced age, and valvular surgery.

Atrial fibrillation may lead to significant *hypotension* if the ventricular rate is too rapid for adequate filling or if the patient relies on an "atrial kick" to maintain cardiac output. An organized atrial contraction is required to fill the stiff ventricles and provide adequate stroke volume in patients with ventricular hypertrophy or with diastolic dysfunction.

Acute intraoperative atrial fibrillation in mitral stenosis is particularly problematic, especially at high ventricular rates, as the time for diastolic filling is reduced even further from baseline. The goal is to control tachycardia by using beta-blockers or calcium channel blockers. If the patient is unstable, synchronized electrical cardioversion should be performed.

Prevention of *postoperative atrial fibrillation* is best achieved with *perioperative beta-blocker therapy*, with the most benefit seen in high-risk patients undergoing high-risk surgery.

Stable atrial fibrillation is managed with a combination of rate control with rhythm conversion and/or anticoagulation. Rate control is usually achieved with a beta-blocker (e.g., metoprolol) or calcium antagonist (e.g., diltiazem). Converting atrial fibrillation to sinus rhythm can be achieved either chemically (e.g., amiodarone) or by synchronized electrical cardioversion.

The *risk of stroke is increased* when patients convert to sinus rhythm 48 hours after the onset of atrial fibrillation. Thrombi are prone to form in the atria due to stasis and may embolize to the systemic or pulmonary circulation when sinus rhythm is restored. *Three weeks of full anticoagulation therapy is required before chemical or electrical conversion can be attempted.* Alternatively, transesophageal echocardiography (TEE) is a highly effective technique to identify clots in the atria, especially at the left atrial appendage, prior to

Essential Clinical Anesthesia Review: Keywords, Questions and Answers for the Boards, ed. Linda S. Aglio, Robert W. Lekowski, and Richard D. Urman. Published by Cambridge University Press. © Cambridge University Press 2015.

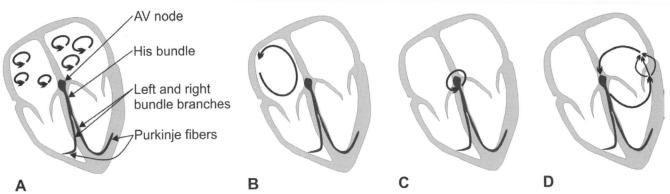

Figure 154.1 Simplified mechanisms of common supraventricular tachycardias. (A) AF is caused by multiple reentry wavelets that provide high-frequency impulses to the atrioventricular (AV) node that are conducted in an erratic fashion. (B) Atrial flutter is caused by a larger reentry circuit within the atrium that provides impulses to the AV node at a rate of approximately 300 beats per minute. Conduction is often regular and limited by a 2:1 or 3:1 blockade due to the refractory period of the AV node. (C) AV nodal reciprocating tachycardia (AVNRT) is entertained by two pathways within the AV node that have different refractory periods and conduction velocities. One premature atrial contraction can suddenly initiate this circular pattern of activation (paroxysmal tachycardia), thus activating the ventricles in a rapid regular fashion. (D) AV reentry tachycardia (AVRT) requires an accessory pathway through which excitation can be conducted back to the AV node. Anterograde conduction through the AV node and then circling back through the accessory pathway causes a regular tachycardia with a narrow QRS. Alternatively, conduction may proceed down the accessory pathway first and return retrogradely through the AV node causing a wide-complex tachycardia. (Adapted from Vacanti et al. 2011. *Essential Clinical Anesthesia*, Cambridge University Press, p. 961.)

cardioversion. However, cardioversion should not be delayed in the presence of cardiovascular collapse.

Atrial flutter results from a macro-reentry phenomenon with an excitatory wavefront circling through the right atrium. The ventricular rate may appear regular as the AV node blocks conduction of every second (2:1) or third (3:1) atrial beat. The EKG tracing has the characteristic "saw-tooth" pattern with a lack of P waves. Usually, the atrial rate is 300 beats per minute and the ventricular rate is 150 beats per minute.

Multifocal atrial tachycardia (MAT) (wandering atrial pacemaker) is uncommon and mostly seen in the critically ill patient with electrolyte abnormalities or COPD. By definition, multifocal atrial tachycardia should have at least three distinctly different P wave morphologies and a ventricular rate of greater than 100 beats per minute.

Sinus tachycardia is defined as a regular heart rate greater than 100 beats per minute in an adult with presence of P wave on EKG. It is typically not pathologic. Common causes are pain, anxiety, fever, and intravascular volume depletion.

In *atrioventricular nodal reciprocating tachycardia (AVNRT)*, there are two distinct electrical pathways in the AV node. One has a short refractory period and slow conduction and the other has a longer refractory period with faster conduction. An irregular atrial contraction (e.g., premature atrial contraction) can activate the slow pathway if the fast pathway is still in the refractory period. The impulse then *circles around the AV node* and activates the fast pathway causing tachycardia in the 140 to 250 beats per minute range. Generally, the QRS complex is normal in contour and duration, and P waves are buried in the QRS complex.

Atrioventricular reentry tachycardia (AVRT) has a normal AV node and a separate accessory pathway between the atria and ventricles. Both pathways can conduct in either direction. In *orthodromic AVRT*, the electrical impulse travels down the AV node as usual; however, it returns to the atria via the accessory pathway and forms a loop back through the AV node. The QRS complex is narrow as conduction is through the His bundle. In *antidromic AVRT*, the impulse travels from the atria to the ventricles via the accessory pathway and returns to the atria by retrograde conduction though the AV node. The QRS complex is wide because the His bundle is not utilized.

If the patient has anterograde conduction through an accessory pathway at a normal heart rate, the upstroke of the QRS complex may be slurred, resulting in a *delta wave. A delta wave combined with a short PR interval is Wolff–Parkinson–White (WPW)*. In WPW, AV nodal blocking drugs such as calcium antagonists and beta-blockers should be avoided, as they can increase conduction through the accessory pathway, leading to unstable tachyarrhythmias.

The *management of supraventricular tachyarrhythmias* is targeted at either stimulating vagal parasympathetic tone to the AV node (e.g., carotid massage) or blocking AV nodal conduction (e.g., metoprolol). *If the patient is hemodynamically unstable, synchronized electrical cardioversion is the most appropriate therapy.*

Questions

1. A patient is in atrial fibrillation with a ventricular rate of 170, a blood pressure of 70/40, and altered mental status. What is the most appropriate next step in management?

   a. diltiazem infusion with bolus

   b. adenosine 6 mg IV push

   c. electrical cardioversion

   d. amiodarone 150 mg IV loading dose

2. In which of the following supraventricular tachycardias is the site of abnormal conduction contained within the AV node?

   a. atrial fibrillation
   b. atrioventricular nodal reciprocating tachycardia
   c. multifocal atrial tachycardia
   d. sinus tachycardia

3. Which of the following is a contraindication to carotid massage for a supraventricular tachycardia?

   a. carotid stenosis
   b. recurrent laryngeal nerve injury
   c. left ventricular hypertrophy
   d. concomitant beta-blocker therapy

Answers

1. c. If the patient demonstrates signs of instability (e.g., hypotension, altered mental status, impaired end-organ perfusion, etc.) the most appropriate next step is synchronized cardioversion. It is important to synchronize to reduce the possibility of an R on T phenomenon, whereby the electrical stimulus occurs during the heart's refractory period and can potentially lead to a ventricular arrhythmia.

2. b. In atrioventricular nodal reciprocating tachycardia (AVNRT), there are two distinct electrical pathways in the AV node. The other three choices originate in the atria above the AV node.

3. a. Carotid massage in the setting of carotid stenosis can potentially dislodge plaque or debris into the cerebral circulation leading to a transient ischemic attack or stroke.

Further reading

Vacanti, C. A., Sikka, P. K., Urman, R. U., Dershwitz, M., and Segal, B. S. (eds) (2011). *Essential Clinical Anesthesia*. New York, NY: Cambridge University Press, pp. 960–965.

Link, M. (2012). Evaluation and initial treatment of supraventricular tachycardia. *New England Journal of Medicine* 367(15), 1438–1448.

155

Cardiac failure in the intensive care unit

Krishna Parekh and David Silver

Keywords

Cardiogenic shock
Myocardial oxygen consumption
Intra-aortic balloon counterpulsation
Pulmonary artery catheter
NIPPV
Diuretics
Volume overload
Vasodilators
Inotropes

Cardiogenic shock is the decrease in oxygen delivery to tissue due to a reduction in cardiac output. This is distinct from other shock states in which peripheral tissue hypoxia occurs despite an increase in cardiac output. In addition to a reduction in cardiac output, cardiogenic shock also results in an increase in systemic vascular resistance and pulmonary congestion. Etiologies of cardiogenic shock may include myocardial ischemia, valvular disease, arrhythmias, congenital cardiac defects, and non-ischemic cardiomyopathy.

Myocardial oxygen consumption increases with increased ventricular filling pressures (preload), increased heart rate, and increased afterload. Ino- and chronotropic agents used to augment end-organ perfusion can additionally increase myocardial oxygen consumption. *Diuretics* and *vasodilators* can be useful in this situation to reduce myocardial ischemia. In the setting of ischemic cardiogenic shock, tissue perfusion can be restored with PCI or CABG.

Intra-aortic balloon counterpulsation (IABP) therapy reduces myocardial oxygen consumption while increasing coronary perfusion and cardiac output. It has not, however, been shown to reduce mortality in patients with acute ischemic cardiogenic shock in whom early revascularization is planned. It can also be used to support circulation in patients being weaned from cardiopulmonary bypass. The balloon is inflated during diastole, resulting in increased coronary perfusion, and deflated during systole, reducing afterload and improving cardiac output. Contraindications to IABP placement include aortic valve insufficiency and aortic pathology (severe atherosclerosis, dissection, aneurysm).

Central venous lines may be used to measure central venous pressure (CVP), and thus to approximate right ventricular end-diastolic pressure, RVEDP. *Pulmonary artery catheters (PAC)* may measure CVP, cardiac output, pulmonary artery occlusion pressure (usually consistent with left ventricular end-diastolic pressure, LVEDP), and mixed venous oxygen saturation. These data have historically been used to guide fluid, inotrope, and vasopressor management. However, evidence increasingly suggests that while PAC use is associated with an increased number of interventions, patient outcomes are not improved, and may be worse. As a result, PAC use has declined dramatically over the past decade, and in many institutions has been entirely replaced by echocardiography and by various commercially available noninvasive cardiac output monitors.

Noninvasive positive pressure ventilation, NIPPV (continuous positive airway pressure [CPAP] or bilevel positive airway pressure [BiPAP™]) provide effective short-term support of ventilation and oxygenation in acute respiratory insufficiency, as with pulmonary edema secondary to congestive heart failure. However, patients on NIPPV have a significant risk of pulmonary aspiration. If aspiration risk is a particular concern, or if oxygenation or ventilation remain inadequate following institution of NIPPV, the patient should be intubated in a timely manner.

Diuretics can be used to reduce symptoms of *volume overload*, and reduce LVEDP. Electrolytes must be closely monitored.

Nitroglycerin is a vasodilator that produces venodilation > arteriodilation. The physiologic result of nitroglycerin administration includes decreased preload and LVEDP, decreased ventricular wall tension, and improved myocardial perfusion (via dilation of the coronary arteries).

Sodium nitroprusside is another vasodilator that produces both venous and arterial dilation. Its administration can be associated with the development of *methemoglobinemia and cyanide toxicity*. Patients who develop tachyphylaxis to nitroprusside or a new metabolic acidosis should be monitored closely for cyanide toxicity.

Essential Clinical Anesthesia Review: Keywords, Questions and Answers for the Boards, ed. Linda S. Aglio, Robert W. Lekowski, and Richard D. Urman. Published by Cambridge University Press. © Cambridge University Press 2015.

Dobutamine and *milrinone* are inodilators, which augment cardiac contractility, but may cause hypotension via vasodilation. *Epinephrine* increases heart rate and contractility via β effects, but also increases systemic vascular resistance via α receptor agonism. All inotropic agents may increase myocardial oxygen demand, which can exacerbate ischemia and arrhythmias.

Questions

1. Which of the following vasodilators is associated with cyanide toxicity?

   a. nitroglycerin
   b. nitroprusside
   c. sildenafil
   d. hydralazine
   e. labetalol

2. Cardiogenic shock results in which of the following hemodynamic changes?

   a. increased LVEDP, decreased CO, decreased SVR
   b. increased LVEDP, increased CO, increased SVR
   c. increased LVEDP, decreased CO, increased SVR
   d. decreased LVEDP, decreased CO, decreased SVR
   e. decreased LVEDP, decreased CO, increased SVR

3. Pulmonary artery catheters may provide all of the following information EXCEPT for which?

   a. temperature
   b. cardiac output
   c. mixed venous saturation
   d. systemic vascular resistance
   e. systolic blood pressure

4. Myocardial oxygen consumption is decreased by which of the following?

   a. milrinone
   b. IV fluid bolus
   c. vasopressin
   d. dobutamine
   e. intra-aortic balloon pump

Answers

1. b.
2. c.
3. e.
4. e.

Further reading

Theiele, H., Zymer, U., and Neumann, F-J. et al. (2012). Intraaortic balloon support for myocardial infarction with cardiogenic shock. *New England Journal of Medicine* 367, 1287–1296.

Sandham, J. D., Hull, R. D., Brant, R. F. et al. (2003). A randomized, controlled trial of the use of pulmonary-artery catheters in high-risk surgical patients. *New England Journal of Medicine* 348, 5–14.

Chapter

156

Sedation in the surgical intensive care unit

Krishna Parekh and David Silver

Keywords

Sedation holidays
Sedation scales
Delirium
Analgesia
Opioids
Propofol
Benzodiazepine
Propofol infusion syndrome
Dexmedetomidine

Sedation of critically ill patients must balance patient comfort (synchrony with the ventilator, tolerance of tracheal tubes/catheters/drains, and anxiolysis) and the achievement of overall goals of care (decreased ventilator and ICU time, decreased morbidity and mortality). *Sedation holidays*, which generally entail a nurse-driven protocol of daily sedation lightening, are used in ICUs to this end. *Sedation scales* in the ICU, such as the Richmond Agitation Sedation Scale (RASS), Ramsay, and the modified Glasgow Coma Scale, may help avoid oversedation.

Sedative-hypnotics, such as *propofol*, and *benzodiazepines*, such as midazolam and lorazepam, are most commonly used to provide sedation to critically ill patients. Both propofol and benzodiazepines are GABA receptor agonists and may be deliriogenic. *Propofol infusion syndrome* is a rare but serious complication first described in children, which includes refractory bradycardia, renal failure, rhabdomyolysis, hyperlipidemia, and metabolic acidosis. Patients at risk include those receiving 4 mg/kg/h for over 48 h. *Lorazepam toxicity* can occur due to the preparation of the injectable form in propylene glycol, accumulation of which results in an anion gap metabolic acidosis.

The alpha2-adrenergic receptor agonist *dexmedetomidine* provides anxiolysis and analgesia without causing respiratory depression, and is nondeliriogenic. Dexmedetomidine is not yet available in a generic form, and is quite expensive compared with alternative drugs.

Adequacy of sedation should be closely monitored in patients receiving neuromuscular blockade, and amnestics (such as propofol or midazolam) should be administered to ensure the patient is not awake and paralyzed.

In recent years, a dramatic change in the approach to ICU sedation has led to most (nonparalyzed) patients receiving little or no sedation. This is very well tolerated, and leads to reduced delirium and improved long-term outcomes. Patients should continue to receive analgesics as needed, especially after undergoing surgical procedures.

Delirium occurs commonly in ICU patients, and is identified by the acute onset of waxing and waning levels of consciousness and cognition. The *CAM-ICU* questionnaire has been identified as a useful tool for diagnosing delirium in the ICU. Delirium is associated with an increase in morbidity and mortality. Treatment of delirium includes avoidance of causative medications (opioids, benzodiazepines, and most other sedatives), frequent reorientation and establishment of normal sleep–wake cycles, and the use of antipsychotic medications such as *haloperidol*.

Analgesia is critical in the management of ICU patients, for both acute and chronic pain. Regional anesthesia, including neuraxial and peripheral nerve blocks, can be used in appropriate patient populations. Infused or injected regional medications may include local anesthetics, opioids, or a combination of the two.

Opioids (commonly fentanyl, morphine, or hydromorphone) may be provided enterally or parenterally, using intermittent dosing, continuous infusions, or patient-controlled analgesia (PCA) techniques. Continuous infusions should be limited to carefully monitored patients and to those who are significantly opioid-tolerant. The *visual analog scale* (VAS) is a subjective tool used to quantify pain and assess adequacy of pain management.

Questions

1. Delirium in the ICU can be treated with which of the following?
   a. propofol
   b. morphine

Essential Clinical Anesthesia Review: Keywords, Questions and Answers for the Boards, ed. Linda S. Aglio, Robert W. Lekowski, and Richard D. Urman. Published by Cambridge University Press. © Cambridge University Press 2015.

c. dexmedetomidine

d. haloperidol

e. midazolam

2. Propofol infusion syndrome is associated with all of the following EXCEPT for which?

a. tachycardia

b. renal failure

c. metabolic acidosis

d. hyperlipidemia

e. rhabdomyolysis

Answers

1. d.

2. a.

Further reading

Barash, P. G., Cullen, B. F., Stoelting, R. K. et al. (2009). *Clinical Anesthesia*, 6th edn. Philadelphia, PA: Lippincott Williams & Wilkins.

Vacanti, C. A., Sikka, P. K., Urman, R. U., Dershwitz, M., and Segal, B. S. (eds) (2011). *Essential Clinical Anesthesia*. New York, NY: Cambridge University Press.

Longnecker, D. E., Brown, D. L., Newman, M. F., and Zapol, W. M. (2012). *Anesthesiology*, 2nd edn. McGraw-Hill.

Chapter

157 Weaning from mechanical ventilation

Marc Philip T. Pimentel and James H. Philip

Keywords

Rapid shallow breathing index (RSBI)
Spontaneous breathing trial (SBT)
Pressure support ventilation (PSV)
Synchronized intermittent mandatory
    ventilation (SIMV)
Tube compensation
Proportional assist
Mandatory minute ventilation
Airway pressure release ventilation
Pressure-regulated volume control and/or volume
    support

Patients in the intensive care unit often require mechanical ventilation, and the process of weaning the patient from the ventilator can be protracted. No single parameter is best for guiding the weaning process. Taken individually, minute ventilation, vital capacity, maximum inspiratory pressure, and even arterial blood gas measurements are unreliable for weaning patients from the ventilator. One of the more widely used measures is the *rapid shallow breathing index* (RSBI), which is the ratio of the respiratory rate to the tidal volume (breaths per minute, per liter of tidal volume). Patients with an RSBI less than 105 breaths/min/l tend to be more successful when weaning from the ventilator. Nevertheless, the patient's overall clinical picture is most helpful to predict successful ventilator weaning.

Weaning strategies should be tailored to each patient's individual clinical needs. In general, the amount of mechanical ventilation is reduced until the patient is able to tolerate breathing without the ventilator, or with minimal support. A *spontaneous breathing trial* (SBT) is recommended to assess readiness for extubation. During an SBT the patient is connected to a fresh gas source but ventilation is unassisted. Patients who are able to tolerate a 2 hour SBT should be considered for extubation. Other factors to consider before extubation include the following: reversal of the reason for

needing mechanical ventilation, adequate oxygenation, hemodynamic stability, and reasonable inspiratory effort.

Certain modes of ventilation may be more suitable or more tolerable for different patients. *Pressure support ventilation (PSV)* reduces the work of breathing by assisting each patient-initiated breath with a specified inspiratory pressure. Patients must have consistent respiratory rates and tidal volumes for weaning by *PSV. Synchronized intermittent mandatory ventilation (SIMV)* delivers baseline minute ventilation and also allows for patient-initiated breaths. SIMV is ineffective as a weaning mode in the ICU and is associated with ventilatory dyssynchrony and respiratory muscle fatigue, although it is used in the OR.

Other, less common modes of ventilation may also be useful during the weaning process. *Tube compensation* reduces the work of breathing by providing flow to overcome the

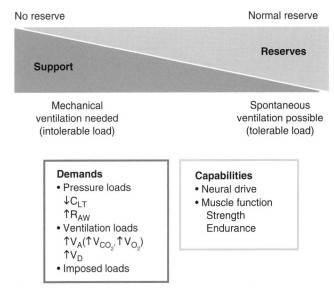

Figure 157.1 Determinants of need for mechanical ventilatory support. (Adapted from Vacanti et al. 2011. *Essential Clinical Anesthesia*, Cambridge University Press, Figure 158.1.)

Table 157.1 Nonrespiratory factors in weaning patients from mechanical ventilation

Category	Factor	Mechanism	Clinical presentation
Cardiac status	Acute left ventricular failure	Increased preload because of increased venous return and decreased pulmonary capillary compression as intrathoracic pressure is reduced	Patient fails weaning, often after initially doing well for 30 to 60 minutes; may develop acute respiratory and/or metabolic acidosis, hypoxemia, hypotension, chest pain, and cardiac dysrhythmias
Acid–base status	Acute alkalosis in patient with underlying carbon dioxide (CO_2) retention	Loss of preexisting metabolic compensation for hypercapnia; inability to sustain required V_E and WOB	Patient with COPD or other cause of chronic respiratory acidosis before acute insult fails weaning after several days of ventilation to a PCO_2 lower than the patient's pH-compensated level
	Respiratory alkalosis	Depression of ventilatory drives by hypocapnia and alkalemia	PCO_2 rises and pH falls during weaning attempt; patient is said to fail weaning if some arbitrary change in these values (e.g., 10 mm Hg increase in PCO_2) is used as a criterion for failure
	Metabolic acidosis	Increase in ventilatory demand to compensate for respiratory alkalosis	Patient may be unable to sustain required increase in V_E and WOB to maintain a lower PCO_2 to compensate for a lower HCO_3^-
Metabolic status	Hypophosphatemia and hypomagnesemia	Ventilatory muscle weakness	Patient fails weaning because of rapid shallow breathing, respiratory distress, and acute respiratory acidosis; maximal inspiratory pressure is decreased
	Hypothyroidism	Decreased ventilatory drive with possible ventilatory muscle weakness	Rare cause of weaning failure that occurs because of acute respiratory distress
Drugs	Narcotics, sedatives, tranquilizers, and hypnotics	Depression of ventilatory drive	Patient fails weaning because of acute respiratory acidosis in the absence of tachypnea and respiratory distress
	Neuromuscular blocking agents	Ventilatory muscle weakness; delayed clearance in patient with renal insufficiency	Patient fails weaning because of rapid shallow breathing, respiratory distress, and acute respiratory acidosis; maximal inspiratory pressure is reduced
		Ventilatory muscle weakness caused by acute myopathy, especially in patients who have received high-dose systemic corticosteroids	Same as above; may have elevated muscle enzymes; can last for weeks or months
	Aminoglycosides	Neuromuscular blockade	Very rare cause of weaning failure that occurs because of rapid shallow breathing, respiratory distress, and acute respiratory acidosis; maximal inspiratory force is reduced
Nutrition	Overfeeding	Increased CO_2 production, especially with excessive carbohydrate calories	Patient fails weaning because of excessive ventilatory demand (high V_E requirement to keep PCO_2 normal); unusual cause of weaning failure unless very large caloric loads are administered
	Malnutrition	Effects of acute illness; preexisting nutritional deficiencies	May contribute to ventilatory muscle weakness, decreased ventilatory drive, impaired immunologic function, fluid retention, depression; distinguishing this from other factors is difficult
Psychological status	Agitation: "psychological ventilator dependence"	Anxiety, fear, delirium, ICU psychosis, or influence of preexisting personality factors	Patient becomes agitated and panicky during attempt to reduce or discontinue ventilatory support; can be said to cause weaning failure when other factors are absent

Table 157.1 (cont.)

Category	Factor	Mechanism	Clinical presentation
	Lack of motivation	Depression, effects of drugs, organic brain dysfunction, or influence of preexisting personality factors	Patient refuses to participate in care (e.g., mobilization, bronchial hygiene, physiologic measurements); flat affect and immobility in bed; considered when other factors are absent

V_E, minute ventilation; WOB, work of breathing; PCO_2, partial pressure of carbon dioxide; pH, hydrogen ion concentration; HCO_3^-, bicarbonate. (Adapted from Pilbeam, S. P. and Cairo, J. M. 2006. *Mechanical Ventilation: Physiological and Clinical Applications*, 4th edn. Philadelphia: Mosby Publications, pp. 461–462; Vacanti, C. A., Segal, B. S., Sikka, P. K., et al. 2011. *Essential Clinical Anesthesia*. New York: Cambridge University Press, Table 158.2.)

resistance of the airway device. *Proportional assist* allows the ventilator to measure the patient's effort and change the level of assistance accordingly. *Mandatory minute ventilation* decreases assistance when the patient meets a minute ventilation threshold. *Airway pressure release ventilation* maximizes alveolar recruitment by keeping lungs inflated at a high pressure, with only a short period for exhalation. *Pressure-regulated volume control* delivers a pressure-controlled breath based on previous breaths, in order to meet a tidal volume goal, which may produce larger tidal volumes at lower peak pressures.

Questions

1. A patient recovering from MRSA pneumonia is being weaned on PSV (inspiratory pressure 5 cm H_2O, PEEP 5 cm H_2O), resulting in tidal volumes of 600 ml at 15 breaths per minute. Based on the RSBI, is the patient appropriate for a spontaneous breathing trial?
   a. No, because RSBI is <100.
   b. No, because RSBI is >100.
   c. Yes, because RSBI is <100.
   d. Yes, because RSBI is >100.

2. A patient with severe ARDS requires substantial PEEP of 20 cm H_2O to maintain a PaO_2 of 60 mm Hg. Overnight, the PEEP requirement increases to 30 cm H_2O. The patient is then noted to have worsening hypotension with blood pressure 66/34 and heart rate 150 beats per minute. Jugular venous distension is noted. Lung sounds are absent in the left lung field. What should the next few steps include?
   a. pressors for worsening pneumonia
   b. chest tube placement for tension pneumothorax
   c. chest radiograph for endobronchial tube position
   d. echocardiogram for left heart failure

3. A 65-year-old man with resolving community-acquired pneumonia is being weaned from the ventilator on PSV (inspiratory pressure 5 cm H_2O, PEEP 5 cm H_2O). His ABG shows pH 7.32, PCO_2 50 mm Hg, and PO_2 34 mm Hg. Tidal volume is 240 ml with respiratory rate 24 breaths per minute. What should be the next step?
   a. nothing, Extubate the patient
   b. increase inspiratory pressure and PEEP
   c. increase inspiratory pressure and decrease PEEP
   d. decrease inspiratory pressure and increase PEEP

Answers

1. c. The RSBI in this patient is calculated as follows: 15 breaths per minute/0.6 l tidal volume = 25. An RSBI under 105 suggests that the patient is appropriate for weaning from the ventilator.

2. b. The excessive application of PEEP can lead to pulmonary barotrauma and tension pneumothorax. High intrathoracic pressures from the PEEP and a building tension pneumothorax lead to a decrease in venous return to the heart and hypotension with tachycardia. The treatment for tension pneumothorax includes timely decompression with a chest tube.

3. b. The patient's ABG indicates respiratory acidosis with hypoxemia. Increasing the inspiratory pressure may improve the patient's ventilation, and increased PEEP may relieve the patient's hypoxemia.

Further reading

MacIntyre, N. (2007). Discontinuing mechanical ventilatory support. *Chest* 132(3), 1049–1056.

MacIntyre, N. (2005) Respiratory mechanics in the patient who is weaning from the ventilator. *Respiratory Care* 50(2), 275–286.

Chapter

158

Acute lung injury and acute respiratory distress syndrome

Beverly Chang and Gyorgy Frendl

Keywords

Acute lung injury (ALI)
Acute respiratory distress syndrome (ARDS)
Low tidal volume ventilation

ARDS is a spectrum of respiratory failure states that form as a reaction to a primary insult to the body. These are *diagnoses of exclusion*. These states are characterized by *acute, diffuse lung inflammation* leading to *increased pulmonary vascular permeability* and decreased area available for gas exchange.

Up to 10% to 20% of patients in the ICU meet the criteria for ARDS. Early mortality is usually due to the underlying cause of ARDS; late mortality commonly due to nosocomial pneumonia and sepsis. In 2012, under the new Berlin definition, the term "acute lung injury" was taken out of the definition and replaced by mild ARDS.

Clinical symptoms

- *acute* symptoms present within *seven days* after an inciting event
- dyspnea, respiratory distress
- hypoxemia
- decreased breath sounds, crackles on examination

Definitions
Acute Respiratory Distress Syndrome (ARDS)

- *PaO_2/FiO_2 ≤300.*

or

- *SpO_2/FiO_2 (S/F ratio) ≤235.*
- *Bilateral infiltrates on CXR.*
- Under the new definition, heart failure no longer needs to be excluded, as these patients can still have lung injury. The new criteria states that ARDS is respiratory failure not fully explained by cardiac failure or fluid overload.

Table 158.1 Severity of ARDS

ARDS severity	PaO_2/FiO_2	Mortality
Mild ARDS	200–300 mm Hg	27%
Moderate ARDS	100–200 mm Hg	32%
Severe ARDS	≤100 mm Hg	45%

Note: the PaO_2 is measured in mm Hg and the FiO_2 is expressed as a decimal between 0.21 and 1.

Pathophysiology

This is not a primary disease process but is the result of a reaction toward a direct or indirect insult to the lungs. This leads to systemic inflammation from the release of inflammatory mediators causing capillary and alveolar endothelium damage. There is protein extravasation into the lung parenchyma. As air spaces become filled with cellular debris, proteinous fluid and surfactant is lost. This leads to pulmonary edema, decreased area for gas exchange, decreased lung compliance, and increased pulmonary arterial pressure.

Oxygen delivery is determined by the following formula:

$$DO_2 = 10 \times CO \times (1.34 \times Hgb \times SaO_2 + 0.003 \times PaO_2)$$

Stages of lung injury

Exudative phase – this occurs during the first seven to ten days of presentation:

- early lung injury
- *inflammation* predominates
- characterized by a *protein-rich pulmonary edema*
- surfactant is inactivated
- widespread atelectasis
- elastases damage the framework of the lung
- procoagulant environment → capillary thrombosis
- some patients recover completely from this phase

Essential Clinical Anesthesia Review: Keywords, Questions and Answers for the Boards, ed. Linda S. Aglio, Robert W. Lekowski, and Richard D. Urman. Published by Cambridge University Press. © Cambridge University Press 2015.

Fibroproliferative phase – some patients recover after the exudative phase, others progress to this next stage of the disease:

- characterized by *chronic fibrosing alveolitis*
- increased alveolar dead space
- low lung compliance
- persistent hypoxemia
- if severe: pulmonary hypertension and right ventricular failure

Recovery phase:

- improvements in lung compliance and oxygenation
- pulmonary function may return to normal
- chest X-ray improves
- long-term recovery and prognosis vary between patients

Common causes

- *sepsis* is the most common cause
- aspiration – one-third of patients with clinical evidence of aspiration will develop ARDS
- pneumonia
- severe trauma
- massive transfusion = >15 units of packed RBC
- transfusion related acute lung injury – defined as respiratory distress within six hours after completion of transfusion of any blood product
- lung transplant and hematopoietic stem cell transplant
- drug and alcohol overdose
  - aspirin, cocaine, opioids, phenothiazines, and tricyclic antidepressants
- genetic determinants

Complications of ARDS

- barotrauma – can present as pneumothorax, less common with low tidal volume ventilation
- delirium
- nosocomial infection, especially ventilator-associated pneumonia (VAP)
  - loss of airway defenses (cough reflex, ciliary reflexes) due to endotracheal tube
  - pulmonary edema is a growth medium for bacteria
  - patients are usually somewhat immunosuppressed and malnourished
- DVT
- GI bleed due to stress ulcers
- poor nutrition

Treatment

Low tidal volume ventilation

This is based on the ARDSnet Trial published in May 2000 in the *New England Journal of Medicine*, which proposed the idea that smaller tidal volumes *prevent overdistension* of the alveoli in the remaining healthy parts of the lung. Patients were shown to have significantly *more ventilator-free days* and have increased chances of being *off the ventilator by day 28*. There was significant *reduction in nonpulmonary organ failure*.

Permissive hypercapnia is usually well tolerated and may be necessary in order to ventilate and oxygenate patients. Patients oftentimes need sedation and some even a brief (less than 48 h) muscle relaxation to improve oxygenation. Recent studies indicate that prone positioning may also benefit these patients.

Application:

1. Calculate ideal body weight.
2. Start with tidal volume (TV) of 8 ml/kg and set a rate that meets minute ventilation requirements.
3. Decrease TV to 6 ml/kg over next three hours.
4. Increase respiratory rate as TV increases.
5. Use a minimum of 5 of peak end-expiratory pressures (PEEP).
6. Wean the FiO_2 down to 40% by using PEEP to maximize oxygenation goals.
7. Check plateau pressure every four hours or with each change in PEEP with a goal of ≤30 cm H_2O.
8. Goal PaO_2 of 55–80, O_2 sat 88–95%.
9. Mode of ventilation does not matter; however, volume mode may ensure low tidal ventilation.

   - Use assist control over partially assisted modes.
10. Elevate head to prevent VAP.

Treat refractory hypoxemia by:

1. optimizing FiO2, PEEP
2. increasing I:E ratio

Paralysis

Neuromusclar blockers may be beneficial in patients with severe gas exchange abnormalities for short periods (<48 h). However, there is no strong data to indicate that it has mortality benefits. It may improve oxygenation but also cause undesirable effects such as prolonged weakness. These risks and benefits have to be considered when deciding whether to initiate paralytic agents or not.

Table 158.2 Calculation of ideal body weight

Male (kg) = 50 + 2.3 × (height in inches – 60)
Female (kg) = 45.5 + 2.3 × (height in inches – 60)

Table 158.3 FiO_2/PEEP combinations to achieve oxygenation goal of PaO_2 55–80 mm Hg or SpO_2 88–95%

FiO_2	0.3	0.4	0.5	0.6	0.7	0.8	0.9	1.0
PEEP	5	5 to 8	8 to 10	10	10 to 14	14	14 to 18	18 to 24

Esophageal balloon manometry

This can be used to calculate transpulmonary pressures (= airway pressure – pleural pressure).

This is used in instances where total airway pressures are high, to demonstrate that transpleural pressures are not dangerously elevated. Transpulmonary pressure can be adjusted by titrating PEEP to an end-expiratory transpulmonary pressure of 0 to 10 cm H_2O.

Other potential treatments (none have been shown to have mortality benefits):

- cyclic "sighs"
- use of chest weights or sandbags
- high-frequency oscillatory ventilation
- airway pressure release ventilation

Pharmacologic interventions

- The use of steroids remains controversial. Systemic steroids administered 14 days after onset of ARDS appears to be harmful. However, early steroid use requires further study:
  - ARDSnet investigators (2006) showed no mortality benefit with methylprednisolone
  - Meduri and colleagues (2007) showed reduction in ventilation time, ICU stay, and ICU mortality.
- Exogenous surfactant – no mortality benefit.
- Nitric oxide – no mortality benefit (for adult ARDS patients).
- Prostacyclin – not shown to improve outcomes.
- Antioxidants via dietary oil supplementation – conflicting evidence.
- Statins – may reduce proinflammatory mediators – does not improve outcomes.
- Macrolide antibiotics – antimicrobial and anti-inflammatory effects – need to be further studied.
- Beta-agonists – no direct benefits.

Fluid management

Conservative fluid management to minimize pulmonary edema has been shown to improve oxygenation and ventilator-free days, although no mortality benefit was seen. *Limit fluid intake as much as possible.*

Transfusion

Transfusion of packed RBC and other blood products are a recognized risk factor for the development of ALI/ARDS in critically ill patients (note TRALI: transfusion-related acute lung injury). Poor outcomes have been associated with aggressive transfusion strategies.

Monitoring

Pulmonary artery catheters are *not recommended*. The ARDS-net trial showed twice as many catheter-related complications and no outcome benefit in the pulmonary catheter group.

Nutritional support

ARDS patients are very catabolic. Enteral feedings are preferred.

Benefits of enteral feedings include fewer intravascular infections, less GI bleeding and maintenance of the intestinal mucosal barrier, and decreased bacterial translocation.

Avoid overfeeding to prevent excessive carbon dioxide production. The end-products of carbohydrate metabolism are ATP, CO_2, and water. This can lead to CO_2 retention and respiratory failure, or inability to wean from the ventilator.

Outcomes

Overall mortality is 30–50%. Cardiopulmonary function usually returns to normal within six months with normal lung volumes and PFT on six-month follow-up. Many survivors have *persistent neurocognitive and emotional deficits* after recovery that persist for years and result in decreased quality of life. Many complain of persistent muscle weakness, fatigue, and abnormal exercise endurance. Most patients are able to return to work.

Questions

1. A 55-year-old male presents to the ED with increasing shortness of breath five days after discharge from a cholecystectomy. Temp 102.2, HR 104, RR of 30, BP 87/50. ABG showed pH 7.32, CO_2 55, bicarbonate 20, and O_2 saturation of 93%. CXR showed bilateral pulmonary infiltrates. What is the most appropriate first action?
   a. start antibiotics
   b. start an IV and bolus fluids
   c. intubate the patient and initiate low tidal volume ventilation
   d. obtain cultures
   e. start the patient on BiPap

2. A 6-year-old 60 kg female presents to the ED with shortness of breath and hypoxia requiring intubation. After admission to the ICU, CXR showed bilateral infiltrates with pulmonary pleural effusion. ARDS is diagnosed. Which ventilator settings should be used?
   a. pressure support with 15 mm Hg
   b. volume control with tidal volumes of 360 ml and PEEP of 5 mm Hg
   c. pressure control with inspiratory pressures of 35 mm Hg with resulting TV of 600–700 ml
   d. hyperventilate patient to $PaCO_2$ of 30

3. Which is NOT in the definition of moderate ARDS?
   a. bilateral pulmonary infiltrates on CXR
   b. echo with LV hypertrophy and EF of 40%
   c. $PaO_2/FiO_2 \leq 200$
   d. SpO_2/FiO_2 (S/F ratio) ≤ 235

Answers

1. b. The first step should be to establish IV access and provide fluids to maintain hemodynamic stability. The next step is to obtain cultures and start antibiotics. Airway management should be determined by patient's clinical picture. If respiratory failure appears to be imminent, then patient should be intubated, otherwise a trial of BiPap can be used.

2. b. An ideal tidal volume of 6 ml/kg is approximately 360 ml for this patient. Either pressure control or volume control may be used; however, volume control may control tidal volumes more consistently.

3. b. Under the new guidelines, congestive heart failure does not need to be ruled out, as these patients can still have concurrent lung injury.

Further reading

Vacanti, C. A., Sikka, P. K., Urman, R. U., Dershwitz, M., and Segal, B. S. (eds) (2011). *Essential Clinical Anesthesia*. New York, NY: Cambridge University Press.

Hansen-Flaschen, J. and Siegel, M. (2013). Acute respiratory distress syndrome: clinical features and diagnosis. www.uptodate.com/contents/acute-respiratory-distress-syndrome-clinical-features-and-diagnosis.

Siegel, M.D. (2013). Acute respiratory distress syndrome: epidemiology; pathophysiology; pathology; and etiology. www.uptodate.com/contents/acute-respiratory-distress-syndrome-epidemiology-pathophysiology-pathology-and-etiology

Siegel, M.D. (2013). Supportive care and oxygenation in acute respiratory distress syndrome. www.uptodate.com/contents/supportive-care-and-oxygenation-in-acute-respiratory-distress-syndrome.

Siegel, M.D. (2013). Acute respiratory distress syndrome: prognosis and outcomes. www.uptodate.com/contents/acute-respiratory-distress-syndrome-prognosis-and-outcomes

Siegel, M.D. and Hyzy, R. C. (2013). Mechanical ventilation in acute respiratory distress syndrome. www.uptodate.com/contents/mechanical-ventilation-in-acute-respiratory-distress-syndrome

Siegel, M.D. (2013). Novel therapies for the acute respiratory distress syndrome. www.uptodate.com/contents/novel-therapies-for-the-acute-respiratory-distress-syndrome.

Sud, S., Friedrich, J. O., Taccone, P. et al. (2010). Prone ventilation reduces mortality in patients with acute respiratory failure and severe hypoxemia: systematic review and meta-analysis. *Intensive Care Medicine* 36, 585.

Ashbaugh, D. G., Bigelow, D. B., Petty, T. L., and Levine, B. E. (1967). Acute respiratory distress in adults. *Lancet* 2, 319.

Bernard, G. R., Artigas, A., Brigham, K. L. et al. (1994). The American-European Consensus Conference on ARDS. Definitions, mechanisms, relevant outcomes, and clinical trial coordination. *American Journal of Respiratory Critical Care Medicine* 149, 818.

Artigas, A., Bernard, G. R., Carlet, J. et al. (1998). The American-European Consensus Conference on ARDS, part 2. Ventilatory, pharmacologic, supportive therapy, study design strategies, and issues related to recovery and remodeling. Acute respiratory distress syndrome. *American Journal of Respiratory Critical Care Medicine* 157, 1332.

Rubenfeld, G. D., Caldwell, E., Peabody, E. et al. (2005). Incidence and outcomes of acute lung injury. *New England Journal of Medicine* 353, 1685.

Chapter 159

Nosocomial infections

Beverly Chang and Gyorgy Frendl

Keywords

Nosocomial infections
Ventilator-associated pneumonia
Catheter-related bloodstream infections

Nosocomial infections, or *health care-associated infections,* are infections acquired in acute or chronic health care settings (hospitals, rehabilitation or chronic care facilities). These infections significantly increase the cost and duration of hospital care and are all *preventable.*

The two most serious are (1) ventilator-associated pneumonia (VAP) and (2) catheter-related bloodstream infections (CRBSI). Others include urinary tract infections and wound infections.

Ventilator-associated pneumonia
Incidence

- **5–20%** of mechanically ventilated patients develop VAP.
- The mortality of VAP is **25–50%**.

Definitions

Hospital-acquired pneumonia is an infection that occurs >48 hours after admission and is not present at the time of admission.

Ventilator-acquired pneumonia is a form of hospital-acquired pneumonia that develops after >48 hours of mechanical ventilation. This is one of most common ICU infections.

Health care-associated pneumonia is a type of pneumonia that occurs in a nonhospitalized patient who has had extensive health care contact via:

- IV therapy, wound care, or IV chemo within the last 30 days
- hospitalization of two or more days within the last 90 days
- hospital visit or hemodialysis visit within the last 30 days

Compared to other patients with similar severity of illness, patients with VAP have longer hospital stays, increased time on the ventilator, and higher mortality.

VAP is estimated to increase the cost of care by *$40,000* per case.

Etiology

VAP develops after more than 48 hours with an endotracheal tube in place. The presence of the tube *disrupts cough reflexes, mucociliary clearance,* and creates a *direct pathway* for bacteria from the upper airway to access the lungs.

Aspiration of oral contents is the most common route of infection. Other routes include direct extension from other sites of infection, hematogenous spread, and inhalation of contaminated aerosols.

Risk factors

- *mechanical ventilation* – most significant risk factor
- age >70 years
- chronic lung disease
- depressed consciousness
- aspiration
- chest surgery
- presence of an intracranial pressure monitor or nasogastric tube
- H_2 blocker or antacid therapy
- transport from the intensive care unit (ICU) for diagnostic or therapeutic procedures
- previous antibiotic exposure, particularly third-generation cephalosporins
- re-intubation or prolonged intubation
- hospitalization during the fall or winter season
- mechanical ventilation for acute respiratory distress syndrome
- frequent ventilator circuit changes
- paralytic agents
- underlying illness

Clinical symptoms

Symptoms include fever, leukocytosis in the mechanically ventilated patient, increased oral or tracheal secretions, change in

Essential Clinical Anesthesia Review: Keywords, Questions and Answers for the Boards, ed. Linda S. Aglio, Robert W. Lekowski, and Richard D. Urman. Published by Cambridge University Press. © Cambridge University Press 2015.

respiratory parameters, and increased need for mechanical support.

Microbiology of VAP

The oropharyngeal flora of critically ill patients differ dramatically compared to those of healthy patients. In critically ill patients, *gram-negative bacteria* and *Staphylococcus aureus* colonization occurs. These are the most common causative organisms of VAP. Up to 75% of patients will be colonized within 48 hours of admission.

In healthy individuals, *streptococci* and *anaerobes* form the predominant oral microbiome.

The primary route of infection is through *microaspiration* of colonized bacteria. 45% of healthy, patients routinely aspirate during sleep and this number increases in severely ill patients, even with an ETT in place.

Organisms

- gram-negative bacilli – *E. Coli, Klebsiella, Enterobacter, Pseudomonas, Acinetobacter*
- gram-positive cocci – *Streptococcus, Staphlococcus aureus*
- anaerobes – aspiration, recent abdominal surgeries
- virus and fungal infections less common
- *multidrug-resistant organisms* – defined as resistant to at least two, three, four, or eight antibiotics used to treat infections

Diagnosis

This is most commonly a *clinical diagnosis*. Chest X-rays are often an unreliable source for diagnosis. There is *no gold standard diagnostic test*.

When VAP is suspected, a lower respiratory specimen should be taken from a tracheal aspiration or a bronchoscopic or nonbronchoscopic bronchoalveolar lavage.

Culture can take two to three days to complete and VAP cannot be confirmed or excluded until that time.

Treatment

Treatment should begin as soon as there are convincing clinical signs of infection and VAP is suspected.

Initial antibiotic therapy should be broad spectrum and cover the typical nosocomial organisms that cause VAP. This includes *mostly gram-negative organisms* but *gram-positive organisms* are becoming more common (*Staph*). Start with a *combination of two classes of antibiotics* – one that targets gram-negative organisms and one that *covers methicillin-resistant staphlococcus aureus (MRSA)*. For gram-positive, linezolid or vancomycin is recommended. This should be tailored down to specific organisms once culture data are known.

Duration of treatment should be *14 to 21 days*; however, some patients may benefit from a short *7- to 8-day course* for uncomplicated VAP.

Prevention

Avoid intubation – consider noninvasive positive pressure ventilation (CPAP, biPAP) if patient is deemed an appropriate candidate. Intubation increases the risk of pneumonia *6- to 21-fold*.

Orotracheal intubation is preferred to nasotracheal intubation.

Minimize the duration of mechanical ventilation. Use daily spontaneous breathing trials to assess for possible extubation.

Prevent aspiration:

- maintain head of bed elevation above 30°
- continual subglottic suctioning
- avoid supine positioning
- consider silver-coated endotracheal tube
- avoid gastric distension

Decontaminate oropharynx – gingival and dental plaque can become colonized. Chlorohexidine is preferred.

Decontamination of GI tract – nystatin.

Avoid histamine receptor blockers and proton pump inhibitors for patients who are not at increased risk for developing stress ulcers.

Avoid changing the ventilator circuit unless absolutely necessary.

Catheter-related bloodstream infections

The majority of nosocomial bloodstream infections are catheter related. The mortality of these infections is 12% to 25%.

Incidence

Up to 80,000 central venous catheter-related bloodstream infections occur in the ICU per year.

There is a higher risk of peripheral catheter infection in *lower extremities* compared to higher extremities.

Table 159.1 Rates of catheter-related bloodstream infections (CRBSI) per 1,000 catheter days from a systemic review of 200 prospective studies

Peripherally inserted midline catheters	0.2
Peripheral intravenous catheters	0.5
Peripherally inserted central catheters	1.1
Cuffed and tunneled central venous catheters	1.6
Arterial catheters for hemodynamic monitoring	1.7
Noncuffed central venous catheters	
Nonmedicated and tunneled	1.7
Nonmedicated and nontunneled	2.7
Pulmonary artery catheters	3.7

(Maki, D. G., Kluger, D. M., and Crnich, C. J. (2006). The risk of bloodstream infection in adults with different intravascular devices: a systematic review of 200 published prospective studies. *Mayo Clin Proc* 81(9): 1159–1171. Note: studies were unable to adjust for severity of illness of patients.)

Mechanisms of infection

- *colonization of skin* at catheter entry site and organisms migrate along catheter itself
- *contamination of catheter hub or stopcock*
  - these two account for the majority of infections
- seeding of catheter from infection at a distant site
- contamination of intravenous infusates

Clinical symptoms

- fevers – most sensitive but poor specificity
- rigors
- hemodynamic changes/instability – hypotension, tachycardia
- blood cultures positive for *S. aureus*, coagulase-negative *Staphococci* or *Candida* with the absence of other identifiable source
- clinical improvement within 24 hours after catheter removal is suggestive

Microorganisms

- gram-positive organisms are the most common
  - *S. aureus* – MRSA
  - *coagulase negative Staphococcus* (such as *S. epidermidis*) – most common, many can be methicillin-resistant
  - these two are the most common organisms
- *Enterococci*
- *Candida*
- assorted gram-negative bacteria

Diagnosis

Definitive diagnosis is made via *blood cultures*. Two sets need to be drawn from two separate venopuncture sites. Additional samples may be drawn from the catheter site.

If there is a multiport catheter, only a sample from one port is needed. *Lumens of catheters are often colonized* and sending cultures from the catheter sites alone will lead to high rates of false positives.

Negative cultures drawn from catheters have *great negative predictive value*.

Quantitative blood culture compares the colony count from the catheter sample to the peripheral sample. If the catheter sample is ≥3× higher than the peripheral sample, a catheter-related infection should be suspected.

Time to positivity of blood cultures of the catheter samples vs. the peripheral vein – this may help to distinguish a line-related infection. Growth in the catheter specimen two hours prior to peripheral cultures is suggestive of catheter-related infection (sensitivity 85%, specificity 91%).

The catheter tip can be sent for culture. A positive tip sample in the absence of bacteria does not require antibiotic therapy.

Roll plate – this technique examines the outside of the line only and does not look at the internal lumen, which is often colonized.

If there is one blood culture positive for coagulase-negative *Staphylococcus*, repeat blood cultures before starting antibiotics.

If there is one positive catheter-drawn culture for coagulase-negative *Staphylococci* or gram-negative *Bacilli* and peripheral cultures are negative, there is most likely a colonized catheter. However, there may be increased risk of CRBSI if this catheter is left in place. Device removal should be considered.

Diagnostic criteria

- same organism cultured from catheter tip and at least one peripheral blood culture
- same organism cultured from at least two blood samples (i.e., one drawn from the catheter and one from peripheral vein)

Treatment

Start treatment immediately if there is high index of suspicion. Do not wait for cultures to come back. If possible, *remove the catheter.*

Vancomycin is the *first-line* agent, as gram-positive organisms are the most common. This can be broadened to gram-negative coverage in critically ill or immunocompromised patients.

The duration of therapy depends on the clinical situation but for uncomplicated infections, *10 to 14 days* (day one is the first day of the first negative blood culture). Patients with persistent bacteremia should be treated for at least *four to six weeks*.

Fungal CRBSIs are rare and treatment should be reserved for high-risk patients.

Risk factors include:

- TPN
- prolonged broad spectrum antibiotic use
- hematologic malignancy
- bone marrow or solid organ transplant
- femoral catheterization
- *Candida* colonization

An exchange of an infected catheter over a guidewire is not an effective strategy for managing CRBSI infections.

Treatment is not required if:

- there is a positive catheter tip culture without clinical signs of infection
- there are positive blood cultures from catheter-drawn samples with negative peripheral blood samples
- there is phlebitis without evidence of infection

Prevention

Catheter-related infections are *almost entirely preventable*.

Use *maximum barrier precautions for all placements* – sterile gloves, surgical mask, hat, gown, large sterile drape.

Table 159.2 Type of catheter and reported risk of infection

Peripheral venous catheter	>3–4 days
Central venous catheter	>6 days
Pulmonary artery (Swan–Ganz) catheter	>3–4 days
Arterial catheter	>4–6 days

Cleaning skin with *chlorhexidine* has been shown to be superior to providine-iodine.

Clean all hubs and stopcocks prior to use.

Ensure proper hand hygiene before line insertion and before handling of stop cocks and ports.

Location of catheter insertion affects rates of infection: femoral (highest rates of infection) > internal jugular > *subclavian*. Recent studies suggest that these rates can be reduced to minimal with meticulous site care for all locations.

The longer a catheter stays in, the higher the risk of bloodstream infection. However, *routine replacement of catheters have not been shown to decrease risks.*

Remove catheters when not needed

Replace peripheral venous catheters every four days. Do not routinely replace CVC, PA, or arterial catheters.

Ideally a patient with CRBSI will be given a period of antibiotic treatment before a new line is inserted to reduce the risk of seeding the new line.

Several studies have showed decreased incidence of catheter-related infections with the use of antibacterial impregnated catheters.

Antibiotic lock technique – this involves filling the catheter with an antibiotic for several hours to prevent colonization of the intraluminal surface of the catheter.

Daily chlorhexidine bathing of ICU patients.

No topical antibiotic ointment or cream at insertion site is recommended.

Questions

1. A 35-year-old male with 80% total body surface area burns is admitted to the ICU for continued burn care and respiratory support. Patient was admitted with high fevers and during the course of his illness continued to spike fever up to 39.6°C. On the fifth day after admission, the patient was noted to have increased secretions from his endotracheal tube that required increased frequency of suctioning. FiO$_2$ was increased from 40% to 60% due to a fall in PaO$_2$ from 106 to 76. CXR showed some blunting of the right costophrenic angle but otherwise no infiltrates. What should be the next course of action?
   a. Start empiric vancomycin and cefotetan.
   b. Continue to monitor respiratory status.
   c. Order a chest CT.
   d. Perform a bronchalveolar lavage and send samples for culture.
   e. Pan-culture (blood, urine, sputum, BAL).

2. Please select the FALSE statement below in regards to catheter-related bloodstream infections:
   a. They are almost entirely preventable.
   b. Full barrier precautions including sterile gowns, masks, gloves, and drapes should be used during each line placement.
   c. Providine-iodine has been shown to be superior to chlorhexidine as a skin preparation agent.
   d. Antifungals should be a part of the treatment regimen for all critically ill patients.
   e. Internal jugular site infections are higher than subclavian-placed catheters.

Answers

1. d. Based on the clinical symptoms consisting of fevers, hypoxia, and required increased ventilatory support, ventilator pneumonia needs to be considered. Although given the findings, antibiotics should be empirically started, the first course of action is to establish a diagnosis. Early VAP may not show up on imaging. Cultures should be taken, however, given the most likely site of infection with the current symptoms. A BAL is the most important culture to take.

2. c. Cleaning skin with *chlorhexidine* has been shown to be superior to providine-iodine.

Further reading

Thomas, M. D. (2013). Epidemiology, pathogenesis, microbiology, and diagnosis of hospital-acquired, ventilator-associated, and healthcare-associated pneumonia in adults. www.uptodate.com/contents/epidemiology-pathogenesis-microbiology-and-diagnosis-of-hospital-acquired-ventilator-associated-and-healthcare-associated-pneumonia-in-adults.

Thomas, M. D. (2013). Risk factors and prevention of hospital-acquired, ventilator-associated, and healthcare-associated pneumonia in adults. www.uptodate.com/contents/risk-factors-and-prevention-of-hospital-acquired-ventilator-associated-and-healthcare-associated-pneumonia-in adults.

American Thoracic Society; Infectious Diseases Society of America (2005). Guidelines for the management of adults with hospital-acquired, ventilator-associated, and healthcare-associated pneumonia. *American Journal of Respiratory and Critical Care Medicine* 171, 388–416.

Kollef, M. H. (2004). Prevention of hospital-associated pneumonia and ventilator-associated pneumonia. *Critical Care Medicine* 32(6), 1396–1405.

No authors listed (1994). Guideline for prevention of nosocomial pneumonia. Centers for Disease Control and Prevention. *Respiratory Care* 39(12), 1191–1236.

Mermel, L. A., Allon, M., Bouza, E. et al. (2009). Clinical practice guidelines for the diagnosis and management of intravascular catheter-related infection: 2009. Update by the Infectious Diseases Society of America. *Clinical Infectious Diseases* 49, 1.

Chaiyakunapruk, N., Veenstra, D. L., Lipsky, B. A., and Saint, S. (2002). Chlorhexidine compared with providine-iodine solution for vascular catheter-site care: a meta-analysis. *Annals of Internal Medicine* 136, 792.

O'Grady, N. P., Alexander, M., Dellinger, E. P. et al. (2002). Guidelines for the prevention of intravascular catheter-related infections. Centers for Disease Control and Prevention. *MMWR Recommendations and Reports* 51, 1–29.

Safdar, N., Fine, J. P., and Maki, D. G. (2005). Meta-analysis: methods for diagnosing intravascular device-related bloodstream infection. *Annals of Internal Medicine* 142, 451–466.

Deshpande, K. S., Hatem, C., Ulrich, H. L. et al. (2005). The incidence of infectious complications of central venous catheters at the subclavian, internal jugular, and femoral sites in an intensive care unit population. *Critical Care Medicine* 33, 13–20.

Lai, K. K. (1998). Safety of prolonging peripheral cannula and i.v. tubing use from 72 hours to 96 hours. *American Journal of Infection Control* 26, 66–70.

Collin, J., Collin, C., Constable, F. L., and Johnston, I. D. (1975). Infusion thrombophlebitis and infection with various cannulas. *Lancet* 2, 150–153.

Raad, I., Umphrey, J., Khan, A. et al. (1993). The duration of placement as a predictor of peripheral and pulmonary arterial catheter infections. *Journal of Hospital Infection* 23, 17–26.

Band, J. D. and Maki, D. G. (1979). Infections caused by arterial catheters used for hemodynamic monitoring. *American Journal of Medicine* 67, 735–741.

Chapter

160

Septic shock and sepsis syndromes

Beverly Chang and Gyorgy Frendl

Systemic inflammatory response syndrome
Sepsis
Severe sepsis
Septic shock
Early goal-directed therapy
Critical illness-related steroid insufficiency

Sepsis is defined as the presence of infection with systemic manifestations of infection. It is a systemic host response to infection.

Millions of patients are diagnosed annually in the United States with septic shock. 60% of patients with severe sepsis are ≥65 years of age. Overall *mortality is approximately 20% to 50%. Mortality remains elevated up to one year* after the sepsis episode. Patients who survive have long-term *decreased quality of life.*

Rapid diagnosis and treatment is vital to the prevention and reversal of organ injury and is likely to influence outcomes. Unfortunately, when clinical evidence of sepsis manifests, the disease process is already well established. Severely ill patients should be routinely screened for sepsis to increase early identification and treatment.

Definitions and clinical findings

Systemic inflammatory response syndrome (SIRS) results from an inflammatory response to a noninfectious insult. It requires two or more of the following:

- temperature >38°C or <36°C
- heart rate >90 bpm or two standard deviations above normal age value
- respiration >30 breaths/min or PCO_2 >32 mm Hg
- white cell count >12,000/mm³ or <4,000
- >10% immature neutrophils

Sepsis: SIRS with a confirmed infectious source. Requires two SIRS criteria with a proven site of infection.

Severe sepsis: sepsis with evidence of organ dysfunction or tissue hypoperfusion. As more organ systems fail, the potential for reversal of the disease process decreases. Timely treatment is extremely important.

- urine output <0.5 ml/kg/h for more than 1 h
- creatinine >2 mg/dl
- lactate >2 mmol/l
- bilirubin >2 mmol/l
- decreased capillary refill or mottling
- change in mental status
- platelets <100,000 platelets/µl
- coagulation abnormalities (INR >1.5; PTT >60 s)
- DIC
- acute respiratory distress syndrome
- cardiac dysfunction

Septic shock: sepsis-induced hypotension that persists despite fluid resuscitation.

- *Hypotension* is defined as SBP <90 mm Hg, MAP <70 mm Hg, or decrease of >40 mm Hg of SBP from baseline.
- A type of *vasodilatory shock* due to *decreased systemic vascular resistance.*

Multiple organ dysfunction syndrome: progressive organ dysfunction, the severe end of the spectrum of SIRS and sepsis.

- *Primary* – from a direct insult that causes organ dysfunction.
- *Secondary* – organ dysfunction due to host's response to an insult and not a direct result of the insult itself.

Pathogenesis

Sepsis is a *systemic disease* of the microcirculation and endothelium. The recognition of a bacterial antigen in the bloodstream initiates an *inflammatory* and *procoagulant* process. Sepsis occurs when the inflammatory response spreads beyond the immediate, local environment and becomes generalized. The excess proinflammatory mediators cause *widespread*

Essential Clinical Anesthesia Review: Keywords, Questions and Answers for the Boards, ed. Linda S. Aglio, Robert W. Lekowski, and Richard D. Urman. Published by Cambridge University Press. © Cambridge University Press 2015.

cellular injury, tissue ischemia, and alter the rate of apoptosis. There is also *activation of the complement system.*

System-based effects of sepsis

Cardiovascular – hypotension (nitric oxide-mediated vasodilation).

Lung – endothelial injury causes microvascular permeability resulting in pulmonary and interstitial edema → V/Q mismatch.

GI – disruption of normal gut barrier causing translocation of bacteria into circulation.

Liver – liver failure causes reticuloendothelial system failure, which is responsible for clearing bacterial products from circulation, resulting in a build up of bacterial components.

Kidney – acute renal failure – unknown etiology but proposed to be due to acute tubular necrosis, hypoperfusion.

CNS – encephalopathy.

Heme/immune system

- *Subendothelial injury* generates thrombin, which potentiates the systemic inflammatory and procoagulant state.
- *Microvascular thrombosis and ischemia* cause vascular autoregulatory collapse, increased oxygen demand, and interferes with perfusion and oxygen delivery. Organ failure and death can ensue. The body compensates by shunting blood from nonessential vascular beds to vital organs – compensated shock. After organ reserves are depleted, systemic organ failure begins.

Organisms

Gram-positive organisms are the most commonly isolated, but all organisms can cause these syndromes.

Diagnosis

First step of treatment is to *identify the source of infection*. Two or more *blood cultures* should be drawn via venopuncture. Additional cultures can be drawn from catheter lumens. Do not delay antibiotics for cultures if these cannot be drawn within 45 minutes of arrival.

Collect *sputum, urine, wound, and CSF (if clinically indicated)* cultures.

Draw lactate levels.

Order imaging studies based on clinical indication.

Treatment

Treatment guidelines are based on the Surviving Sepsis Campaign.

The goals of care are:

- early initiation of supportive care
- support circulation, perfusion – arterial line, central line
- support breathing – intubation

- identify the source of infection
- initiate source control and control of the inflammatory response

Summary of National Quality Forum/Surviving Sepsis Campaign Management Bundles/ Milestones – SEPSIS 0500

To be completed within three hours of presentation

1. Measure lactate level.
2. Obtain blood cultures prior to antibiotic administration.
3. Administer broad spectrum antibiotic (within one hour).
4. Administer 30 ml/kg crystalloid for hypotension or for lactate >4 mmol/l.

To be completed within six hours of presentation

5. Apply vasopressors if unresponsive to appropriate fluid resuscitation (goal MAP >65 mm Hg).
6. If hypotension is sustained after initial fluid resuscitation
   - measure and follow CVP trend
   - measure and follow central venous oxygen saturation ($ScvO_2$).
7. If lactate is elevated, remeasure and aim for normalizing lactate.

Early goal-directed therapy

To be *started within six hours* of severe sepsis presentation with evidence of tissue hypoperfusion. Achieving the following targets has been shown to reduce 28 day mortality by 15% to 17%:

- *central venous pressure 8–12 mm Hg*
  - for ventilated patients or patients with restrictive lung disease, higher CVP thresholds of 12 to 15 mm Hg should be used
- *MAP >65 mm Hg*
- urine output *>0.5 ml/kg/h*
- superior vena cava oxygenation saturation of *70%* or mixed venous O_2 saturation *>65%*
- consider blood transfusion if venous saturation is unresponsive to fluid alone despite CVP of 8 to 12 mm Hg

Antibiotic therapy

Broad spectrum antibiotics should be initiated *within one hour of arrival. Do not delay antibiotics for cultures (beyond 45 minutes).*

Only 5% of severe sepsis cases are due to fungal infection. There is no need for empiric fungal coverage unless otherwise indicated (TPN, immunocompromised patients, positive fungal cultures, transplant patients).

Patients should be assessed daily to evaluate for possible de-escalation of antibiotics. Empiric antibiotics should not be administered for more than three to five days.

Treatment depends on suspicion of *Pseudomonas* infection. If *Pseudomonas is not* suspected:

- vancomycin plus a third-generation cephalosporin, a beta-lactam/beta-lactamase inhibitor or a carbapenem

If *Pseudomonas is* suspected:

- vancomycin and two of the following:
  - ceftazidime, cefepime
  - imipenem, meropenem
  - piperacillin-tazobactam, ticarcillin-clavulanate
  - ciprofloxacin
  - gentamicin, amikacin
  - aztreonam

The duration of therapy should typically be *7 to 10 days*. Tailor the duration to clinical improvement.

Fluid resuscitation

The presence of hypotension with systemic acidosis indicates the presence of anaerobic metabolism and requires urgent fluid and/or vasopressor resuscitation. Use lactate as a target for resuscitation if levels are elevated.

Crystalloids should be used as the initial fluid of choice. Albumin should be used if substantial amounts of crystalloids are anticipated to be needed. Hydroxyethyl *starches should not be used* for resuscitation.

For patients with acute respiratory distress syndrome a conservative fluid strategy should be used to prevent further lung injury.

Vasopressor and inotropic therapy

If hypotension persists despite adequate fluid resuscitation, vasopressors can be started. *IV fluid is the first-line treatment* for hypotension. Vasopressors are the second line.

Norepinephrine is the first choice vasopressor. Epinephrine and *vasopressin* can be added if additional agents are needed. Vasopressin has been shown to have a moderate benefit in the 0.04 to 0.08 U/min range in early sepsis; however, it should not be used as the sole agent. *Phenylephrine* is usually only used as a temporizing agent.

Dopamine should only be used in select patients with a low risk of tachyarrhythmias. Low-dose dopamine should not be used for renal protection.

Conventional markers for perfusion are unreliable because sepsis is a disease of the microcirculation. Trends of hemodynamic values and monitors are more important.

Lactate is often used as a monitoring tool for patients with sepsis. It is considered a late, insensitive marker of ischemia that does not reflect regional or organ-specific events. The *presence of lactate does not always indicate ischemia.*

The *absence of lactic acid also does not exclude the presence of tissue ischemia. Lactate is often artificially elevated due to sepsis* itself because of disordered pyruvate dehydrogenase activity. Different treatments can also change levels of lactate

(i.e., induction of aerobic glycolysis by vasopressor therapy). Lactate may also increase with adequate perfusion due to the washout effect with restoration of perfusion.

Dobutamine should be administered (or added to vasopressors) when the following are present:

- myocardial dysfunction (elevated cardiac filling pressures with low cardiac output)
- ongoing signs of tissue hypoperfusion despite achieving adequate intravascular volume and mean arterial pressure

Source control

Specific anatomical diagnosis (nidus) of infection should be sought (e.g., necrotizing soft tissue infection, peritonitis with intra-abdominal infection, cholangitis, intestinal infarction, etc.) or ruled out, and emergent source control should be sought as rapidly as possible (*Crit Care Med.* 2008; 36: 296). Surgical drainage (if required) should be undertaken within 12 hours of the diagnosis for source control.

Management of mechanical ventilation of sepsis-induced ARDS

Acute respiratory distress syndrome (ARDS) refers to a spectrum of respiratory states that form as a primary insult to the body. ARDS can form as a primary or secondary reaction. This disease process is characterized by diffuse lung inflammation, increased pulmonary vascular permeability, causing pulmonary edema and resulting in impaired gas exchange.

Early identification of ARDS, like sepsis, is the key to improved outcomes. Treatment is generally supportive, providing low tidal volumes with high positive end-expiratory pressures to maintain oxygenation while preventing further injury to the lungs.

Ventilator settings: tidal volumes should be weaned to 6 ml/kg of predicted body weight. Positive end-expiratory pressures should be used and plateau pressures should be ≤30 cm H_2O.

Head of the bed should be elevated by 30 to 45 degrees in mechanically ventilated patients.

Prone positioning should be used in patients with PaO_2/FiO_2 ≤100 mm Hg. Neuromuscular blockers should not be used for more than 48 hours for patients with a PaO_2/FiO_2 <150 mm Hg. When used, train-of-four monitoring should be used to titrate the medications.

The routine use of pulmonary artery catheters is *not recommended*.

Steroid therapy

The hypothalamus secretes corticotropin-releasing hormone → adrenocorticotropic hormone (ACTH) is secreted from the anterior pituitary → cortisol is secreted from the adrenal gland. During critical illness, the hypothalamic–pituitary–adrenal

(HPA) axis is activated and diurnal variation in cortisol secretion is lost. The loss of cortisol binding globulin causes *increases in free cortisol. Standard assays that measure total plasma cortisol and not free cortisol may underestimate cortisol levels.*

Serum cortical levels vary among patients presenting with septic shock. The presence of suboptimal cortisol production during septic shock is also termed *critical illness-related corticosteroid insufficiency.*

The *decision to start steroids is controversial* due to the variability in response to therapy. Also biologically active free cortisol is not measured from these tests, so it is often unclear whether treatment is actually indicated.

Clinical trials have demonstrated mixed results. There is no data to suggest that steroids are beneficial in mild septic shock. Recent reviews indicate that patients with refractory shock to fluids and vasopressors, the addition of steroid therapy may improve hemodynamic stability and reversal of shock. However, there is not a clear mortality benefit.

Current Surviving Sepsis Guidelines recommend continuous intravenous infusion of hydrocortisone of 200 mg per day (without fludrocortisone) for only those patients with *septic shock* whose tissue perfusion and hemodynamic stability is not restored by fluids and vasopressor therapy (no mortality benefit: *N. Engl. J. Med.* 2008; 358: 111). ACTH stimulation test is not necessary prior to treatment. Treatment should be tapered once vasopressors have been weaned off. There is no clear protocol for weaning steroids due to the rebound effect of decline in cardiovascular improvement and increased inflammation with decreasing dose.

Bicarbonate therapy

Sodium bicarbonate should not be used to improve hemodynamic parameters with a pH of ≥ 7.15. Although bicarbonate may be useful temporarily in reducing ventilatory needs, no evidence has shown any survival benefits. Bicarbonate administration can be associated with hypernatremia and fluid overload, an increase in lactate and PCO_2, and a decrease in ionized calcium. The effects of bicarbonate on hemodynamic parameters in patients with lower pH have not been studied.

Blood product administration

After the acute phase of fluid resuscitataion, transfuse only to keep hemoglobin concentration between 7 and 9 g/dl, especially if hypotension has been unresponsive to fluids.

FFP should not be transfused to correct coagulation abnormalities unless there are clinical signs of bleeding.

Administer platelets prophylactically when counts are $<10,000/mm^3$ in the absence of bleeding.

- Transfuse when counts are $<20,000/mm^3$ if the patient is at high risk of bleeding.
- Maintaining platelet count of $>50,000$ is recommended for active bleeding or invasive procedures.

Metabolic management

Hyperglycemia and insulin resistance are commonly found in critically ill patients. Maintain glucose between *140 and 180 mg/dl* and avoid hypoglycemia. Insulin should be initiated when more than two consecutive glucose measurements are greater than 180 mg/dl.

Stress ulcer prophylaxis

Stress ulcer prophylaxis should be given to patients with bleeding risks. Patients without any risk factors do not require prophylaxis. When used, proton pump inhibitors are preferred to histamine blockers.

Nutrition

Oral or enteral feedings should be started within *48 hours* of diagnosis. This has advantages of maintaining the integrity of cut mucosa and preventing bacterial translocation. The use of intravenous glucose and enteral feeding is recommended over the use of total parenteral nutrition in the first seven days of diagnosis. Several studies have highlighted the potential infectious complications of parental nutrition. A low caloric feeding is recommended in the first week and can be advanced as tolerated.

Questions

1. SIRS criteria encompasses all except which of the following?
   a. temperature $<36°C$
   b. heart rate >100 bpm
   c. respiration >20 breaths/min or $PCO_2 >32$ mm Hg
   d. white cell count $>15,000/mm^3$
   e. immature neutrophils 10%

2. Which is the most important step to take after sepsis is identified?
   a. initiation of antibiotics
   b. IV fluid resuscitation
   c. insertion of arterial line
   d. insertion of central line
   e. draw blood cultures prior to initiating antibiotic therapy

3. What is TRUE about steroid use in sepsis?
   a. Steroid therapy should be started with diagnosis of sepsis.
   b. Steroids have been shown to be beneficial in mild septic shock.
   c. IV hydrocortisone may be considered in patients with septic shock refractory to IV fluids and vasopressors.
   d. Fludrocortisone supplement should be added to IV hydrocortisone for steroid replacement in critical illness adrenal insufficiency.

Answers

1. c. SIRS criteria include:
   - temperature >38°C or <36°C
   - heart rate >90 bpm or two standard deviations above normal age value
   - respiration >30 breaths/min or PCO_2 >32 mm Hg
   - white cell count >12,000/mm³ or <4,000
   - immature neutrophils >10%

2. a. Once sepsis has been identified, the most important step is to initiate antibiotics within one hour of presentation. If possible, cultures should be drawn prior to antibiotic initiation but never delay administration of antibiotics beyond one hour for cultures. For patients presenting with septic shock with evidence of hypotension and tissue hypoperfusion, first step of management should be IV access and fluid resuscitation. Similarly, antibiotics should be given within one hour of presentation.

3. c. Current Surviving Sepsis Guidelines recommend initiating a continuous infusion of hydrocortisone only for patients with septic shock refractory to fluids and vasopressors. ACTH stimulation tests are not necessary prior to initiation of hydrocortisone. There are no current recommendations as to whether fludrocortisones should be administered as well.

Further reading

Dellinger, R. P., Levy, M. M., Rhodes, A., Annane, D., Gerlach, H. et al. (2013). Surviving Sepsis Campaign Guidelines Committee including the Pediatric Subgroup. Surviving sepsis campaign: international guidelines for management of severe sepsis and septic shock: 2012. *Critical Care Medicine* 41(2), 580–637.

Neviere, R. (2013). Sepsis and the systemic inflammatory response syndrome: definitions, epidemiology, and prognosis. www.uptodate.com/contents/sepsis-and-the-systemic-inflammatory-response-syndrome-definitions-epidemiology-and-prognosis.

Schmidt, G. and Mandel, J. (2013). Management of severe sepsis and septic shock in adults. www.uptodate.com/contents/management-of-severe-sepsis-and-septic-shock-in-adults.

Neviere, R. (2013). Pathophysiology of sepsis. www.uptodate.com/contents/pathophysiology-of-sepsis.

Kaufman, D. and Mancebo, J. (2013). Corticosteroid therapy in septic shock. www.uptodate.com/contents/corticosteroid-therapy-in-septic-shock.

No authors listed (1992). American College of Chest Physicians/Society of Critical Care Medicine Consensus Conference: definitions for sepsis and organ failure and guidelines for the use of innovative therapies in sepsis. *Critical Care Medicine* 20, 864–874.

Levy, M. M., Fink, M. P., Marshall, J. C. et al. (2003). SCCM/ESICM/ACCP/ATS/SIS International Sepsis Definitions Conference. *Critical Care Medicine* 31(4), 1250–1256.

Annane, D., Bellissant, E., and Cavaillon, J.M. (2005). Septic shock. *Lancet* 365, 63–78.

Dellinger, R. P., Levy, M. M., Carlet, J. M. et al. (2008). Surviving Sepsis Campaign: international guidelines for management of severe sepsis and septic shock: 2008. *Critical Care Medicine* 36,296–327.

Hollenberg, S. M., Ahrens, T. S., Annane, D. et al. (2004). Practice parameters for hemodynamic support of sepsis in adult patients: 2004 update. *Critical Care Medicine* 32, 1928–1948.

Rivers, E., Nguyen, B., Havstad, S. et al. (2001). Early goal-directed therapy in the treatment of severe sepsis and septic shock. *New England Journal of Medicine* 345, 1368–1377.

Rhodes, A. and Bennett, E. D. (2004). Early goal-directed therapy: an evidence-based review. *Critical Care Medicine* 32, S448–S450.

Brun-Buisson, C, Doyon, F., Carlet, J. et al. (1995). Incidence, risk factors, and outcome of severe sepsis and septic shock in adults. A multicenter prospective study in intensive care units. French ICU Group for Severe Sepsis. *Journal of the American Medical Association* 274, 968–974.

Chapter

161

Anesthetic management of the brain-dead organ donor

Allison Clark and Lisa Crossley

Keywords

Brain death pathophysiology
Organ donor: bradycardia Rx
Organ donor: treatment of DI
Glascow Coma Scale: definition
Intraoperative management: organ donor

Brain death is defined as the absence of brainstem reflexes, motor responses, and respiratory drive in a comatose patient. Injury must be irreversible and not attributed to hypothermia, drug intoxication, or metabolic abnormalities.

The diagnosis of brain death requires two separate physical examinations performed at least six hours apart and may be confirmed by a number of tests, including electroencephalography.

By definition, *bradycardia* in the brain-dead patient is *unresponsive to atropine* and may require electronic pacing.

Diabetes insipidus (DI) may ensue in up to 80% of brain-dead patients. Diagnostic features of DI are presented in Table 161.1. Treatment of DI includes matching urine output (UOP) with hypotonic crystalloid infusion and may require desmopressin acetate (DDAVP) if hourly UOP exceeds 200 ml. Electrolyte abnormalities should be closely monitored and corrected.

The *Glascow Coma Scale* (GCS) is a tool utilized to assess neurologic status in the brain-injured patient and includes best *eye opening, motor, and verbal responses.* The GCS is depicted in Table 161.2.

Management goals include ensuring normoxia and normocarbia, optimizing tissue perfusion with careful fluid management and vasopressor therapy, treatment of electrolyte abnormalities, and prevention of hypothermia.

Table 161.1 Diagnostic features of DI, from: Vacanti et al., 2011. *Essential Clinical Anesthesia*, Cambridge University Press, p. 1005.

Urine output	$\geq$5 ml/kg/h
Urine specific gravity	1005
Urine osmolarity	<300 mOsm/L
Serum osmolarity	>310 mOsm/L
Hypernatremia	$\geq$155 mmol/L
Hypovolemia	
Hypokalemia	
Hypomagnesemia	
Hypophosphatemia	
Hypocalcemia	

Table 161.2 Glasgow Coma Scale

	1	2	3	4	5	6
Eyes	Does not open eyes	Opens eyes in response to painful stimuli	Opens eyes in response to voice	Opens eyes spontaneously	N/A	N/A
Verbal	Makes no sounds	Incomprehensible sounds	Utters inappropriate words	Confused, disoriented	Oriented, converses normally	N/A
Motor	Makes no movements	Extension to painful stimuli	Abnormal flexion to painful stimuli	Flexion/withdrawal to painful stimuli	Localizes painful stimuli	Obeys commands

N/A, not applicable.

Questions

1. Which of the following is not compatible with the diagnosis of brain death?
   a. positive apnea test
   b. Glasgow Coma Scale score of 3
   c. temperature 32°C
   d. absent gag reflex

2. Which of the following will not increase the heart rate of the brain-dead patient?
   a. atropine
   b. epinephrine
   c. dobutamine
   d. electronic pacing

3. Which of the following is the best first-line treatment for the brain-dead patient with DI?
   a. dextrose saline infusion
   b. hypertonic saline infusion
   c. hypotonic saline infusion
   d. DDAVP

4. A patient arrives to the ED following MVA. He opens his eyes to pain, is making incomprehensible signs, and displays abnormal flexion to painful stimuli. This patient's GCS is which of the following?
   a. 3
   b. 6
   c. 7
   d. 9

Answers

1. c. Diagnosis of brain death requires normothermia.
2. a. Bradycardia in the brain dead is unresponsive to atropine, whereas response to direct inotropes such as epinephrine or dobutamine, as well as to electronic pacing, is normal.
3. c. Hypotonic saline is the first-line therapy for DI, whereas DDAVP may be required as second-line therapy. Hypertonic saline would be contraindicated in this hypernatremic state. Dextrose-containing solutions are avoided in the brain-injured patient.
4. c. See the Table 161.1.

Further reading

Pasternak, J. and Lanier, W. (2008). Diseases affecting the brain. In Hines, R. and Marschall, K. (eds) *Stoelting's Anesthesia and Co-Existing Disease*, 5th edn. Philadelphia, PA: Churchill-Livingstone, pp. 199–238.

Walz, J. and Heard, S. (2011). Anesthetic management of the brain-dead organ donor. In Vacanti, C. A., Sikka, P. J., Urman, R. D., Dershwitz, M., and Segal, B. S. (eds) *Essential Clinical Anesthesia*. Cambridge, MA: Cambridge University Press, pp. 1002–1006.

Williams, M. and Rogers, S. O. (2011). Principles of trauma management. In Vacanti, C. A., Sikka, P. J., Urman, R. D., Dershwitz, M., and Segal, B. S. (eds) *Essential Clinical Anesthesia*. Cambridge, MA: Cambridge University Press, pp. 1007–1009.

Principles of trauma management

Hanjo Ko and Robert W. Lekowski

Keywords

Golden hour
ABCDE
Tension pneumothorax
Flail chest
Glasgow Coma Scale
Conduction
Convection
Evaporation

The golden hour

Refers to the limited time available to intervene effectively to salvage life and limb. The golden hour calls for the immediate prioritization and management of the trauma patient according to ATLS principles.

In order to prioritize the management of trauma patients, the *ABCDE* mnemonic was developed in descending order of importance:

- A: airway and cervical spine protection.
- B: breathing.
- C: circulation and hemorrhage control.
- D: disability and neurologic status.
- E: exposure and environmental aspects.
- Other principles: treat injuries that have the greatest risk to life first. Lack of definitive diagnosis should never impede the application of an indicated treatment. A detailed history is not essential in the evaluation and treatment of the injured patient.

Tension pneumothorax

Patients who present with a:
- deviated trachea
- hypotension

- distended neck veins
- absent breath sounds

Tension pneumothorax should be suspected. A tension pneumothorax can be transiently decompressed with the placement of a 14-gauge angiocatheter in the second intercostal space in the midclavicular line. Following this, a thoracotomy tube has to be placed.

A flail chest

- Multiple contiguous rib fractures along two lines (that are either located bilaterally or in anterior and posterior positions on one side of the chest).
- Rib fractures, especially in the elderly, carry a significant rate of morbidity and mortality.

Glasgow Coma Scale (GCS)

A summation score based on best eye opening, best motor, and best verbal responses. The GCS can be altered by systematic factors such as drug intoxication, hypoxia, and hypotension. (See Table 161.1 in previous chapter for full details of the Glasgow Coma Scale.)

Hypothermia in trauma patients

- increases mortality
- worsens coagulopathy
- conduction, convection, and evaporation are important sources of heat loss:
    - *conduction* is heat loss through direct contact between objects (e.g., wet clothes)
    - *convection* is a process of conduction during which one of the object is in motion (e.g., wind chill)
    - *evaporation* is heat loss from converting water from a liquid to a gas (e.g., perspiration and respiration)

Essential Clinical Anesthesia Review: Keywords, Questions and Answers for the Boards, ed. Linda S. Aglio, Robert W. Lekowski, and Richard D. Urman. Published by Cambridge University Press. © Cambridge University Press 2015.

Questions

1. Which is the main mechanism of heat loss?

   a. radiation

   b. convection

   c. conduction

   d. evaporation

2. Which of the following statements regarding tension pneumothorax is FALSE?

   a. Classic signs (decreased breath sound, deviated trachea) are very uncommon.

   b. Most common signs are hypotension, tachycardia, oxygen desaturation, and narrowed pulse pressure.

   c. Under anesthesia, airway pressure is decreased.

   d. In the setting of hemodynamic instability, needle decompression should be established without further diagnostic interventions.

Answers

1. a. Radiation accounts for 67%, evaporation 17%, and conduction/convection approximately 16% each.

2. c. A rise in airway pressure is seen with a tension pneumothorax.

Further reading

Vacanti, C. A., Sikka, P. K., Urman, R. U., Dershwitz, M., and Segal, B. S. (eds) (2011). *Essential Clinical Anesthesia*. New York, NY: Cambridge University Press, Chapter 163.

Venous thromboembolic disease in the critically ill patient

Andrea Girnius and Annette Mizuguchi

Keywords

Deep venous thrombosis (DVT)
DVT: pathophysiology
DVT: prevention
DVT: diagnosis
DVT: perioperative
Pulmonary embolus: diagnosis
Pulmonary embolus: treatment
ABG: pulmonary embolism

Virchow's Triad, which consists of hypercoagulability, venous stasis, and endothelial dysfunction, describes factors necessary for the formation of a venous thrombus. Immobility is a major factor predisposing patients in the ICU to thrombosis.

ICU patients with DVT may have an underlying *hypercoagulable state*, such as factor V Leiden or prothrombin gene mutation, but most patients with DVT do not have an identifiable cause of hypercoagulability.

Methods of *preventing* DVT include compression devices (prevent blood stasis and promote fibrinolysis) and chemical prophylaxis with heparin or LMWH. The best prophylaxis is early ambulation, but this is impractical in many ICU patients.

Diagnosis of DVT: clinical signs include unilateral leg swelling, Homan's sign (pain with forced foot extension).

Duplex ultrasonography is the most commonly used test to *diagnose DVT*. Criteria used to diagnose DVT are: (1) non-compressibility of the vein, (2) presence of echogenic material in lumen, (3) loss of plasticity and augmentation of spontaneous flow, and (4) venous distension. For proximal vein DVT, sensitivity is 97%, specificity is 94%, negative predictive value is 99%. Sensitivity decreases to 73% for calf DVT. Only patients with a high pretest probability should be tested.

Other less common *diagnostic tests* include contrast venography (gold standard, but rarely used) and MRI (sensitivity 92%, specificity 95%).

Pulmonary embolism (PE), a sequelae of DVT, can present subtly or can cause circulatory collapse. *Signs/symptoms* of PE include dyspnea, tachypnea, chest pain, palpitations, tachycardia, hypoxia, hypotension, and sudden fall of $ETCO_2$ (in mechanically ventilated patients or intraoperatively).

Hemodynamically significant PE: acute pulmonary outflow obstruction decreases blood flow to the lungs, causing hypoxemia. This results in hypoxic pulmonary vasoconstriction and further increases PA pressure and RV afterload. This then leads to RV strain, increased RV wall tension, and depressed RV function. Cardiac output and blood pressure become decreased due to RV failure.

PE can be *diagnosed* by imaging studies. Pulmonary angiography is the gold standard; however, *CT angiography* has been shown to have a comparable sensitivity and specificity, is much less invasive, and is easier to perform. Contrast nephropathy is a major concern for angiography in critically ill patients and adequate hydration before a dye load is very important.

Other *diagnostic studies* include V/Q scan, which uses scintigraphy to compare relative ventilation and perfusion of different parts of the lung. It is commonly used in patients with renal insufficiency. The results can be difficult to interpret.

D-dimer is a blood test that measures fibrin split products. It is very sensitive (>95%) for PE, but not specific. It is useful because of its high negative predictive value. However, ICU patients are likely to have elevated D-dimers for many reasons, so it is not a very useful test in this population.

EKG classically shows S1Q3T3 (S Wave in Lead I, Q Wave in Lead III, T Wave Inversion in Lead III) in PE, but this is seen in less than 20% of cases. *ABG* is usually not very helpful but can show hypoxia and hypocarbia (respiratory alkalosis) due to hyperventilation.

Treatment of DVT and PE in most cases is aimed at preventing clot propagation or a second embolism. *Anticoagulation* is the mainstay of treatment, with intravenous heparin as first-line therapy. Hospitals use weight-based nomograms and monitor therapy using activated partial thromboplastin time (aPTT).

In patients with contraindications to anticoagulation, *vena cava filters* can be placed as a physical barrier to embolization. They significantly decrease rates of embolization, but long-

Essential Clinical Anesthesia Review: Keywords, Questions and Answers for the Boards, ed. Linda S. Aglio, Robert W. Lekowski, and Richard D. Urman. Published by Cambridge University Press. © Cambridge University Press 2015.

term can increase rates of repeat DVT and postphlebitic syndrome when left in place. Therefore they should be removed as soon as there is no further contraindication to anticoagulation.

In patients with hemodynamically significant PE, other *treatment options* include thrombolysis and embolectomy. Thrombolysis can be achieved with systemic or catheter-directed alteplase (tPA). However, many ICU patients have contraindications to thrombolysis due to the high bleeding risk.

Embolectomy can be used to relieve pulmonary outflow obstruction if the following criteria are met: (1) hemodynamic instability (SBP <90, drop in SBP <40 mm Hg for >15 minutes, vasopressor requirement), (2) subtotal or total filling defect in left and/or right main pulmonary artery, and (3) major contraindication to thrombolysis (including recent surgery).

Perioperative management of anticoagulation for DVT/PE depends on length of time since the event. The risk of recurrent DVT goes down significantly in the initial three months after the event. In the first three months or in high-risk patients, patients are instructed to stop their coumadin five days before surgery and receive a "bridge" with LMWH. The last therapeutic LMWH dose would be the day before surgery. Postoperatively, both LMWH and coumadin are started on postoperative day 1 to ensure almost uninterrupted anticoagulation. If it has been longer than three months after the initial DVT, only prophylactic measures are indicated.

Questions

1. Which is the best initial test to evaluate for DVT in a critically ill patient?
   a. Homan's sign
   b. duplex ultrasonography
   c. MRI
   d. contrast venography
   e. D-dimer

2. A 65-year-old male is admitted to the ICU immediately after exploratory laparotomy with small bowel resection for incarcerated hernia. He is currently intubated. On postoperative day 1 he develops sudden tachycardia, hypoxia, and hypotension requiring vasopressors. Echocardiography reveals right heart strain and elevated pulmonary artery pressures. CT angiography reveals a large filling defect in the distal right main pulmonary artery. Which is the most appropriate treatment at this time?
   a. expectant management
   b. thrombolysis
   c. inferior vena cava filter
   d. embolectomy
   e. anticoagulation with heparin

3. Which of the following is NOT true about vena cava filters?
   a. They do not prevent DVT propagation.
   b. They are effective at preventing clot embolization.
   c. They do not increase rates of long-term repeat DVT and postphlebitic syndrome.
   d. They are indicated when a patient has a contraindication to anticoagulation.
   e. They should be removed as soon as there is no longer a contraindiction to anticoagulation.

Answers

1. b. Duplex ultrasonography is quick, easy, does not expose the patient to radiation, and is very sensitive for proximal DVT. It is a good initial test in a patient with a high pretest probability. Physical examination, including Homan's sign, is not sensitive or specific, and other imaging modalities are not significantly superior to ultrasonography.

2. d. This patient has evidence of hemodynamic instability and right heart failure due to his pulmonary embolus, as well as a large filling defect in a main pulmonary artery. All of these together are indications for pulmonary embolectomy.

3. c. Vena cava filters have been found to reduce pulmonary embolism but they also increase the rate of postphlebitic syndrome and repeat DVT. Therefore they are most useful when a patient has a contraindication to anticoagulation and should be removed once that contraindication is no longer present.

Further reading

Williams, M., Shimizu, N., and Gates, J. D. (2011). Venous thromboembolic disease in the critically ill patient. In Vacanti, C. A., Sikka, P. J., Urman, R. D., Dershwitz, M., and Segal, B. S. (eds) *Essential Clinical Anesthesia*. New York: Cambridge University Press, pp. 1010–1015.

Roizen, M. F. and Fleisher, L. A. (2010). Anesthetic implications of concurrent diseases. In Miller, R. D. et al. (eds) *Miller's Anesthesia*, 7th edn. Philadelphia: Elsevier, pp. 1067–1150.

Decousus, H., Leizorovicz, A., Parent, F. et al. (1998). A clinical trial of vena caval filters in the prevention of pulmonary embolism in patients with proximal deep-vein thrombosis. Prevention du Risque d'Embolie Pulmonaire par Interruption Cave Study Group. *New England Journal of Medicine* 338, 409–415.

Chapter

164

Traumatic brain injury

Whitney de Luna and Linda S. Aglio

Keywords

Glasgow Coma Scale: use and limits
Glasgow Coma Scale: criteria
Head trauma: acute management
Increased intracranial pressure: diagnosis
Increased intracranial pressure: intraoperative and
  pharmacologic management
Barbiturate coma: indications
Monitoring: barbiturate coma
Head trauma: anesthetic and fluid management
CSF: sustained hyperventilation
Traumatic brain injury: cerebral perfusion pressure
Brain injury and edema
Post-traumatic diabetes insipidus
Brain death: definition; criteria and pathophysiology

The *Glasgow Coma Scale (GSC)* is composed of scores for eye, verbal, and motor responses and is *used to evaluate neurological status*. Scores range from 3 (deep coma/brain-dead state) to 15 (fully awake patient) and are indicative of the level of brain injury:

- mild (GCS 14)
- moderate (GCS 9 to 13)
- severe (GCS 3 to 8)

Table 161.1 (in Chapter 161) illustrates how to score eye/verbal/motor responses. *GCS scores are limited by the subjectivity of clinicians, sedation, intubation (modified scoring available), and pediatric patients (modified scoring available).*

Acute management of head trauma

1. Determination of whether injury requires surgical intervention (based on examination/radiological imaging).
2. Prevention of secondary brain injury (i.e., beyond injured region) through normalization of intracranial pressure (ICP), cerebral perfusion pressure (CPP), and oxygen delivery. Endpoints: MAP >80, PaO$_2$ >95, ICP <20–25 mm Hg, CPP 50–70 mm Hg.

Increased intracranial pressure

Normal ICP is 5 to 15 mm Hg. Initiate treatment at ICP 20 to 25 mm Hg.

Reduction of ICP can be achieved by:

1. Elevating head of bed to 30 degrees with neutral head position.
2. Acute hyperventilation – may be used emergently with impending herniation but should be stopped when other therapies are in place. Hypoventilation raises PaCO$_2$ and ICP. While hyperventilation will lower ICP, it may also decrease CBF.
3. Sedation/analgesia – use as needed. Will blunt sympathetic responses from pain or endotracheal intubation. Propofol may also be used so that neurological checks can be performed easily, due to its short half-life.
4. Mannitol bolus of 0.25 to 0.5 g/kg q 4–6 h as needed to improve CBF and oxygen delivery while decreasing ICP. Synergistic with furosemide administration.
5. CSF drainage through ventriculostomy catheter.
6. Hypertonic saline – adjunct/alternative to mannitol. There is a lower risk of rebound intracranial hypertension and renal failure than mannitol. Risk of hypernatremia, hyperosmolality, or hyperchloremic acidosis from long-term administration.
7. *Therapeutic barbiturate coma*:
   - *Indicated for refractory ICP elevation*. Not for regular use in TBI because of cardiovascular depressant effects – only for hemodynamically stable TBI patients with refractory ICP already on maximal medical/surgical therapy. Also not routinely administered given to side effect profile (e.g., hypotension, global oligemic hypoxia, hypokalemia, respiratory depression, hepatic/renal dysfunction.
   - *Monitoring* includes EEG, arterial blood pressure, PA catheter, blood chemistries. Barbiturates are titrated to burst suppression according to EEG monitoring, after which a constant infusion of barbiturates can be maintained.

Essential Clinical Anesthesia Review: Keywords, Questions and Answers for the Boards, ed. Linda S. Aglio, Robert W. Lekowski, and Richard D. Urman. Published by Cambridge University Press. © Cambridge University Press 2015.

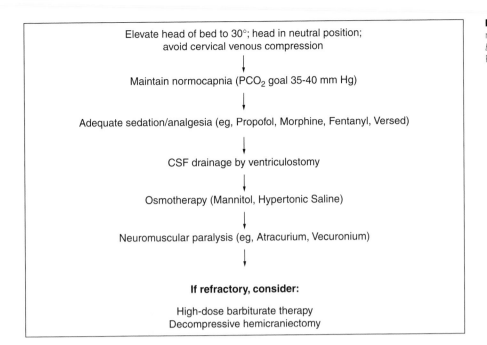

Figure 164.1 Step-wise protocol for ICP management. (Adapted from Vacanti et al. 2011. *Essential Clinical Anesthesia*, Cambridge University Press, p. 1019.)

8. Decompressive hemicraniectomy – remove overlying bone and open dura to increase intracranial vault.

CSF: sustained hyperventilation

Hyperventilation reduces brain volume by decreasing CBF through cerebral vasoconstriction. For every 1 mm Hg change in $PaCO_2$, CBF changes by 1 to 2 ml/100 g/min. Duration of effectiveness for lowering ICP may be as short as four to six hours, depending on the pH of the CSF. Target $PaCO_2$ is 30 to 35 mm Hg. Cerebrovasculature must be reactive to CO_2, which may be impaired in ischemia, trauma, tumor, and infection.

Anesthetic management of head trauma

General management includes resuscitation, airway management, fluid/electrolyte balance, and ICP control to avoid secondary brain injury.

Induction with sodium thiopental 3 to 6 mg/kg or propofol 1 to 2 mg/kg IV if patient is hemodynamically stable. This decreases CBF, CBV, and ICP. Etomidate at 0.2 to 0.3 mg/kg decreases $CMRO_2$/CBF with less effect on blood pressure.

Intubation should be performed with in-line neck stabilization and back-up laryngeal masks/fiberoptic scope. Fentanyl at 3 to 5 μg/kg IV may be used to blunt hemodynamic response to laryngoscopy and intubation. Assume full stomach – rapid sequence induction with cricoid pressure. Administer lidocaine at 1.5 mg/kg IV 90 seconds prior to laryngoscopy to prevent increase in ICP.

Intraoperatively, avoid hypotension from blood loss/anesthetic drugs with volume expansion. $PaCO_2$ should be maintained between 30 and 35 mm Hg and PaO_2 >60 mm Hg. Emergence should be without hypertension, coughing, or bucking.

Intraoperative management of fluids and ICP

The goal is to avoid cerebral ischemia/hypoxia through oxygen delivery. TBI patients require aggressive fluid resuscitation – hypotension systolic <90 mm Hg at any point will worsen prognosis. Fluid management for TBI patients is achieved with a mix of colloids and crystalloids to maintain colloid oncotic pressure during large-volume resuscitation.

Use inotropes/vasopressors (i.e., dopamine or norepinephrine) as adjuncts. Vasoconstriction effects may impair local CBF – despite improving CPP.

Previously described therapies to reduce ICP should be used throughout the perioperative period (positional therapy when possible, osmotherapy, analgesia, and sedation).

Traumatic brain injury: cerebral perfusion pressure

Normal cerebral perfusion pressure can range from 40 to 160 mm Hg due to autoregulation and is impaired following TBI. CBF is proportional to CPP in TBI, so CPP should be between 50 and 70 mm Hg. Low CPP will begin a feedback loop wherein pial arteries will dilate to increase CBV. This will further increase ICP, leading to a lowering of CPP.

Post-traumatic diabetes insipidus

Caused by trauma to the neurohypophysis. Symptoms include postoperative hypotension, tachycardia, hypernatremia, high output of urine without glycosuria, and polydipsia. Treat with fluid replacement (monitor urine output and hypernatremia) and hormone replacement (intranasal desmopressin if urine output >300 ml/h).

Brain death

Brain death is the irreversible cessation of cerebral and brain-stem function.

Criteria for brain death:

1. Coma = absence of response to stimulus (movement, withdrawal, grimace, blinking).
2. Negative apnea test ($PaCO_2$ >20 mm Hg above baseline when disconnected from ventilator).
3. Dilated, unresponsive pupils.
4. Absence of brainstem reflexes. Reversible medical conditions must be ruled out.

Brain edema related to trauma: classified as vasogenic or cytotoxic edema. Vasogenic – functional breakdown of endothelial cell layer leading to protein and ion transfer into interstitial brain compartments. Cytotoxic – intracellular water accumulation from increased cell membrane permeability due to ionic pump failure from energy depletion.

Brain death pathophysiology: related to effects of brain edema. Edema increases ICP, which decreases cerebral blood flow (CBF) if ICP exceeds arterial blood pressure. Direct cellular injury from absence of blood flow and hypoxia leads to cerebral acidosis and brain swelling. Finally, herniation and aseptic necrosis occur.

Questions

1. Which is true regarding mannitol therapy?
   a. reduces ICP by reducing intracranial water content
   b. reduces ICP by expanding plasma volume and decreasing plasma viscosity
   c. can precipitate acute renal failure
   d. may work in conjunction with furosemide
   e. all of the above

2. Which statement is correct regarding hyperventilation after TBI?
   a. Hyperventilation ($PaCO_2$ <30 mm Hg) should be used during the first 24 hours after severe TBI.
   b. Hyperventilation has no significant role unless the patient is deteriorating quickly.

   c. Chronic prophylactic hyperventilation therapy is effective for several days after the initial injury.
   d. Hyperventilation has no effect on brain ischemia.
   e. None of the above.

3. Which patient has a Glasgow Coma Scale (GCS) score of 13?
   a. Eye opens to pain, inappropriate verbal responses, withdraws from pain.
   b. Eyes open spontaneously, incomprehensible speech, withdraws from pain.
   c. Eyes open spontaneously, oriented, movement to painful stimulus.
   d. Eye opening to speech, makes confused conversation, obeys commands.
   e. Opens eye to pain, inappropriate verbal responses, withdraws from pain.

Answers

1. e. Originally thought to reduce ICP by reducing intracranial water content, mannitol is now understood to expand plasma volume and decrease plasma viscosity. It will also increase CBF and decrease ICP through autoregulatory vasoconstriction. Furosemide is known to inhibit the production of CSF and may potentiate the effects of mannitol.

2. b. Hyperventilation should only be used in emergency situations as a temporizing measure to control ICP and should be discontinued once there is evidence of cerebral edema. While hypoxemia is associated with increased morbidity/mortality, the use of prophylactic hyperventilation therapy during the first 24 hours after severe TBI may compromise cerebral perfusion, since TBI patients already have reduced CBF. Likewise, chronic hyperventilation therapy should also be avoided.

3. d. Using the scoring system: eyes opening to speech (3), makes confused conversation (4), obeys commands (6) equalling a total of 13.

Further reading

Bullock, M. R., ed. (2007). Guidelines for the Management of Severe Traumatic Brain Injury, 3rd edn. *Journal of Neurotrauma* www.braintrauma.org/pdf/protected/

Guidelines_Management_2007w_bookmarks.pdf.

Vacanti, C. A., Sikka, P. K., Urman, R. U., Dershwitz, M., and Segal, B. S. (2011). *Essential Clinical Anesthesia,*

1st edn. Cambridge University Press, pp. 1016–1023.

Miller, R. D. (2010). *Miller's Anesthesia.* Philadelphia, PA: Churchill-Livingstone/ Elsevier, pp. 2296–2299.

Chapter

Burn management

165

Christopher Voscopoulos and Joshua Vacanti

Keywords

Pathophysiologic changes associated with burn injury
Burn shock
Hypermetabolic phase of burn recovery
The rule of nines
Lund and Browder burn diagrams
Assessment of burn depth
Electrical burns
Inhalation injury
Parkland Formula
Burn resuscitation endpoints
Curling ulcers
Infection in burn patients
Blood loss during surgical excision of burns

Pathophysiologic changes associated with burn injury are extensive and effect all organ systems. Tissue trauma caused by burn injury leads to local and systemic inflammation characterized by the release of the inflammatory mediators, including histamine, free oxygen radicals, and prostaglandins, and contributes to burn shock.

Burn shock is a systemic condition directly related to the disruption of the integument's ability to regulate water balance, and is characterized by generalized capillary leak, intravascular volume depletion, and myocardial dysfunction. These pathophysiologic changes coupled with direct evaporated losses at the sites of burn injury necessitate large-volume resuscitation.

The *hypermetabolic phase of burn recovery* becomes evident clinically with resolution of burn shock and restoration of capillary integrity. Resting metabolic rates can double and may remain elevated for up to 9–12 months depending on the size of the burn injury.

The *rule of nines* is a commonly used method for estimating the extent of body surface area effected by burn injury. The head receives a percentage score of 9. Likewise, each upper extremity, the anterior thorax, the posterior thorax, the anterior abdomen, and the posterior abdomen each account for 9%

Table 165.1 Systemic effects of burn injury

System	Pathophysiologic changes and complications
Respiratory	Airway edema Reduced pulmonary and chest wall compliance Bronchospasm Pneumonia, pulmonary edema, and ARDS
Cardiovascular	Hypovolemia Myocardial dysfunction and decreased cardiac output (early) Increased cardiac output and hypertension (late)
Renal	Decreased renal blood flow (early) Increased renal blood flow (late) Myoglobinemia
Metabolic	Increased metabolic rate Impaired thermoregulation Protein catabolism Electrolyte imbalances (from resuscitation and topical antibiotics)
Gastrointestinal	Curling ulcers Ileus and delayed gastric emptying Impaired intestinal barrier
Hematologic	Hemoconcentration (initially) Chronic anemia (later) Thrombocytopenia (dilutional and consumptive) Coagulopathy and disseminated intravascular coagulopathy (in severe cases)
Infectious	Postburn sepsis
Neurologic	Encephalopathy Acute and chronic pain Cyanide and carbon monoxide poisoning
Skin	Increased fluid and heat loss Need for escharotomy in severe cases Contracture and scar formation
Pharmacologic	Altered pharmacokinetics and pharmacodynamics Increased tolerance to sedatives and opioids Altered response to muscle relaxants

(*Essential Clinical Anesthesia*, 1st edn. 2011. Cambridge University Press, p. 1024, Table 166.1.)

Essential Clinical Anesthesia Review: Keywords, Questions and Answers for the Boards, ed. Linda S. Aglio, Robert W. Lekowski, and Richard D. Urman. Published by Cambridge University Press. © Cambridge University Press 2015.

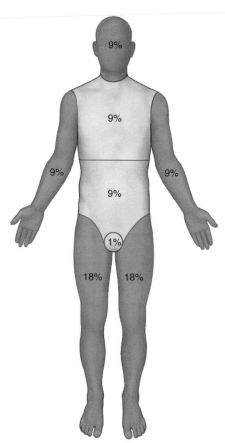

Figure 165.1 The rule of nines for estimating total body surface area. Note: not accurate for all age groups. (Adapted from Vacanti et al. 2011. *Essential Clinical Anesthesia*, Cambridge University Press, Figure 166.1.)

Table 165.2 Burn resuscitation endpoints

Arousable and comfortable
Warm extremities
Systolic blood pressure: for infants, 60 mm Hg; for older children, 70–90 + 2 × age (y); for adults, mean arterial pressure >65 or within 20% of baseline
HR 80–150 bpm (age-dependent)
Urine output 0.5 ml/kg/h
Lactate levels <2 mmol/l

(*Essential Clinical Anesthesia*, 1st edn. 2011. Cambridge University Press, Table 166.3.)

of the body's surface area. Each lower extremity accounts for 18% of its surface area, and the groin accounts for 1% (see Figure 165.1). Although this methodology provides reasonable estimates for adults, it underestimates burn surface in children.

Lund and Browder burn diagrams provide an alternative method for assessing the extent of burn injury. Evidence suggests that these may produce more accurate estimates of burn surface area in children. In the Lund and Browder burn chart, age brackets are separated into six different columns: ages 0, 1, 5, 10, 15, and adults. Head size is proportionately greater in younger patients; this ratio decreases with age. In contrast, the thigh and leg are relatively smaller by percentage in children.

Assessment of burn depth has classically included the terms first, second, or third degree. This has generally been replaced by a new system that describes thermal injury as superficial, superficial partial-thickness, deep partial-thickness, and full thickness. This system helps clarify the level of injury and the involvement of the epidermis, papillary dermis, reticular dermis, subcutaneous fat, and the fascia, muscle, or bone.

Electrical burns are a distinct class of burn injury. Electrical burns often result in massive amounts of tissue destruction that may not be predicted by the burn size alone. Although direct thermal injury may occur at contact points, where current enters and exits the body, the skin provides excellent insulation while electrical current travels across muscle fibers. The skin surface often appears intact, and may conceal widespread muscle damage and necrosis. Morbidity also occurs

from arrhythmias induced by electrical current. Extensive deep tissue damage can result in myoglobinuria and acute renal failure, and compartment syndrome.

Inhalation injury may be suspected by direct observation of residual soot in the airway. Indirectly, carboxyhemoglobin levels in the blood may suggest the diagnosis. Because edema formation occurs in nonburned tissues after major thermal injury, and often worsens during prolonged resuscitation, obstructive respiratory failure is common. Since inhalation injury carries a high mortality, early intubation may be indicated. Some studies suggest that mortality in pure inhalational burn injury may exceed 40%. Airway management may be difficult owing to mucosal edema, and the need for a surgical airway must be anticipated. Inhalational injury places patients at increased risk for pneumonia, noncardiogenic pulmonary edema, and acute respiratory distress syndrome, often leading to a lung-protective ventilation strategy and low-tidal volume ventilation (6 ml/kg) during mechanical ventilation.

The Parkland Formula estimates the volume of crystalloid required for resuscitation over a 24-hour period. The percentage of total body surface area burned is multiplied by weight in kilograms and then quadrupled. This volume of lactated Ringer's solution is infused over 24 hours starting at the time of injury, with one half of this amount administered over the first eight hours and one quarter given over each of the next eight-hour periods. As a general rule, burns involving less than 15% body surface area are not associated with extensive capillary leak and can be managed with 1.5 times the maintenance rate. Importantly, the Parkland Formula only serves as a means of estimating fluid requirements.

Formulas for estimating fluid requirements after major thermal injury only approximate fluid requirements, and *burn resuscitation endpoints* should be used in a flexible manner. Resuscitative effort should be tailored to specific surrogates of organ perfusion (see Table 165.2). Urine output is the most widely used metric to guide volume replacement and should be the focus of any resuscitation strategy.

Curling ulcers are peptic ulcers that occur secondary to hypovolemia in burn patients and result in ischemic changes in the gastric mucosa. The incidence of these ulcers decreases significantly with proper volume resuscitation, enteral feeding, and gastric acid prophylaxis during mechanical ventilation.

Infection is the leading cause of morbidity and mortality in burn patients. Because of disruptions in the skin, microbial agents easily enter the systemic circulation, leading to sepsis, which has an incidence in burn patients estimated to be between 8% to 42.5%. Gram-positive skin flora are commonly implicated early, followed late in the first week by nosocomial gram-negative bacteria or bacteria associated with the gastro-intestinal or respiratory systems. Yeast and fungi are late colonizers. Topical antimicrobials provide high concentrations of drug at the wound surface, reduce the levels of wound flora, and delay the interval between injury and colonization. Possible agents are gentamicin sulfate, mafenide acetate, nitrofurazone, providine-iodine, silver nitrate, and silver sulfadiazine.

Blood loss during surgical excision of burns can be as high as 3.5% to 5% of the blood volume for every 1% of excised burn area. Blood loss should be aggressively replaced, with an emphasis on avoiding hypothermia, coagulopathy, and acidosis.

Questions

1. The Parkland Formula is best used in which patient groups?
   a. pediatric patients with greater than 15% burns
   b. adults with less than 15% burns
   c. adults with superficial burns
   d. adults with greater than 15% burns

2. To reduce the risk of infection in burn patients:
   a. Enteral antibiotics should be used prophylactically to prevent wound infection.
   b. Prophylactic intravenous antibiotics should be used for the first two weeks of treatment.
   c. Prophylactic intravenous antibiotics should be used for 24 hours postoperatively following grafting.
   d. Topical antibiotic should be used prophylactically to prevent wound infection.

3. Mortality in burn patients is highest secondary to which of the following?
   a. hypovolemic shock
   b. cardiac arrhythmias
   c. acute renal failure
   d. infection

Answers

1. d. As a general rule, burns of <15% TBSA in adult patients are not associated with extensive capillary leak or other symptoms of burn shock, and can be managed with 1.5 times the standard maintenance rate. The Parkland Formula is more accurate in estimating the fluid needs of adult burns >15%. Lund and Browder burn diagrams are used to estimate fluid requirements and guide resuscitation in pediatric patients.

2. d. Topical antimicrobials deliver higher concentrations of drug at the wound surface, reduce the levels of wound flora, and delay the interval between injury and colonization.

3. d. Infection is the leading cause of morbidity and mortality in burn patients.

Further reading

Alvarado, R., Chung, K. K., Cancio, L. C., and Wolf, S. E. (2009). Burn resuscitation. *Burns* 35(1), 4–14.

Bittner, E. A., Grecu, L., and Martyn, J. A. J. (2008). Evaluation of the burn patient. In Longnecker, D. E. et al. (eds) *Anesthesiology*. New York: McGraw-Hill.

Bittner, E. A., Grecu, L., and Martyn, J. A. J. (2008). Management of anesthesia for the burn patient. In Longnecker, D. E. et al. (eds) *Anesthesiology*. New York: McGraw-Hill.

Ipaktchi, K. and Arbabi, S. (2006). Advances in burn critical care. *Critical Care Medicine* 34(Suppl.), S239–S244.

Latenser, B. A. (2009). Critical care of the burn patient: the first 48 hours. *Critical Care Medicine* 37, 2819–2826.

Sheridan, R. (2002). Burns. *Critical Care Medicine* 30(Suppl.), S500–S514.

Vacanti, C. A., Sikka, P. K., Urman, R. U., Dershwitz, M., and Segal, B. S. (2011). *Essential Clinical Anesthesia*, 1st edn. Cambridge University Press.

El-Helbawy, R. H. and Ghareeb, F. M. (2011). Inhalation injury as a prognostic factor for mortality in burn patients. *Annals of Burns and Fire Disasters* 24(2), 82–88.

Mann, E. A., Baun, M. M., Meininger, J. C., and Wade, C. E. (2012). Comparison of mortality associated with sepsis in the burn, trauma, and general intensive care unit patient: a systematic review of the literature. *Shock* 37(1), 4–16.

Dai, T., Huang, Y. Y., Sharma, S. K. et al. (2010). Topical antimicrobials for burn wound infections. *Recent Patents on Anti-infective Drug Discovery* 5(2), 124–151.

Chapter
166

Common ethical issues in the intensive care unit

Christopher Voscopoulos and Joshua Vacanti

The four principles
Autonomy
Beneficence
Nonmaleficence
Justice
Paternalism
Competence and decisional capacity
Substituted judgment
Designated health care proxy agents
Advanced care directives
Living wills
Synthetic judgment
Informed consent

With respect to medical ethics, *the four principles* are generally regarded as the standard framework around which to approach ethical dilemmas in the ICU. These principles, which include autonomy, beneficence, nonmaleficence, and justice, can be applied to the doctor–patient relationship and should be considered in the context of patient care.

Autonomy describes the right of patients to dictate those medical interventions they will accept and those that they will reject.

Beneficence refers to the obligation of physicians to do or promote the most possible good for patients.

Nonmaleficence is the companion concept to beneficence that is summarized by the Latin aphorism *primum non nocere*, which when translated means "above all, do no harm."

Justice refers primarily to distributive justice, in which the obligation of the physician, or more widely the health care delivery system, is to ensure that care is delivered fairly, equitably, and appropriately to all individuals.

Paternalism describes the notion whereby physicians initiate care based on their determination of what is in "the best interest of the patient."

Competence and decisional capacity refer to a cognitive or physical issue, which should preclude patients from making decisions regarding their own care, although both terms differ

with respect to their precise definition. These categories of patients include those that lack *competence*, such as patients with delirium, dementia, or depression, or those patients who lack *decisional capacity*, such as patients that are sedated.

Substituted judgment describes a situation where a patient does not possess decisional capacity. In this case, the goal of care should be to extend as accurately as possible that person's autonomy through a surrogate decision maker.

A *designated health care proxy agent* is someone preselected by a patient to make medical decisions for them when they cannot. Ideally this person should have an understanding of the patient's long-term wishes and have participated in discussions with the patient regarding future goals for health care with respect to varying medical scenarios.

Advanced care directives are detailed documents completed by patients prior to losing decisional capacity that include statements outlining a patient's medical wishes.

Living wills are a specific type of advanced care directive, and describe a patient's medical wishes in specific terms (e.g., no chest compressions, no mechanical ventilation, no feeding tubes, etc.).

Synthetic judgment describes medial decision making in instances where patients have not completed an advanced care directive, and have no known living relatives or close friends who might act as a surrogate decision maker. In this case, all efforts should be made to try and determine what the patient's wishes might be based on available information. This should be done in close consultation with the hospital ethics liaison and the legal department.

Informed consent refers to a physician's ethical duty to acquaint a patient or proxy with information regarding the risks and benefits of proposed treatments. Several standards have been proposed to describe methods of proper informed consent as follows:

- Reasonable person standard: the principle that a health care provider is required to inform a patient of all the facts, risks, and alternatives that a reasonable person in a similar situation would find important in deciding whether or not to proceed with a proposed treatment course.

Essential Clinical Anesthesia Review: Keywords, Questions and Answers for the Boards, ed. Linda S. Aglio, Robert W. Lekowski, and Richard D. Urman. Published by Cambridge University Press. © Cambridge University Press 2015.

- Standard of care: a diagnostic or treatment process that is generally accepted by the medical community to be the appropriate course of care.
- Subjective standard: the notion that each patient, based on their background and belief systems, needs specific information to make an informed decision. It requires the physician to empathize with the patient in an effort to reconcile the patient's own values with the treatment options available to them.
- Waiver of consent: a document relieving a person or organization required to obtain consent from actually getting that consent.

Questions

1. Which are the four principles of medical ethics?
   a. autonomy, self-determination, justice, and good will
   b. beneficence, nonmaleficence, self-determination, and paternalism
   c. autonomy, beneficence, nonmaleficence, and justice
   d. beneficence, justice, self-determination, and nonmaleficence

2. Someone designated by a patient to make medical decisions for them when they cannot is called which of the following?
   a. designated health care proxy
   b. designated health care proxy agent
   c. substituted judgment proxy
   d. substituted judgment proxy agent

3. Which of the following would not interfere with a patient's competence or decisional capacity?
   a. depression
   b. intubation
   c. biventricular assist devices
   d. delirium

Answers

1. c. Beauchamp and Childress described the four ethical principles as autonomy, beneficence, nonmaleficence, and justice.
2. b. A designated health care proxy agent is someone designated by a patient to make medical decisions for them when they cannot. A health care proxy refers only to the papers that delegate the medical decision making to another person.
3. c. Competence and decisional capacity differ in terms of their precise definition, but neither an incompetent patient nor a patient lacking decisional capacity should dictate his or her own medical care. Examples include patients with delirium, dementia, depression, or those who are intubated.

Further reading

Applebaum, P. S. (2007). Assessment of patients's competence to consent to treatment. *New England Journal of Medicine* 357, 1834–1840.

Beauchamp, T. L. and Childress, J. F. (1994). *Principles of Biomedical Ethics*, 4th edn. New York: Oxford University Press.

Englehardt, H. T. (1996). *The Foundations of Bioethics*, 2nd edn. New York: Oxford University Press.

Vacanti, C. A., Sikka, P. K., Urman, R. U., Dershwitz, M., and Segal, B. S. (2011). *Essential Clinical Anesthesia*, 1st edn. Cambridge University Press.

Chapter 167

Bronchopleural fistula

Yuka Kiyota, George P. Topulos, and Philip M. Hartigan

Keywords

Bronchopleural fistula (BPF)
Causes of BPF
Predisposing factors for BPF
Preoperative evaluation of BPF
Intraoperative management of BPF
Postoperative management of BPF
High-frequency jet ventiation

Bronchopleural fistula (BPF) is a pathologic connection between an airway and the surrounding pleural cavity. It is usually managed conservatively. Surgery is indicated when the conservative management fails.

Causes of bronchopleural fistula (BPF)

- breakdown of suture/staple line following lung resection
- rupture of cavity (cyst, abscess, bulla, bleb)
- erosion of bronchial wall by infection (empyema, pneumonia, tuberculosis)
- erosion of bronchial wall by neoplasm
- penetrating trauma
- pulmonary infarction
- iatrogenic

Predisposing factors for BPF

- radiation exposure
- infection
- right-sided pneumonectomy
- residual neoplasm
- a long bronchial stump without coverages (reinforcing flap)
- prolonged intubation

Goals of BPF management during the perioperative period

Management strategies depend on the size, location, and acuity of the BPF. Early dehissence of a bronchial pneumonectomy stump requires immediate surgical repair. Delayed postpneumonectomy stump leaks require that the associated empyema be addressed (drainage, antibiotics, Clagett window, etc.) prior to closure. More limited distal parenchymal air leaks may be managed conservatively. The following general principles apply to all:

- minimization of airflow across the fistula
- adequate gas exchange in the unaffected lung
- avoidance of tension pneumothorax
- protection against contamination of the remaining lung
- control of infection

Preoperative evaluation of BPF

- Evaluation of the size and location of the BPF:
  - a continuous, persistent leak indicates a large fistula
  - utilize radiographic or bronchoscopic information if available
  - measurement of difference between the inspired tidal volume and the expired tidal volume (intubated patients).
- Evaluate safety of transport to the OR:
  - large air leaks may require ICU transport ventilator for sufficient flows
  - placing chest tube on "water seal" rather than continuous suction may improve ventilation during transport
  - trial of transport ventilation prior to departing ICU is prudent.

Essential Clinical Anesthesia Review: Keywords, Questions and Answers for the Boards, ed. Linda S. Aglio, Robert W. Lekowski, and Richard D. Urman. Published by Cambridge University Press. © Cambridge University Press 2015.

- If the patient does not have a chest tube, discuss this with the surgeon prior to positive pressure ventilation.
- Raising the head of the bed and tilting the patient "fistula-side down" reduces the chances of cross-contamination.
- Establish a plan for rapid lung isolation and ventilation.

Intraoperative management of BPF

- Early lung isolation is indicated except for very small BPFs.
- If a large BPF is anticipated, a mask induction while maintaining spontaneous ventilation, followed by intubation with DLT and OLV should be considered (or alternatively, an IV induction with immediate lung isolation during apnea):
  - DLT should be advanced under fiberoptic guidance to assure that bronchial lumen does not further disrupt stump BPF (right DLT for left BPF and vice versa)
  - DLT allows bronchoscopic evaluation of BPF via tracheal lumen.
- When ventilating both lungs, minimize tension on and airflow through the fistula by reducing mean airway pressures with small tidal volumes and rapid respiratory rates (*high-frequency jet ventilation* can be advantageous in this aspect).

Postoperative management of BPF (following Clagett window or BPF repair)

- Resume spontaneous breathing as positive pressure ventilation may stress the repair.
- If the patient cannot be extubated, ventilatory pressures must be minimized.
- If a large air leak remains, a patient may need to remain on OLV or both lungs ventilated independently on separate ventilators in the ICU.
- Pressure-controlled ventilation may be useful to avoid high peak airway pressures, which may stress stump repairs. It also provides higher flows early in the inspiratory cycle to better overcome air leaks.
- Suction on the chest tube should be minimized.

High-frequency jet ventilation (HFJV)

- Theoretically reduces air leaks due to lower mean and inspiratory airway pressures and tidal volumes (but controversial).
- Inadequate CO_2 elimination in some studies of BPF patients.
- Less effective in patients with noncompliant lungs such as acute respiratory distress syndrome (ARDS) or pulmonary fibrosis.

Questions

1. All are TRUE statements about management of patients with BPF EXCEPT for which?
   a. If the patient does not have a chest tube, it is generally indicated to place one prior to the surgery.
   b. High-frequency jet ventilation's theoretical benefit in the management of BPF is its lower tidal volume and lower inspiratory pressure, minimizing air leaks.
   c. As opposed to spontaneous ventilation, early initiation of positive pressure ventilation offers advantage for minimizing the air leak from BPF in a patient with a large BPF.
   d. Patients with large BPFs are usually managed surgically.

2. All are TRUE statements except for which?
   a. Radiation exposure is a predisposing factor to develop BPF postoperatively.
   b. Volume-controlled ventilation is the better mode for ventilation, as the expiration is flow-triggered rather than time-triggered.
   c. It is usually best to resume spontaneous ventilation to reduce the leak in many cases.
   d. Intraoperatively, early lung isolation is indicated for patients with BPF.

Answers

1. c. In a patient with a large BPF, a mask induction with spontaneous ventilation is considered.
2. b. Pressure-controlled ventilation more reliably limits peak inspiratory pressures that may stress proximal BPF repairs.

Further reading

Ng, J.-M. and Gerner, P. (2011). Chapter 168. Bronchopleural fistula. In Vacanti, C. A., Sikka, P. J., Urman, R. D., Dershwitz, M., and Segal, B. S. (eds) *Essential Clinical Anesthesia*. New York: Cambridge University Press, pp. 1043–1045.

Ng, J.-M. (2012). Chapter 31. Bronchopleural fistula. In Hartigan, P. M. (ed) *Practical Handbook of Thoracic Anesthesia*. New York: Springer, pp. 497–510.

Inhaled nitric oxide

Chapter 168

Yuka Kiyota and Stanton Shernan

Keywords

Nitric oxide
Toxicity of nitric oxide

Nitric oxide (NO)

- Colorless and odorless with a short half-life (a few seconds in vivo).
- A free radical produced endogenously or provided by exogenous sources.
- Main action includes vasorelaxation and bronchodilation.
- Inhaled NO binds rapidly to hemoglobin and induces selective pulmonary vasodilation.
- Inhaled low-dose NO: V/Q match improves and PaO_2 increases.
- Inhaled high-dose NO: may decrease pulmonary artery pressure without systemic vascular resistance or systemic blood pressure.

Mechanism: inhaled NO stimulates guanylate cyclase to synthesize cyclic guanosine monophosphate (cGMP), which then activates cGMP-dependent protein kinase, leading to vascular relaxation. In the presence of oxygenated hemoglobin, NO is rapidly metabolized to nitrate with formation of methemoglobin. Rapid metabolization of NO is primarily responsible for its effects on selective pulmonary vasodilation and relative sparing of systemic vasodilation (systemic hypotension).

Clinical use:

- NO improves oxygenation and decreases the requirement of ECMO in patients with persistent pulmonary hypertension of the newborn (PPHN).
- Definitive use of NO in the ARDS population and in patients during or after cardiac surgery complicated by pulmonary hypertension and right ventricular dysfunction is yet to be determined.

Toxicity of nitric oxide

- Mainly from methemoglobinemia as well as NO_2 formation.
- Gas phase of NO and NO_2 should be monitored closely while inhaled NO is given to the patient.
- Methemoglobin level should be monitored, especially in patients breathing 80 ppm or more NO.
- Administer at the lowest dose NO concentration to produce the desired physiologic effect.
- Abrupt discontinuation of NO can result in "rebound" pulmonary hypertension.

Question

1. All are FALSE statements except for which?
   a. As NO has a very short half-life, toxicity is not a clinical concern.
   b. Use of NO in patients with ARDS has been proven to decrease overall mortality.
   c. NO has been proven to be effective in reducing the requirement of ECMO in neonates with PPHN.
   d. NO's main actions include vasodilation and bronchoconstriction.

Answer

1. c. Major toxicity concern includes methemoglobinemia and NO_2 formation. There has not been enough data to suggest NO's effect on decreased mortality outcome in the ARDS population yet. NO's main actions are vasodilation and bronchodilation.

Further reading

Vacanti, C. A., Sikka, P. K., Urman, R. U., Dershwitz, M., and Segal, B. S. (2011). Chapter 169. Inhaled nitric oxide. In *Essential Clinical Anesthesia*, 1st edn. Cambridge University Press.

Block, K. D., Ichinose, F., Roberts, J. D. Jr, and Zapol, W. M. (2007). Inhaled NO as a therapeutic agent. *Cardiovascular Research* 75(2), 339–348.

Skin and collagen disorders

Richard Hsu and Christopher Chen

Keywords

Hereditary angioedema
Ehlers–Danlos syndrome
Systemic lupus erythematosus
Epidermolysis bullosa
Osteogenesis imperfecta
Marfan syndrome

Hereditary angioedema (HAE)

This is an autosomal dominant disorder with acute episodic nonpitting edema of the eyes, lips, larynx, mouth, tongue, face, genitalia, and bowels. Airway edema occurs secondary to swelling in the larynx, which may lead to asphyxiation and death. Abdominal pain is likely due to peristaltic movement of the swelling bowel with some component of obstruction.

The leakage of plasma from postcapillary venules into the dermal layers of the skin plays a role in the pathophysiology of this disorder. Type 1 is characterized by low C1 inhibitor, Type 2 has nonfunctioning C1 inhibitor, and Type 3 has no clear deficiency in the complement/kinin system, but patients still present with HAE symptoms.

Treatment in the acute phase involves epinephrine, glucocorticoids, narcotics, purified C1 inhibitor, and/or ε-aminocaproic acid (EACA). These can all abort attacks and be used in the perioperative setting. Short-term prophylaxis involves FFP, androgens, and plasmin inhibitors. Long-term prophylaxis utilizes danazol, stanozolol, and methyltestosterone. Antihistamines are ineffective.

Ehlers–Danlos syndrome (EDS)

This is a group of more than ten different types of inherited disorders, all involving genetic defects in collagen metabolism and connective tissue synthesis and structure. All types share common joint hypermobility, skin fragility, bruising, poor wound healing, scarring, joint pain, and arthritis.

- Type IV (vascular) is the most severe form: associated with spontaneous rupture of the bowel, uterus, or major blood vessels, cervical spine or airway trauma, preterm labor and excessive bleeding with delivery.
- Type VI: scoliosis is common.
- Type VIII: gum disease is common.

Cardiac manifestations include cardiac conduction abnormalities and valvular defects (e.g., mitral valve prolapse, mitral regurgitation). There is an increased risk for perioperative endocarditis, therefore consider prophylactic antibiotics in the presence of cardiac murmurs. There is also a high bleeding risk, so avoid airway trauma, and take caution with arterial and central venous line placement, as well as regional anesthesia.

Systemic lupus erythematosus (SLE)

This is a chronic multisystem autoimmune disease involving antinuclear antibodies (i.e., anti-dsDNA antibodies). Anesthetic management depends on disease stage, and anesthetic considerations are varied. Patients on chronic steroid therapy will need perioperative stress-dose treatment. Rheumatoid and inflammatory conditions (e.g., scleroderma, CREST, antiphospholipid syndrome) may make IV access difficult. If the esophagus is fibrosed, Sellick's maneuver (application of cricoid pressure) may not be effective. Stiff temporomandibular joints may create difficulty with mouth opening during direct laryngoscopy. In general, patients should be kept warm to avoid exacerbation of Raynaud's phenomenon. Also, parturients may have coexisting pulmonary hypertension.

Epidermolysis bullosa (EB)

There are three major types that are differentiated by the location of the lesions:

- EB simplex (keratin mutations): intraepidermal skin separation.
- Junctional EB (various mutations): separation in the lamina lucida and basement membrane zone.

Essential Clinical Anesthesia Review: Keywords, Questions and Answers for the Boards, ed. Linda S. Aglio, Robert W. Lekowski, and Richard D. Urman. Published by Cambridge University Press. © Cambridge University Press 2015.

- Dystrophic EB (Type VII collagen mutation): separation in the sublamina densa basement membrane zone.

Avoid intramuscular medication in patients with EB. Take caution with skin monitors (e.g., EKG leads, tape/Tegaderm, BIS monitoring), and use artificial tears and ointment to avoid eye tape or patches. Intubation, suction, temperature probe placement, and any other instrumentation must be done with great care. Epidural and spinal anesthesia have been reported to be successful in EB patients, but local anesthetic skin infiltration is contraindicated. Succinylcholine can cause fasciculation-induced tissue damage, and nondepolarizing agents are unpredictable.

Osteogenesis imperfecta (OI)

This is a rare autosomal dominant disease where mutations in Type I collagen cause osteomalacia, excess fractures, short stature, scoliosis, basilar skull deformities, blue sclerae, hearing loss, easy bruising, and increased laxity of ligaments and skin. Increased thyroxine levels are found in 50% of OI patients and are associated with increased O_2 consumption and body temperature. However, there is no clear relationship between OI and malignant hyperthermia. Fractures may present as cervical spine deformities, or result from an inflated blood pressure cuff or succinylcholine-induced fasciculations. Hypoxemia may occur due to restriction and decreased compliance from kyphoscoliosis and pectus excavatum. Regional anesthesia has been administered successfully to avoid tracheal intubation.

Marfan syndrome

This is an autosomal dominant disorder caused by a mutation in matrix glycoprotein fibrillin 1, characterized by cardiovascular, skeletal, and ocular connective tissue abnormalities.

Cardiac manifestations abound. Aortic dilatation and dissection due to aortic media weakness is the most life-threatening manifestation. Monitor with periodic echocardiography and control hypertension tightly. Severe aortic regurgitation is a late finding. Mitral and/or tricuspid prolapse is common due to thickening of the AV valves. Antibiotic prophylaxis for bacterial endocarditis is common. Bundle branch blocks are a common conduction abnormality.

Bony manifestations include craniofacial deformities, dislocation of joints (e.g., atlanto-axial joint, temporomandibular joint), and thoracolumbar scoliosis, which can compromise pulmonary function. Lumbosacral dural ectasia is seen in 63% to 92% of patients, which may cause an erratic spread of intrathecal local anesthetics. Instead, continuous spinal, epidural, or combined spinal–epidural anesthesia (instead of single-shot spinal anesthesia) allows for titration to an adequate level for cesarean section.

Questions

1. A parturient with which of the following skin/collagen disorders would require regular monitoring with echocardiograms throughout the pregnancy?
   a. hereditary angioedema
   b. systemic lupus erythematosus
   c. osteogenesis imperfecta
   d. Marfan syndrome

2. Which would be a good agent to treat an acute attack in a patient with hereditary angioedema?
   a. antihistamines
   b. danazol or stanozolol
   c. epinephrine
   d. fresh frozen plasma

Answers

1. d. Risk of aortic dissection is the most life-threatening cardiac consideration in Marfan syndrome. According to the National Marfan Foundation, an echocardiogram should be performed prior to pregnancy and should be repeated a minimum of three times during pregnancy – once in each trimester – and once during the two months following pregnancy. In women whose aortic root diameter prior to pregnancy is close to 4 cm, more frequent echocardiograms are recommended (approximately every six to eight weeks) to identify any sudden increase in aortic size.

2. c. The angioedema in HAE is *not* responsive to antihistamines. Instead, epinephrine, glucocorticoids, narcotics, purified C1 inhibitor, and/or ε-aminocaproic acid (EACA) can all be used to abort attacks acutely.

Further reading

Vacanti, C. A., Sikka, P. K., Urman, R. U., Dershwitz, M., and Segal, B. S. (2011). Chapter 170. Inhaled nitric oxide. In *Essential Clinical Anesthesia*, 1st edn. Cambridge University Press.

Keane, M. G. and Pyeritz, R. E. (2008). Medical management of Marfan syndrome. *Circulation* 117(21), 2802–13.

Chapter

170

Anesthesia for aesthetic surgery

Richard Hsu and Maksim Zayaruzny

Keywords

Local anesthetic toxicity: diagnosis and treatment

Liposuction

Two similar techniques, "superwet" and tumescent, both involve infiltrating the surgical area with a mixture of normal saline or lactated Ringer's solution with a low concentration of lidocaine. Total doses of lidocaine frequently exceed maximum recommended dose on a "per kilo" basis. Complications include hyper- or hypovolemia, pulmonary embolism, hypothermia, and lidocaine toxicity. The risk of lidocaine toxicity increases when more than one body region is being treated with liposuction (e.g., lower extremity in addition to head and neck).

Rhytidectomy ("facelift")

This involves the removal of excess facial skin and tightening of underlying tissues on the patient's face and neck. A variety of anesthetic techniques can be employed. Dexmedetomidine may be used in addition to standard anesthetic techniques to allow the patient to breathe spontaneously on room air while providing sedation and analgesia.

Blepharoplasty

Removing or repositioning excess tissue reshapes the eyelids. Local anesthesia and/or IV sedation may be used to allow the procedure to be performed in the office setting.

Rhinoplasty

A common procedure involving the surgical reshaping of the nose. General or local anesthesia, depending on the extent of the planned operation, may be used safely. Local anesthetics can provide analgesia and lower opioid requirements.

Local anesthetic toxicity

May occur with exceeding maximum recommended dose, inadvertent intravascular injections, or rapid absorption in a highly vascular area. Adhering to the maximum dosing recommendations, careful aspiration before injection of local anesthetics, and careful patient monitoring reduce the risk of clinically significant toxicity.

Mild toxicity may manifest as circumoral tingling, metallic taste, and tinnitus. Increased toxicity is usually accompanied by the neurologic symptoms, including changes in mental status, speech slurring or visual disturbances, or seizures. Severe toxicity may be manifest or be accompanied by sudden loss of consciousness, seizures, and cardiovascular collapse, including sinus bradycardia, conduction blocks, ventricular tachyarrhythmias, or asystole.

Bupivacaine toxicity may initially manifest as sudden cardiovascular collapse before any of the neurologic symptoms develop.

Prilocaine may induce methemoglobinemia. If recognized, treat with methylene blue injections.

Immediate management:

- STOP injecting the local anesthetic.
- Call for help.
- ABC:
  - maintain and secure the airway if necessary
  - give 100% O_2 and ensure adequate ventilation
  - confirm or establish IV access.
- Control seizures: benzodiazepine, propofol in small incremental doses.
- CPR if cardiovascular collapse occurs.

Cardiovascular collapse may be refractory to standard treatment, especially in the case of bupivacaine toxicity. Consider cardiopulmonary bypass or treatment with lipid emulsion.

Treatment with lipid emulsion:

- IV bolus of Intralipid® 20% 1.5 ml/kg over one minute.
- Continue CPR.

Essential Clinical Anesthesia Review: Keywords, Questions and Answers for the Boards, ed. Linda S. Aglio, Robert W. Lekowski, and Richard D. Urman. Published by Cambridge University Press. © Cambridge University Press 2015.

- Start IV infusion of Intralipid® 20% at 0.25 ml/kg/min.
- Repeat the bolus injection twice at five-minute intervals if adequate circulation has not been restored.
- Increase infusion to 0.5 ml/kg/min if adequate circulation has not been restored, and continue infusion until a stable and adequate circulation has been restored.

Note that recovery from local anesthetic-induced cardiac arrest may take more than one hour. Propofol is *not* a suitable substitute for Intralipid®. Take blood samples into a plain and heparinized tube to measure local anesthetic and triglyceride levels.

Questions

1. During injection of 0.25% bupivacaine for a regional block, a patient develops a widened complex ventricular tachyarrhythmia and loses consciousness. What is the first step in management?
   a. Start bag-mask ventilation with a nearby Ambu bag at 15 l/min O$_2$.
   b. Start IV bolus of Intralipid® 20% 1.5 ml/kg over one minute.
   c. Stop injecting the local anesthetic.
   d. Call a code blue.

2. Which is the recommended maximum dose of lidocaine with epinephrine added?
   a. 3 mg/kg
   b. 4.5 mg/kg, not to exceed 300 mg
   c. 7 mg/kg
   d. 11 mg/kg

Answers

1. c. Cessation of the primary cause for this clinical scenario is of utmost priority; otherwise, ongoing resuscitation efforts will be undermined and perhaps futile.
2. c. Familiarity with maximum doses of local anesthetics used in clinical practice is essential for patient safety.

Further reading

Vacanti, C. A., Sikka, P. K., Urman, R. U., Dershwitz, M., and Segal, B. S. (2011). Chapter 171. Inhaled nitric oxide. In *Essential Clinical Anesthesia*, 1st edn. Cambridge University Press.

Taghinia, A. H., Shapiro, F. E., and Slavin, S. A. (2008). Dexmedetomidine in aesthetic facial surgery: improving anesthetic safety and efficacy. *Plastic and Reconstructive Surgery* 121, 269–271.

Chapter

171

Intra-abdominal hypertension and abdominal compartment syndrome

Kelly G. Elterman and Suzanne Klainer

Keywords

Abdominal compartment syndrome: diagnosis
Abdominal compartment syndrome: management
Abdominal compartment syndrome: physiologic effects
Intra-abdominal hypertension: definition and diagnosis
Intra-abdominal pressure measurement

Abdominal compartment syndrome (ACS) is *defined as intra-abdominal hypertension (IAH) with resultant organ dysfunction*

Causes of IAH include blunt and penetrating trauma, burns, major abdominal surgery, large fluid resuscitation, refractory ascites, ruptured AAA, intraperitoneal hemorrhage, ovarian tumors, and liver transplantation. Forceful abdominal closure under tension may also cause IAH.

IAH is defined as an *intra-abdominal pressure (IAP) greater than 12 mm Hg*. ACS is defined as an IAP of *20 mm Hg or higher, with evidence of organ dysfunction*. IAH is often present prior to the appearance of clinical signs of ACS.

ACS is classified as primary, secondary, or recurrent. *Primary ACS is due to an intra-abdominal process. Secondary ACS is due to an extra-abdominal process. Recurrent ACS is ACS that redevelops in a patient who was previously successfully treated.*

IAPs can be measured either directly, via a catheter in the abdominal cavity, or more commonly, indirectly, via transduction of pressure within intra-abdominal organs. *The bladder is the most frequently used organ for indirect IAP measurement.* The transducer should be zeroed at the level of the pubic symphysis.

ACS diagnosis is clinical. Imaging is not sensitive, and often not helpful.

Classic clinical manifestations include tense abdomen, elevated IAPs, decreased cardiac output, difficult ventilation with increased peak airway pressures, hypoxia and hypercarbia, and renal dysfunction. All organs can be affected.

Table 171.1 Grading system for ACS

Grade	Pressure, mm Hg	Possible organ dysfunction
I	7–11	Splanchnic hypoperfusion
II	11–18	Elevated airway pressure, reduced cardiac output, oliguria
III	18–25	Hypotension, hypercarbia, hypoxia, anuria, increased intracranial pressure
IV	>25	Multiple organ failure

(Havens, J. M., Watkins, J. F., and Rogers, S. A. 2011. Intra-abdominal hypertension and abdominal compartment syndrome; From Vacanti et al. 2011. *Essential Clinical Anesthesia*, Cambridge University Press, p. 1061)

Cardiovascular effects – diaphragmatic elevation compresses the heart, *reducing ventricular compliance and contractility. Preload is decreased* due to IVC compression. *SVR increases* as a result of sympathetic stimulation. Ultimate outcome is *decreased cardiac output. CVP and PCWP are typically elevated, despite hypovolemia.* Hypovolemic patients with IAH tend to have worse outcomes than normovolemic patients. Of note, hypervolemia, as may occur with aggressive resuscitation, is a risk factor for ACS. The mean resuscitation volume associated with ACS is 25 L.

Pulmonary effects – diaphragmatic elevation compresses the lungs, and can result in *hypoxia, hypoventilation, atelectasis, edema, increased alveolar dead space, and intrapulmonary shunt fraction.* Increases in pleural pressure are directly proportional to intra-abdominal pressures. Hypoxia and edema are worsened by fluid resuscitation and systemic inflammation, which may accompany ACS. Patients with ACS are also at increased risk for pulmonary infection.

Renal effects – oliguria is common, resulting from *renal hypoperfusion,* and may occur with an IAP of 15 mm Hg. *Kidney perfusion decreases due to congestion as a result of decreased venous outflow, as well as arterial vasoconstriction as a result of sympathetic and renin-angiotensin system*

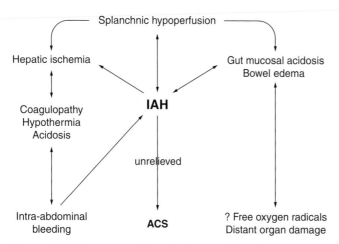

Figure 171.1 Intra-abdominal hypertension and abdominal compartment syndrome. (From Vacanti et al. 2011. *Essential Clinical Anesthesia*, Cambridge University Press, p. 1062.)

activation in the setting of decreased cardiac output. Levels of renin, aldosterone, and ADH typically double. Urine sodium and chloride decrease. If decompression is not achieved urgently, *hypoperfusion may result in acute tubular necrosis.*

Gastrointestinal effects – *mesenteric blood flow is reduced with an IAP of 10 mm Hg, and decreased mucosal perfusion occurs at 20 mm Hg. Mucosal hypoperfusion leads to sloughing, loss of the barrier with resultant bacterial translocation, and ultimately sepsis and/or multiorgan system failure.* Concomitant hypovolemia or hemorrhage compounds mucosal hypoperfusion and may accelerate these effects. Compression of intestinal veins results in edema, which increases intra-abdominal pressure and creates a vicious cycle. Hypoperfusion worsens, resulting in *lactic acidosis,* which is compounded by the liver's decreased ability to clear lactate in this state. *Metabolic acidosis may become refractory,* despite adequate resuscitation. Increasing lactate and base deficit are associated with increased mortality.

CNS effects – *elevated ICP and decreased CPP have been shown to occur with IAH in animals.* Decrease in ICP has been noted to occur in humans following abdominal decompression. Although unproven, ICP is likely increased due to decreased venous drainage associated with IAH, and CPP is likely decreased due to the combination of decreased cardiac output and increased ICP.

Anesthetic considerations

Cardiovascular – potent inhalational agents and volume depletion worsen hemodynamic effects of IAH. Organ perfusion is decreased in IAH, and perfusion may worsen as a result of vasodilation with use of inhalational agents. *Sudden hypotension upon correction of intra-abdominal hypertension is common,* and should be treated with IVF and vasopressors as necessary.

Pulmonary – pulmonary dysfunction associated with ACS may require *increasing PEEP, peak airway pressures, and*

elevated plateau pressures to maintain ventilation. In extreme cases, significant tidal volume may be lost in circuit expansion. In most cases, pulmonary function improves immediately after abdominal decompression; however, the severity of lung injury and progression of organ failure may continue to increase for 48 hours after decompression, particularly in burn patients.

Renal – urine output should be closely monitored. *Volume resuscitation should be carefully managed, with the goal of normovolemia.* Aggressive resuscitation should be avoided, as it may worsen hypoperfusion and multiple organ function.

Gastrointestinal – aggressive attempts at correcting metabolic acidosis with fluid resuscitation may paradoxically increase IAP, further decrease perfusion, and worsen end-organ damage.

Management

It is important to realize that the detrimental effects of IAH begin to occur before clinical signs emerge. Not all patients with IAH have the same clinical course, therefore there is no specific IAP at which intervention is mandated. Some base the decision to intervene on IAP, others on clinical dysfunction.

Another consideration is *abdominal perfusion pressure, defined as MAP – IAP.* One group found that APP <50 mm Hg predicted mortality more so than MAP or IAP alone.

Surgical decompression is a mainstay of treatment. Recurrent ACS after decompression should alert the clinician to the possibility of intra-abdominal bleeding. Without intervention, the cycle of hypoperfusion and increased IAP results in death (mortality approaches 100% without intervention).

If definitive closure cannot be accomplished after decompression, the abdomen may be temporarily closed using a Bogota bag, which is a 3 L genitourinary bag sutured to the abdominal fascia. Definitive closure should be delayed until the patient is hemodynamically stable, and all metabolic derangements have normalized.

Questions

1. Which is the definition of abdominal compartment syndrome?
   a. intra-abdominal pressure greater than or equal to 20 mm Hg with organ dysfunction
   b. intra-abdominal pressure greater than or equal to 15 mm Hg with organ dysfunction
   c. intra-abdominal pressure greater than or equal to 20 mm Hg with or without organ dysfunction
   d. intra-abdominal pressure greater than or equal to 15 mmHg with or without organ dysfunction

2. The most common method of measuring intra-abdominal pressure is via which of the following?
   a. intraperitoneal catheter
   b. central venous line
   c. bladder catheter
   d. rectal tube

3. Which of the following statements regarding abdominal compartment syndrome is most likely true?
   a. Cardiac output increases due to increased preload, as evidenced by elevated CVP.
   b. Pulmonary dysfunction may persist for several hours after surgical decompression.
   c. The associated metabolic acidosis should be treated with fluid administration until it corrects.
   d. Surgical intervention is not always necessary.

Answers

1. a. Intra-abdominal hypertension is defined as an IAP $\geq$20 mm Hg.
2. c. Intra-abdominal pressure is most frequently measured using a bladder catheter.
3. b. If a patient develops pulmonary dysfunction in the setting of intra-abdominal hypertension or abdominal compartment syndrome, it may take up to 48 hours for pulmonary function to improve, even after surgical decompression.

Further reading

Havens, J. M., Watkins, J. F., and Rogers, S. A. (2011). Intraabdominal hypertension and abdominal compartment syndrome. In Vacanti, C. A., Sikka, P. J., Urman, R. D., Dershwitz, M., and Segal, B. S. (eds) *Essential Clinical Anesthesia*. New York: Cambridge University Press, p. 1061.

Cullen, D. J., Coyle, J. P., Teplick, R. et al. (1989). Cardiovascular, pulmonary, renal effects of massively increased intra-abdominal pressure in critically ill patients. *Critical Care Medicine* 17, 118–121.

Schein, M. and Ivatury, R. (1998). Intra-abdominal hypertension and the abdominal compartment syndrome. *British Journal of Surgery* 85, 1027–1028.

Burch, J. M., Moore, E. E., Moore, F. A., and Franciose, R. (1996). The abdominal compartment syndrome. *Surgical Clinics of North America* 76, 833–842.

Ivatury, R. R., Diebel, L., Porter, J. M., and Simon, R. J. (1997). Intra-abdominal hypertension and the abdominal compartment syndrome. *Surgical Clinics of North America* 77, 783–800.

Chapter

172

Carbon monoxide and cyanide poisoning

Iuliu Fat and Devon Flaherty

Keywords

Carbon monoxide
Hyperbaric oxygen therapy
Cyanide

Carbon monoxide (CO) is an odorless, tasteless, colorless, nonirritating gas formed by hydrocarbon combustion. Exposures to smoke in a dwelling fire or to automobile exhaust are the most common mechanisms of poisoning. Endogenous CO can also be produced by the breakdown of methylene chloride, a halogenated hydrocarbon, which can be inhaled from the vapors of paint thinner, super glues, or spray paint. Patients who smoke also have a higher baseline CO level as compared to nonsmokers. Volatile anesthetics can react chemically with certain carbon dioxide (CO_2) absorbents, such as Baralyme® or soda lime, which are components of the anesthesia machine. Standard pulse oximetry (SpO_2) cannot properly screen for CO exposure, as it cannot differentiate between carboxyhemoglobin and oxyhemoglobin. An accurate SpO_2 and CO level can be assessed with CO-oximetry of arterial or venous blood.

Pathophysiology

CO produces tissue hypoxia by impairing oxygen transport and interfering with cytochrome oxidase function, causing cellular hypoxia. CO binds avidly to Hb, forming carboxyhemoglobin (COHb) with an affinity 240 times greater than that of oxygen. The tight binding of CO to Hb decreases the affinity and binding of oxygen to Hb, resulting in a leftward shift of the oxygen–hemoglobin dissociation curve. There is a reduction of oxygen transport by CO-bound Hb and a subsequent decreased release of oxygen to tissues. CO binds to mitochondrial cytochrome oxidase and reduces cellular respiration by disrupting mitochondrial function, uncoupling oxidative phosphorylation, and decreasing adenosine triphosphate (ATP) production. The net effects are profound tissue hypoxia, anaerobic metabolism, and lactic acidosis with a normal PaO_2.

Table 172.1 Clinical findings in CO poisoning

Estimated CO concentration, ppm	COHb, % of total Hb	Symptoms
<35 ppm (cigarette smoking)	5	None, or mild headache
0.005% (50 ppm)	10	Slight headache, dyspnea on vigorous exertion
0.01% (100 ppm)	20	Throbbing headache, dyspnea with moderate exertion
0.02% (200 ppm)	30	Severe headache, irritability, fatigue, dimness of vision
0.03%–0.05% (300–500 ppm)	40–50	Headache, tachycardia, confusion, lethargy, collapse
0.08%–0.12% (800–1200 ppm)	60–70	Coma, convulsions
0.19% (1900 ppm)	80	Rapidly fatal

(Vacanti, C., Segal, S., Urman, R. (eds) 2011. *Essential Clinical Anesthesia*. New York: Cambridge University Press, p. 1068.)

Manifestations

The clinical findings of CO poisoning are highly variable and largely nonspecific.

Cardiac manifestations include chest pain, arrhythmias, heart failure, and hypotension. Patients are often tachypneic due to lactic acidosis. Skin manifestations can include a characteristic "cherry red" blood color, which occurs when COHb levels exceed 40%. Up to 40% of patients with significant CO exposure will have neurologic sequelae. Higher concentrations of CO produce more severe symptoms.

Treatment

Tobacco smokers

Patients should be advised to stop smoking for at least 24 to 48 hours preoperatively. The baseline level of COHb in chronic smokers can be as high as 10% to 15%. The level decreases rapidly with abstinence (4 h half-life) and eventually causes a normalization of the oxyhemoglobin dissociation curve within 48 hours of smoking cessation.

Fire/burn/industrial exposure

The first step in the treatment of an industrial exposure to CO is to administer 100% oxygen by a nonrebreather mask. More serious exposures require intubation to achieve a PaO_2 of greater than 300 mm Hg in order to quickly displace CO bound to Hb. Patients with an altered mental status or those whose PaO_2 has not improved significantly with the administration of 100% oxygen may require endotracheal intubation. *Hyperbaric oxygen therapy* (HBO) is another treatment option that exposes patients to 100% oxygen under supraatmospheric conditions. HBO dramatically reduces the half-life of carboxyhemoglobin. The half-life of carboxyhemoglobin (COHb) is approximately 90 minutes when breathing 100% normobaric oxygen and approximately 30 minutes during HBO therapy.

Carbon monoxide exposure from anesthesia gas breakdown

Desiccated carbon dioxide absorbers found on anesthesia machines can put patients at risk for CO exposure. In particular, Baralyme® and soda lime, which contain strong bases, will react with volatile anesthetics to create CO. For a given minimum alveolar concentration (MAC), the amount of CO produced when using Baralyme® or soda lime is greatest in the presence of desflurane, followed by enflurane, isoflurane, halothane, and sevoflurane. Also, there is increasing evidence that using volatile anesthetics in the presence of desiccated carbon dioxide absorbers may result in exothermic reactions. This can lead to fires and the production of toxic products (e.g., carbon monoxide, compound A, methanol, formaldehyde). Although fires have only been reported in association with sevoflurane exposed to desiccated Baralyme®, there is significant evidence that toxic products can be produced upon exposure of volatile anesthetics to other desiccated absorbents containing strong bases, particularly potassium and sodium hydroxide.

Cyanide poisoning

Cyanide is a mitochondrial toxin that is among the most lethal poisons known to man. Cyanide is present in a variety of forms including a volatile liquid or flammable colorless gas, such as hydrogen cyanide, or as a crystal, such as sodium or potassium cyanide. It is used in the manufacturing of plastics, paper, fabrics, dyes, and pesticides. Inhalation exposure may occur during house or industrial fires. Certain foods, such as cassava, bitter almond, pits of stone fruits, and lima beans, also contain cyanide. Cyanide has a very high affinity for ferric iron in the mitochondrial cytochrome oxidase. This binding blocks respiration and oxidative phosphorylation, resulting in the production of lactic acidosis, high mixed venous oxygen saturation, and cellular death. The oxygen content, SaO_2, and carrying capacity of the blood may be unaffected. The diagnosis of cyanide poisoning is difficult because there are no pathognomonic signs.

Manifestations

Initially, the victim may complain of shortness of breath and chest tightness, and exhibit tachycardia and hypertension. Other nonspecific symptoms include dizziness, excitement, nausea, vomiting, headache, and weakness. If the poisoning is more severe, obtundation, coma, severe acidosis, and hypotension ensue. Cyanide levels greater than 0.5 mg/l are considered toxic. Cyanide is normally detoxified in the body by the action of the mitochondrial enzyme rhodanese. Rhodanese converts cyanide into thiocyanate, a less toxic substance that is excreted by the kidneys.

Treatment

The treatment of cyanide poisoning involves three strategies: binding of the cyanide, induction of methemoglobinemia, and use of sulfur donors. The administration of nitrites will convert hemoglobin to methemoglobin. Cyanide avidly binds to the iron moiety on methemoglobin, converting methemoglobin into cyanmethemoglobin. As a result, the induced methemoglobin scavenges free cyanide, thus preventing it from complexing with mitochondrial cytochromes. Methemoglobin can be induced before IV access is obtained by having the victim inhale vapors from crushed amyl nitrite pearls for 15 to 30 seconds with a 30-second rest between doses. Each pearl lasts approximately two to three minutes. Inhalation will produce a methemoglobin level of approximately 5%. When IV access is established, 300 mg of sodium nitrite (10 ml of a 3% solution) in adults is given over five minutes while monitoring for hypotension, to convert additional Hb to methemoglobin. Sodium nitrite (150 mg) can be administered again in two hours (in adults) if the methemoglobin level is less than 20%. Methemoglobin levels must be monitored. Sodium thiosulfate (the usual adult dose is 12.5 g) is also administered IV over 10 to 20 minutes as part of the antidote strategy, because thiosulfate acts as a receptor for the cyanide radical, yielding thiocyanate. One half of this dose may be repeated in two hours if cyanide toxicity persists. Sodium thiosulfate converts cyanmethemoglobin to the less toxic thiocyanate, which is then excreted in the urine. However, in cases of renal failure thiocyanate levels can rise, leading to toxicity. Hydroxocobalamin is also used to treat cyanide toxicity because the cobalt moiety binds with intracellular cyanide to form cyanocobalamin.

Questions

1. All of the following are FALSE statements about carbon monoxide except for which?

   a. It is an odorless, tasteless, irritating gas.
   b. The diagnosis of intoxication is made by pulse oximetry.
   c. It is formed by hydrocarbon combustion (e.g., automobile exhaust).
   d. It has an affinity for hemoglobin 100 times greater than oxygen.

2. Choose the best answer regarding cyanide.

   a. It is a slow-acting poison.
   b. Intoxication occurs solely via inhalation.
   c. Treatment is aimed at induction of methemoglobinemia and binding of cyanide.
   d. Rhodanese is a precursor of cyanide.

Answers

1. c. Carbon monoxide is an odorless, tasteless, nonirritating gas formed by hydrocarbon combustion. Pulse oximetry cannot detect the difference between carboxyhemoglobin and oxyhemoglobin. CO affinity for Hgb is 200 to 300 times that of oxygen.

2. c. Treatment of cyanide intoxication involves binding of cyanide, induction of methemoglobinemia, and the use of sulfur donors. Cyanide is a fast-acting poison. Intoxication occurs via inhalation or ingestion.

Further reading

Centers for Disease Control and Prevention (CDC) (2005). Unintentional non–fire-related carbon monoxide exposures in the United States, 2001–2003. *MMWR Morbity and Mortality Weekly Report* 54(2), 36–39.

Fang, Z. X., Eiger, E. I., Laster, M. J. et al. (1995). Carbon monoxide production from degradation of desflurane, enflurane, isoflurane, halothane, and sevoflurane by soda lime and Baralyme. *Anesthesia and Analgesia* 80, 1187–1193.

Moklesi, B., Leikin, J., Murray, P., and Corbridge, T. C. (2003). Adult toxicology in critical care. Part II: specific poisoning. *Chest* 123, 897–922.

Weaver, L. K., Hopkins, R. O., Chan, K. J. et al. (2002). Hyperbaric oxygen for acute carbon monoxide poisoning. *New England Journal of Medicine* 347(14), 1057–1067.

Chapter

173

Chemical and biologic warfare agents: an introduction for anesthesiologists

Joyce Lo and Laverne D. Gugino

Keywords

Organophosphate poisoning: diagnosis and treatment
Acetylcholinesterase inhibitors: muscarinic, nicotinic, and central effects
Anticholinesterase toxicity treatment: atropine, pralidoxime chloride, pyridostigmine
Pseudocholinesterase
Echothiophate clinical implications
Cyanide toxicity and treatment
Botulinum toxin

Table 173.1 The TOXALS system for provision of advanced life support in a contaminated zone

Assessment (patient and site)
Airway
Breathing IPPV (intermittent positive pressure ventilation)
Circulation–control of hemorrhage and cardiac abnormalities
Disability (AVPU scale–patient Alert or reacts or Vocal or Painful stimuli or is Unreactive)
Drugs and antidotes
Decontamination
Evacuation

(From: Vacanti et al. 2011, *Essential Clinical Anesthesia*, p. 1071, Table 174.1)

Chemical and biologic warfare (CBW) agents are chemical substances and living organisms that cause mass injury and death. Effective management of crisis situations in which CBW agents have been employed may help to limit the loss of life. As such, anesthesiologists play a key role in the management of these victims. Early steps in patient management include triage and use of the advanced life support for acute toxic injury (TOXALS system) introduced by the International Trauma Anesthesia and Critical Care Society.

Nerve agents (e.g., sarin, VX) are organophosphate compounds that are inhaled or rapidly absorbed across skin and mucous membranes. Organophosphate agents develop a stable irreversible covalent bond (known as "aging") with the active sites on cholinesterases. Their primary toxic effect is due to the *inhibition of acetylcholinesterase*, which results in a build up of acetylcholine with overstimulation of muscarinic and nicotinic receptors. The time required for irreversible binding of nerve agents to acetylcholinesterase varies depending on the particular agent. *Pseudocholinesterase* (or butyrylcholinesterase) is responsible for the metabolism of esters such as succinylcholine, procaine, tetracaine, etc., and is also inhibited.

Signs of *organophosphate poisoning* and *anticholinesterase toxicity* can be grouped into muscarinic, nicotinic, and central effects. *Muscarinic effects* include salivation, lacrimation, urination, diarrhea, vomiting, miosis, glandular hypersecretion, ciliary body spasm, sweating, bradycardia, heart block, and bronchospasm. *Nicotinic effects* include fasciculations,

paralysis, and anomalous tachycardia due to ganglionic stimulation in the sympathetic system. *Central effects* include apprehension, dizziness, ataxia, seizures, coma, and respiratory depression.

Aside from chemical warfare agents, other forms of irreversible anticholinesterases include organophosphate-containing pesticides (e.g., parathion), insecticides, and the ophthalmic drug, echothiophate. *Echothiophate* is available in topical drop form for the treatment of glaucoma and can continue to be effective two to three weeks after use. Therefore knowledge of echothiophate use is important in avoiding prolonged action of succinylcholine and other drugs requiring *pseudocholinesterase* for metabolism.

In the *treatment of anticholinesterase toxicity*, the first step should be removal of contaminated clothing and rinsing with soap and water. If an organophosphate has been ingested, vomiting and gastric lavage should be attempted. Airway evaluation must immediately be considered as the muscarinic side effects, such as laryngospasm, bronchospasm, and hypersecretion, may precipitate respiratory compromise and necessitate noninvasive or invasive ventilation. Early aggressive treatment with atropine may be helpful in limiting the need for intubation.

Atropine is the drug of choice in the *treatment of anticholinesterase toxicity*. It is effective in countering muscarinic receptor-mediated effects and is able to cross the blood–brain

Essential Clinical Anesthesia Review: Keywords, Questions and Answers for the Boards, ed. Linda S. Aglio, Robert W. Lekowski, and Richard D. Urman. Published by Cambridge University Press. © Cambridge University Press 2015.

barrier and may be helpful with the management of some central effects of acetylcholine excess such as seizures and respiratory depression. However, atropine has no effect at the neuromuscular junction or on nicotinic receptors. Atropine should initially be given as a 1 to 2 mg IV bolus and repeated every three to ten minutes as needed, and titrated to improvement of muscarinic symptoms, in particular to the resolution of airway secretions and improved oxygenation. Signs of atropinization (e.g., increased heart rate and dilation of initially constricted pupils) will be seen with treatment and should not limit dosing. An atropine infusion may also be started, and repeat dosing may be required for days until complete recovery. In situations in which intubation is necessary, it may be prudent to avoid succinylcholine given the risk of prolonged paralysis.

Pralidoxime chloride (2-PAM-Cl) is a cholinesterase reactivator that has been used in the setting of organophosphate poisoning. Its action is primarily seen at the neuromuscular junction and therefore is useful in reversing paralysis before irreversible binding to acetylcholinesterase occurs. Muscarinic effects of acetylcholinesterase poisoning are not reversed by pralidoxime, so atropine must also be administered. Benzodiazepines should be used to treat seizures due to the central effects of acetylcholine excess.

Reversible anticholinesterases include neostigmine, physostigmine, pyridostigmine, and edrophonium. *Pyridostigmine* produces only a mild parasympathetic response and it may be used as a pretreatment prior to potential high-level organophosphate exposure. It is a quaternary compound that is unable to cross the blood–brain barrier and is able to limit organophosphate coupling to acetylcholinesterase by binding approximately 40% of the enzyme. The pyridostigmine-bound enzymes return to 90% of normal 12 hours after a dose; however, victims of organophosphate exposure may develop cholinergic crisis with depolarizing block during this time and require life support measures.

Other types of chemical warfare agents include mitochondrial agents, lung-damaging agents, and vesicants. *Cyanide toxicity* occurs with exposure to hydrogen cyanide, which inhibits adenosine triphosphate (ATP) production by inactivating the mitochondrial enzyme cytochrome oxidase and disrupting oxidative metabolism. Hydrogen cyanide has an almond odor and metallic taste and causes dyspnea and hyperventilation, which increases the inhaled amount of agent. Victims develop a metabolic acidosis, loss of consciousness, seizures, and respiratory arrest.

In the *treatment of cyanide toxicity*, 100% oxygen should be administered to facilitate oxidative metabolism. Cyanide is reduced to thiocyanate in the liver by enzymes, including rhodanese, and is then excreted by the kidneys. This reaction is dependent on sodium thiosulfate, which can be administered to promote this reaction. Thiocyanate toxicity can occur in the setting of renal failure but is less harmful than cyanide toxicity. Amyl nitrate and sodium nitrate convert hemoglobin to methemoglobin, and cyanide subsequently will combine with methemoglobin to form cyanomethemoglobin. Hydroxycobalamin is another treatment, as it combines with cyanide to form cyanocobalamin (vitamin B_{12}), which is then eliminated in urine. Additional supportive care and ventilatory support should be provided.

Lung-damaging agents, including chlorine, phosgene, and isocyanates, all trigger inflammatory reactions resulting in pulmonary edema and acute respiratory distress syndrome. While there are no defined treatments for these agents, observation is warranted in all patients who have been exposed given the likely need for invasive ventilation. Mustard gas is the best known vesicant, with a latency period of two to four hours. Initial symptoms of blurred vision, ocular pain, and lacrimation progress to erythematous and edematous skin, burns, bullae, and necrosis. Leukopenia and respiratory failure may occur, requiring intubation. Victims may benefit from treatment with sodium thiosulfate, vitamin E, and steroids.

Some organisms produce toxins that may be exploited for use in chemical warfare. *Botulinum toxin* irreversibly inhibits acetylcholine release and causes dry mouth, bulbar weakness, muscular paralysis, and respiratory failure. An antitoxin is available for treatment, and ventilatory support may be required. Saxitoxin is a marine toxin that, when inhaled, acts on motor neurons and blocks the voltage-gated sodium channel, resulting in neurologic symptoms and cardiorespiratory failure. Treatment is supportive. Ricin is extracted from castor seeds and inhibits cellular protein synthesis. Therefore victims develop symptoms such as diarrhea, altered mental status, cardiorespiratory failure, and multisystem organ failure. Again, treatment is supportive.

Victims contaminated with biologic agents should be decontaminated and treated with similar precautions as those contaminated with chemical agents. Biologic agents require aerosolization for effective massive dispersal and, luckily, few organisms are able to withstand this. A notable exception is spore-forming anthrax. After initial inhalation exposure, victims experience malaise, fever, and a nonproductive cough for a few days while the toxin is released into the bloodstream. Once in the bloodstream, patients develop necrotizing, hemorrhagic mediastinitis and multiorgan failure, with a high frequency of hemorrhagic meningitis. Antibiotic and prophylactic therapy may both be lifesaving. Other organisms (e.g., smallpox, cholera, etc.) also carry the threat of being utilized as vehicles for terrorist attack and practitioners should consult updated guidelines and recommendations for management.

Questions

1. Which is the drug of choice for treatment of anticholinesterase toxicity?
   a. pralidoxime
   b. atropine
   c. pyridostigmine
   d. echothiophate
   e. edrophonium

2. Treatment of cyanide toxicity includes all of the following EXCEPT?
   a. methylene blue
   b. hydroxycobalamin
   c. amyl nitrate
   d. sodium thiosulfate
   e. sodium nitrate

Answers

1. b. Atropine is the drug of choice in the treatment of anticholinesterase toxicity and may reverse some central and muscarinic effects but has no effect on nicotinic receptors.

2. a. Sodium thiosulfate is a sulfur donor in the conversion of cyanide to thiocyanate. Amyl nitrate and sodium nitrate will increase the amount of methemoglobin available to combine with cyanide and form cyanomethemoglobin. Hydroxycobalamin combines with cyanide to form cyanocobalamin. Methylene blue is not indicated in the treatment of cyanide toxicity.

Further reading

Baker, D. J. (1996). Advanced life support for acute toxic injury (TOXALS). *European Journal of Emergency Medicine* 3(4), 256–262.

Baker, D. J. and Nurok, M. (2011). Chemical and biologic warfare agents: an introduction for anesthesiologists.

In Vacanti, C. A., Sikka, P. J., Urman, R. D., Dershwitz, M., and Segal, B. S. (eds) *Essential Clinical Anesthesia*. New York: Cambridge University Press, pp. 1070–1074.

Murray, M. (2009). Disaster preparedness. In Barash, P. G. (ed) *Clinical Anesthesia*, 6th edn. Philadelphia: Lippincott Williams & Wilkins, pp. 1559–1577.

Anesthesia for robotic surgery

Michael Vaninetti, Joyce Lo, and Assia Valovska

Keywords

Surgical cart
Operative console
Muscle relaxation in robotic surgery
Abdominal robotic surgery
Carbon dioxide insufflation: complications
Cardiothoracic robotic surgery
Single-lung ventilation
Thoracic robotic surgery
Urologic robotic surgery
Robotic prostatectomy: contraindications

Surgical robots have mechanical limbs, which are used to assist in a variety of surgical procedures. The anticipated benefits of robotic surgery include increased range of motion of surgical implements, shorter recovery, reduced pain, and improved cosmetic results.

The surgical robotic system consists generally of a *surgical cart*, which is the base station from which the operating limbs extend into the patient, and the *operative console*, where the surgeon sits and manipulates sensor-equipped graspers. The movements of the sensor-equipped graspers are exactly replicated in the operative field by the surgical robotic limbs. An example of a typical operating room utilizing a robotic system is depicted in the Figure 174.1.

Muscle relaxation during robotic surgery is critical, as the robotic arm is rigid and therefore patient movement can cause severe injury.

As in laparoscopic surgery, endotracheal intubation is recommended for robotic surgery because of insufflation of the surgical field and increased ventilatory pressures often necessary to overcome insufflation pressure. Endotracheal intubation also offers the most precise control over CO_2 management, the most commonly used gas for insufflation.

Abdominal robotic surgery

Commonly performed abdominal robotic procedures include cholecystectomy, Nissen fundoplication, Heller myotomy, bariatric surgery, and colectomy. Because of the proximity of the surgical cart to the patient's head and upper body, care must be taken to ensure that the robot does not contact the patient inadvertently, causing injury to the patient. The robot must be fully disengaged from the patient before bed adjustments can be made, or in the event of an airway or anesthesia emergency. Abdominal insufflation pressures should generally not exceed 20 mm Hg. *Complications of carbon dioxide insufflation* during robotic surgery include vascular injury or injury to organs due to trocar placement, cardiac arrhythmias due to hypercarbia or increased vagal tone, subcutaneous emphysema, pneumothorax or pneumomediastinum, and carbon dioxide embolism. Ventilator adjustments must be made to prevent hypercarbia and prevent barotrauma.

Cardiothoracic robotic surgery

Robot-assisted cardiothoracic surgeries include atrial septal defect closures, mitral valve repairs, patent ductus arteriosus ligations, totally endoscopic coronary artery bypass grafting, minimally invasive atrial fibrillation surgery, and left ventricular pacemaker lead placement. Single-lung ventilation is necessary, often for prolonged periods of time, during robotic-assisted cardiothoracic surgery. Severe lung disease and resultant inability to tolerate prolonged *single-lung ventilation* is an important contraindication to consider preoperatively. The anesthesiologist for these procedures must be well-versed in both cardiac and thoracic anesthesia techniques, including intraoperative transesophageal echocardiography (TEE), double-lumen endotracheal tube placement, single-lung ventilation (see Table 174.1) and management of cardiopulmonary bypass. Insufflation of the thoracic cavity is often required for visualization of the surgical field, which can alter venous return. Hypovolemia should be corrected prior to or concurrently with thoracic insufflation, and extra care should be taken for hemodynamic control in patients with altered LV function.

Essential Clinical Anesthesia Review: Keywords, Questions and Answers for the Boards, ed. Linda S. Aglio, Robert W. Lekowski, and Richard D. Urman. Published by Cambridge University Press. © Cambridge University Press 2015.

Thoracic robotic surgery

Currently performed robotic-assisted thoracic surgeries include Heller myotomy, resection of esophageal and mediastinal masses, esophagectomy, thymectomy, and pulmonary lobectomy. Similar to cardiothoracic surgery, robotic thoracic surgery often involves insufflation of the thorax, reducing venous return and thus necessitating adequate volume status.

Table 174.1 Single-lung ventilation strategy

1. Use $FiO_2 = 1.0$.
2. Begin single-lung ventilation with pressure-control ventilation, maintaining a plateau pressure <30 cm H_2O.
3. Adjust respiratory rate so that $PaCO_2$ approaches 40 mm Hg.
4. Check arterial blood gases periodically.
5. Apply continuous positive airway pressure to nonventilated lung.
6. Apply positive end-expiratory pressure to ventilated lung.

FiO_2, fraction of inspired oxygen content.
(Adapted from Vacanti, C. A., et al. (eds). 2011. *Essential Clinical Anesthesia.* Cambridge University Press, pp. 1076.)

Supine or slight lateral decubitus (15 to 30 degrees) positioning is optimal for exposure of anterior mediastinal structures, whereas full lateral decubitus is preferable for hilar masses or lobectomies. Posterior mediastinal exposure may require nearly prone positioning.

Robot-assisted urologic surgery

Urologic procedures commonly performed using robotic systems include radical prostatectomy, radical cystectomy, radical and simple nephrectomy, live donor nephrectomy, pyeloplasty, and adrenalectomy. Robot-assisted radical prostatectomy (RARP) has become the most commonly performed robotic surgery. Transfusion rate, positive surgical margin rate, urinary continence recovery, and erectile function with RARP seem to compare favorably with laparoscopic or traditional retropubic approaches. A prolonged supine lithotomy position is required for RARP. Care should therefore be taken to avoid common peroneal nerve injury (see Chapter 97, Urology). Important *contraindications to RARP* include previous hernia surgery, previous abdominal surgery, and previous prostate surgery.

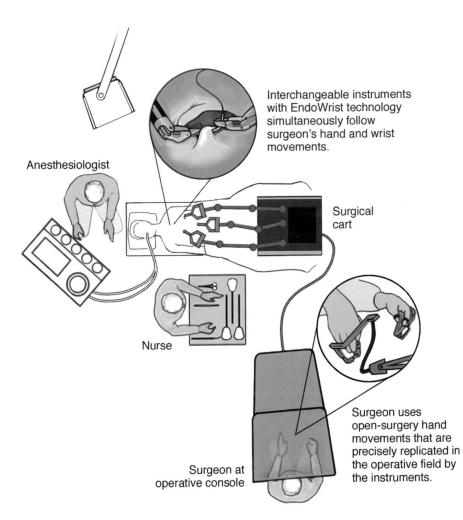

Figure 174.1 Operating room schematic of the use of a robotic surgical system in cholecystectomy surgery. (Courtesy of Intuitive Surgical, Inc, Sunnyvale, CA; Adapted from Vacanti et al. 2011. *Essential Clinical Anesthesia*, Cambridge University Press, p. 1077.)

Interchangeable instruments with EndoWrist technology simultaneously follow surgeon's hand and wrist movements.

Anesthesiologist

Surgical cart

Nurse

Surgeon uses open-surgery hand movements that are precisely replicated in the operative field by the instruments.

Surgeon at operative console

Questions

1. In comparison to more traditional open or laparoscopic techniques, robotic surgery may offer all of the following advantages EXCEPT?

   a. reduced recovery time
   b. reduced operative time
   c. improved cosmetic results
   d. reduced pain

2. A supine or slight lateral decubitus positioning would be most appropriate for which of the following robotic-assisted procedures?

   a. thymectomy
   b. esophagectomy
   c. pulmonary lobectomy
   d. hilar mass excision

3. Robotic-assisted radical prostatectomy appears to confer all of the following advantages over laparoscopic and open approaches EXCEPT?

   a. reduced transfusion rate
   b. reduced positive surgical margin rate
   c. improved intraoperative hemodynamic stability
   d. improved urinary continence recovery

Answers

1. b. Robotic surgery has been shown to decrease postoperative recovery time, decrease postoperative pain, and improve surgical cosmetic result, but has not been shown to reduce operative time.

2. a. Supine or slight lateral positioning is preferable for thymectomy. Full lateral positioning is most commonly used for hilar mass excision or pulmonary lobectomy. Full lateral to nearly prone positioning may be required for esophagectomy.

3. c. Robotic-assisted radical prostatectomy appears to reduce transfusion rate, reduce the rate of positive surgical margins, and improve recovery of urinary continence over laparoscopic and open approaches. It has not been shown to improve intraoperative hemodynamic stability.

Further reading

Nishanian, Ervant (2011). Anesthesia for robotic surgery. In Vacanti, C. A., Sikka, P. J., Urman, R. D., Dershwitz, M., and Segal, B. S. (eds) *Essential Clinical Anesthesia*. New York: Cambridge University Press, pp. 1075–1082.

Lanfranco, A. R., Castellanos, A. E., Desai, J. P., and Meyers, W. C. (2004). Robotic surgery: a current perspective. *Annals of Surgery* 239, 14–21.

Atug, F., Castle, E. P., Woods, M., Davis, R., and Thomas, R. (2006). Robotics in urologic surgery: an evolving new technology. *International Journal of Urology* 13, 857–863.

Chapter 175

Human immunodeficiency virus, methicillin-resistant *Staphylococcus aureus*, and vancomycin-resistant *Enterococcus*

Benjamin Kloesel and Michaela K. Farber

Keywords

Human immunodeficiency virus (HIV)
Acquired immunodeficiency syndrome (AIDS)
Highly active antiretroviral therapy (HAART)
Protease inhibitors (PI)
Nucleoside analog reverse transcriptase inhibitors (NRTI)
Non-nucleoside analog reverse transcriptase inhibitors (NNRTI)
Methicillin-resistant *Staphylococcus aureus* (MRSA)
Vancomycin-resistant *Enterococcus* (VRE)

Human immunodeficiency virus (HIV) is transmitted through contaminated blood after contact with mucous membranes, wounds, transfusions, intravenous drug use, through sexual contact, and from mother to child during gestation, delivery, or breastfeeding. After inoculation, seroconversion occurs after two to three weeks. Initial symptoms resemble flu and can include fever, fatigue, myalgias, pharyngitis, and generalized lymphadenopathy. The term *AIDS* is reserved for individuals with HIV infection and presence of at least one AIDS-defining diagnosis.

HAART is effective therapy; available drugs fall into six classes: (a) *protease inhibitors*, (b) *nucleoside analog reverse transcriptase inhibitors (NRTIs)*, (c) *non-nucleoside analog reverse transcriptase inhibitors (NNRTIs)*, (d) fusion inhibitors, (e) entry inhibitors, and (f) integrase inhibitors.

Main issues in the care of a patients with HIV include: (a) HIV-related end-organ dysfunction, (b) medication interaction between HAART and other drug classes, and (c) risk of occupational exposure to HIV for operating room personnel (risk of developing HIV after needle-stick injury with contaminated blood is 0.3%).

Organ system-based problems in HIV patients:

- Cardiac: pericarditis (most common), myocarditis, endocarditis (HIV, coxsackie B, HSV, CMV, *Cryptococcus*, *Toxoplasma gondii, Aspergillus, Candida*); cardiomyopathy; myocardial infarction (even at younger age).
- Pulmonary: opportunistic infections leading to pneumonia and lung parenchyma destruction; pneumothorax; airway obstruction caused by lymphadenopathy; *Pneumocystis jirovecii* pneumonia.
- Renal: HIV-associated nephropathy; nephrotic syndrome.
- Hepatic: LFT elevation; hepatitis.
- Gastrointestinal: stomatitis and esophagitis (*Candida*); HIV-related diarrhea.
- Neurological: cerebral toxoplasmosis; primary central nervous system lymphoma; progressive multifocal leukoencephalopathy; primary HIV encephalopathy (AIDS dementia); aseptic meningitis; infectious meningitis (*Cryptococcus*, HIV, *Tuberculosis*); vacuolar myelopathy; peripheral neuropathy; autonomic dysfunction.
- Hematological: decreased protein C and S levels leading to hypercoagulability; anemia (decreased erythropoiesis); thrombocytopenia; Kaposi sarcoma.
- Endocrine: adrenal insufficiency; glucose intolerance.

Adverse effects of HIV medication:

- protease inhibitors: nausea/vomiting/diarrhea (common); strong inhibitors of CYP450 (prolonged action of opiates, benzodiazepines, lidocaine, digoxin, amiodarone); premature atherosclerosis; diastolic dysfunction; dyslipidemias; hyperbilirubinemia; LFT elevation; hyperglycemia
- NRTI: nausea/vomiting/diarrhea (common); lipoatrophy; lactic acidosis; peripheral neuropathy; pancreatitis; myopathy
- NNRTI: dizziness/insomnia (common); some NNRTIs are inducers, some are inhibitors of CYP450 (resistance or sensitivity of opiates and benzodiazepines); CNS toxicity; LFT elevation/hepatic failure
- fusion inhibitors: injection-site irritation

Essential Clinical Anesthesia Review: Keywords, Questions and Answers for the Boards, ed. Linda S. Aglio, Robert W. Lekowski, and Richard D. Urman. Published by Cambridge University Press. © Cambridge University Press 2015.

- entry inhibitors: LFT elevation
- integrase inhibitors: hyperlipidemia; myopathy; rhabdomyolysis

HIV patients often receive *prophylactic medications* to protect them from opportunistic infections. These also have significant adverse effect profiles:

- inhaled pentamidine for *Pneumocystis jirovecii* prophylaxis (cough, dyspnea, bronchospasm)
- TMP/SMX for *Pneumocystis jirovecii* and *Toxoplasmosis* prophylaxis (can potentiate anticoagulant effect of warfarin, acute hemolytic anemia, agranulocytosis, aplastic anemia)
- dapsone for *Pneumocystis jirovecii* and *Toxoplasmosis* prophylaxis (severe hemolysis in patients with glucose-6-phosphate dehydrogenase deficiency, methemoglobinemia)
- atovaquone for *Pneumocystis jirovecii* prohylaxis (nausea, vomiting, LFT elevation)
- azithromycin/clarithromycin for *Mycobacterium avium* complex prophylaxis (QT prolongation, hepatotoxicity)

Having a positive HIV serum viral load is not a contraindication to *neuraxial anesthesia or epidural blood patch* in HIV patients. HIV is detectable in the CSF early after infection.

Pain in HIV patients is often underrecognized and undertreated. Pain can arise directly from the disease process itself, from associated processes such as tumors and opportunistic infections, or as an adverse effect from treatment with antiretroviral medications.

Methicillin-resistant Staphylococcus aureus (MRSA) most commonly presents as bacteremia, but can also cause pneumonia, cellulitis, osteomyelitis, endocarditis, and septic shock. The organism is resistant against all penicillins, cephalosporins, and carbapenems. Available antibiotics that are effective for treatment include vancomycin, clindamycin, linezolid, daptomycin, and quinopristin/dalfopristin. Agents with lower activity include doxycycline, tigecycline, levofloxacin, moxifloxacin, and trimethoprim/sulfamethoxazole.

Strains of *vancomycin-intermediate S. aureus (VISA) and vancomycin-resistant S. aureus (VRSA)* are an emerging problem.

Vancomycin-resistant Enterococcus (VRE) is an increasing problem in ICU patients. The organism is resistant to penicillins, cephalosporins, clindamycin, carbapenems, and vancomycin. Available antibiotics that are effective for treatment include daptomycin, linezolid, quinopristine/dalfopristine, and tigecycline.

Questions

1. A 27-year-old HIV-positive patient presents for colonoscopy. He is maintained on HAART with tenofovir (NRTI), emtricitabine (NRTI), ritonavir (PI), and darunavir (PI). He receives 2 mg of midazolam and 100 μg of fentanyl for the procedure, which is completed successfully within 15 minutes. You are called to the recovery unit an hour after the procedure. The patient's vital signs are stable but he remains unarousable to voice. Painful stimuli elicit a withdrawal reaction. What should you do next?
   a. Obtain a head CT for concern of CNS lesion or bleed.
   b. Consider administration of flumazenil and/or naloxone.
   c. Draw a blood sample and check lactic acid levels.
   d. Induce general anesthesia and intubate the patient.

2. A critically ill patient in the ICU is found to have a right lower lobe pneumonia. Culture of a bronchoalveolar lavage grows VRE. Which of the following antibiotics is the best choice for this patient?
   a. linezolid
   b. cefipime
   c. daptomycin
   d. vancomycin

Answers

1. b. Given the patient's use of two protease inhibitors with resultant inhibition of CYP450, and the use of relatively high doses of midazolam and fentanyl for a short procedure, the most reasonable first step would be a trial of antagonists.
2. a. Only linezolid and daptomycin possess antibacterial activity against VRE; daptomycin is inactivated by surfactant and therefore a poor choice for pneumonia.

Further reading

Madan, K. (2011). Chapter 176. Human immunodeficiency virus, methicillin-resistant *Staphylococcus aureus* and vancomycin-resistant *Enterococcus*.

In Vacanti, C. A., Sikka, P. J., Urman, R. D., Dershwitz, M., and Segal, B. S. (eds) *Essential Clinical Anesthesia*. New York: Cambridge University Press.

Leelanukrom, R. (2009). Anaesthetic considerations of the HIV-infected patients. *Current Opinion in Anesthesiology* 22(3), 412–418.

Chapter

176

Alternative medicines and anesthesia

Syed Irfan Qasim Ali and Richard D. Urman

Keywords

CAM
Bleeding
Garlic
Ginseng
Ginkgo biloba
St. John's Wort
Echinacea
Fish oil
Flax seed
Glucosamine

Introduction

Alternative medicine uses nonprescription herbs or supplements to replace traditional medications. Examples are naturopathy and homeopathy in the Western world, and Chinese medicines (including acupuncture) and Ayurveda (Indian subcontinent) in the Eastern world. Alternative medicine can include massage, dietary modifications, exercise, acupuncture, minor surgery, and aromatherapy (uses volatile plant materials, known as essential oils, and other aromatic compounds for the purpose of altering a person's mind, mood, cognitive function, or health).

Homeopathy is a medical science developed by Dr. Samuel Hahnemann (1755–1843), a German physician. It is based on the principle that "like cures like." In simple words, it means that any substance that can produce symptoms in a healthy person, can cure similar symptoms in a person who is sick.

Following is some data from the National Institutes for Health (NIH) about complementary and alternative medicine (CAM):

- 38.3% of the US population is using alternative medicines, according to 2007 data.
- 27 million patients are at increased risk of drug interactions due to combinations with herbs and supplements.
- Even more disconcerting is the fact that 40% to 69% of these patients mixing prescription medications with

nonvitamin dietary supplements do not report this use to their physicians.

Regulations

The US Food and Drug Administration (FDA) and the Center for Food Safety and Applied Nutrition (CFSAN) regulate dietary supplements. Because dietary supplements are usually extracts, they are not patented or regulated in the US, but are regulated in European countries.

Reporting of adverse effects from supplement use is voluntary via the FDA Med Watch site. It has been suggested, however, that this only captures approximately 1% of adverse events associated with these products. The FDA process to ban retail sales of ephedra in 2004 took many years and followed 16,000 reports of adverse effects and 150 deaths of ephedra users.

A study of ayurvedic herbal medicine products produced in South Asia and purchased in the Boston area showed that 20% of these products contained potentially harmful amounts of lead, mercury, and/or arsenic. Other contaminants reportedly found in supplements include bacteria, pesticides, and glass.

Harmful reactions to supplements

The potential for drug interactions is higher in anesthesia than in other areas of medicine, because the risk of adverse events increases exponentially with the number of drugs a patient receives.

Table 176.1 Most commonly used alternative medicines

Fish oil	Chondroitin aloe
Glucosamine	Garlic
Coenzyme Q10	Kava kava
Echinacea	St. John's Wort
Flax seed oil/pills	Saw palmetto
Ginseng	Valerian
Combination herbal pills	Goldenseal
Ginkgo biloba	

Tables 176.2–176.5 illustrate common herbs with serious adverse reactions important for modern-day anesthesiologist to know.

Common supplements in the perioperative period

Gingko (*Gingko biloba*)

Commonly used as a memory enhancer and in Alzheimer's disease. Due to its antiplatelet effect it can cause spontaneous

Table 176.2 Supplements causing decreased platelet aggregation

Bilberry	Fish oil
Bromelain	Flax seed oil
Feverfew	Garlic
Don quoi	Ginger
Ginkgo biloba	Grape seed

Table 176.3 Supplements inhibiting clotting

Chamomile	Feverfew
Dandelion root	Horse chestnut
Dong quoi	Vitamin E
Chondroitin	

Table 176.4 Supplements causing potential potentiation of anesthetics

Valerian	Hops
Kava kava	Passion flower
St. John's wort	

Table 176.5 Supplements causing miscellenous adverse effects

Agent	Adverse effects
Weight loss supplements, licorice	Hypotension/hypertension
Licorice, goldenseal, milk thistle	Arrhythmias/electrolyte disturbances/ volume depletion
Kava kava, *Echinacea*, black cohosh	Hepatotoxicity
Ginseng, glucosamine	Hypoglycemia
Coenzyme Q10	Insomnia, increased sensitivity to insulin (causing hypoglycemia), decreased sensitivity to warfarin (requiring higher doses)
Aloe	Oral intake can cause liver and kidney damage
Chondroitin	May cause spread or recurrence of prostate cancer

bleeding. Recommended to discontinue one week prior to surgery.

Feverfew (*Tanacetum parthenium*)

Used for prevention and treatment of migraine headaches. Its antiplatelet activity can cause *bleeding*, plus some patients may experience withdrawal symptoms and need to be treated with benzodiazepines. Recommended to discontinue at least two weeks before surgery to allow enough time for weaning.

Ginger (*Zingiber officinale*)

Used for motion sickness and nausea, despite all studies showing it to be ineffective for PONV. It inhibits thromboxane synthetase and can cause *bleeding*. Recommended to be discontinued one week prior to surgery.

Glucosamine

Used in combination with chondroitin for osteoarthritis. In diabetic patients, it may increase insulin resistance, but in nondiabetic persons its structural similarity to human insulin may lead to hypoglycemia. Recommended to be discontinued 24 hours prior to surgery.

Valerian (*Valeriana officinalis*)

Used for insomnia, it increases activity at GABA receptors. There are case reports of interaction with barbiturates, and there could be possible potentiation of anesthetic action. Recommended to be discontinued one to two weeks prior to surgery.

Goldenseal (*Hydrastis canadensis*)

Used to improve digestion, treat ulcers, and act as a natural antibiotic. It causes sodium depletion and potentiates diuretic effects of other drugs. It also inhibits the P450 cytochrome system. Recommended to be discontinued two weeks prior to surgery.

Ginseng (*Panax ginseng*)

Used as a stimulant, to protect the body against stress, to restore homeostasis, and to treat some menopausal symptoms. It has steroid-like effects and may cause hypoglycemia, Stevens–Johnson syndrome, and decreased blood concentrations of warfarin and ethanol. It inhibits platelet aggregation. Recommended to be discontinued one week prior to surgery.

Garlic (*Allium sativum*)

Used to stave off symptoms of heart disease due to its lipid-lowering and vasodilatory effects. Garlic causes a dose-related inhibition of platelet aggregation. Recommended to be discontinued one week prior to surgery.

St. John's wort (*Hypericum perforatum*)

Proven benefit for the short-term treatment of mild to moderate depression. It inhibits the reuptake of serotonin, norepinephrine, and dopamine. Serotonin syndrome has been reported in patients combining St. John's wort with certain selective serotonin reuptake inhibitors. Also induces cytochrome P450. Recommended to be discontinued five days prior to surgery.

Kava kava (*Piper methysticum*)

Used for anxiety and muscle relaxation. Potentiates GABA receptors thereby potentiating anesthetic actions. Also inhibits thromboxane synthetase. Some case reports of hepatic failure are also reported. Recommended to be discontinued 24 hours to two weeks prior to surgery.

Saw palmetto (*Serenoa repens*)

Found to be useful for benign prostatic hypertrophy. There is one case in the literature of intraoperative hemorrhage in a patient taking this supplement. Recommended to be discontinued 24 hours to two weeks before surgery.

Echinacea (*Echinacea purpura*)

Used for colds because of immunostimulating effects without any evidence supporting this. It should be avoided in patients requiring perioperative immunosuppression, such as transplant patients. It has been found to potentiate the hepatotoxic effects of other drugs, and it inhibits the P450 cytochrome system. Recommended to be discontinued 24 hours to two weeks prior to surgery.

According to the American Society of Anesthesiologists (ASA) statement, all herbs and supplements should be discontinued two weeks before surgery.

Questions

1. During a total abdominal hysterectomy, the surgeon notices more than expected bleeding and oozing. Which of the following supplements may be responsible for this finding?
   a. valerian
   b. St. John's wort
   c. kava kava
   d. ginseng

2. Which best explains the American Society of Anesthesiologists (ASA) statement about herbal medicines and supplements in the perioperative period?

   a. All should be discontinued two weeks before surgery.
   b. All should be continued until the day of surgery.
   c. All should be stopped 24 hours before surgery.
   d. All should be discontinued one week before surgery.

3. Which of following supplements may decrease the MAC during surgery?
   a. valerian
   b. garlic
   c. ginger
   d. flax seed

4. In a 72-year-old man with no medical problems who is taking glucosamine for OA, which of the following abnormalities may be present due to glucosamine?
   a. hypoglycemia
   b. hyperglycemia
   c. increased risk of bleeding
   d. decreased MAC

5. In the United States herbal medicines and supplements are regulated by which organization?
   a. the Food and Drug Administration (FDA)
   b. the Center for Food Safety and Applied Nutrition (CFSAN)
   c. both (a) and (b)
   d. none of the above

Answers

1. d. Ginseng inhibits platelet aggregation. Recommended to discontinue one week prior to surgery.
2. a. According to the ASA statement, all herbs and supplements should be discontinued two weeks before surgery.
3. a. Valerian is used for insomnia, it increases activity at GABA receptors. There are case reports of interaction with barbiturates, and there could be possible potentiation of anesthetic action. Recommended to discontinue one to two weeks prior to surgery.
4. a. Glucosamine in diabetic patients may increase insulin resistance, but in nondiabetic persons its structural similarity to human insulin may lead to hypoglycemia. Recommended to discontinue 24 hours prior to surgery.
5. d. Because these products are usually extracts, they are not patented or regulated in the United States; but they are regulated in European countries.

Further reading

Vacanti, C. A., Sikka, P. K., Urman, R. U., Dershwitz, M., and Segal, B. S. (2011). *Essential Clinical Anesthesia*, 1st edn. Cambridge University Press, Chapter 177.

Kaye A. D., Kucera, I., and Sabar, R. (2004). Perioperative anesthesia clinical considerations of alternative medicines. *Anesthesiology Clinics of North America* 22, 125–139.

Chapter

177

Anesthesia in high altitudes

Stephanie Yacoubian, Syed Irfan Qasim Ali, Felicity Billings, and Richard D. Urman

Keywords

Partial pressure of oxygen at high altitudes
Oxygen cascade and aerobic threshold limit
Cheyne–Stokes breathing
Oxygen transport at high altitudes
High altitude pulmonary edema (HAPE)
Hyperbaric oxygen therapy
Acute motion sickness (AMS)
High altitude cerebral edema (HACE)
High altitude: other physiologic changes
High altitude: anesthetic implications
Vaporizer output at high altitude

Partial pressure of oxygen at high altitudes

The atmosphere contains 21% oxygen at sea level and also at high altitude, but at high altitudes (e.g., Denver, CO) the partial pressure of oxygen is lower. Thus the partial pressure of oxygen (PO_2) decreases at high altitude due to a decrease in atmospheric pressure.

Example:

PO_2 at 760 mm Hg (sea level) $\times$ 0.21 = 160 mm Hg

PO_2 at 540 mm Hg (e.g., Denver, CO) $\times$ 0.21 = 113 mm Hg

Increased 2,3-diphosphoglycerate in red blood cells shifts the oxygen dissociation curve to the right, leading to increased oxygen delivery and unloading in tissues.

Respiratory alkalosis (secondary to hyperventilation) shifts the oxygen dissociation curve to the left. This increases oxygen's affinity to red blood cells and favors uptake through the alveolar circulation.

Decreased alveolar PO_2 stimulates peripheral chemoreceptors, leading to increased ventilation and increase in O_2 delivery.

Mixed venous blood of a person at high altitude has the same PO_2 because of the following compensatory mechanisms.

1. Hyperventilation (primary mechanism), which may increase alveolar oxygen tension by 25% to 30%.

2. Decreased tissue metabolism due to decreased availability of oxygen.

3. Adjustment of oxygen transport characteristics:
   - increase in pulmonary oxygen diffusion capacity by three- to four-fold
   - increase in pulmonary capillary blood flow
   - increase in lung volume and surface area of alveolar membrane
   - increase in blood supply to upper lobes of lung.

Oxygen cascade and aerobic threshold limit

The oxygen gradient drops from alveolar oxygen to the value seen at the mitochondrial level. The gradient is less steep in a person breathing at high altitudes. The final PO_2 in mitochondria is about 1.5 mm Hg. The aerobic threshold limit is likely to be a mitochondrial PO_2 equal to about 1 mm Hg.

Cheyne–Stokes breathing

Most often occurs during sleep. May be seen as a symptom in persons breathing at high altitudes. It is defined as periodic breathing where periods of hyperpnea alternate with periods of apnea (3–15 seconds). This pattern may disappear with acclimatization, use of acetazolamide, or descent to a lower altitude.

Oxygen transport at high altitudes

Physiologic adaptations to high altitudes start around two to three weeks and it may take months to complete.

The decrease in partial pressure of oxygen stimulates the kidney to produce more erythropoietin, which leads to a rise in hemoglobin (15 g/dl to 22 g/dl). The hematocrit increases from 45% to 65% as plasma volume drops by 10% to 20%, secondary to intravascular fluid shifts into the interstitial compartment.

Hypoxia leads to an increase in sympathetic output, which contributes to an increase in cardiac output, mostly due to an increase in heart rate. Stroke volume decreases due to a

Essential Clinical Anesthesia Review: Keywords, Questions and Answers for the Boards, ed. Linda S. Aglio, Robert W. Lekowski, and Richard D. Urman. Published by Cambridge University Press. © Cambridge University Press 2015.

decrease in preload. Systemic blood pressure rises as a result of peripheral vasoconstriction.

High altitude pulmonary edema (HAPE)

A noncardiogenic pulmonary edema seen at high altitudes in the setting of an elevation in pulmonary artery pressures. Possible mechanisms:

1. Decreased barometric pressure and partial pressure of O_2 leading to pulmonary vasoconstriction and elevated pulmonary artery pressure (PAP).
2. Patchy pulmonary vasoconstriction with some parts of the lungs receiving overperfusion cause fluid leakage, plus elevated PAP and increased blood viscosity, leading to capillary endothelial damage and fluid leakage.
3. Fibrin thrombin formation in the lungs due to an increase in plasma fibrinogen levels.
4. Increased production of oxygen free radicals, causing oxidation of alveolar intracellular lipids and mitochondrial cell membranes.

HAPE is characterized by a normal ventricular function and presence of any two of the following symptoms and signs.

Symptoms: dyspnea at rest; decreased exercise performance; chest congestion; cough (pink frothy sputum)

Signs: lung crackles; tachycardia; tachypnea; cyanosis

A neurogenic pulmonary edema can also be seen in the setting of a massive sympathetic surge, with blood shifting from the high-resistance systemic circulation to the lower-resistance pulmonary circulation.

Treatment of HAPE: (1) urgent descent to a lower altitude; (2) management of pulmonary edema with supplemental oxygen, diuretics, calcium channel blocker (i.e., nifedipine), morphine, noninvasive/invasive positive pressure ventilation; (3) hyperbaric oxygen therapy; (4) steroids; (5) phosphodiesterase inhibitor (tadalafil).

It is important to monitor respiratory rate and effort along with volume status, especially in the setting of treatment with opioids and diuretics.

Hyperbaric oxygen therapy (HBOT)

HBOT involves breathing 100% oxygen at 1.5 to 3 atmospheres, in an enclosed chamber. It can be used in the setting of hypoxia in high altitudes as well as in decompression sickness, wound healing/gangrene, carbon monoxide poisoning, and brain abscesses, to list a few examples. Its application is expanding in the literature.

Acute motion sickness (AMS)

This condition is seen with rapid ascent to high altitudes thought to occur secondary to a hypoxia-induced subclinical cerebral edema. It is self-limiting and resolves within a week.

AMS presents as a throbbing generalized bilateral headache accompanied with anorexia, nausea, dizziness, fatigue, or insomnia. Treatment includes supplemental oxygen, analgesics, antiemetics, steroids, and acetazolamide. Descent to a lower altitude is recommended as long as possible.

High altitude cerebral edema (HACE)

HACE is a severe form of AMS and is considered a medical emergency with a high risk of mortality. It results in a vasogenic and cytotoxic cerebral edema secondary to hypoxia. Symptoms are similar to AMS, in addition to gait ataxia, mental status alterations, hemiparesis, or coma. Treatment requires urgent descent to normal altitudes. Medical management includes: supplemental oxygen, steroids, acetazolamide, diuretics (e.g., furosemide), high carbohydrate diet, and hyperbaric chamber.

High altitude: other physiologic changes

- Hypothermia: platelet dysfunction, cold injuries, cardiac arrest.
- Immune suppression: ineffective healing and increased risk of infection.

High altitude: anesthetic implications

High altitude may exacerbate the respiratory-depressant effects of benzodiazepines and opioids. If not treated or prevented, hypothermia may potentiate the effect of induction agents and muscle relaxants due to decrease in drug metabolism. Ketamine may be the drug of choice due its analgesic effects and respiratory preservation. There is increased risk of perioperative bleeding due to high venous pressure, vasodilation, and increased capillary density. Tobacco smoking increases carboxyhemoglobin levels, further impairing oxygen delivery. Alcohol, caffeine, and diuretics should be used with caution, as they increase diuresis and can aggravate dehydration.

Nitrous oxide loses potency at high altitudes. It also limits inspired oxygen concentration and may further increase pulmonary artery pressures. Therefore nitrous oxide is not recommended during anesthetics at high altitudes.

Delivery of inhaled anesthetics at high altitude

Except for the Tec 6 Plus desflurane vaporizer (GE Healthcare), all other vaporizers do not need to be dialed up in order to adjust and compensate for the drop in atmospheric pressure at high altitudes.

Tec 6 vaporizer

The *Tec 6 vaporizer* will deliver the dialed volume percentage at higher altitudes, but as soon as desflurane is exposed to the ambient pressure at high altitude, its partial pressure will decrease. Therefore, the Tec 6 vaporizer has to be dialed up to deliver the same partial pressure of desflurane at higher altitude. Therefore, final dial setting (Tec 6) = dial setting required × 760 mm Hg/ambient pressure (mm Hg).

Causes of delayed emergence

Causes include hypothermia, hypoxia, and any of the high altitude-related pathologic (cardiopulmonary, central) conditions.

Questions

1. Which of the following cardiovascular changes will a person acclimatize to after spending two weeks hiking at 6,000 feet?
   a. Plasma volume will increase.
   b. Cardiac index will increase.
   c. Pulmonary artery pressure will remain unchanged.
   d. Oxygen-carrying capacity will decrease.

2. You are delivering anesthesia at a bariatric center in Denver. The anesthesia machine has a Tec 6 Plus desflurane vaporizer (GE Healthcare). How are you going to proceed in order to assure that your patient receives the appropriate MAC of desflurane anesthetic?
   a. This vaporizer can compensate for the lower atmospheric pressure and therefore there is no need to adjust the dial setting.
   b. This vaporizer has to be dialed down to deliver the same partial pressure of desflurane at high altitudes.
   c. This vaporizer can not be used at high altitudes. It is appropriate to ask the hospital for another bypass vaporizer.
   d. This vaporizer has to be dialed up in order to deliver the same partial pressure of desflurane at high altitudes.

3. For HAPE (high altitude pulmonary edema), all of the following are possible treatments options except for which?
   a. calcium channel blocker
   b. beta-blocker
   c. loop diuretics
   d. dexamethasone

4. At high altitude which of the following physiologic changes are present?
   a. respiratory acidosis

   b. hypertension
   c. increase in 2, 3-diphosphoglycerate
   d. increased preload

Answers

1. b. Cardiac index will increase. CI = CO/BSA. Hypoxia leads to an increase in sympathetic output, which leads to an increase in HR, hence CO (CO = SV × HR). This increases the incidence of congestive heart failure. Pulmonary artery pressure increases. Oxygen-carrying capacity increases as hemoglobin levels go up. Plasma volume decreases and contributes to a rise in hematocrit and a drop in cardiac preload.

2. d. The Tec 6 Plus vaporizer is the only type of contemporary vaporizer that needs to be adjusted up while delivering anesthesia at high altitudes in order to assure appropriate partial pressure of gas in the system. For example:
   At 760 mm Hg, inspiratory pressure of 1% isoflurane = 7.6 mm Hg.
   At 540 mm Hg (Denver, CO), inspiratory pressure of 1% isoflurane = 5.4 mm Hg.
   The output of an inhaled anesthetic from all except the Tec 6 vaporizer depends on the ratio of the vapor pressure of agent/atmospheric pressure. The carrier gas passing through the bypass vaporizer will pick up more gas at higher altitude than at sea level. The actual output is therefore higher than the set dial percentage. For example:
   Isoflurane (sea level) = 1:3 (240 mm Hg/760 mm Hg).
   Isoflurane (Denver, CO) = 1:2 (240 mm Hg/525 mm Hg).
   All current vaporizers, except for the Tec 6 Plus, are temperature-and pressure-compensated. In case of the Tec 6, the lower ambient pressure at high altitude will lead to a drop in partial pressure of desflurane.
   Final dial setting (Tec 6) = dial setting required × 760 mm Hg/ambient pressure mm Hg.

3. b. Calcium channel blockers are used for pulmonary vasodilation. Diuretics are sometimes used for prophylaxis, and dexamethasone is used to reduce inflammation. Beta-blockers are not used for HAPE.

4. c. At high altitude respiratory alkalosis, not respiratory acidosis, is present, and 2, 3-diphosphoglycerate is increased.

178

Medical informatics and information management systems in anesthesia

Syed Irfan Qasim Ali and Richard D. Urman

Keywords

AIMS
Areas impacted by anesthesia information
    management system
Benefits of informatics in anesthesia
Massachusetts General Hospital Utility Multi-
    Programming System (MUMPS)
MEDLINE
Medical informatics

Medical informatics is the application of information science to health care. It focuses on using information technology to optimize the storage and retrieval of health information, and can also include individual patient-level data for use in routine clinical care (such as the reporting of laboratory results) or large data sets, including thousands of patients, to facilitate the performance of health outcomes research.

Medical informatics began in the 1950s with the advent of computers and the microchip. The earliest use of computers in medicine took place at the US National Bureau of Standards. The National Library of Medicine started *MEDLINE* in 1965, and, at approximately the same time, the *Massachusetts General Hospital Utility Multi-Programming System (MUMPS)* was developed in Boston.

Anesthesia information management systems (AIMS) are a specialized form of electronic health records that allow the automatic and reliable collection, storage, and presentation of patient data during the perioperative period. In addition, most AIMS also allow end users to access information for management, quality assurance, and research purposes.

Widespread adoption of *AIMS*, which have been in existence since the 1970s, has been hindered primarily by the financial barriers associated with implementation of these systems. As a result of these hurdles, only an estimated 5% of US operating rooms in 2006 had an AIMS. Adoption has accelerated recently, driven primarily by a need to address increased regulatory reporting requirements and a desire to improve routine clinical documentation.

Areas impacted by anesthesia information management systems

Impact on patients

- More accurately records patient responses to anesthesia.
- Improves availability of historic records.
- Allows an anesthesiologist to focus on the patient, rather than charting.

Impact on the practice of anesthesia

- Improves quality assurance functionality due to more accurate and complete records.
- Allows quick searches for specific occurrences or rare events across multiple cases.
- Provides a means to track individual provider performance over time.
- Assesses patient outcomes through integration with other hospital databases.
- Makes available accurate, high-resolution charts for educational purposes.
- Provides legal protection through more accurate, unbiased information.

Impact on departmental management

- Facilitates accurate and timely billing.
- Allows analysis of supply costs by patient, provider, or type of surgery.
- Can assist with concurrency and other regulatory compliance issues.
- Satisfies The Joint Commission requirements for comprehensive, legible records.
- Provides ready verification of ACGME case requirements for residents-in-training programs.
- Most systems can generate point-of-care alerts for patient allergies or drug–drug interactions. In fact, the Anesthesia Patient Safety Foundation has both endorsed and

Essential Clinical Anesthesia Review: Keywords, Questions and Answers for the Boards, ed. Linda S. Aglio, Robert W. Lekowski, and Richard D. Urman. Published by Cambridge University Press. © Cambridge University Press 2015.

advocated the use of AIMS because of the ability of the technology to provide high-quality data.

Specific benefits of AIMS in peer-reviewed literature

Cost and billing improvements

- Controlling and reducing anesthesia drug costs.
- Improving capture of anesthesia-related charges.
- Impact on hospital reimbursement.

Decision support and provider education

- Clinical decision support.
- Training and provider education.

Patient safety and quality assurance

- Increased patient care and safety.
- Enhancement of clinical quality improvement programs.
- Support of clinical risk management.
- Monitoring for diversion of controlled substances.

Data quality and clinical research

- Enhancement of clinical studies.
- Improved intraoperative record quality.

Questions

1. Which of the following parameters are least likely to be recorded by AIMS (anesthesia information management system) automatically?
   a. arterial BP reading
   b. end-tidal sevoflurane concentration
   c. fresh gas flow
   d. tidal volume

2. Name the first computerized medical informatics system developed by the National Library of Medicine.
   a. MUMPS
   b. MEDLINE
   c. AIMS
   d. Medical Media

Answers

1. c.
2. b.

Further reading

Vacanti, C. A., Sikka, P. K., Urman, R. U., Dershwitz, M., and Segal, B. S. (2011). *Essential Clinical Anesthesia*, 1st edn. Cambridge University Press, Chapter 182.

Miller, R. (2011). *Basics of Anesthesia*, 6th edn. Philadelphia: Elsevier, Chapter 4.

Chapter 179

Hypertrophic cardiomyopathy and prolonged QT interval

Thomas Hickey and Linda S. Aglio

Keywords

Hypertrophic cardiomyopathy (HCM)
HOCM anesthetic management
HOCM: hypotension treatment
Congenital long QT syndrome: management
Methadone: QT interval
QT prolongation with antiemetics

Overview: Hypertrophic cardiomyopathy (*HCM*) is an autosomal dominant disorder with an incidence of 1:500. Diagnostic features include unexplained LV wall thickness $\geq$15 mm, systolic anterior motion (SAM) of the mitral valve, and left ventricular outflow tract (LVOT) obstruction represented by increased LVOT to aorta pressure gradient (i.e., >30 mm Hg). Asymmetric LV hypertrophy is typical, with the anterior ventricular septum most affected. Major concerns include increased risk of ventricular arrhythmias, outflow tract obstruction, diastolic dysfunction, and increased susceptibility to ischemia.

Congenital long QT syndrome (LQTS) can be dominant, recessive, or spontaneous; the implicated genes (LQT1, LQT2, LQT3) code for ion channels and have been named for the syndrome. Incidence is 1:5,000. Deafness is often a part of congenital LQTS. LQTS is characterized by prolonged QTc (>470 ms in males, >480 ms in females) and can include syncope or cardiac arrest, likely caused by torsades de pointes. History of these symptoms in a patient or in family members should at least prompt an EKG; T-wave alternans (beat-to-beat T-wave amplitude variation) is considered pathognomonic. Female gender, QTc >500, and widened T waves predict an increased risk of sudden death. Various medications can cause the acquired LQTS (typically antibiotics, antiarrhythmics, antiemetics).

Hypertrophic obstructive cardiomyopathy (HOCM) anesthetic management: LVOT obstruction is not only due to the bulging septum but also to the malformed mitral valve apparatus. The obstruction is dynamic, worsened by any decrease in ventricular size. Hence, decreases in preload and afterload are

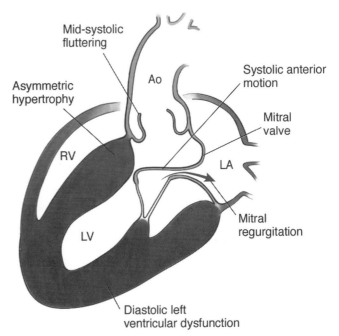

Figure 179.1 Features of HCM.

likely to exacerbate outflow tract obstruction. Hyperdynamic states may also worsen obstruction, bringing the septum and leaflet closer together via the Venturi effect. Systolic anterior motion describes the pulling of the anterior mitral valve leaflet towards the septum during systole. Medical management with β-blockers or calcium channel blockers tends to improve symptoms of exertional dyspnea and atypical angina. Both agents reduce heart rate, prolonging diastole with improved ventricular filling. Refractory symptoms may indicate septal myomectomy to relieve the outflow obstruction. ICD placement is recommended in patients with prior arrest, prior VT, and possibly in those with prior myomectomy.

HOCM: hypotension treatment. Hemodynamic collapse in HCM is often precipitated by cessation of β-blockade or calcium channel blocker, decreased preload (as in hemorrhage, sepsis, diuretics, dehydration), decreased afterload, and/or arrhythmia.

Essential Clinical Anesthesia Review: Keywords, Questions and Answers for the Boards, ed. Linda S. Aglio, Robert W. Lekowski, and Richard D. Urman. Published by Cambridge University Press. © Cambridge University Press 2015.

Note that standard treatments for heart failure could exacerbate the obstruction. For severe cases, immediate fluid resuscitation and *phenylephrine* are indicated. For less severe cases, β-blockade and less aggressive fluid resuscitation (i.e., PO) may be sufficient.

Congenital long QT: management. β-blockade with consequent sympathetic suppression is the cornerstone and results in a dramatic decrease in ten-year mortality (50% to 5%). ICDs can be considered if symptoms persist despite medical management. Stressors, including loud noises, should be avoided. Electrolytes should be maintained in the normal range. Pain control and anxiolysis should be adequate. Opioids are used to blunt the sympathetic response to laryngoscopy. Some texts recommend isoflurane or propofol for maintenance. QT interval should be monitored and defibrillation equipment immediately available. In cases of torsades, withdrawal of offending drugs, correction of electrolytes, and magnesium (30 mg/kg magnesium sulfate bolus followed by 2 mg/kg infusion) are recommended. Refractory torsades may respond to transvenous pacing or cardioversion.

Methadone: QT interval. Methadone causes a dose-dependent increase in QT interval and should be given with caution to patients with known or suspected LQTS, or who are on other prolonging drugs (including cocaine). Patients should get a pretreatment EKG, follow-up at 30 days, then annual follow-up at a minimum.

QT prolongation with antiemetics: haloperidol and droperidol are members of the butyrophenone class of dopamine receptor antagonists and are known to prolong the QT interval. Both are effective antiemetics but are generally avoided given this side effect. Droperidol in particular has a "black box warning" concerning QT prolongation. 5-HT3 antagonists (i.e., ondansetron) also prolong the QT interval.

Questions

1. A 23-year-old patient without medical history is seen preoperatively before scheduled cholecystectomy. A recent resting TTE to investigate a new systolic murmur identified anterior ventricular septal thickness of 18 mm. There were no other abnormalities noted on echo. EKG was remarkable for downsloping ST segments and T-wave inversions in the anterolateral leads. She does endorse a history of at least one premature sudden death in a first-degree relative. If the suspected diagnosis is confirmed, which of the following would confer the highest disease-related mortality in this patient?

   a. stroke
   b. heart failure
   c. sudden cardiac death (SCD)
   d. infective endocarditis

2. A 63-year-old patient without medical history is seen preoperatively before scheduled thyroidectomy. She takes only a multivitamin. On review of systems, she endorses likely prior syncopal and presyncopal episodes that appear to have been precipitated by exercise. She also recalls that she had a sister who died of sudden cardiac death at age 22. Resting EKG is normal sinus rhythm with a QTc of 494. If the suspected diagnosis is confirmed, which of the following interventions would result in the greatest mortality benefit in this patient?

   a. verapamil
   b. furosemide
   c. amiodarone
   d. propranolol

Table 179.1 Medications that may trigger torsades de pointes

Antibiotic	Antiarrhythmic
Chloroquine	Amiodarone
Clarithromycin	Bepridil
Erythromycin	Disopyramide
Halofantrine	Dofetilide
Pentamidine	Ibutilide
Sparfloxacin	Procainamide
	Quinidine
Pain	Sotatol
Levomethadyl	
Methadone	**Antipsychotic**
	Chlorpromazine
Miscellaneous	Haloperidol
Cisapride	Mesoridazine
Droperidol	Pimozide
	Thioridazine

(Adapted from Arizona CERT list of drugs that are generally accepted to have a risk of causing torsades de pointes. Visit www.torsades.org for complete list.)

Answers

1. c. Annual mortality in patients with HCM is approximately 1%. Sudden death is most common in young patients; heart failure and stroke are most common in older patients.

2. c. As above, β-blockade is the cornerstone therapy for LQTS and confers an impressive mortality benefit. Amiodarone would be on a list of medications to be avoided in patients with LQTS, as it can prolong the QT interval.

Further reading

Vacanti, C. A., Sikka, P. K., Urman, R. U., Dershwitz, M., and Segal, B. S. (2011). *Essential Clinical Anesthesia*, 1st edn. Cambridge University Press, Chapter 180.

Index

Figures and tables are denoted in bold typeface.

pulmonary fibrosis transplant
    indications, 287
pulmonary function test, **276**
pulmonary hypertension
    and COPD, 10
    lung transplantation, 289
    obstetrics, 396
    transplant indications, 287
pulmonary resection, 282–284,
    283
pulmonary system
    ACS and IAH effects, 525–526
    and CHF, 26
    and elderly patients, **43**, 43
    and liver disease, 31
    aspiration, 143–145, **144**
    changes during pregnancy,
    382
    circulation, **274**
    MAC effects, 121
    preoperative assessment, 5
pulmonary vascular obstructive
    disease, 414
pulmonary vascular resistance
    (PVR), 414–415, **415**
pulmonary venous obstruction,
    290
pulse oximeter, 101
pulse pressure variation
    physiology, 89–90
PVD. See peripheral vascular
    disease
pyloric stenosis, **412**, 412
pyridostigmine, 532

quality assurance (management),
    429

radiation
    non-OR, 426
    safety, 439
radiofrequency lesioning, 460
ranitidine, 144
rapid sequence induction, 68,
    376
rapid shallow breathing index,
    487
rebreathing, 82
recurrent laryngeal nerve, **63**,
    63
red blood cell transfusion, 217
regional anesthesia
    epidural, 190–191
    lower extremity nerve blocks,
    197–199
    pediatric pain, 418
    spinal, 187–188
    spinal column anatomy,
    183–185
    tourniquets, 369–370
    ultrasound nerve blocks,
    192–193
    upper extremity nerve blocks,
    194–196
regression analysis, **442**, 442–443

remote location anesthesia
    office, 425–426
    outside the OR, 425–426
renal anesthesia
    kidney transplantation,
    319–320
    pancreas transplantation, 320
renal conditions assessment, 5–6
renal system
    abdominal aortic aneurysm,
    271
    ACS and IAH effects, 525–526
    and elderly patients, 43
    and liver disease, 31
    CHF, 26–29
    effect of muscle relaxants on,
    138
    physiology, 314
renin, 314
renin-angiotensin, **348**
replacement fluid, **202**, **203**, **204**
rescue therapy, 147
respiratory system
    cardiac failure insufficiency,
    483
    effects of spinal anesthesia,
    188
    failure, 174
    neonatal, 401
    physiology, **274**, 274–276, **275**,
    276
respiratory variation-based
    indicators, 89
restrictive lung disease, **13**
retinal ischemia, 172
retinopathy
    obstetrics, 397
    of prematurity, 411
retrobulbar block, 361
rheumatoid arthritis, **372–373**,
    397
rhinoplasty, 523
rhytidectomy, 523
right-to-left intracardiac shunt,
    284
risk. See also complications
    abdominal surgery aspiration,
    322
    atrial fibrillation, 480
    COPD, 10–11
    criteria for pneumonectomy,
    284
    for POCD, **181**
    from patient positioning,
    172–173
    intraoperative awareness, 113
    management in a practice, 430,
    434
    management in OR, **158**,
    438–439
    patient assessment, **3**, 3–6
    PONV, 179
    postoperative bleeding, **263**
    preoperative assessment, 4
    statistical, 443

robots
    laparoscopic surgery, 332
    surgical, **534**, 534–535
rocuronium, 138
ropivacaine, 162
rule of nines (burns), 513–514,
    515

sacrum anatomy, 184
safety
    electrical, **85**, 85, **91**
    fire hazard, **158**, 438–439
    in anesthesia practice, 217–429
    needle, 438
    patient, 436
    radiation, 439
    WAGs, 438
saw palmetto, 541
scavenging gas delivery systems,
    75
schizophrenia, 53–54
sciatic nerve blck
    lower extremity, 197, **198**
    orthopedic surgery, 367, **371**
scoliosis, 373
second gas effect, 119
sedation levels (MAC), **133–169**
seizure disorders, 45–46, 394
selective serotonin receptor
    antagonists, 147
selective serotonin reuptake
    inhibitors (SSRIs), **52**, 52
sensitivity (statistical), **441**, 441
sepsis
    and ARDS, 491
    ICU, 499–502
serotonin syndrome, **52**, 52
serotonin–norepinephrine
    reuptake inhibitors (SNRIs),
    52, 52
sevoflurane
    and PONV, 423
    inhalation anesthetic, 115
shunts
    respiratory system, 275
    right-to-left intracardiac,
    284
SIADH. See syndrome of
    inappropriate antidiuretic
    hormone
sickle cell, 406
single-lung transplantation
    indications, 287
single twitch block, **104**
sitting position
    and nerve damage, 172
    neurosurgery, 306
skin and collagen disorders,
    521–522
sleep apnea, 5, 362, 408
smoking
    and carbon monoxide
    poisoning, 529
    and COPD, 11
sniffing position, 64

soda lime breathing equipment,
    82
SOFA score, **478**
somatic pain, **448**, 448, 469
somatosensory evoked
    potentials, 306
specificity (statistical), **441**, 441
spina bifida, 411
spinal anesthesia
    adverse neurologic effects,
    188
    anticoagulation guidelines, **188**
    cesarean delivery, **388**
    effects of, 187–188
    equipment, 188
    pediatric, 408
    pros and cons of using, **187**
    types of, 188
spinal column anatomy,
    183–185, **184**, **185**
spinal cord injury
    acute, 47
    chronic, 47–48
    urologic procedures, 316
spinal surgery, 375–377
splenectomy, 323
spontaneous breathing trial, 487
St. John's wort, 540
statistics, **441**, 441–443, **442**
stellate ganglion block, **458**, 463
stenosis, **396**, 396, **412**, 412
stereoselectivity, 127
steroid injections
    complications with, 462–463
    sepsis, 502
Stewart hypothesis, 206
stimulation techniques
    for pain, 461
    peripheral nerve, 461
stress (diabetic), 34
stroke volume index, 90
subarachnoid bleed, 97
subarachnoid hemorrage, 308
subcutaneous pain therapy, 460
substance abuse
    alcohol, 57
    amphetamine, 58
    cocaine, 57–58
    hallucinogens, 59
    marijuana, 59
    opioids, 57
    tobacco, 56
substituted judgment, 516
succinylcholine (SCh)
    and IOP, 360
    and MG, 355
    and muscular dystrophy, 358
    in neonatals, 403
    muscle relaxant, 137–138, 140
sugammadex, 141
superior hypogastric plexus
    block, 458
superior laryngeal nerve, **63**, 63
superior vena cava syndrome,
    296